Miriam Lucio Mc Mahon
CPR
First aids

A
Massage Therapist's
Guide to
Pathology

A
Massage Therapist's
Guide to
Pathology

SECOND EDITION

Ruth Werner, LMP, NCTMB

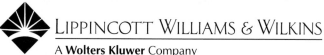

LIPPINCOTT WILLIAMS & WILKINS
A **Wolters Kluwer** Company

Philadelphia • Baltimore • New York • London
Buenos Aires • Hong Kong • Sydney • Tokyo

Editor: Peter Darcy
Managing Editor: Eric Branger
Marketing Manager: Christen DeMarco
Project Editor: Jennifer Ajello
Designer: Armen Kojoyian
Cover Illustration: Terry Watkinson
Cover Designer: Armen Kojoyian
Compositor: Graphic World
Printer: Courier-Westford

530 Walnut Street
Philadelphia, Pennsylvania 19106

351 West Camden Street
Baltimore, Maryland 21201-2436 USA

Printed in the United States of America

Library of Congress Cataloging-in-Publication Data

Werner, Ruth (Ruth A.)
    A massage therapist's guide to pathology / Ruth Werner.—2nd ed.
        p. cm.
    Includes index.
    ISBN 0-7817-3293-X
        1. Massage therapy. 2. Physiology, Pathological. 3. Diseases. I. Title.

    RM721 .M366 2002
    615.8'22—dc21   2002016270

To purchase additional copies of this book, call our customer service department at **(800) 638-3030** or fax orders
to **(301) 824-7390**. For other book services, including chapter reprints and large quantity sales, ask for the Special
Sales department.

For all other calls originating outside of the United States, please call **(301)714-2324**.

Visit Lippincott Williams & Wilkins on the Internet: **http://www.lww.com**. Lippincott Williams & Wilkins customer service representatives are available from 8:30 am to 6:00 pm, EST, Monday through Friday, for telephone
access.

03 04
3 4 5 6 7 8 9 10

DEDICATION

*This book is dedicated to the memory
of my grandmother, Dora C. Beckhard,
who probably never got a massage in her life—
but she sure could have used one.*

—RW

Preface to the Second Edition

Dear Students and Practitioners,

This book is a compilation of years of teaching and doing massage, collaboration with dozens of professionals in the field, a variety of printed resources, hundreds of articles about ongoing research, and *lots* of feedback on the strengths and weaknesses of the first edition. I have done my best to make it a useful, accurate source of information so that bodyworkers can make informed choices when designing treatments for clients who may not be perfectly healthy.

Why Do Massage Therapists Need to Know About Pathology?

We all know that the demographics of the average massage client are changing. Every year the percentage of the population that receives massage goes up; every year more people perceive massage as a health care modality rather than (or in addition to) as an occasional indulgence.

The result is that today massage therapists can expect to see clients who struggle with various simple and complex health issues. These clients may seek massage as a special treat, but they are just as likely to be using massage as part of an integrated, proactive, carefully constructed health care plan. This puts a burden on the shoulders of massage therapists which we have never had before. When we work with clients whose bodies may not have the capacity to keep up with the kinds of changes some types of bodywork bring about, we run the risk of doing more harm than good.

What shape might that harm take? It might be as simple as overtreating a tight muscle so that a client is sore for longer than strictly necessary. It might be as complex and dangerous as dislodging a fragment of a silent deep vein thrombosis, thus opening the door to a life-threatening pulmonary embolism. The high incidence of cardiovascular disease in the United States has tremendous implications for massage. Atherosclerotic plaques often accumulate in the carotid arteries (a location highly vulnerable to disruption), which could subsequently lead to a cerebrovascular accident. Rising statistics for type 2 diabetes should raise concerns about circulatory impairment and numbness in the lower extremities. The close physical contact involved with massage provides a potent environment for the spreading of contagious diseases, including herpes, hepatitis B, fungal infections, and others. These are threats every massage therapist should be trained to recognize. This is just a short list of problems that could be caused or exacerbated by undertrained massage therapists.

Carefully, knowledgeably applied massage has found an important place in hotels, spas, and salons—but also in cancer wards, hospice centers, senior citizen homes, drug rehabilitation clinics, and other settings where the health of the clientele is far from perfect. The only way to work safely in these environments is to engage in a thorough education about the physiology of a healthy human body and the consequences of diseases and disorders that interrupt normal processes. This background is absolutely fundamental to the training of any bodywork professional and is critical for the maintenance of public safety.

The positive power of informed touch is irrefutable. When massage therapists and other bodyworkers have the tools to make educated decisions about how to structure their sessions for maximum benefit with minimum risk, they can help not only themselves, but whole communities of clients who otherwise would be out of their reach.

What Is Massage, and How Do We Make Decisions About It?

This looks like a simple question, but it is not. Massage can range from being an intense, intrusive, rock'em-sock'em assault on soft tissues, to being a subtle invitation to positive change delivered through pathways of energy sensed only at the most subjective levels of experience. Both ends of the spectrum (and every place in between) have value for the promotion of health and impact on human experience. I have used the terms "massage" and "bodywork" to mean the application of informed, educated touch with the consent and participation of the receiver, for the purpose of allowing or promoting positive changes to occur in the receiver's physical and/or energetic state.

For massage therapists or bodyworkers to evaluate whether their skills are applicable to the needs of a particular client, they must have a thorough knowledge of three things: how the human body works when it is healthy; how the body works in the context of disease or dysfunction; and how a particular bodywork modality may influence those processes, either for good or for ill. When these questions can be answered clearly, the therapist is in a position to turn positive intention into positive action.

For the purposes of this text I have loosely classified bodywork into two different but complementary camps. One involves mechanical types of massage that work through the physical manipulation of skin, fascia, muscles, tendons, ligaments, and fluid flow. The other includes reflexive and energetic types of bodywork that address the flow of energy and/or the parasympathetic nervous system response to create an environment conducive to positive change. In simplified terms, the mechanical approach to bodywork *enacts* change; the reflexive/energetic approach *invites* change. Some modalities defy categorization, of course; manual lymph drainage and other lymph drainage techniques, for instance, work to mechanically influence the direction of lymph flow, but they also enlist the parasympathetic response to encourage the lymphatic capillaries to open fully. Craniosacral therapy influences the flow of cerebrospinal fluid (a mechanical goal), but does so through feather-light touch and reflexive parasympathetic affect. Ultimately, most therapists use both mechanical and reflexive/energetic intention; one could hardly touch another body without doing so!

Delineating approaches becomes useful when we evaluate whether massage is appropriate for certain clients who are not healthy. Modalities that have at their core the intention of *enacting* change on blood and lymph flow (e.g., Swedish and sports massage), carry a risk of potential overtreatment in the context of disorders that involve fluid restriction—conditions like congestive heart failure, kidney disorders, or advanced cirrhosis, among many others. Other modalities that enlist internal reaction rather than external force are usually safer to use in these circumstances. Although overtreatment with these modalities is certainly possible, it is far less likely to happen and the repercussions are generally less dangerous.

Conditions that are contagious and that spread through close physical contact may contraindicate *any* kind of bodywork, regardless of whether the intention is for mechanical or reflexive/energetic action.

Some readers have requested that a part of this text be devoted to a discussion of specific modalities and to what conditions they may most effectively be applied. I resist this request for several reasons. The main one is that I am no expert on most of the thousands of bodywork techniques that have been developed in the millennia since people discovered that the sensation of touch is both pleasurable and healthful. Furthermore, new techniques are developed practically daily, each with its own specialized applications and accompanying cautions; the moment a person tries to write something down about this topic, it is automatically obsolete. In addition, to list *some* modalities without listing *all* of them runs the risk of leaving out information that may be extremely valuable. Therefore, it comes to this: each practitioner of each bodywork modality must research *how* that modality influences processes during health and disease, and must apply that information in a conservative, knowledgeable way to achieve the best possible results with his or her clients.

Statements about the applicability of massage in this text generally refer to modalities that intend to mechanically influence tissues or fluid flow ("circulatory" techniques like Swedish or sports massage) and modalities that work energetically or reflexively ("noncirculatory" techniques that could include multitudes of skills like polarity, reflexology, craniosacral therapy, Touch For Health, trigger point work, ad infinitum). To categorize bodywork in this way may seem simplistic to some practitioners, but please understand that that is not at all my intention. It is my job to lay out some guidelines about how bodywork fits in the context of disease; it is the reader's job to evaluate that information and decide how and when those guidelines may be stretched.

A Nod to Political Correctness

In this book the terms "therapist" and "practitioner" are synonymous and refer to the person performing bodywork. The people who have conditions are called "patients" in the context of medical care and "clients" in the context of receiving massage. Patients or clients are referred to as "he" or "she" depending on what statistics indicate is the more likely gender to experience the condition. Thus, although it is possible for a woman to have hemophilia, for instance, the large majority of hemophiliacs are male and patients are therefore referred to as males. When there is no particular gender-related risk factor, patients or clients have been referred to as males or females more or less randomly.

Is This the Definitive Text?

This text is more complete and more up-to-date than the first edition of *A Massage Therapist's Guide to Pathology*, but it still cannot be a permanent, definitive massage pathophysiology text. Readers of the first edition will see how our understanding of some conditions has remained static over the past several years, but some others have substantially changed; it will always be so. We all anticipate that future research will reveal much more about massage and disease, perhaps even research that some of you will conduct.

A Final Note

One of the items on my personal agenda in writing this book is to share with you the wonder of the human body. It is amazing that we work as well as we do. It is even more miraculous that we can recover from injury and disease. As massage practitioners we work to create an internal environment in our clients that fosters healing and recovery. Having conscious intention in our work makes us even better at achieving this goal. My purpose in writing this book is to help each practitioner develop that specific sense of intention: we should know *why* we are doing what we are doing every minute that we are working with a client.

So, happy reading. Do more research if it interests you, and remember that some of the questions dealt with here will probably never be completely answered. What we think we know now may someday be revised or proved wrong. Isn't that terrific?!

Ruth Werner
Fall 2001

How To Use This Book

One of the best definitions of health I have ever heard is, "Health is the ability to adapt to changes in the environment." In other words, health is not a noun; it is a verb. Health means being able to cope with changes in external conditions, but even more, being healthy means being able to adapt to changes in the *internal* environment of the body. Health is not simply the absence of infection or injury; it is an active state of adjustment and counter-adjustment that allows the body to function under a broad variety of circumstances. When that ability to adapt is compromised, when a person's homeostatic processes are threatened, then the whole organism becomes weak and vulnerable to sickness, to disease.

The term "pathology" (from the Greek *pathos*, "disease," and *logos*, "science") is the study of the nature and causes of disease as related to structure and function of the body. This discipline can be divided into two specialties: *anatomic pathology* (the examination of tissues removed from cadavers or living people for the diagnosis of disease), and *clinical pathology* (also known as laboratory medicine: a broad field involving chemistry, histology, microbiology, hematopathology, immunopathology, and other specialties). Thus, pathology can be viewed as the laboratory study of cell and tissue changes associated with disease and/or injury.

Patho*physiology*, on the other hand, involves the study of functional or physiologic changes in the body that result from various disease processes. It explains the processes within the body that create the signs and symptoms of a disorder and examines how normal functions are altered by disease.

Massage therapy is intimately involved with anatomic and histologic changes associated with disease and injury. More importantly, we work with how these diseases or conditions change the way our clients function. Therefore, massage therapists need to be familiar with the principles of pathophysiology to be able to judge whether our work is appropriate for each client. This book is designed to assist in the formation of that judgment.

Massage therapists challenge homeostasis. We create changes in the internal environment of our clients' bodies. We influence the diameter of blood vessels and the direction of fluid flow. Massage changes the chemical balance of the body, reducing some types of hormones while increasing others, shifting neurotransmitter secretion, and altering the protein levels in interstitial tissues. Our first job, before we ever touch a client, is to determine whether that person is capable of adjusting to the changes massage precipitates.

This book has been written for two audiences: massage students who are learning about the body in health and disease for the first time, and practicing therapists working with a wide variety of people who may present a broad spectrum of disorders. It is written to present a wealth of complicated, interrelated, and convoluted material in an orderly fashion, but it can also provide easy reference and quick answers to the practitioner who needs to make a fast, well-informed decision.

The conditions that have been chosen to appear in this book are here for one of two reasons: either they occur frequently enough that practicing massage therapists will probably encounter them at some point, or because massage may have such a profound effect on certain conditions that practitioners are obligated to be well-informed about them.

Some controversy exists over what constitutes a disease rather than just a symptom; the dividing line between the two sometimes seems completely arbitrary. Although "jaundice" is sometimes considered a disease, it is really a description of the yellow skin and mucous membranes that occur when the liver is malfunctioning: it is, in fact, just a symptom. At a very basic level most "diseases" could be considered to be *symptoms* of other underlying problems. These are usually simple but insidious situations like inadequate sleep, too much stress, poor nutrition, or genetic predisposition. These issues, after all, determine the body's susceptibility to a variety of environmental triggers or infectious agents. So an argument could be made that the common cold is not really a disease at all; it is a symptom of a compromised immune system that is vulnerable to infection because of lack of sleep, stress, and poor nutrition. In this book no particular division is drawn between conditions that could be labeled symptoms and those that could be labeled diseases; we have simply followed medical convention and traditional terminology, and, when necessary, clarified how those terms may be used within each section.

The material is presented by body system, following the order most anatomy and physiology texts use. Each chapter begins with a brief overview of how the system works to provide the context for a discussion of what happens when things break down. Then the disorders are arranged by category, so that related conditions will appear together in the text. Each section is accompanied by an "In Brief" box that presents the basic information in abbreviated form. Each section contains information about the condition, including, where applicable, the demographics of the disorder, the etiology and progression of the disease, signs and symptoms, the standard medical approach to diagnosis and treatment, and the applicability of massage.

Each condition is said to "indicate" or "contraindicate" massage. Where bodywork is contraindicated, guidelines are provided to explain whether this is a local caution, in other words, only the affected area must be avoided, or whether this is a systemic situation, in which case the client needs to be referred to a primary care physician or needs to reschedule his or her appointment. Further qualifications list whether some bodywork modalities are more appropriate than others, or they describe specific phases or stages of healing when massage can be most helpful.

Many of the conditions in this book list massage as "indicated," at least at some stage of the healing process. I want to make very clear that to call massage "indicated" does *not* imply that massage will *fix* something that is wrong. We all know that at times massage can certainly influence the healing process for the better: the subacute stage of a sprained ankle, for instance. In other circumstances massage may have no effect on the severity of a condition whatsoever, for instance, with fibroid tumors. Massage is called "indicated" for both of these situations, which in this case, simply means that massage will not make the situation any worse.

Diseases and dysfunctions, like everything else in the body, are interconnected. References are therefore made within each section to other related conditions, even though they may not be listed under the same body system. It will be worthwhile to review those references to obtain the most thorough understanding of the relationships between different kinds of disorders.

Additional elements are included here to round out the central information in each section. Sidebars often examine the history or statistics of various conditions. "Watch for This" boxes provide a "compare and contrast" opportunity for conditions that are easily confused with each other. Finally, case histories that are based on interviews with clients, massage therapists, and other individuals are supplied to give a human face to abstract discussions.

Study aides have been included in the form of chapter objectives at the beginning of each chapter and review questions at the end of each chapter. A reader may claim mastery of this material when he or she can answer these questions and independently recreate the material included in the "In Brief" boxes.

For teachers using this book we have created a web site with valuable resources for instruction. Visit the Connection web site (http://connection.lww.com/go/werner) to access instructor materials that can be downloaded quickly. The site includes a test bank, images from the book, chapter questions and answers for each chapter, and PowerPoint slide presentations for each chapter.

Every possible effort has been made to make this material as accurate as possible. However, it needs to be said that *nothing* in this book is meant to act as a substitute for a doctor's advice. Massage therapists and bodyworkers with questions about the applicability of their work should consult with their clients' health care team for the best possible results. This consultation cannot occur without the consent of the client. Therefore, the most fruitful relationships happen when a client, the massage therapist, and the other members of the health care team are all informed of each others' activities and all work together toward the same goals.

Acknowledgments

No book is written in a vacuum, although it may sometimes seem that way. Many people contributed to the development of this work, and it is important—for me, anyway—to recognize them publicly and with gratitude.

To Brian Utting, LMP, teacher, boss, Big Kahuna, commissioner of the original work, and source of inspiration to constantly strive to do something that might be too hard (and to this day one of the most influential people in my life);

To Suzanne Carlson, RN, LMP, who first made it clear to all of us how important it was to know this material—years before we were required to;

The two of you formed the germinal material from which this work grew. My thanks and admiration will always be with you.

To the students of the Brian Utting School of Massage, the Myotherapy College of Utah, the Ogden Institute of Massage Therapy, and those I have encountered in my travels with this material;

I am so grateful to you all. You continue to teach me far more than I could ever hope to teach you, and I dearly hope that it never, ever stops.

To all the people I pestered and bugged and cornered and button-holed to look at this, or comment on that, or talk to me about the other;

To the very special people who allowed themselves to be interviewed for case histories in the first and second editions;

Your generosity will provide a service to many people for many years. Thank you with all my heart.

Finally, to my family: Curtis, Nathan, and Lily Anne Rose;

Writing a book does not always fit easily into family life. But every time I wanted to quit (and there were more than a few), I realized that with all of you watching, I couldn't possibly. You have kept me on task through thick and thin, and I will be grateful forever. Remember that I love you, all the time, every minute, no matter what.

R. Werner
Fall 2001

Table of Contents

Integumentary System Conditions

1

CHAPTER OBJECTIVES

After reading this chapter, you should be able to . . .

- Tell why broken skin contraindicates massage.
- Name three differences between acne and boils.
- Name three variations on fungal infections of the skin.
- Name what kind of bacteria are associated with boils.
- Name what kind of bacteria are associated with erysipelas.
- Name two dangers associated with widespread burns.
- Name three dangers associated with long-term use of corticosteroid creams.
- Name the ABCDE's of melanoma.
- Name the cardinal sign of non-melanoma skin cancer.
- Name a feature that distinguishes plantar warts from calluses.

INTRODUCTION

Function and Construction of the Skin

Massage practitioners speak in a language of touch. The messages practitioners send are invitations to a number of different possibilities: to enjoy a state of well-being, to heal and repair what is broken, or to reacquaint a client with his or her own body. All this happens through the skin, a medium equipped like no other tissue in the body to take in information and respond to it, mostly on a subconscious level. The goal of massage practitioners is to anticipate these reactions and set the stage for them in a way that is most beneficial for their clients.

Functions of the Skin

A student once said that the purpose of skin is to keep our insides from falling out. That is true, but that is not all skin does; its functions are manifold. Among them are several devices to keep the body healthy and safe, all wrapped up in one tidy 18-to-30–pound package.

Protection

The skin keeps pathogens out of the body, just by being intact, and it discourages their growth on its surface by secreting the acidic lubricants otherwise needed for keeping hair-shafts oiled. Furthermore, by constantly sloughing off dead cells, it sloughs off potential invaders, too.

The skin is the first line of defense against invasion, and the superficial fascia is especially well supplied with immune system cells that are constantly on patrol for potential sources of infection. These mast cells and other nonspecific white blood cells can create an extreme inflammatory response very quickly. When these defense mechanisms become hyperactive, they can cause certain types of rashes and other skin problems. For more details on hypersensitivity reactions, see the introduction to Lymph and Immune Conditions (Chapter 5).

Homeostasis

The skin protects us from fluid loss, a top homeostatic priority and one of the functions most dangerous to lose when the skin is damaged. The skin is the membrane that connects inner bodies to the outside world. It helps to maintain a constant internal temperature despite what is happening outside the body, because blood supply to the skin far exceeds the need for local nutrition; capillaries dilate or constrict according to what is needed at the time. The fat in the subcutaneous layer also acts as insulation.

Sensory Envelope

With as many as 19,000 sensory receptors in every square inch of skin, it is obvious that this is the organ (or tissue, or membrane, or system— depending on the source of information) that tells us the most about our environment. Eyes and ears appear to be indispensable, but look how far Helen Keller got with just her skin to take in information. Massage therapists must develop the skill of becoming conscious of the subtle information their hands pick up when they touch their clients, and must understand that every sensation created on a client's skin is also causing ripples of reactions all through the client's body.

Absorption and Excretion

To a small extent, the skin does absorb and excrete. Fat-soluble materials can be absorbed through the capillaries in hair shafts. Some massage oil is also absorbed in this way. Compounds like dimethyl sulfoxide (DMSO) are completely absorbed in a phenomenon called transcutaneous absorption.

The skin can help to excrete metabolic wastes, but it does so only as a last-ditch option. When the liver, colon, or especially kidneys are so congested that they cannot handle any more waste products, sweat can carry noxious chemicals out of the body.

Construction of the Skin

Skin varies from being very thin (on the lips) to remarkably thick (on the heels). It remodels according to stresses put on it. Callus formation is an example of this phenomenon: extra thick, extra hard epidermis on places that really take a beating.

The construction of the skin is important to understand, because it has relevance for how disease occurs and how easily it might spread. Three basic layers of tissue define the skin, and within those layers are more layers (Fig. 1-1). The subcutaneous tissue is probably familiar: it is also called superficial fascia. The dermis, or "true skin," is the location of hair shafts, oil and sweat glands, and some nerve endings. The outermost layer of dermis, the basal layer, lies just deep to the epidermis. It has the best capillary supply, and this is where new skin cells are born. Pigment cells (called melanocytes) are here; these protect people from harmful ultraviolet (UV) rays. Some of the worst diseases are born here too, for reasons described later in this chapter. New cells are produced near the bottom of the epidermis and migrate toward the top, dying of starvation and becoming keratinized, or scaly, in the process, which takes about 1 month. By the time they get to the surface, they are long dead and are sloughed off to become the major ingredient of household dust.

The epidermis is made of epithelium. Epithelium heals faster than any other type of tissue, which is good because no other tissue type is as vulnerable to damage as skin. It would be nice if the central nervous system healed as readily as the skin does, but consider the priorities: compare the number of neurologic traumas a person is likely to experience to the number of cuts, scrapes, scratches, tears, and punctures he or she will endure. Nevertheless, healing quickly has its disadvantages. Cells that have instructions to replicate at the drop of a hat sometimes replicate without the hat dropping, and that causes trouble.

Rules for Massage

Skin conditions have a special relevance for massage therapists, because we are in a position to notice lesions and blemishes that clients often do not know are there. That is why it is especially important to be able to recognize most common skin conditions, at least as far as being able to recommend that clients investigate them further with their doctors. Many skin conditions contraindicate massage because they might be contagious. Beyond that danger, the one cardinal rule for skin conditions and massage is: *if the intact state of the skin has been compromised in any way, the client is a walking invitation for infection.* Open skin, broken skin, scabbed skin, and any skin that allows access to the blood vessels inside is a red flag for massage practitioners. No matter how much a person scrubs, pathogens will always be present on the skin. By considering any compromised area of skin at least a local contraindication, practitioners take the responsibility to ensure that their microorganisms do not jump into their clients' vulnerable spots. At the same time, practitioners can prevent *clients'* pathogens from jumping into the tiny cracks in the practitioner's skin.

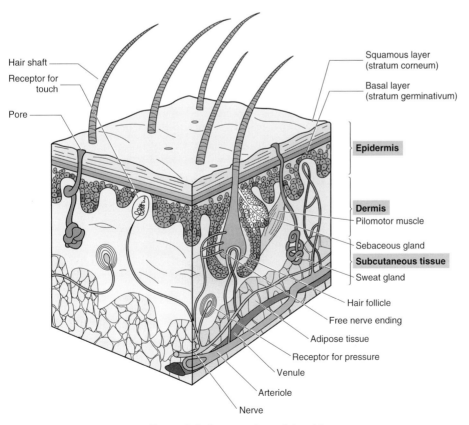

Figure 1-1. Cross section of the skin.

Integumentary System Conditions

Contagious Skin Disorders
    Boils
    Erysipelas
    Fungal Infections
    Herpes Simplex
    Impetigo
    Lice and Mites
    Warts

Non-Contagious Inflammatory Skin Disorders
    Acne
    Dermatitis/Eczema
    Hives

Neoplastic Skin Disorders
    Moles
    Psoriasis
    Skin Cancer

Skin Injuries
    Burns
    Decubitus Ulcers
    Open Wounds and Sores
    Scar Tissue

Other Conditions
    Ichthyosis

Contagious Skin Disorders

BOILS IN BRIEF

What are they?
Boils are localized bacterial infections of the skin. The causative agent is usually *Staphylococcus aureus*.

How are they recognized?
Boils involve painful, red, hot pustules on the skin. They may occur singly or in interconnected clusters called carbuncles.

Is massage indicated or contraindicated?
Boils contraindicate massage at least locally, and care should be taken to make sure the infection is not systemic (screen the client for other symptoms such as swelling, fever, or discomfort other than at the site of the lesion). The bacteria that cause boils are extremely virulent and communicable. The sheets of a client with boils should be isolated and treated with bleach.

BOILS
Boils are also called **furuncles**, from the Latin *furunculus*, which means "petty thief." The association between petty thievery and boils is obscure, unless one refers the extreme irritation caused by both.

Boils

Definition: What Are They?

Boils, also called *furuncles*, are localized staphylococcus infections of the skin.

Etiology: What Happens?

Boils are staphylococcus infections of sebaceous glands that are clogged by dirt, dead skin cells, or other debris. They have much in common with another skin infection, acne, but the variety of staphylococcus associated with boils is more aggressive than most. It does not simply take advantage of a stagnant pool of oil; it actively attacks living tissue. The bacterium that usually causes boils is *S. aureus*, which is a particularly virulent, aggressive variety.

Signs and Symptoms

Boils are large and painful infections. They usually occur one at a time or in small groups (Fig. 1-2, Color Plate 1). A cluster of boils connected by channels under the skin is called a *carbuncle* (Fig. 1-3, Color Plate 2). In the early stages, boils are hard, small, and red. As they mature, they may grow to the size of a golf ball. They soften in the middle and accumulate pus; this is the site where drainage usually takes place.

Treatment

As long as the infection stays localized boils are not dangerous, although they are *extremely* painful. Conservative treatment begins with hot compresses, which sometimes help them to burst and then drain, relieving the pressure and therefore the pain. If compresses do not work, doctors may lance the boil. Antibiotics are sometimes prescribed, but they tend to be slow acting and have the best effect for people who are plagued with a recurring problem.

It is important never to try to squeeze or pop a boil. It could force the infection deeper into tissues or spread the bacteria over the surface of the skin. Boils also carry a risk of complications brought about by the possibility of the staph bacteria invading other parts of the body or even other bodies altogether.

Chronically repeating boils may indicate a compromised immune system. They may also be a warning sign for *diabetes* (Chapter 8) or kidney problems.

Massage?

This is a local infection with extremely virulent, hardy bacteria. A client who has a boil with no signs of systemic infection may receive massage, but not on or near the lesion. If signs of systemic infection are present (fever, swelling at nearby lymph nodes, discomfort anywhere other than the site of the boil), it will be necessary to reschedule the massage. The sheets of a client who has a boil require special treatment: they must be isolated and washed with extra bleach to ensure that any staph bacteria are eradicated.

Erysipelas

Definition: What Is It?

Originally called St Anthony's Fire, erysipelas is a streptococcal infection of the cells in the skin. "Erys" means *red*, referring to the characteristic red patches an infection of this kind can cause.

Etiology: What Happens?

Colonies of bacteria are always growing on the skin—under the fingernails, between the toes, everywhere. It is virtually impossible to remove all the bacteria from a living person's skin. These colonies include both staphylococcus and streptococcus bacteria. Staph is usually responsible for small, localized infections like boils and pimples; it seems to have an affinity for sebum. Once strep gets under the skin, the local infection may become systemic, involving first the lymphatic and then the circulatory systems. The redness that characterizes this condition is caused by the enzymes produced by strep bacteria that break down and kill skin cells.

Strep bacteria must gain access to the body through some portal of entry. In many cases it can be difficult to identify exactly where the bacteria gained entry. Sometimes it is possible to trace the infection to a specific cut or scratch, athlete's foot (see *Fungal Infections* in this chapter), an insect bite, or some other skin injury.

Signs and Symptoms

Erysipelas begins with a tender, red swollen area (Fig. 1-4, Color Plate 3). It is unclear why, exactly, but erysipelas usually begins on the face or the lower leg. The wound soon shows signs of infection, which can include red streaks running toward the nearest set of lymph nodes. If the infection starts on the face, a raised red, hot, tender area develops and may spread laterally across the bridge of the nose. It looks like the "butterfly rash" pattern sometimes seen with *lupus* (Chapter 5). One hallmark of erysipelas is a sharp margin between involved and uninvolved skin; the red edges are usually very clear.

When the infection has thoroughly engaged the lymph system, symptoms include fever, chills, and systemic discomfort. Facial infections are particularly dangerous because of the risk of intracranial spreading through lymphatics. If erysipelas is left untreated, the

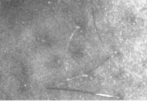

Figure 1-2. Single boil

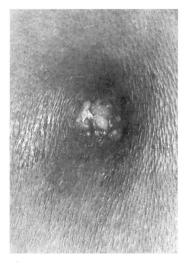

Figure 1-3. A group of interconnected boils is called a carbuncle

bacteria may get past the lymph system and enter the circulatory system, leading quickly, and perhaps fatally, to septicemia, or blood poisoning.

Treatment

Not so long ago, streptococcus was streptococcus. A person was diagnosed with an infection like strep throat or erysipelas, given penicillin, and sent home. Those days are gone forever. As good as penicillin is, strep bacteria are smarter and have mutated into myriad different drug-resistant forms faster than new antibiotics have been created to kill them. If a person is diagnosed with a strep infection now, antibiotics prescriptions are likely to take a catch-as-catch-can approach, shooting bullets until one of them finds the target. This is why doctors sometimes change prescriptions in the middle of treatment if a patient is not seeing results, that is, if the streptococcus is simply unaffected by whatever drug the patient is taking, and a different drug is required.

ERYSIPELAS
This term comes from the Greek roots *eryth*, for "redness" (think of *erythema* or *erythrocyte*) and *pello*, for "skin." Red skin with a sharply demarcated border is a hallmark of erysipelas.

Massage?

This is a condition involving a highly contagious bacterial infection, skin damage, and the risk of blood poisoning if it should find its way into the circulatory system. It systemically contraindicates massage until all signs of infection have been eradicated.

Fungal Infections
Definition: What Is It?

The nomenclature for the range of fungal infections people can get is dizzying. Fungal infections of human skin, also called *mycoses*, can involve several different types of fungi (*dermatophytes*). *Dermatophytosis*, then, is another term for mycosis. The lesions the infections create are called *tinea*. To top it all off, the generic term *ringworm*, although misleading because no worms are involved, is frequently used to refer to several types of tinea.

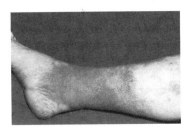
Figure 1-4. Erysipelas

Etiology: What Happens?

Dermatophytes live on keratin, the protein that fills dead epithelial cells on the surface of the skin. They thrive in warm, moist places like skin folds between toes or around the groin. They tend to infect people with depressed or sluggish immune systems. Fungal infections are transmitted via touch: either skin-to-skin or skin-to-anything that has some fungus on it, like massage sheets, locker room benches, or the family hairbrush. Dogs and cats can also transmit fungal infections to humans. It takes anywhere from 4 to 14 days for lesions to appear. During that time the carrier is infectious, which makes this condition very hard to control.

Signs and Symptoms

Tinea infections vary considerably depending on where they appear. Some varieties of dermatophytes fluoresce under black lights; others do not. Several varieties of tinea affect human skin. The following are descriptions of the most common ones.

- *Tinea corporis*, or *body ringworm*, is relatively common and very contagious, so it deserves special attention. It generally begins as one small round, red, scaly, itchy patch of skin on the trunk. Scratching spreads the fungus to other parts of the body, and so other lesions appear. They heal from the center first, and they soon take on the appearance of red circles, or rings, that may gradually increase in size, as the fungus spreads out for new food sources (Fig. 1-5, Color Plate 4).

- *Tinea capitis*, or *head ringworm*, inhabits the scalp. Lesions here result in itchiness and flaking (like really bad dandruff). If scratching and secondary infection result in scar tissue, temporary or permanent hair loss may occur. This variety is as contagious as body ringworm.

- *Tinea pedis*, or *athlete's foot*, usually focuses its attention on the skin between the toes (Fig. 1-6, Color Plate 5). Athlete's foot affects about 20% of the population to some degree. It burns and itches and carries the additional complication of weeping blisters; cracking, peeling skin; and the possibility of infection. Athlete's foot can even lead to *lymphangitis* (Chapter 5) or *erysipelas* (this chapter).

  One variety of athlete's foot fungus presents as dry, scaly, itchy lesions on the heel and sole of the foot. This is called a "moccasin distribution."

  Athlete's foot thrives in the growth medium provided by closed shoes. If a person has athlete's foot, it is especially important to make sure his or her feet are always as dry as possible, since these fungi, like most others, love warm, dark, moist places.

- *Tinea cruris*, or *jock itch*, is probably the least contagious of the group, but it does not occur exclusively around the groin. It can also be found on the upper thigh and buttocks; lesions may appear which a client is not aware of, but which massage therapists must avoid carefully (Fig. 1-7, Color Plate 6). Many cases of jock itch are actually caused by yeast infections (see *candidiasis*, Chapter 7).

- *Other varieties of tinea*. These include *tinea manus*, *tinea barbae*, *tinea versicolor*, and *tinea unguium*. Tinea manus, or hand ringworm, usually appears on the palm or between the fingers. It often occurs when a person also has athlete's foot. Tinea barbae affects the bearded area of the face; it is often misdiagnosed as bacterial folliculitis (a variety of *boils*, this chapter). Tinea versicolor is a fungal infection frequently picked up from the sand on Caribbean beaches. It creates variegated pigmentation on the skin. Tinea unguium is a fungal infection that invades the skin under finger and toenails. It has another name: *onychomycosis*.

Treatment

Treatment for fungal infections can sometimes be frustrating. Dermatophytes, like some viruses and bacteria, have mutated into many different varieties of the originals, each one more resistant to standard fungicides than the last. What's more, they somewhat resem-

---

FUNGAL INFECTIONS IN BRIEF

What are they?
Fungal infections of human skin, also called *mycoses,* are caused by fungi called *dermatophytes*. When dermatophytes colonize the skin, the characteristic lesions are called *tinea*. Thus, within this heading several different types of tinea are listed.

How is it recognized?
Most tinea lesions begin as one reddened, circular, itchy patch. Scratching the lesions may help to spread them to other parts of the body. As they get larger, they tend to clear in the middle and keep a red ring around the edges. Athlete's foot, another type of mycosis, usually involves moist blisters and cracking between the toes. If it affects the nails they will become yellow, thickened, and pitted.

Is massage indicated or contraindicated?
Fungal infections contraindicate massage at least locally in all phases. If the affected areas are very limited (e.g., only the feet are involved or only one or two small, covered lesions are present), massage may be administered to the rest of the body. If a large area is involved, and especially if the infection is acute (i.e., not yet responding to treatment), then massage is a systemic contraindication.

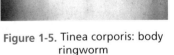

Figure 1-5. Tinea corporis: body ringworm

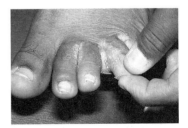

Figure 1-6. Tinea pedis: athlete's foot

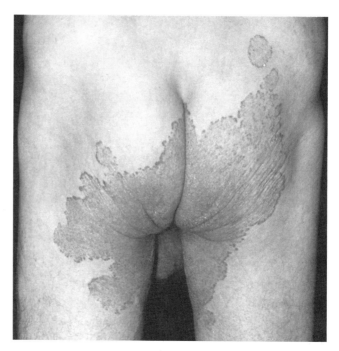

Figure 1-7. Tinea cruris: jock itch

ble the body's own proteins, which makes it difficult for the immune system to tag it and slow to fight it off. External applications of fungicide are the normal treatment, unless the infection is under the nail. In this case, internal doses of fungicides may be prescribed. Persons treating athlete's foot need to remember to treat their shoes as well, or they will be reinfected continually with the fungus.

Prevention

Where any kind of dermatophytosis is concerned, an ounce of prevention is worth a pound of cure. The best way for a massage therapist to avoid getting ringworm is to

RINGWORM
Delores G.

In June 1994, I was working hard in massage school. I was living in a house where some stray kittens were close by. I wanted to pet them, so I brought them some food. They came out, and I got to pet them while they were eating.

I was sitting down next to them with my knees up. I had shorts on. I was petting them with my left hand, and then I held my legs with the same hand when I was done. I also folded my arms, so my left hand touched my right bicep.

About 9 days later there were specific round red spots, the size of a half-dollar, on my left calf, and then on my right arm. It wasn't until I remembered petting the kittens that I realized where they came from. About a week after the spots appeared they started really burning and keeping me awake.

Having ringworm was awful. It turns out that I had massaged only two people between being exposed and being diagnosed, so it didn't spread through the class, but I had to wait until I was cleared up before I could work again. I sat out of practices, which was really depressing, *plus* it was spreading all over me, from my right arm to my right breast, and on my other calf.

I treated it by showering and then putting tea tree oil and anti-fungal vaginal cream all over me. I did that for 2 or 3 weeks before it started clearing up. It was all cleared up in 4 weeks. I waited an extra week just to be sure, so I missed a total of 5 weeks of massage.

When I got ringworm I was extremely run down from school, which probably made me susceptible. My teacher said it was interesting that my body chose ringworm as the thing that would slow me down, but it worked!

know what it looks like and to stay away from it. It is also particularly important to maintain one's own health. This gives the body every chance of fighting off any fungal attack.

Massage?

Fungal infections contraindicate massage in every phase (including the invisible gestation period, which can make it difficult). If it is a small infestation (just one or two lesions), it can be considered a *local* caution as long as the lesions are covered and the therapist does a 10% bleach rinse afterward. For clients with athlete's foot that shows blistering, weepy skin, the feet are a local contraindication. The decision might also depend on the therapist's own state of health; if the therapist is feeling run down and vulnerable, this may not be the week to work on someone with ringworm.

Herpes Simplex
Definition: What Is It?

Among the several different viruses in the herpes family that affect humans, two closely related herpes simplex viruses are especially common. These viruses cause painful blisters around the outside of the mouth and lips (oral herpes) or around the genitals, thighs, and buttocks (genital herpes).

When the herpes simplex viruses were first documented, it was found that the virus that caused oral herpes (Type I) was different from the one associated with genital herpes (Type II). Since then, a large amount of crossover has been noted, and so the delineation between a Type I and a Type II herpes infection has lost much of its significance.

Demographics: Who Gets It?

Estimates of the incidence of herpes simplex vary. Up to 60% of all sexually active adults may carry genital herpes; the number is probably higher for oral herpes. About 30 million people in the United States experience at least one outbreak of some variety of herpes simplex every year. Men and women are affected equally.

Etiology: What Happens?

Oral herpes is transmitted through oral or respiratory secretions. Genital herpes is transmitted through genital mucous secretions during any skin-to-skin contact. In any case, a person's first outbreak, which usually occurs 2 to 20 days after exposure, is called *primary* herpes. All subsequent outbreaks are called *recurrent* herpes.

A primary herpes outbreak may be almost unnoticeable. Most cases of oral herpes are picked up during childhood, and the new carrier may never be aware of his or her infection. In some cases, however, the primary infection may be extreme. It may be accompanied by fever, swollen glands, and painful sores that may last from 2 to 6 weeks.

One of the distinguishing features of the herpes virus is that it is never fully eliminated from the body. After the primary outbreak, the virus goes into hiding. There it waits for

---

HERPES SIMPLEX IN BRIEF

What is it?
Herpes simplex is a viral infection resulting in cold sores or fever blisters on the face or around the mouth, or blisters around the genitals, thighs, or buttocks.

How is it recognized?
Herpes simplex outbreaks are often preceded by 2 to 3 days of tingling, itching, or pain. Then blisters appear gathered around a red base. The blisters gradually crust and disappear, usually within 2 weeks.

Is massage indicated or contraindicated?
Any kind of herpes simplex in the acute stage locally contraindicates massage. Massage is also inappropriate if the client is showing any signs of systemic infection. The sheets of clients with active herpes simplex must be isolated and bleached. Massage for clients with a history of herpes but no active or prodromic symptoms may be appropriate, but therapists should be aware that no visible lesions need to be present for the virus to be present on the skin.

HERPES

The name for this collection of viruses, some of which spread on the skin, comes from the Greek word *herpo*, which means "to creep." This is also the root word of *herpetology:* the study of snakes.

an appropriate trigger, which could be a fever, a systemic infection, a sunburn, stress, a menstrual period, or some other factor. When the virus reactivates, a recurrent outbreak occurs, usually at or near the site of the original infection.

Communicability

The herpes virus is famous for its communicability. Unlike many pathogens, the herpes virus can remain dormant and healthy outside of a host body for hours at a time; exactly how long is a matter of some debate. This means that the face pad that an infected client used may now pass the virus to another client. Face cloths and towels are also potentially dangerous. Even leaving aside the strong possibility of infecting other people, herpes is notorious for spreading to other parts of the body. Touching a cold sore and then touching the eye can result in a painful and dangerous herpetic infection of the cornea (herpes keratitis).

One of the most dangerous aspects of a herpes infection is that a patient could be shedding the virus even from skin that has no visible lesion. This means that all it takes to catch herpes from another person is skin-to-skin contact with live virus. *No sore or break in the skin is necessary.*

Signs and Symptoms

Whether oral or genital, herpes simplex usually presents itself in the same way: the affected area may experience some pain or tingling a few days before an outbreak (the "prodromic" stage), then a blister or cluster of blisters appears on a red base. The blisters erupt and ooze virus-rich liquid all around the area (Fig. 1-8, Color Plate 7). The blisters scab over after a week or 10 days, ending the most dangerous phase for spreading the disease. Altogether, the outbreak lasts about 2 to 3 weeks.

The following are some differences in the ways genital and oral herpes present themselves:

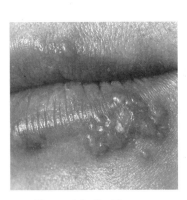

Figure 1-8. Oral herpes

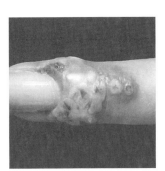

Figure 1-9. Herpes Whitlow

- *Oral herpes* tends to erupt when immunity is otherwise depressed (they are called "cold sores" or "fever blisters" because they often occur when a person is fighting off some other infection), during hormonal changes as in pregnancy or menstruation, after prolonged exposure to sunlight, or in response to emotional stress. They appear most often on the lips and on the skin around the mouth. They may be a lifelong problem.

  Oral herpes lesions usually appear on or around the mouth, but it is possible for them to appear elsewhere on the body as well. Of special concern to massage therapists is a variety called *herpes Whitlow*, which is an outbreak of lesions around the nail beds of the hands (Fig. 1-9, Color Plate 8). *Herpes gladiatorum* is a variety of herpes simplex picked up from athletic mats by wrestlers.

- *Genital herpes* outbreaks also correspond to depressed immunity and general stress levels, but they do seem to run a course of appearing with less and less frequency until finally they simply never come back. As stated above, these blisters appear on the genitals, but they can also be found on the thighs, buttocks, and even on the skin over the sacrum. People who have herpes and are immune-suppressed tend to experience outbreaks over larger areas of the body than others. The lesions are usually quite painful, but if they are inside the vaginal canal a woman may be unaware of them, which has important implications for communicability. Genital herpes outbreaks are sometimes accompanied by systemic symptoms such as fever, muscular aching, swelling in the inguinal lymph nodes, and difficult or painful urination.

Complications

Secondary infection is a common complication of herpes lesions. Immune-suppressed persons (especially patients who have undergone organ transplants or those with acquired immune deficiency syndrome [AIDS]) are especially susceptible to infections. Vaginally delivered newborns of mothers with active genital herpes may suffer blindness or even brain damage. Genital herpes has also been statistically connected with higher rates of cervical cancer, so infected women are wise to have frequent Pap smears. The herpes simplex virus has also been linked to *encephalitis* and *meningitis* (Chapter 3).

Treatment

Herpes is a viral infection, which means there's little to do for it but wait for it to be over. Acyclovir is one anti-viral drug that may suppress viral activity, but it will not prevent future outbreaks. Prevention is the main thrust for treatment of this condition; this means isolating towels, bedding, and clothing as well as avoiding sexual contact while lesions are present. Keeping as healthy as possible between outbreaks is an important way to reduce the frequency and severity of herpes episodes.

Massage?

Obviously, acute herpes outbreaks contraindicate massage. If a client has a history of herpes, it is important to explain why it is a bad idea to receive a massage during the prodromic stage or during an outbreak. Even after a lesion has scabbed over, herpes is at very least a local contraindication. Because this virus can survive outside a host for hours, the sheets of any client with herpes should be considered "hot" and be isolated in a closed container and either professionally sterilized or receive extra bleach in the wash cycle.

Clients who have active herpes outbreaks are not good candidates to receive massage. Likewise, massage therapists who have active herpes outbreaks need to respect their clients' health by not exposing them to the virus. Scabbed-over cold sores may be very itchy. Massage therapists need to take special care not to inadvertently brush their face with their sleeves, wrists, or hands and then touch a client with a contaminated surface.

When is a Mouth Sore *Not* Herpes?

Oral herpes causes the familiar lesions we call "fever blisters" or "cold sores," but not all sores around the mouth are caused by the herpes virus.

- Angular stomatitis is a condition involving painful, irritated cracks around the corners of the mouth. This is often associated with denture-wearers who may drool while they sleep. The accumulation of saliva around the corners of their mouths provides a rich growth medium for the yeast that causes these lesions.

- Aphthae, or "canker sores," are lesions that occur inside the mouth, often on the gums and cheeks. These are small, painful ulcers whose cause is unknown. Aphthae may be virally related, but they are not contagious.

Impetigo

Definition: What Is It?

Impetigo is a bacterial infection that is especially common in children. Lesions usually occur around the nose and mouth, sometimes appearing inside the nostrils or ear canals. Although it usually begins somewhere on the head, impetigo can infect the skin anywhere on the body.

This infection is caused by both staphylococcus and streptococcus bacteria.

Signs and Symptoms

Impetigo begins as a rash with small blisters or pustules filled with clear or murky fluid. These often occur where the skin has been damaged by some other injury. When the blis-

IMPETIGO
This comes from the Latin words *im* and *peto*, which mean "to rush up, attack." This may refer to the invasive and extremely infectious nature of this type of infection.

ters pop, a characteristic honey-colored crust forms (Fig. 1-10, Color Plate 9). Impetigo is itchy and is most common in hot, humid climates or in dry, cold areas in the winter when lips and noses become chapped and vulnerable to infection.

Treatment

Mild impetigo can be treated with topical antibiotic cream. If the blisters have spread over much of the body, and especially if other signs of systemic infection (i.e., fever and chills) are present, then oral antibiotics are prescribed. Very rarely, the infection can complicate into *erysipelas* (this chapter) or *glomerulonephritis* (Chapter 9).

Prevention

Impetigo often appears where the skin has already been damaged: scabbed-over mosquito bites, chapped lips or noses, cuts, and sores. The first step in prevention is to stop any kind of infection from developing at these sites. Chapped skin should be treated with lubricant to prevent damage. All other wounds should be cleaned thoroughly and treated with anti-bacterial ointment.

Impetigo is an extremely contagious condition, and since it is both very itchy and most common in children, special precautions are recommended to prevent its spread. First, the patient must be discouraged from touching or scratching the lesions; impetigo can easily be spread to other parts of the body this way. Second, the lesions must be kept clean and dry, and crusts removed as soon as possible, since they harbor bacteria in the moisture underneath. Third, the patient's bedding and towels must be strictly isolated while he or she is infected. Children with impetigo are encouraged to stay home from school and avoid contact with other children for 1 to 3 days after they begin treatment.

Massage?

This contagious bacterial infection of the skin involves virulent pathogens that can be drug-resistant. Impetigo systemically contraindicates massage until the lesions have completely healed.

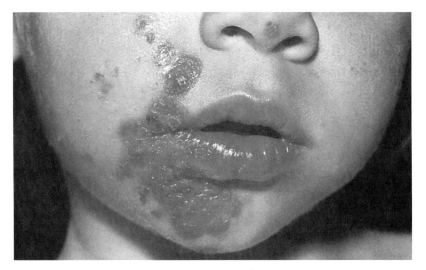

Figure 1-10. Impetigo

Lice and Mites

Mites

Definition: What Are They?

Tiny mites called *Sarcoptes scabiei* are the cause of skin lesions called scabies (Fig. 1-11). The female mites burrow under the skin in warm, moist spots where they drink blood, defecate and urinate, and lay eggs. The mites' waste is highly irritating, which causes an itchy allergic reaction in most hosts. If scratching damages the skin, the risk of secondary infection is high.

How Do They Spread?

Mites spread readily through close personal contact or through contact with something someone else has worn or lain on—like massage sheets.

Signs and Symptoms

Scabies-causing mites are too small to see with the naked eye, so a visual diagnosis is based on the trails they leave behind. Sometimes their burrows are visible. They look like reddish or grayish lines around the areas scabies favor: the groin, the axilla, elbows, the palms of the hands, and between fingers (Fig. 1-12, Color Plate 10). Mites like skin folds, although they also colonize the skin around the belt line. Other signs of mite infestation are the irritated blisters and pustules that arise from allergic reactions to their waste and secondary bacterial infection.

This condition is itchiest at night, when the mites are most active, but many skin irritations seem to itch more at night, simply because when a person is trying to sleep there are fewer distractions. The itching caused by mites, however, has a distinctive unrelenting quality. Where eczema or mosquito bites might itch intermittently and then subside, scabies itching gets continually worse.

Diagnosis

Scabies lesions can sometimes be hard to diagnose. Just a few mites can cause a great deal of irritation. People can be so miserable with their infestation that they cannot eat or sleep, but the skin tests sometimes do not show an actual bug, so a definitive diagnosis is difficult to make. It is typically based on the nature of the rash, the person's history, and the possibility of exposure.

Treatment

Mites, like other parasitic infestations, are treated by bathing with a pesticidal soap. This treatment can be harsh on the skin, and so must be used carefully. The mites die within several hours of being separated from human contact, so washing and then isolating bedding, towels, and clothing for that length of time will help to prevent further outbreaks. It is not necessary to fumigate the home, because scabies mites never stray far from their hosts.

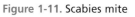

LICE AND MITES IN BRIEF

What are they?
Lice and mites are tiny animals that drink blood. They are highly contagious and spread through close contact with skin or infested sheets or clothing.

How are they recognized?
- The mites that cause scabies are too small to see, but they leave itchy trails where they burrow under the skin. They prefer warm, moist places such as the axillae or between fingers.
- Head lice are easy to see, but they can hide. A more dependable sign is their eggs: nits are small white, rice-shaped flecks that cling strongly to hair shafts.
- Pubic lice look like tiny white crabs.

All three of these parasites create a lot of itching.

Is massage indicated or contraindicated?
All three infestations contraindicate massage, until the parasites have been completely eradicated. If a massage therapist is exposed to any of these animals, every client he or she works on subsequently is also exposed, even before the therapist shows any symptoms.

Parasitic infestations are something every massage therapist fears. Bodyworkers are so very vulnerable to whatever is crawling around on clients' skins. Here, as in all things fearful, the best defense is information.

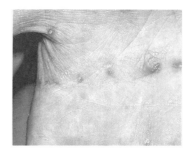

Figure 1-11. Scabies mite

Figure 1-12. Scabies lesions

Massage?

Massage is out of the question. If a massage therapist thinks he or she might have been exposed to mites, that patient's sheets should be considered "hot" (requiring isolation from other sheets and washing with extra bleach), and the therapist should consult a doctor about treatment immediately. The symptoms of scabies sometimes do not show up for 4 weeks or more; it takes that long to build up enough toxins to be irritating. Nevertheless, the therapist is certainly contagious the whole time; anyone he or she works on could become infested too. This caution holds true for the next two parasites as well.

SCABIES
Valerie

Valerie was a massage student. She worked with a variety of people, including fellow students, friends, and her student internship group, people with AIDS.

One day Valerie noted that she had some areas on the outsides of her elbows that were slightly but persistently itchy during the day. They gradually developed red bumps. Ironically, this occurred while Valerie was studying skin conditions in her massage course. "It's natural to convince yourself that you have symptoms for a lot of things. I knew something was going on, and it seemed like it *could* be scabies, but my symptoms were different from anything I'd seen described," she said. The itching was not particularly worse at night and there were no tracks or typical signs of infestation. Even the site of infestation was unusual: scabies mites usually go for warm, moist protected areas like skin folds on the *insides* of elbows, but not the outsides.

Eventually Valerie went to her general practitioner, who pronounced her condition a "mystery rash" and suggested a corticosteroid cream to limit the itchiness. In a way, Valerie was relieved by this diagnosis. "You never want to think you have scabies," she said. When her husband also developed symptoms, however, he went straight to a dermatologist, who immediately diagnosed scabies and prescribed enough pesticidal soap for both of them.

The cream was applied all over the body up to the chin; evidently scabies do not infest the head or face. "That night after I washed off the cream, I was really, really, *really* itchy, and then for 4 or 5 weeks my skin was raw and uncomfortable." The cream itself can create symptoms that mimic a scabies infestation for weeks at a time. This can lead to a condition called "scabiosis," in which a person is convinced that they need to medicate for scabies again and again, although they are not really infested. Scabiosis can become a life-threatening condition if the patient repeatedly self-medicates.

Six to eight weeks passed between the onset of Valerie's symptoms and a final diagnosis. During this time Valerie had continued to work on friends and clients as well as to receive massage from other students. Two other classmates were finally infested and diagnosed. "The first few days (after we knew it was scabies) were full of panic and fear. Within a couple of days of people getting over their fear and paranoia there was a lot of support. People had the attitude that this is just one of the things that can happen when you're a bodyworker."

Head Lice

Definition: What Are They?

Head lice are insects that live in head hair and suck blood from the scalp. Having lice is a condition called *pediculosis*. Lice are quite a bit larger than mites and can easily be seen without a microscope (Fig. 1-13). Their saliva is very irritating, which causes itching and the accompanying complication of possible infection.

How Do They Spread?

Lice jump. They also like hats. They thrive in classrooms and batters' helmets that are shared by little league teams. A person does not need close contact to someone who is infected to catch lice; *no* contact is needed. All a person needs to do is try on an infested hat at the local hat store, hang a coat on the same hook that an infested person used, or take a ride in a car with an infested headrest.

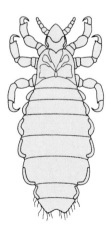

Figure 1-13. Head louse

Signs and Symptoms

If a client has lice the actual parasites may or may not be obvious; they are quite mobile and can hide. They lay eggs called *nits* (the source of the term "nit-pick"). Nits cling to hair shafts and look like tiny grains of rice. They hatch after about 1 week. If nits are dark, they may not yet have hatched. White nits are usually the empty eggshells that are still sticking to the hair. Nits are a prime diagnostic feature for pediculosis; anything else of that size and color (like dandruff) would brush out easily.

Lice lay their eggs right at the base of the hair shaft, mostly behind the ears and along the base of the neckline. One way to determine how long an infestation has been present is to observe how far the nits have grown away from the scalp.

A person with an active infestation of lice will experience itchiness and the sensation of movement on the scalp. Rigorous scratching can damage the skin and open the door to secondary infection or *dermatitis* (this chapter).

Treatment

Again, repeated applications of pesticidal shampoo to kill adults and eggs is the first step in treating lice. Some types of lice are becoming resistant to standard pesticides, so it is now recommended that applications of the medicine be followed by systematically combing every section of hair with a fine-toothed comb.

Persons averse to bathing in the toxic pesticides that are prescribed for lice infestations may choose to "smother" the lice with petroleum jelly or mayonnaise. These treatment options are slightly less effective than medicated shampoos, and so it is especially important to combine them with the systematic removal of nits with a nit comb.

Washing bedding, towels, and clothing is also necessary, as well as thoroughly cleaning hats, hairbrushes, combs, and anything else that comes in contact with the head. Washing items at 130°F and drying them on high heat for 20 minutes is considered sufficient. Dry cleaning nonwashable items is also effective. Anything else that might harbor lice (stuffed animals, soft toys, etc.) should be tied in a dry cleaning bag and isolated for 2 weeks.

Massage?

Clients who know that they have head lice should not receive massage. If a therapist suspects that he or she has been exposed, precautionary measures should be taken at once.

Pubic Lice

Definition: What Are They?

Pubic lice are a breed apart from their head-hair–loving relatives. They are tiny insects that look a lot like their nickname: *crabs* (Fig. 1-14). "Crabs" are a bit less discerning in their tastes: they like pubic hair in the groin best, but they will also live in armpit hair and body hair. They will even be found in eyebrows and eyelashes.

How Are They Spread?

Pubic lice are usually spread through sexual contact, but infested massage sheets can spread them, too. They do not jump, however, and they do not spread as easily as head lice. Of all the parasites being discussed, these may be the hardest to catch.

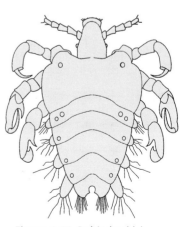

Figure 1-14. Pubic (crab) louse

Signs and Symptoms

Pubic lice look like tiny white crabs, about 1 millimeter across. They also leave nits, but they are so small they are just barely visible. Like all the infestations discussed, the primary symptom is itching.

Treatment

Pubic lice are the least contagious of the animals discussed here, but they can be spread through personal contact or contact with infested sheets. Crab lice carriers must follow the same protocols as head lice carriers. The sheets of any massage client suspected of a crab infestation should be isolated from all others and sterilized as soon as possible.

Massage?

Infestations of pubic lice, head lice, mites, and any other parasitic infestation of the skin contraindicate massage.

Parasitic infestation carries a powerful social stigma that is negatively (and inaccurately) associated with poverty and poor hygiene. It must be remembered that any individual (including massage therapists) could have this problem, and people in touch professions are in a position to cause a lot more damage with it than anyone else. Therefore, massage therapists must be respectful and remember that it could happen to anyone.

Warts

Definition: What Are They?

Warts are fascinating. Most of them are small, benign neoplasms caused by the human papilloma virus, which targets the keratinocytes, the same cells affected by squamous cell carcinoma. These protein-producing cells then produce a great amount of extra keratin, which is the material that makes our epithelial cells hard and scaly. The result: *verruca vulgaris*.

Etiology: What Happens?

Warts affect young children occasionally, adults rarely, and teenagers mercilessly. Most adults who get warts are probably somehow immune-suppressed. Warts can be contagious if the edges are roughened; the virus is contained in the blood and in the shedding skin cells. They are usually self-limiting, that is, they tend to go away on their own. In that sense they are a viral infection in slow motion: the virus slowly enters the body, it slowly takes over a few skin cells, and they slowly respond. Slowest of all, the body finally vanquishes this not very threatening invader, and that's the end of it. In very healthy people they can be expected to clear within 1 year. For others it can take longer.

Signs and Symptoms

Warts look like hard, cauliflower-shaped growths on the skin (Fig. 1-15, Color Plate 11). They are usually more of a nuisance than anything else, but when they occur on the bot-

---

WARTS IN BRIEF

What are they?
Warts are neoplasms that arise from the keratinocytes in the epidermis; they are caused by extremely slow-acting viruses.

How are they recognized?
Typical warts (verruca vulgaris) look like hard, cauliflower-shaped growths. They usually occur on the hands. They can affect anyone, but teenagers are especially prone to them.

Is massage indicated or contraindicated?
Massage is a local contraindication for warts. The virus is contained in the blood and shedding skin cells, and it is possible to get warts from another person.

tom of the feet (*plantar warts*) they can seriously impair function. In this case (and sometimes when they occur on the palm of the hands) the warts grow *inward*, creating a sensation of always stepping on something hard that never goes away (Fig. 1-16, Color Plate 12).

Verruca vulgaris is the most common kind of wart, but it is worth looking at some of the other types. Sixteen different subtypes of warts have been identified; only a few will be discussed here.

- *Plane warts.* These are small, brown, smooth warts that are most often seen on the faces of children.
- *Flat warts.* These are similar to verruca vulgaris, but they are much smaller and tend to occur in exposed places. Flat warts on the face can be spread by nicks and cuts with shaving.
- *Molluscum contagiosum.* This is also a children's malady, involving small white lumps.

Treatment

If warts are not going away fast enough on their own (and this can sometimes take years), medical intervention may be necessary. Drug stores sell preparations that claim to be effective, but they must be used with great caution to avoid damage to surrounding tissues. The common ingredient in most of these products is salicylic acid.

A standard medical approach is to freeze warts off with liquid nitrogen. However, if any of the virus remains in the body, the warts will probably recur. Other treatment op-

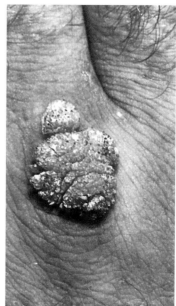

Figure 1-15. Warts

⚠ Plantar Warts Versus Callus

Plantar warts often look like a simple callus: the thick skin that grows on areas of the feet is subject to much wear and tear. The problem is that although people may file or snip off their calluses with no ill effects, to do the same with a plantar wart is to risk having that wart virus spread all over the foot and lead to more growths until it becomes difficult to walk.

Massage therapists are in a unique position to observe their clients' feet and notice the subtle differences between plantar warts and calluses.

	Plantar Warts	**Callus**
Location	Could be anywhere on the plantar surface of the foot; usually *not* bilateral.	Appears in areas of wear and tear, especially the back of the heels and the lateral aspect of the feet; callus usually grows in a similar pattern on both feet
Appearance	May be white but with darker speckling under the thickened skin: this is the capillary supply for the wart	Thick, white skin
Sensation	Very hard and unyielding: like stepping on a stone	No particular sensation

WATCH FOR THIS

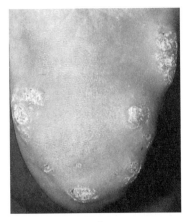

Figure 1-16. Plantar warts

tions include electrosurgery, carbon dioxide lasers, injections, and excision. These interventions will be particularly important for someone struggling with plantar warts that make it difficult to walk.

Wart treatment seems to be especially suggestible. If a person believes that a treatment will work, it is far more likely to be successful. This has led to some interesting approaches to wart management. One of the best came from a student who said, "Take a potato and cut it in six pieces. Bury each of the pieces in a different place, and *don't tell anyone where you hid them.* The wart will go away in a couple of weeks. Mine did."

Massage?

Consider warts a local contraindication. As stated above, the virus is found in the shedding skin cells around the lesion. Further, warts are often caught and torn around the edges, and if the skin is not intact, the client is a walking invitation for infection.

Non-Contagious Inflammatory Skin Disorders

ACNE IN BRIEF

What is it?
Acne is a bacterial infection of sebaceous glands usually found on the face, neck, and upper back. It is closely associated with adolescence or liver dysfunction that results in excess testosterone in the system.

How is it recognized?
It looks like raised, inflamed pustules on the skin, sometimes with white or black tips.

Is massage indicated or contraindicated?
Acne locally contraindicates massage, because of the risk of spreading infection, causing pain, and exacerbating the symptoms with the application of an oily lubricant.

Acne

Definition: What Is It?

Acne is a condition in which a person becomes susceptible to small, localized skin infections. They usually appear on the face, neck, and upper back.

Demographics: Who Gets It?

Many people have painful, awkward memories of adolescence thanks to this condition. When individuals make the transition from childhood to adulthood, their bodies start to secrete the hormones (some estrogen, but mostly testosterone) that are responsible for more than sexual maturity; they also sponsor mood swings, teenage rebellion, and excess sebum production. This change in hormone levels accounts for the high incidence of acne among teenagers. Adults can get acne too, although not necessarily because of excessive testosterone production.

Up to 80% of all people experience acne at one time or another. This makes it one of the most common diseases in the world.

Etiology: What Happens?

The process of developing acne is complicated, with many contributing factors. This is a condition often associated with puberty, but it is not exclusive to teens. A brief discussion of several of the contributing factors for teens and adults follows.

Factor 1: Testosterone Production   When a person enters puberty, one of the changes that occurs is the sudden secretion of high levels of androgens (male hormones that are secreted by both males and females). High levels of testosterone cause sebaceous glands, the oil glands that lubricate hair shafts, to shift into high gear. At this point, it is especially important that sebaceous ducts to the surface of the skin stay clear. If any tiny particle like a bit of duct lining or a flake of dead skin obstructs the duct, sebum rapidly accumulates behind the blockage.

Factor 2: Bacterial Activity   The pooling of oil in hair shafts is an invitation to the colonies of bacteria that grow on the skin. Staphylococcus may cause some acne lesions, but the majority of them are due to a special microbe: *Propionibacterium acnes. P. acne* produces enzymes that exacerbate inflammation and cause bacteria to clump together. This leads to more colonization of the sebaceous ducts.

Soon a localized infection leads to a pustule, a pimple, or some other type of acne lesion. These blemishes usually appear on the face, upper neck, and upper back in the sebaceous glands that lubricate tiny, almost invisible hair shafts.

Factor 3: Stress   Stress can upset endocrine balance and slow the activity of immune system cells. ("Stress" and "adolescence" are also practically synonymous.) If the macrophages stationed in the superficial fascia are sluggish, they cannot fight the bacteria that want to colonize the sebaceous glands. Furthermore, once the infection has subsided, those same suppressed macrophages are slower to consume the residual dead bacteria and white blood cells, which means it takes longer for pimples to fade.

Factor 4: Liver Congestion   When acne affects adults, it is often because liver congestion makes it difficult to neutralize the normal amounts of testosterone in the system. This leads to excess sebum production, bacterial colonization of sebaceous glands, and all the signs of acne. What causes liver congestion? It varies from person to person, but generally high-fat diets, smoking, drugs, and chemical pollutants are the most common culprits for most people. *Hepatitis* (Chapter 7) or other disorders can also severely compromise liver function.

Factor 5: Hormonal Imbalance   Hormonal changes that accompany the menstrual cycle or the beginning or ending of birth control pill prescriptions may lead to acne in mature women.

Signs and Symptoms

The symptoms of acne are probably familiar to most people. It can be locally painful but is not generally associated with systemic infection (Fig. 1-17, Color Plate 13).

Bacterial infections of the skin can cause several different types of acne lesions:

- *Pimples* are infections trapped below the surface of the skin; they involve raised, red, painful bumps or papules.
- *Cysts* are infections trapped deep in the dermis. They can protrude into the subcutaneous layer. Cysts may or may not be inflamed.
- *Open comedones* are also called "blackheads." These infections are superficial and the passage into the hair follicle is open to the air. This allows the trapped sebum to oxidize and turn dark. Blackheads are not, as popular belief would have it, trapped particles of dirt.
- *Closed comedones* are also called "whiteheads" or pustules. They are superficial infections that are covered with a thin layer of epithelium that traps the sebum and pus.

Treatment

Working with diet and other life habits to cleanse the liver and make its filtering job easier often results in clearer skin as well as a host of other benefits. Massage of the abdomen

ACNE

The root of this word is probably the result of a copyist's error. The original Greek work, *akme*, means "point of efflorescence." This describes a process in which a crystalline substance gradually changes to a powder as it dries.

and liver may support this process, but it is erroneous to claim that massage reliably clears up acne—too many other factors are involved in the process.

For teenagers with acne, the best advice is the most difficult to follow: *don't touch the face.* Touching, scratching, and popping acne lesions do little except to spread the bacteria and present the possibility of permanent scarring.

When medical help is requested for acne, interventions usually take a two-pronged attack: topical steroids are applied for their anti-inflammatory properties, and antibiotics are administered internally to fight the bacteria. The disadvantage here is that a long-term course of antibiotics can play havoc with intestinal flora and the immune system. One alternative is a line of drugs called retinoids, which are effective for acne but have a list of troubling side effects including joint pain and hair loss. Retinoids are also contraindicated if the patient may be pregnant during treatment, because they are highly implicated in birth defects.

Massage?

Massage of the abdomen and liver can sometimes yield good results. However, massage on the lesions themselves is out of the question. Pimples are *infections* and they involve a compromised shield: the skin is no longer intact, which means massage can make the infection worse. Also, the excellent blood supply to the skin creates at least the possibility, if not the likelihood, that the infection could spread. Finally, the lubricant can also block sebaceous glands, further aggravating an already irritable situation.

Wiping down an acne-prone client with alcohol after an oily treatment would seem to make some sense because it can cut right through and remove *all* the oil from the skin. However, the human body has a habit of lashing back from such extreme changes in environment: it will work overtime to replace all the natural oils the alcohol just removed and more. If a client is concerned about the lubricant, the best options are to use a water-based lotion instead of oil or to recommend that they shower with an astringent soap as soon as possible after treatment.

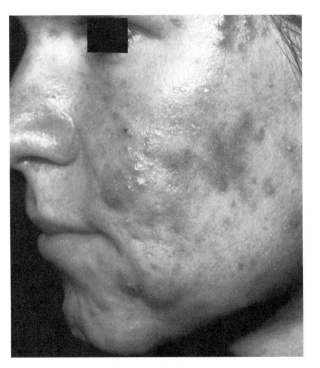

Figure 1-17. Acne

Boils Versus Acne

Boils and acne have a lot in common: they are both localized infections of sebaceous glands in hair follicles, they are both caused by staphylococcus infections, and they both have a red base with a pustule. Nevertheless, boils are far more serious than acne and require different precautions from massage therapists. The following are some differentiating features:

	Boils	Acne
Pattern of appearance	One lesion at a time, or a small interconnected group of pustules	Spread over large areas (the face, back, or neck)
Virulence	Aggressive bacteria that attack living tissue	Less aggressive bacteria that simply take advantage of a hospitable growth medium
Symptoms	Extremely painful	Mildly painful
Communicability	Highly communicable	Not communicable without prolonged contact
Special precautions	At least a local contraindication, but may be systemic if signs of general infection are present; isolate and bleach sheets	Local contraindication; no other precautions necessary

Dermatitis/Eczema

Definition: What is it?

Dermatitis is an umbrella term for skin inflammation, which is about as nonspecific as a diagnosis can get. Many of the conditions in this chapter could be called dermatitis, although by convention the term dermatitis is reserved for disorders that are not infectious in origin. This section focuses on atopic dermatitis and contact dermatitis, with some brief discussions of other types of skin inflammations.

Contact dermatitis is a skin inflammation caused by an *external* irritation or allergen. This separates it from other inflammatory skin conditions that arise from an infection, for instance, *erysipelas* (this chapter) or other internally mediated skin problems like *psoriasis* (this chapter). Atopic dermatitis, or eczema, is a condition connected to hypersensitivity reactions in the skin.

Demographics: Who Gets It?

Statistics on contact dermatitis are unavailable because it is such a general problem and can accompany many other disorders. Eczema is very common. It affects approximately 1 of every 7 infants and young children. Most people grow out of it; its incidence is about 3% of adults.

DERMATITIS/ECZEMA IN BRIEF

What is it?
Dermatitis is an umbrella term for inflammation of the skin. Eczema is a type of *atopic* dermatitis: a non-contagious skin rash usually brought about by an allergic reaction. Contact dermatitis is an inflammation brought about by irritation or allergic responses in the skin.

How is it recognized?
Dermatitis presents itself in various ways, depending on what type of skin reactions are elicited. Exposure to poison oak or poison ivy results in large inflamed wheals; metal allergies tend to be less inflamed and more isolated in area.

Eczema usually appears as very dry and flaky skin (seborrheic eczema) or blistered, weepy skin (dyshidrotic eczema).

Is massage indicated or contraindicated?
The appropriateness of massage depends completely on the source of the problem and the condition of the skin. If the skin is very inflamed or has blisters or other lesions, it contraindicates massage at least locally until the acute stage has passed. If the skin is not itchy and the affected area is highly isolated, as with a metal allergy to a watchband or earrings, massage is only a local caution.

ECZEMA
The root of this word is the Greek *ekzeo*, which means "to boil over." This is a very apt description of many types of eczema.

Etiology: What Happens?

Many types of dermatitis are brought about by an overreaction in the immune system to some irritating substance. These hypersensitivity reactions are discussed in detail in the introduction to the Lymph and Immune System (Chapter 5), but it is useful to look at an encapsulated version here.

The two types of hypersensitivity reactions that create skin symptoms are Type I allergic reactions and Type IV delayed reactions.

Atopic dermatitis, or eczema, is an example of a Type I reaction. These are immune system responses to nonthreatening stimuli. In this situation, nearby mast cells release vasodilating chemicals, including histamine, which create an inflammatory response. The term "atopic" refers to an inherited tendency toward various allergic reactions. Someone with eczema very likely has other family members who struggle with hay fever (see *sinusitis* and *asthma*, Chapter 6.)

Allergic contact dermatitis is a Type IV reaction, mediated by a complex organization of immune system agents. Poison oak, poison ivy, and local skin reactions to metals, soaps, dyes, or latex are examples of contact dermatitis.

Causes of Eczema

Research into the causes of eczema is proceeding, but no single factor has yet been identified.

Some of the possible causes of eczema include the following:

- A deficiency in certain fatty acids has been observed in eczema patients. A lack of linoleic acid can make the skin less able to retain moisture and more susceptible to drying.

- Certain monocytes may malfunction in persons with eczema, which causes a very extreme immune system response to minor stimuli.

- Persons with eczema tend to have elevated levels of immunoglobulin E (IgE), allergy-related antibodies that cause excessive secretion of histamine. Histamine causes many inflammatory reactions, including capillary dilation, red skin, and itching.

Signs and Symptoms of Eczema

Signs and symptoms of eczema vary according to what type is present.

- *Seborrheic eczema.* This is the most common variety. It seems to be genetic and is irritated by stress. Seborrheic eczema is usually red, flaky, and dry, occurring in the creases on the sides of the nose and other skin creases such as knees, elbows, and hands (Fig. 1-18, Color Plate 14). If it occurs on the scalp, seborrheic eczema has another name: dandruff. As long as the skin is dry, intact, and not puffy or itchy, seborrheic eczema indicates massage. Caution must be exercised, however, when verifying that the skin is intact, and a nonirritating lubricant that will not exacerbate the situation should be used.

- *Dyshidrosis.* This is a less common form of eczema, but it is still fairly common. In this condition blisters filled with fluid appear, mostly on hands and feet. It is sometimes described as looking like a combination of *fungal infection* (this chapter) and a contact allergy. It often occurs in response to hot weather or emotional stress.

    Dyshidrosis can be very difficult to treat and can sometimes require systemic steroids. Like seborrheic eczema, dyshidrosis is non-contagious. Unlike the dry

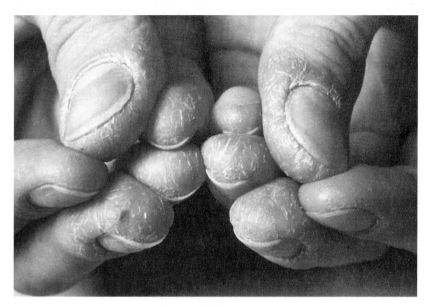

Figure 1-18. Eczema

presentation of eczema, dyshydrosis presents the danger of blisters breaking, which exposes the client to infection. It is therefore a local contraindication for massage.

- *Nummular eczema.* This form of eczema appears in small circular lesions, often on the legs and buttocks.

Causes of Contact Dermatitis

Contact dermatitis can stem from simple irritation or from an allergic reaction. Irritant contact dermatitis usually arises from prolonged contact with some substance that would eventually be irritating to *anyone;* this distinguishes it from allergic contact dermatitis. Irritants that can reliably bring about a reaction include working in water, harsh cleansers, acids and alkalis, and ongoing friction. These stimuli eventually damage even the healthiest skin, but removal from the irritation results in a cessation of symptoms.

Allergic contact dermatitis differs from irritant contact dermatitis because the causative factors create a specific type of allergic response in the skin of the affected person. Some common allergens associated with allergic contact dermatitis include nickel (found in watchbands and earrings), preservatives used in lotions, the adhesive used in many medical bandages, some perfumes and dyes, and latex. Some substances cause an allergic reaction when the affected skin is exposed to sunlight. In this case rashes will break out only where sunlight hits the skin that has been in contact with the allergen, for instance, preservatives in sunscreen.

Signs and Symptoms of Contact Dermatitis

The symptoms of contact dermatitis can vary according to the causative factors. Acute situations are typically locally red, swollen, and itchy or tender, showing exactly where the irritation took place (Fig. 1-19, Color Plate 15). Long-lasting low-grade reactions may not show signs of inflammation, although mild itchiness is common.

Other types of dermatitis show specific patterns but are not related to irritation or contact with allergenic substances:

- *Stasis dermatitis.* This usually appears on the lower legs in association with poor circulation as seen with *diabetes* (Chapter 8) or *heart failure* (Chapter 4). Stasis dermati-

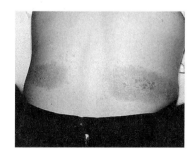

Figure 1-19. Contact dermatitis

tis is very red and may occur with small ulcers where the skin has been deprived of nutrition. It often resembles *erysipelas* (this chapter). Stasis dermatitis implies severe problems with blood flow and therefore contraindicates circulatory massage.

- *Neurodermatitis.* This condition involves a small injury, such as a mosquito bite, that creates an enormous inflammatory response and localized scaly patches of skin. It locally contraindicates massage until the inflammation has subsided.

Complications

Both contact dermatitis and eczema can begin a process by which what begins as a mildly irritating skin problem can exacerbate into a debilitating problem. When a person with dermatitis scratches the mildly itchy lesions, the lesions become stimulated and much itchier. This leads to more scratching, more itchiness, and a vicious circle called the "itch-scratch cycle."

Persons with dermatitis are particularly susceptible to secondary infection because their skin tends to be so irritable. *Impetigo, herpes simplex*, and *fungal infections* (all in this chapter) are all common complications for dermatitis and eczema patients.

Treatment

Self-help measures for people with contact dermatitis and eczema begin with isolating the substances that irritate them and then avoiding them carefully. Persons with eczema must also try to maintain adequate hydration of the skin. This means finding a moisturizer or emollient that does not contain any irritating substances.

The medical treatment of choice for dealing with contact dermatitis and eczema is corticosteroid cream. Cortisol, among other things, is a powerful anti-inflammatory (see side bar), but corticosteroid creams must be used *exactly* as prescribed because:

- Steroid creams can cause their own "steroid rash," or they can quell macrophage action, making users prone to *boils* (this chapter).

- A "backlash" effect can occur: after the use of steroidal creams is stopped, the original complaint can come back in a more extreme version.

- If steroid creams are used over a long period (several months), permanent changes can be brought about by exposure to a substance that melts connective tissue: the skin can become thin, delicate, and easily damaged. (Of course massage would be inappropriate in a case like this.)

- Finally, in a worst case scenario, the adrenal glands can suffer damage, which can be life-threatening.

  Massage practitioners must emphasize how important it is to use medications exactly as they are prescribed: not less, not more. Above all, a person must make the effort to get to the root of the problem, rather than just patching over the symptoms. After all, if a person is allergic to a certain soap, what makes more sense: applying steroid cream daily for months or changing brands?

Massage?

The appropriateness of massage depends entirely on the causes and severity of a client's dermatitis. If the skin is red, hot, puffy, and itchy from a morning walk through poison oak, massage is *not* appropriate. First, the inflammation will be exacerbated by extra blood in the area. Second, the irritating substance (the poison oak oils) can be distributed over more of her body, spreading the inflammation. Acute dermatitis systemically contraindicates massage until all inflammation has subsided.

If, on the other hand, a client is displaying a small, slightly reddened, flaky, circular area on the back of her left wrist (about the place where a wrist watch would usually sit), it may be possible to pursue a line of questioning that will determine that massage probably will not aggravate or spread the irritation, which is probably being caused by an allergy to nickel.

The appropriateness of massage for eczema depends on the type that is present and whether the skin has been compromised to point at which a danger of infection is a problem. For more details, see the individual descriptions above.

Hives

Definition: What Are They?

Hives, also called *urticaria*, are the result of emotional stress or an allergy: an immune response to a substance that is not necessarily threatening to the body.

Etiology: What Happens?

Let's consider someone who is allergic to shellfish. Somehow a shrimp finds its way into his Lemon Grass Soup. Within moments his immune system cells launch a full-scale attack . . . but they don't quite know where to go. In the confusion, specialized cells called mast cells freely distributed in the superficial fascia release histamine. This causes local capillary dilation, extra cell permeability, and *lots* of edema. Hives is an example of a Type 1 hypersensitivity reaction (a true "allergic" reaction).

Histamine release causes a localized inflammatory response (redness) and the edema presses on nerve endings (itching). Some people need an unexpected encounter with an allergen to make this happen, but for others all it takes is an unfamiliar or threatening situation. Hives are very common. It is estimated that up to 20% of all people experience them at some point, although they are more frequent with people who have other allergies. Sometimes students break out in hives when they take a test; some may do it while reading about diseases. Some clients who have never had massage before will get hives the first time they get on a massage table.

Signs and Symptoms

Hives begin as small, raised, reddened areas called wheals that may join to become larger irregular patches (Fig. 1-20, Color Plate 16). The lesions are red around the outside and are sometimes paler in the middle. They are itchy and hot to the touch. They are not contagious but are usually brought about by a food allergy, an insect bite or sting, a reaction to medication, or emotional stress.

HIVES IN BRIEF

What are they?
Hives are an inflammatory skin reaction to an allergen or emotional stressor.

How are they recognized?
Hives range from small red spots to large wheals, which are warm to the touch and itchy. Individual lesions generally subside within a few hours, but successive hives may appear; the cycle can continue for several weeks.

Is massage indicated or contraindicated?
Hives contraindicate massage at least locally. If the lesions cover a large portion of the body, this may be a systemic contraindication. Bringing even more circulation to the skin only makes a bad situation worse.

Stress, Allergies, and Cortisol

Stress can ripple through the body in a number of different chemical ways. Massage therapists study some of these effects because they too have some influence over what chemicals are being released, and that influence should be informed and intentional.

For people who are prone to allergies, long-term stress creates some special problems. Cortisol is the hormone that is specifically related to long-term stress. When it's secreted over a long time, cortisol does some things that can damage the body, like systemically weakening the connective tissues. However, cortisol does one thing that is very, *very* good: it is a powerful anti-inflammatory agent. When people undergo long-term stress, they can become depleted in their cortisol supplies. When cortisol is depleted, the body has only limited resources to quell the inflammatory reaction. For persons subject to allergies, this means that they have a difficult time de-inflaming from immune system attacks against nonthreatening stimuli such as wheat, pollen, cat dander, or anything else. If the immune reaction takes the form of a skin rash, then it may be called dermatitis or eczema.

This is not to say that stress is the only cause of allergies, or even the most important one. It is just to point out that stress can often make allergies *worse*.

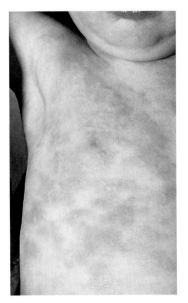

Figure 1-20. Hives

Individual hives usually clear within a few hours, but they may be replaced by other hives. It is common for a person to have ongoing hives for days or weeks.

A rarer version of hives is called *chronic urticaria*. In this situation the cycle of hives appearing, resolving, and being replaced by others lasts for 6 weeks or more. The triggers for these long-lasting episodes can be difficult or impossible to identify; evidence points toward an autoimmune component in chronic urticaria, but this condition is not well understood.

Treatment

Hives are always annoying but seldom really serious. If they require treatment, it is usually in the form of an antihistamine to quell histamine release. Even chronic urticaria is treated this way. Antihistamines for hives are usually prescribed in heavy doses to undo all the work of the mast cells. This can be problematic, as high doses of antihistamines often have a sedative effect.

Angioedema is one variety of hives that can be a medical emergency. These hives are occurring in deeper layers of the skin, usually around the face and throat. The tissue can swell up to the point that breathing becomes difficult. It is rare, but angioedema can be life-threatening, requiring an immediate injection of epinephrine to bring down the swelling and restore ease of breathing.

Massage?

Hives contraindicate massage in the acute phase; there is no benefit to bringing more blood into an area that is already too full. If a client has a history of this kind of problem, it is a good idea to take extra precautions to use an oil or lotion that will not initiate an attack.

Neoplastic Skin Disorders

MOLES IN BRIEF

What are they?
Moles are isolated areas where the pigment cells in the epidermis have produced excess melanin.

How are they recognized?
Moles can range in color from light tan to blackish-blue. Their color is usually uniform throughout. Moles are usually circular or oval.

Are they indicated or contraindicated for massage?
Massage does not help or hurt moles, but massage therapists may be able to see changes in a mole that a client cannot see.

Moles

Definition: What Are They?

Moles, or *nevi*, are benign neoplasms: areas where melanocytes replicate on-site, although without threatening to invade surrounding tissues. The melanocytes produce excessive melanin, the coloring agent for skin.

Signs and Symptoms

Moles are usually smaller than 6 mm (the size of a pencil eraser). They generally appear in a symmetrical shape (circular or oval) and they are unicolored. These features help to distinguish moles from malignant melanoma.

Etiology: What Happens?

Most people are genetically programmed to develop moles, and moles generally appear before age 20. (If any moles appear after this time, it is recommended to consult a dermatologist to rule out melanoma.)

Moles generally begin as flat black or brown marks on the skin. They may become elevated and grow coarse, dark hairs (Fig. 1-21, Color Plate 17). Many people find that as they get older their moles fade and may even disappear.

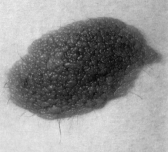

Treatment

A mole is not inherently dangerous, but that can change. Risk factors for moles becoming cancerous are determined by when they appear (anything that appears after age 20 is highly suspect) and how big they are (anything bigger than 6 mm bears watching). About 42% of all large moles appear on the back, where clients cannot see them, but therapists can.

Figure 1-21. Mole

Two types of moles have been identified as having a higher-than-average risk for changing to melanoma: *congenital nevi* (moles that are present at birth, especially when they're quite large) and *dysplastic nevi* (moles that exhibit the ABCDE symptoms described in *skin cancer*; this chapter).

Some doctors suggest removing large moles, just as a precaution. Some doctors recommend tracing a large nevus and then comparing the tracing to the real thing a few times a year. That way the patient can keep an accurate record of any changes.

Massage?

Massage neither hurts nor helps moles (unless they become irritated or torn), but massage practitioners are in a unique position to see what clients may not be able to; the practitioner may be the one to spot the transition from harmless nevus to life-threatening melanoma.

Psoriasis

Definition: What Is It?

The introduction to this chapter discusses how the readiness of epithelium to repair itself is a two-edged sword. On the one hand, the body can heal quickly and thoroughly from most insults to the skin. On the other hand, sometimes the ease of replication in skin cells can cause problems, as with this condition. Psoriasis is a chronic skin disease with occasional acute episodes in which epithelial cells in isolated patches replicate too rapidly. Whereas normal skin cells replace themselves every 28 to 32 days, psoriatic skin cells divide every 2 to 4 days. The result is a pile-up of excess cells that are itchy, red or pink, and scaly. This condition comes and goes, but no permanent cure has been found.

Demographics: Who Gets It?

Statistics on psoriasis vary. It affects between 5 and 7 million Americans, mostly Whites. Between 150,000 and 260,000 new cases are diagnosed every year. Some psoriasis cases have a genetic link. It is most commonly diagnosed in middle years, but it has been seen on tiny babies as well as quite elderly people. Psoriasis affects slightly more women than men.

Other Skin Pigmentations

Age and the uneven distribution of melanin in the skin can give rise to several different types of skin patches. Because massage therapists are health professionals who work closely with the skin, it is important to be familiar with the most common types of marks clients may have.

- *Freckles.* These are simple concentrations of melanin in the skin. They can range from light tan to red but are always darker than the surrounding skin. Most freckles are about the size of a nailhead, although when several blend together they can seem much larger. Fair-skinned people are more susceptible to freckles than others. Freckles often darken when they are exposed to sunlight and fade when they are protected from UV radiation.

- *Lentigos.* These are similar to freckles, but they usually appear on older people and are often much larger than freckles. They are often mistakenly referred to as "liver spots," but they have nothing to do with liver function.

- *Seborrheic keratosis.* These are skin lesions that are very common in older people. They are benign growths on the skin that have a waxy, "pasted on" appearance. They often develop a warty appearance when they have been present for a long while. Seborrheic keratosis blemishes can appear singly or in groups. The chest, back, and face are most often affected; they rarely appear below the waist. When seborrheic keratoses are very dark, they can look like malignant melanoma, although these growths are entirely benign.

- *Port wine stains.* These are a variety of birthmarks that affect blood vessels near the surface of the skin. They are often quite large and are harmless.

PSORIASIS
Psora comes from Greek for "the itch."

PSORIASIS IN BRIEF

What is it?
Psoriasis is a non-contagious chronic skin disease involving the excessive production of new skin cells that pile up into isolated lesions.

How is it recognized?
The most common variety of psoriasis looks like pink or reddish patches, sometimes with a silvery scale on top. It occurs most frequently on elbows and knees, but it can develop anywhere.

Is massage indicated or contraindicated?
The acute stage of psoriasis locally contraindicates massage, because the extra stimulation and circulation massage provides can make a bad situation worse. In subacute stages, massage is appropriate as long as the skin is intact.

Etiology: What Happens?

Psoriasis is not a well-understood disease, and research into its causes and possible cures continues. One theory is that overactive T-cells in the skin create an inflammatory response and the rapid replication of new skin cells. Vitamin D deficiencies in the skin of psoriasis patients have also been observed; vitamin D slows down the replication of skin cells. In about one third of all cases, psoriasis appears within families, leading to the exploration of a genetic predisposition for the disease.

Signs and Symptoms

Plaque psoriasis is a very common condition; most people have at least seen it. It usually takes the form of raised red or pink patches that, if they are present for a long time, develop a white or silvery "scale" on top (Fig. 1-22, Color Plate 18). They have sharply defined edges. The patches, or "plaques", may be itchy but seldom really uncomfortable unless they're in an acute stage, when they can itch and burn severely. Plaques are usually on the knees or elbows but can be found on the scalp, trunk, palms and soles, inside the mouth, and around the genitals as well. Psoriasis can also get under fingernails and toenails, where it can cause pitting and infection and sometimes result in the loss of the nail altogether.

Psoriasis often occurs in cycles of acute flares followed by periods of remission; this is a pattern seen with many diseases involving immune system dysfunction. Psoriatic flares can be triggered by a number of things: physical or emotional trauma, skin damage, sunburn, hormonal changes, prescription drugs related to high blood pressure and depression, or a state of immune suppression. Psoriasis outbreaks may be more common in wintertime because of the combination of dry skin and lack of sunlight.

In its subacute or non-active phase, a slight discoloration may remain on the skin where the lesions tend to appear. This is especially true on the trunk.

Other varieties of psoriasis are less common than plaque psoriasis but can be more serious. They include the following:

- *Guttate psoriasis.* This version is usually triggered by a viral or bacterial infection of the respiratory tract.

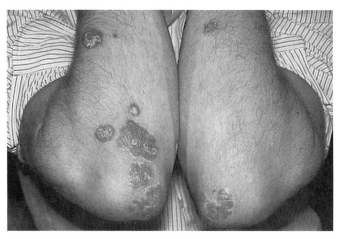

Figure 1-22. Psoriasis

- *Pustular psoriasis.* This involves small, noninfectious pustules in the affected areas.
- *Inverse psoriasis.* This appears at skin folds under the breasts, in the armpits, and around the genitals.
- *Erythrodermic psoriasis.* This version is triggered by sunburn and steroidal anti-inflammatories.

Complications

This is rarely a life-threatening condition, although it can be extreme and uncomfortable in the acute stages. In severe cases profound drying and cracking of the skin can lead to infection, fluid loss, and shock. Complications of psoriasis cause about 400 deaths per year in the United States.

Another complication of psoriasis is a condition called *psoriatic arthritis.* This is a type of joint inflammation that affects approximately 10 to 20% of psoriasis patients. The symptoms are very similar to *rheumatoid arthritis* (Chapter 2). The guidelines for massage and psoriatic arthritis are the same as those for rheumatoid arthritis.

Treatment

For such a common skin condition, psoriasis can be surprisingly difficult to treat. No single treatment is effective for a majority of patients, many of the most effective medications carry a number of serious side effects, and people often build up resistance to medications, making them less effective. Three main avenues are pursued with psoriasis treatments: topical applications, phototherapy, and systemic medications.

Topical medications vary from coal tar (popular because it carries a minimum of side effects, but problematic because it smells bad and stains clothing), to vitamin D ointments, to various strengths of steroid creams. The drawbacks of long-term steroid applications are spelled out in the *eczema* section of this chapter. Other topical treatments include salicylic acid (which is also used to remove warts) to help dissolve and remove plaques, and oatmeal or Epsom salt baths.

Phototherapy involves limited exposure to sunshine, or carefully regulated doses of exposure to UVA or UVB lights. UV exposure stimulates vitamin D production, which in turn inhibits skin cell replication. Too much UV exposure can exacerbate symptoms, however, so this therapy must be used cautiously.

Systemic medications may be steroidal drugs, retinoids to limit sebaceous secretions, or cytotoxic drugs (as in chemotherapy) to limit the activity of those skin cells that have run amok. Psoriasis and cancer have a lot in common in terms of uncontrolled replication, and this option is occasionally successful.

Topical and systemic therapies are often combined with phototherapy. PUVA is a common example. It is a combination of a systemic medication (psoralen) and UV light exposure. PUVA is often successful. Unfortunately, it is also linked to increased chances of contracting basal cell or squamous cell carcinoma as well as some other serious side effects.

Although many types of treatment for psoriasis are available, none of them has shown to be a permanent solution. Patients with very severe cases of psoriasis must frequently change strategies as their skin builds up resistance to treatment.

Massage?

In ancient Greece massage with olive oil was the prescribed treatment for psoriasis. It is now recognized that massage *on* the lesions during an acute outbreak will probably only aggravate the situation by stimulating circulation in an area where too much activity is already taking place. Psoriasis is a local contraindication in the acute phase, but otherwise massage is appropriate. (Of course, it is first necessary to make sure that there has not been any drying or cracking of the skin that would make the client vulnerable to infection.) Psoriasis will not be spread by massage, it is not contagious, and massage may be able indirectly to help deal with some of the internal and external stress factors that can stimulate an outbreak.

SKIN CANCER IN BRIEF

What is it?
Skin cancer is cancer in the stratum basale of the epidermis (basal cell carcinoma [BCC]), cancer of the keratinocytes in the epidermis (squamous cell carcinoma [SCC]), or cancer of the melanocytes (pigment cells) of the epidermis (malignant melanoma).

How is it recognized?
For BCC and SCC, one should look for the cardinal sign: sores that never heal. These sores can resemble blisters, warts, pimples, or simple unexplained bumps and abrasions. They are usually painless but may bleed or become slightly itchy as the cells become active. For malignant melanoma, one should look for a mole that exhibits the ABCDE's of melanoma.

Is massage indicated or contraindicated?
For BCC, which does not tend to metastasize, massage is a local contraindication, as long as the lesion has been diagnosed by a dermatologist. SCC and malignant melanoma carry the risk of metastasis. Therefore, any decisions about massage must be made according to the treatments the client is having, weighing possible benefits with possible risks.

Skin Cancer
Definition: What Is It?

Cancer is the uncontrolled replication of cells into tumors. These tumors can damage surrounding tissues, spread throughout the body, and sometimes be fatal. The tissues that are most vulnerable to cancer are often those that have to tolerate a great deal of wear and tear (skin cells, the epithelium of the lungs, and the inner layer of the colon are good examples). These cells heal easily and rapidly, but sometimes that feature backfires and a situation develops as in skin cancer, where cells that have endured a lifetime of abuse start "healing" in a way that could quite possibly kill.

Demographics: Who Gets It?

Some people wish that sleep could be cumulative, that is, that a person could sleep an extra 14 hours on a weekend and then not be tired for all of the following week. In a certain way, *sunlight* is cumulative. Picture a person playing on the monkey bars when he is 5 years old, roller-blading when he is 10, hiking in the mountains when he is 15, sailing when he is 40, and snorkeling when he is 50. His skin cells are keeping accurate records of exactly how much and how often he has insulted them with too much sun. One day, those skin cells may respond to all that exposure by replicating out of control. This is a particular risk if a person:

- Has pale skin that burns but does not tan.
- Lives in a place with a lot of sunshine.
- Spends a good deal of time outside.
- Is in any way immune-suppressed.
- Is mature and has built up a lifetime of exposure to the sun in the skin cells.

Skin cancer is the most common variety of cancer that humans experience. It is estimated that 40 to 50% of all adults older than 65 years of age will experience some type of skin cancer. Non-melanoma skin cancer will affect about 1.3 million Americans this year. Malignant melanoma will affect 44,000 people and will probably kill approximately 7,300. The good news is that the mortality rate of this disease is going down, largely due to an increased public knowledge of the signs of skin cancer that leads to early diagnosis and effective treatments.

Etiology: What Happens?

Three basic types of skin cancer and one precancerous condition are the most common forms of this disease. They will each be discussed in detail.

Actinic Keratosis: Precancerous Lesions

Definition: What is it?

Also called solar keratosis, this is a precancerous condition that can lead to SCC.

Signs and Symptoms

Brown or red scaly lesions usually appear on the forehead or other areas subject to a lot of sun exposure. These sores form a crust but they do not heal normally. The crust falls off and forms over again (Fig. 1-23, Color Plate 19). This pattern is the single most important sign of non-melanoma skin cancer. It is estimated that 1 person in every 6 will have actinic keratosis (AK) lesions at some time, and 10 to 20% of all untreated AK lesions can develop into SCC, which is a potentially dangerous disease.

Treatment

AK lesions are usually frozen off with liquid nitrogen. They may also be injected with medication, or a topical ointment may be applied. Very large lesions may be excised.

Massage?

Strictly speaking, AK is not a cancerous condition and therefore does not contraindicate massage. However, if a client has AK lesions, he or she should consider having them removed promptly. If there is a history of AK but nothing more serious has developed, massage is appropriate. Undiagnosed skin lesions are a caution for massage therapists, who should recommend that their clients consult their doctors as soon as possible.

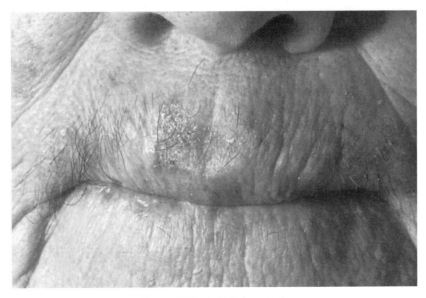

Figure 1-23. Actinic keratosis

Basal Cell Carcinoma

Definition: What Is It?

This is by far the most common type of skin cancer; it accounts for approximately 75 to 90% of all skin cancer cases. Fortunately, it is also the least serious. It is a slow-growing, nonmetastasizing tumor of epithelial cells in the stratum basale of the epidermis. It is not usually dangerous, although if the tumor is left untreated for years it can become life-threatening because of other tissues (e.g., nearby arteries or nerves) that are eroded by the tumor's growth.

Signs and Symptoms

BCC can be tricky to describe, because it looks like all sorts of different things. Typically it appears on the face, around the bridge of the nose or the eyebrow. It looks like a small, hard, pearl-colored lump, with rounded edges, and a soft, sunken middle. The borders are often hard, and they may bleed and form crusts. The middle of the lump is usually soft, with an open sore that may scab but never permanently heals: an ulceration. BCCs are sometimes called "rodent ulcers" (Figs. 1-24–1-26, Color Plates 20–22).

Another type of BCC is particularly common in elderly fair-skinned people who have spent a lot of time in the sun. This variety looks like flat sores, not on the face, but on the back and trunk. Like the typical facial BCCs, these sores do not heal but simply crust, shed the scab, and crust again. This variety of BCC is easily mistaken for seborrheic keratosis, a non-cancerous condition, which is why it is essential that massage therapists refer any client with suspicious lesions for further diagnosis (see sidebar).

Treatment

BCC, because it grows so very slowly and does not metastasize, responds very well to simply being excised (cut out with a knife or a laser). The tumor-producing cells can also be killed off with liquid nitrogen or radiation. Occasionally BCC recurs, so it is wise to keep a close watch for any non-healing sores after an episode.

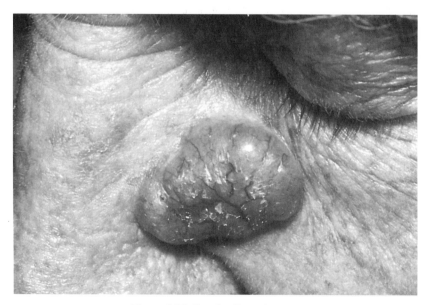

Figure 1-24. Basal cell carcinoma

Massage?

The tumor itself is a local contraindication, of course (*if* it is diagnosed as BCC). This is not something that spreads through the body, or that massage can make worse in any way. If a client fits the profile for the flat sore on the trunk, the practitioner may be the one to spot it in the first place.

Squamous Cell Carcinoma

Definition: What Is It?

This is a malignancy of keratinocytes in the epidermis. Keratinocytes are the cells that produce keratin, the protein that fills up the epithelial cells that are migrating toward the surface of the skin.

Signs and Symptoms

SCC can occur anywhere epidermis grows—on the skin, usually, but occasionally on mucous membranes too. It is especially common on ears, hands, and lower lips, but it can also happen *inside* the mouth, often as a response to pipe-smoking or chewing tobacco and the constant irritation that those habits incur. SCC accounts for about 22% of all skin cancers. It is significantly more dangerous than BCC, since it *can* metastasize through the lymph system and the tumors can infiltrate deeper tissues far more quickly than BCC.

SCC tumors often happen on pre-existing lesions on sun-exposed skin. In other words, they happen where the skin has had to repair itself before. Some but not all SCC lesions begin as AK. They generally start as hard, firm lumps that may look like a wart. The sores appear and *do not heal*. The borders of SCCs are often less distinct than the more self-contained basal cell tumors (Figs. 1-27 and 1-28, Color Plates 23–24).

AK, BCC, and SCC bear one key feature in common: an open sore that never quite heals. Often a crust forms but it does not hold on; inevitably the crust falls off and

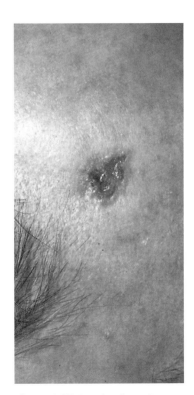

Figure 1-25. Basal cell carcinoma

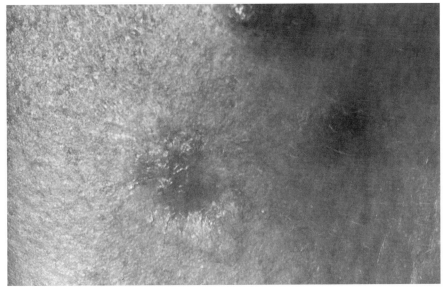

Figure 1-26. Basal cell carcinoma

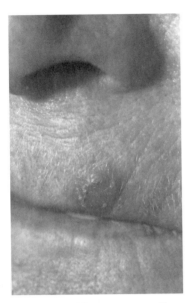

Figure 1-27. Squamous cell carcinoma

starts to form again. All the while, the sore is ulcerating, and the cancer cells are getting a deeper and deeper grip on the underlying tissues. A person who is experiencing this cycle with a sore *anywhere* on the body should *run, not walk* to the nearest dermatologist.

Treatment

As with BCC, SCCs are frozen and or excised. With SCC, however, it is especially important to be sure that *all* the affected tissue is removed, because if any "hot" cells should find their way into the lymph system, the cancer could spread to elsewhere in the body. Therefore, excess tissue is often also taken, which may require postoperative skin grafts. The area may also then be radiated to make doubly sure that all the cancer-causing cells are dead.

Massage?

SCC is not always an aggressive form of cancer but it can be. People undergoing treatment for it may face surgery, skin grafts, radiation, chemotherapy, or any combination of the above. These treatments carry specific cautions for massage that are outlined in the section on *cancer* in Chapter 11. Massage can be appropriate for persons who are fighting cancer, but the therapist must make sure the client and the health care team are fully informed and design a treatment that delivers maximum benefit with a minimum of risk.

Malignant Melanoma
Definition: What Is It?

Melanocytes are the pigment cells that give skin its color. They are located deep in the epidermis. Melanin protects us, as much as it can, from harmful UV radiation from the sun. As in the other cancers discussed here, if melanocytes get *too much* stimulation, they can start replicating without control. This is malignant melanoma.

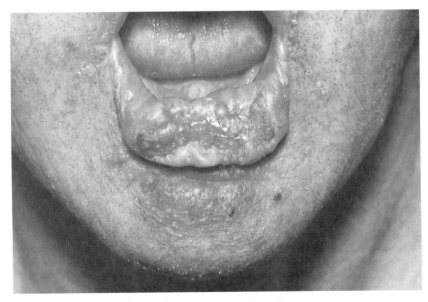

Figure 1-28. Squamous cell carcinoma

Four types of malignant melanoma have been classified: *superficial spreading melanoma*, which is the most common variety, accounting for about 65% of all cases; *nodular melanoma*, which is a rare, highly aggressive variety that grows more on a vertical plane than a horizontal one; *acrolentiginous melanoma*, which can affect younger patients and often appears on the hands or feet, between fingers and toes; and *lentigo melanoma*, which affects mainly elderly patients.

Melanoma is the leading cause of death from skin diseases and the cause of 75% of all deaths from skin cancer. Fortunately, it is also the least common variety of skin cancer, accounting for about 3 to 5% of skin cancer cases. About 1 in every 100 persons in the United States will have malignant melanoma at some time.

Signs and Symptoms

Melanoma often starts from a pre-existing mole, which later in life begins to change; it lightens, darkens, thickens, becomes elevated. Sometimes it is itchy or bleeds around the edges (Fig. 1-29, Color Plate 25). Melanoma does not always start from a mole, however, nor does it always begin in areas that have been exposed to the sun.

Here is a simple mnemonic to remember the key diagnostic features for melanoma:

- *A: Asymmetrical.* Most benign moles are circular or oval. A melanoma has an indeterminate shape.

- *B: Border.* The borders of melanomas are irregular and may be indistinct as it goes into the skin.

- *C: Color.* The colors of most moles are consistent: they are brown or black, but not both. Melanomas are typically multicolored, with brown, black, purple, and possibly blue all mixed together.

- *D: Diameter.* Melanomas are large. Any mole that is bigger than 6 mm across should be examined by a dermatologist.

- *E: Elevated.* Melanomas are usually at least partly elevated from the skin. They may even be big enough to snag on things and bleed.

Because melanoma is a disease of cumulative sun exposure, it rarely happens in young people. Large moles that develop *after* adolescence, however, are highly suspect. Moles in areas that are subject to a lot of irritation are at especially high risk of becoming cancerous.

Men most often get melanoma on the trunk, neck, or head. Women tend to get it on the arms or legs.

Treatment

Treatment for melanoma is generally aggressive. Because this cancer spreads very rapidly, there is literally no time to lose. Once a lesion has been positively identified and staged (evaluated for how far it has progressed), it is usually attacked with every weapon available. Surgical excision involves shaving the tumor layer by layer and examining the surrounding tissues for signs of involvement. A margin of healthy tissue is usually taken

Skin Cancer Statistics

Here's the bad news:

- By the time persons reach 18 years of age, they will have received half or more of their lifetime's exposure to the sun.

- One serious sunburn can increase the risk of skin cancer by up to 50%.

- It is estimated that 1 of every 7 people in the United States will develop some form of skin cancer sometime in their life.

- 40 to 50% of all people in the United States who reach the age of 65 will have some kind of skin cancer at least once.

- Approximately 800,000 new cases of SCC and BCC are diagnosed every year.

- About 34,000 cases of malignant melanoma are diagnosed every year, but since 1973 that incidence has increased by 4% every year.

- Approximately 9300 people died of skin cancer in the United States in 1995.

The good news is that education and vigilance make a big difference in the mortality rates for this disease. Studies done in Queensland, Australia, where melanoma is more common than anywhere else in the world, show that early intervention in the development of malignant melanoma dramatically improves the chances of survival. All types of skin cancer are 100% survivable, if they are caught early enough.

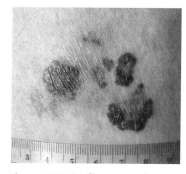

Figure 1-29. Malignant melanoma

along with the cancerous areas to be sure all the mutated cells have been removed. Radiation and examination of nearby lymph nodes follows. Perfusion chemotherapy may be used: the affected limb is tied off with a tourniquet. High doses of chemotherapeutic drugs are then injected and isolated to the affected area. Another treatment intervention is called "biological therapy": doses of man-made interferon and interleukin-2 are injected to help support the body's natural cancer-fighting mechanisms.

Prognosis

The prognosis for malignant melanoma is determined largely by how far the cancerous cells have invaded the skin. Melanoma usually begins by spreading shallowly across the epidermis before invading deeper tissues. If it is caught and removed before it is about 0.7 mm deep, the prognosis is generally hopeful. If it gets up to 4 mm deep, it will probably have already invaded nearby lymph nodes and metastasized through the body. In this case the prognosis is generally poor.

Massage?

Melanoma is an aggressive form of cancer that spreads through the lymph system. Persons undergoing treatment for melanoma may be receiving high doses of chemotherapy or radiation or be dealing with surgery and skin grafts. Cautions for massage revolve around circulatory impact and the side effects of cancer treatments. These are outlined in the section on *cancer* in Chapter 11.

In situations in which cancer is terminal, massage can sometimes be a valuable part of patient care. In hospice situations in which the patient is aware of the risks and is more interested in the quality of life than quantity, massage may be taught to family members and friends who are caring for the dying person.

WATCH FOR THIS

ABCDE's

As public awareness about skin cancer grows, everyone is becoming more cautious about his or her moles. Although most moles are harmless, a small percentage of them become cancerous. This is why it is especially important for massage therapists, who work so intimately with the skin, to be able to recognize some of the key features that distinguish moles from melanoma. The points of comparison listed here refer to the mnemonic ABCDE, which stands for *asymmetrical, border, color, diameter,* and *elevation* (see *skin cancer*, this chapter). A final comparison, age at which the markings appears, has also been included.

	Moles	Skin Cancer
Symmetry	Symmetrical: round or oval	**A**symmetrical
Border	Clearly distinct from nearby skin	**B**orders are irregular, occasionally indistinct, and blended with nearby skin
Color	Unicolored: could be brown, black, purple, or reddish, but usually won't be mixed	**C**olor is mottled and several colors may be mixed together
Diameter	Less than 6 cm (the circumference of a pencil eraser)	**D**iameter is greater than 6 mm
Elevation	May be elevated	May be elevated
Age at which it appears	Before puberty	After puberty

Skin Injuries

Burns

Definition: What Are They?

Most people think about burns in the context of touching a hot iron or brushing a hand across a broiler rack. The world of burns goes beyond household appliances. A person can sustain burn damage from dry heat like irons and broilers, wet heat like hot liquids or steam, electricity, friction (i.e., "rug burn"), radiation, and corrosive chemicals. Any one of these can destroy the proteins in the exposed skin cells, which causes the cells to die. If a significant amount of skin is affected, it is unable to accomplish its protective tasks: it *will not* provide a shield from microbial invasion, it *will not* help to maintain a stable temperature, and, perhaps most importantly, it *will not* provide protection from fluid loss. This opens the door to a number of complications including loss of water, plasma, and plasma proteins, which leads to shock.

Etiology: What Happens?

The severity of burns is determined by how deep they go, how much surface area they cover, and what part of the body has been affected. Losing more than 15% of skin function can put a person at risk of infection, shock, and circulatory collapse. Burns to the face and neck are more serious than to other areas because the resulting inflammation can block breathing passages.

Skin is composed of three layers of tissue. Burns are graded in three levels of severity. This is not entirely coincidental.

First-Degree Burns   This is a sometimes quite painful but relatively mild irritation of the superficial epidermis characterized by redness but no blistering. Diaper rash is an example of a burn due to chemical irritation. Mild sunburn is perhaps the most common example of first-degree burns. Overexposure to the sun damages cells in the epithelium, setting up an inflammatory response. This leads to pain, heat, redness, and swelling (Fig. 1-30, Color Plate 26). Sunburns generally heal in 2 to 3 days, sometimes with flaking and peeling. If the sunburn is more severe it *will* lead to blistering, which is a sign of second-degree burns.

Second-Degree Burns   This is damage that involves all layers of the epidermis and possibly some of the dermis. Symptoms include redness, blisters, edema, and a lot of pain. Still, if the burn area is fairly small it will heal in 1 week (or maybe 1 month if it involves the dermis). The hair shafts and glands usually do not sustain permanent damage, although some superficial scarring may occur. Second-degree burns can come from the sun and from many other things, too, such as steam under pressure, toxic chemicals, or hot glue guns (Fig. 1-31, Color Plate 27).

Third-Degree Burns   These go right down to the bottom of the dermis or beyond, destroying hair shafts, sebaceous glands, erector pilae muscles, sweat glands, and even nerve endings, which paradoxically makes third-degree burns less painful than second-

BURNS IN BRIEF

What are they?
Burns are caused by damage to the skin that causes the cells to die. They can be caused by fire, overexposure to the sun, dry heat, wet heat, electricity, radiation, extreme cold, and toxic chemicals.

How are they recognized?
First-degree burns involve mild inflammation. Second-degree burns also involve blistering and damage at the deeper levels of the epidermis. Third-degree burns go down into the dermis itself and often show white or black charred edges. In the postacute stage serious burns often involve shrunken, contracted scar tissue over the area of skin that has been affected.

Is massage indicated or contraindicated?
Burns contraindicate massage (except, perhaps, mild sunburns) in the acute stage. In the subacute and postacute stages massage may be performed around the damaged area within pain tolerance of the client.

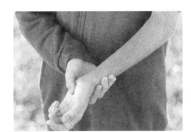

Figure 1-30. First-degree burn

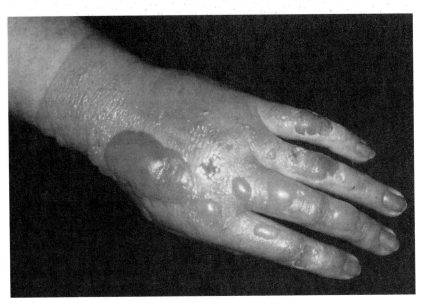

Figure 1-31. Second-degree burn

degree burns. Symptoms include whiteness and/or charring as well as a leathery texture of the skin in the affected area. Third-degree burns are dangerous for all the reasons mentioned above: risk of infection, fluid loss, and shock, especially if a significant percentage of the body surface has been affected. In addition to all this, one of the special problems with third-degree burns is that they tend to contract rapidly, forming a very confining web of scar tissue, even with quickly applied skin grafts (Fig. 1-32, Color Plate 28).

Signs and Symptoms

The symptoms of burn damage depend on what level of skin has been affected. Details about symptoms by degree of damage are listed above.

Treatment

First- and second-degree burns are seldom treated with anything more than soothing lotion and possibly antibiotic cream if the skin has been damaged to the point of not providing protection from infectious agents. Third-degree burns, however, must be treated with more care to minimize the accumulation of binding scar tissue. This often means wound cleansing and debridement: skin brushing to remove debris as well as skin grafts and plastic surgery.

Massage?

The *only* kind of burn that is appropriate for circulatory massage in the acute stage is a very mild sunburn; of course, even then, one must work within pain tolerance. By sloughing off dead cells massage can speed the healing process along, but it is not something to do without a client's permission.

Other burns may be approached in the *subacute* stage as a local contraindication; it is fine to work around the edges *within pain tolerance* to improve elasticity and minimize scar tissue, without running the risk of exposing the client to infection. In this situation it is important to be working with a doctor to establish when the burn is in a subacute stage

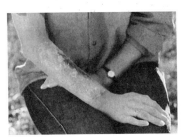

Figure 1-32. Third-degree burn

and to rule out any other tissue trauma that may contraindicate massage. Lymph drainage techniques that specialize in working reflexively to stimulate lymph flow may also be used with recent burn victims.

Massage has been used successfully to reduce the stress associated with treatment for third-degree burns. The pain of debriding damaged skin tissue is often described as worse than the burn itself. When patients receive massage before their wound care sessions, they report lower levels of anxiety, pain, and depression, and their levels of stress-related hormones and pulse rates are appreciably decreased. These benefits set the stage for a less painful, more efficient healing process.[1]

Finally, if burns are obviously long past the acute and subacute stages, that is, no pain remains and all that is left is residual scar tissue, massage is safe. The only caution here is that in serious cases there might have been permanent nerve damage. If that is the case, the client will not be able to feel it if the massage is doing any damage.

Decubitus Ulcers

Definition: What Are They?

This condition, which is also known as *bedsores*, *pressure sores*, and *trophic ulcers* is one massage therapists would most likely see when working in a hospital, a hospice, or some other setting with bed-ridden patients. This problem stems from chronic inadequate blood flow to the skin that stretches over bony or otherwise prominent areas. It almost always occurs in an area that has had constant contact with a surface: usually a bed, sometimes a cast or a splint.

Demographics: Who Gets Them?

The persons most at risk for developing decubitus ulcers are elderly, underweight, male, nonambulatory, and incontinent. This does not preclude other people from developing them, however; anyone who is immobile even for just a few hours can develop pressure sores.

Etiology: What Happens?

Imagine looking microscopically into the skin of an immobilized person. The circulation is not being stimulated by the person or by anyone else. Capillaries are squeezed between bone and bed, and new epithelial cells are starving for nutrition. The cells close to the surface of the skin died long ago, but now the cells in the deeper layers of the epidermis are dying too. Although the damage to deep layers of the skin may be extensive, only small lesions appear at the surface. Bacteria take advantage of the opportunity and begin to attack the weakened skin cells, exposing more of the damaged tissues. Capillaries are too narrow to let anything through, including the white blood cells that would otherwise limit the intruders. Gradually the surface tissue dies, and along with it the possibility of regeneration. Left unchecked, the ulcer can destroy the epidermis, the dermis, and the superficial fascia as well as erode tissues down to the bone (Fig. 1-33, Color Plate 29). Secondary infection of the open wound can lead to blood poisoning and death.

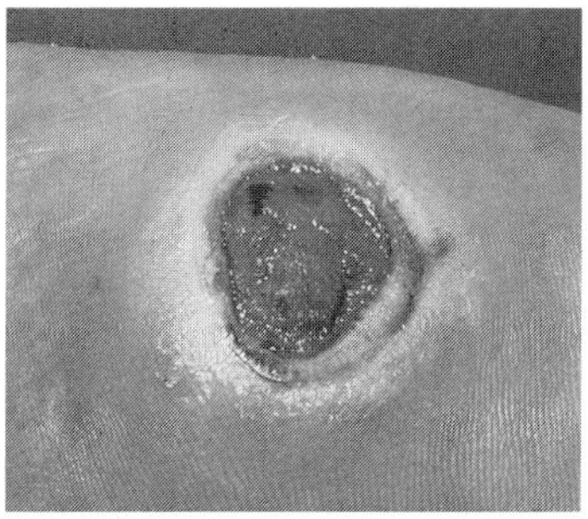

[1]Field T. *Touch Therapy*. London: Churchill Livingstone; 2000:53–58.

DECUBITUS ULCERS IN BRIEF

What are they?
Bedsores, also called decubitus ulcers, are caused by impaired circulation to the skin. Lack of blood supply leads to irreversible tissue death.

How are they recognized?
Unlike other sores, ulcers do not crust over. They remain open wounds that are highly vulnerable to infection.

Are they indicated or contraindicated for massage?
Bedsores indicate massage only *before* they develop. Once the tissue has been damaged it is too late, and they locally contraindicate massage until they have completely healed over.

Figure 1-33. Decubitus ulcer

Signs and Symptoms

The first stage of decubitus ulcers shows a marked change in skin temperature (it can become cooler or warmer than the surrounding area). Localized reddening becomes visible on pale skin, whereas on dark skin the discoloration may appear to be red, purple, or bluish. Pain and itching accompany these changes.

In later stages the lesions turn purple, and then necrosis (or tissue death) begins. Bacteria will probably invade the damaged tissue, which can result in local or systemic infection.

Ulcers on the skin (and anywhere else on the body) differ from other types of sores because they do not go through a normal healing process. Whereas most injuries stimulate the production of new epithelial cells and connective tissue fibers to replace the damaged tissues, the damage incurred by decubitus ulcers prevents this from happening. Ulcers do not even form a crust to cover regenerating epithelium. Of course, eventually they can heal, but not in a normal way. When circulation to the affected area is finally restored, the lesion closes up by having scar tissue grow over the area, but a permanent dip remains where the dead tissue will never grow back.

Bedsores can start in a surprisingly short amount of time. They can be a real danger for people with spinal injuries who may have to travel for hours strapped to a backboard. Bedsores and joint and muscle degeneration are the primary reasons comatose people are moved and turned frequently. Heels, buttocks, the sacrum, and elbows are the most common places for bedsores to appear.

Treatment

Treatment for pressure sores depends on their stage and location. Topical antibiotics and dressings can be effective for some lesions. Bigger, more advanced sores may require debridement and plastic surgery.

The biggest danger regarding bedsores is the possibility of infection, which can be life-threatening for someone who is already bedridden and immune-suppressed. The treatment protocols outlined by the Agency for Health Care Policy and Research include maintaining good nutrition (extra high-protein calories and minerals), avoiding pressure of any kind, and proper cleaning and dressing of the wound.[2]

Public attention to this problem has recently been aroused as the number of elderly patients is rapidly rising, and the cost of treating bedsores tops $8.5 billion a year. Furthermore, the litigation issues around elder care and bedsores are becoming increasingly expensive. Consequently, more efforts are being made to find ways to stop these injuries before they start, since preventing bedsores costs only a fraction of what it takes to treat them.

Massage?

Bedsores happen because circulation is interrupted long enough that cells literally starve to death. It would make sense that massage, with its wonderful influence over circulatory flow, would be an appropriate way to deal with this problem. However, because of the peculiar open sore nature of ulcers and because it is virtually impossible to sterilize hands, massage is not appropriate for bedsores. If a client is at risk for developing bedsores (and does not have other conditions that contraindicate bodywork), the improved skin nutrition that massage can provide could be an excellent preventive measure. If the sore has already begun to fester, a significant danger of infection is present. The latest research shows that even working around the edges of bedsores is risky, so decubitus ulcers are considered a local contraindication.

[2]Rovner S. Treating bedsores with a new approach. *Washington Post*. January 31, 1995.

Open Wounds and Sores
Definition: What Are They?

Many different technical names are used for all the different ways skin can be damaged. Any damaged tissue can be referred to as a *lesion*. The following is a list of common skin lesions:

- *Lacerations* (rips and tears)
- *Incisions* (cuts)
- *Excoriations* (scratches)
- *Fissures* (cracks)
- *Papules* (firm raised areas, like pimples)
- *Vesicles* (blisters)
- *Pustules* (vesicles filled with pus, like whiteheads)
- *Punctures* (any kind of hole)
- *Avulsions* (something has been ripped off, like a finger or an ear)
- *Abrasions* (scrapes)
- *Ulcers* (sores with dead tissue that do not go through a normal healing process).

Knowing these technical terms is important, but not as important as knowing that massage is inappropriate for any condition in which the skin is not entirely intact.

Massage?

These injuries are usually just local contraindications for massage; it is not necessary to reschedule an appointment if a client has a scraped knee. The exception would be if the open wounds or sores were caused by some other systemically contraindicating condition like advanced untreated *diabetes* (Chapter 8) or *mites* (this chapter).

Scar Tissue
Definition: What Is It?

The body's ability to heal itself after injury is one of the wonders of nature. The new material generated to literally "knit" damaged tissue back together is scar tissue.

This discussion is limited to the regenerative capacities of the skin. For information on scar tissue associated with musculoskeletal injuries, see *tendinitis* (Chapter 2).

Etiology: What Happens?

The skin, because it is subject to more wear and tear than any other tissue, has cells with special properties not found anywhere else in the body. If a scrape or abrasion occurs, basal cells detach themselves from the basement membrane and begin to migrate in a single-layered sheet across the wound. When they reach the other side and touch other epithelial cells, an internal code makes them stop moving. (It is the absence of this in-

---

OPEN WOUNDS AND SORES IN BRIEF

What are they?
Open wounds and sores are skin injuries that have not completely healed.

How are they recognized?
Unhealed lesions may be marked by bleeding, crusts, exuding pus, or other signs of regenerative activity.

Are they indicated or contraindicated for massage?
Any opening in the skin is an open invitation for infection. At the very least, open wounds and sores locally contraindicate massage. They may systemically contraindicate massage if they appear as a sign of serious systemic disease.

SCAR TISSUE IN BRIEF

What is it?
Scar tissue refers to the new tissue that is created to replace damaged and dead cells at the site of an injury. Scar tissue on the skin has some different characteristics than scar tissue that develops in deeper layers of fascia and muscle.

How is it recognized?
Scar tissue on the skin often lacks pigmentation and hair follicles.

Is massage indicated or contraindicated?
The acute stage of any injury in which the skin has been damaged contraindicates massage. In the subacute stage massage may improve the quality of the healing process.

ternal code, called *contact inhibition*, which makes cancer cells so dangerous; nothing ever tells them to **stop**.)

Meanwhile, back at the original site, stationary basal cells are duplicating to build up the ranks of migrating cells. When the whole wound has been covered, the new sheet of basal cells begin dividing to form new strata. After enough bulk has accumulated, the crust, or scab, falls off and the cells on the surface become keratinized. Then the wound is healed; access to the blood supply is cut off from the outside world, and it is no longer vulnerable to infection. The whole process can take place within 24 to 48 hours, depending on the size and location of the lesion.

If the injury goes deeper than the dermis, the healing process is more complicated. Fibroblasts in the area are summoned to the site, so beneath all that basal cell activity much fibroblastic activity is also taking place. This "fill-in" connective tissue is called *granulation tissue*. Eventually it changes to become an accumulation of collagenous scar tissue, meant to knit up the fascia, but which may intrude on the superficial layers as well. If the scar tissue does not stay within the boundaries of the original injury, it is called *hypertrophic scar*. Sometimes the fibroblasts are *too* active and produce much more collagen than is necessary. The scar overflows the injury, resulting in a permanently raised mass of tissue. This is called *keloid scar*. Keloid scar can be a very annoying complication of surgery or any kind of deep wound healing, but it is seldom a serious problem.

Collagenous scar tissue differs from normal skin in some important ways: the collagen fibers are much denser, they do not lay down in the same patterns as uninjured tissue, no epidermis covers it, fewer blood vessels supply it, and it will probably be missing hair follicles, normal skin glands, and possibly even sensory neurons.

Treatment

Several treatment options have been developed to minimize the appearance of scar tissue on the skin, but none of them can eradicate the scars themselves. Hypertrophic scar tissue may be injected with cortisone, which dissolves the excess collagen. Keloids are frozen with liquid nitrogen and then treated with cortisone, but they may still recur. Scarred areas that dip into underlying tissues may be injected with collagen to help them "fill out" their normal area. Other options to improve the look and texture of scar tissue include dermabrasion (the skin is mechanically "buffed" to remove excess epithelium), chemical peels (the top layers of epithelium are chemically treated and removed to create more even texture and coloring), punch grafts (small pieces of normal skin are surgically implanted to replace localized scars such as old acne lesions), and laser resurfacing.

When a large surface area of skin has been damaged, it is important to control the amount of scar tissue that accumulates, because large masses of scar can contract into uncomfortable and unsightly areas (see *burns*, this chapter). Skin grafts and some specialized types of gene therapy can control the accumulation of new scar tissue for the best possible long-term results.

Massage?

Obviously, massage is only appropriate in the subacute stage of healing. Why? Because if the skin is not intact, the client is a walking invitation for infection. If someone is healing from a deep wound like a surgery, bodywork around the area may help to keep the skin supple and may inhibit the build-up of hypertrophic scars (see *postoperative conditions*, Chapter 11). If a client has old, deep scar tissue on the skin, sensation in those areas may be reduced. In such a case, the massage therapist should be extra solicitous of client feedback.

Other Conditions

Ichthyosis

Definition: What Is It?

Ichthyosis is a rare disorder in which the skin is pathologically dry. Although it can happen alone, it can also be a symptom of a variety of diseases.

Etiology: What Happens?

Several types of ichthyosis have been identified. It can occur by itself, usually on the legs of elderly people and especially in cold weather when the air is very dry. In this kind of situation it is sometimes called *xeroderma*. Ichthyosis can also be a symptom of some congenital problems associated with birth defects or certain rare neurologic diseases. Other cases are indicators of a variety of other diseases, including *Hodgkin's disease*, *AIDS* (see both in Chapter 5), *hypothyroidism* (see Chapter 8) or Hansen's disease (leprosy).

Signs and Symptoms

Ichthyosis creates distinctive diamond-shaped plates on the skin that resemble fish scales, hence its name, which means "fish condition." Sometimes the affected area may become darker than the surrounding areas (Fig. 1-34, Color Plate 30).

ICHTHYOSIS IN BRIEF

What is it?
Ichthyosis is pathologically dry skin that is much more severe than average dry skin.

How is it recognized?
Ichthyosis creates distinctive diamond-shaped "scales" on the skin, usually on the lower legs.

Is massage indicated or contraindicated?
When ichthyosis appears independently of other conditions, it certainly indicates massage. Massage probably will not provide a permanent solution to this problem, but massage can make it better in the short run. Areas where deep cracking may expose the blood supply should be avoided.

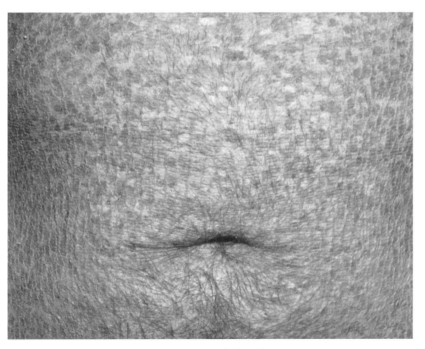

Figure 1-34. Ichthyosis

ICHTHYOSIS:
Ichthys is Greek for "fish." Ichthyosis means, literally, "fish condition." Other terms for this condition are equally descriptive: "alligator skin," "sauriasis" (*sauros* is from the Greek for "lizard," as in dinosaur), "sauroderma," and "sauriosis."

Treatment

The first recourse for persons living with pathologically dry skin is to change their bathing habits. People with ichthyosis need to take special care to preserve the protective coating of sebum on their skin. This is accomplished by bathing less frequently and by applying emollients to the skin while it is still wet. A variety of preparations can be applied to help soften and remove the scales that develop with ichthyosis; these depend on the age of the patient and the cause and severity of the disorder.

Massage?

This is one of the few skin conditions that, in the absence of underlying contraindications, massage can substantially improve. It does so by adding non-irritating oil to the skin and by stimulating the sebaceous glands become active too. The massage therapist should be cautious, however, of skin that is *so* dry it cracks and bleeds, whereupon it becomes, like all compromised skin, an invitation to infection.

Chapter Review Questions: Skin Conditions

1. What is the cardinal rule for massage and skin conditions?

2. A client has eczema on her hands which is extremely dry and flaky. Does this condition indicate or contraindicate massage? Why?

3. A client has severe ichthyosis that is cracked and oozing. Does this condition indicate or contraindicate massage? Why?

4. What does psoriasis have in common with cancer?

5. When working with a client who is prone to acne, is it a good idea to follow the treatment with an alcohol rinse to remove the oil? Why?

6. A client has white flakes that cling to hair shafts and do not brush out. What condition is probably present?

7. A client has a circle-shaped, reddish-pink mark on the back of his upper thigh. What condition may be present?

8. What should be done with this client's massage sheets?

9. In what stage of the development of a decubitus ulcer is massage appropriate?

10. In what situation would an open sore be a systemic rather than just a local contraindication?

Bibliography, Integumentary System Conditions

General References, Integumentary System

1. de Dominico G, Wood E. Beard's Massage. Philadelphia: WB Saunders; 1997.
2. Damjanou I. Pathology for the Health-Related Professions. Philadelphia: WB Saunders; 1996.
3. Travell J, Simons DG. Myofascial Pain and Dysfunction: The Trigger Point Manual. Baltimore: Williams & Wilkins; 1983.
4. Clemente CD. Anatomy: A Regional Atlas of the Human Body. 3rd ed. Baltimore: Urban & Schwarzenburg; 1987.
5. Tortora GJ, Anagnostakos NP. Principles of Anatomy and Physiology. 6th ed. New York: Harper & Row; 1990.
6. Taber's Cyclopedic Dictionary. 14th ed. Philadelphia: FA Davis; 1981.
7. Stedman's Medical Dictionary. 26th ed. Baltimore: Williams & Wilkins; 1995.
8. Memmler RL, Wood DL. The Human Body in Health and Disease. 5th ed. Philadelphia: JB Lippincott; 1983.
9. Juhan D. Job's Body: A Handbook for Bodywork. Barrytown, NY: Station Hill Press; 1987.

10. Mulvihill ML. Human Diseases: A Systemic Approach. 2nd ed. Norwalk: Appleton & Lange; 1987.
11. Kunz JRM, Finkel AJ, eds. The American Medical Association Family Medical Guide. New York, NY: Random House; 1987.
12. Marieb EM. Human Anatomy and Physiology. Redwood City, CA: Benjamin/Cummings; 1989.
13. Field T. Touch Therapy. London: Churchill Livingstone; 2000.

Boils

1. Boils (skin abscesses). MedicineNet, Inc.; 1996–2000. Available at: http://www.MedicineNet.com. Accessed fall 2000.
2. Carbunculosis. Dr.Koop.com, Inc.; 1998–2000. Available at: http://www.Dr.Koop.com. Accessed fall 2000.

Erysipelas

1. Erysipelas. In: *The Merck Manual.* Section 10, Chapter 112, Bacterial infections of the skin. Whitehouse Station, NJ: Merck & Co.; 1995–2000. Available at: http://www.merck.com/pubs/mmanual/section10/chapter112/112a.htm. Accessed fall 2000.
2. Erysipelas. MedicineNet, Inc.; 1996–2000. Available at: http://medicinenet.com. Accessed fall 2000.

Fungal Infections

1. Drugge RJ. Common dermatologic diseases. The Internet Dermatology Society, Inc.; 1995–2000. Available at: http://telemedicine.org/common/common.htm#Fungus. Accessed fall 2000.
2. Fungal infections. MedicineNet, Inc.; 1996–2000. Available at: http://medicinenet.com. Accessed fall 2000.

Herpes Simplex

1. Welcome to the herpes zone. In Life Energy Systems; 1999. Available at: http://www.herpeszone.com. Accessed fall 2000.
2. Genital herpes in women. MedicineNet, Inc.; 1996–2000. Available at: http://medicinenet.com. Accessed fall 2000.
3. Herpes simplex infections (non-genital). MedicineNet, Inc.; 1996–2000. Available at: http://medicinenet.com. Accessed fall 2000.
4. Herpes simplex. American Academy of Dermatology; 1999. Available at: http://www.aad.org/pamphlets/herpes.html. Accessed fall 2000.
5. Siwek J. Herpes infections. *Washington Post Health (Consultation).* July 19, 1994.
6. Weiss R. Should herpes drugs be sold over-the-counter? *Washington Post Health.* May 17, 1994, p. 7.

Impetigo

1. Impetigo. MedicineNet, Inc.; 1996–2000. Available at: http://medicinenet.com. Accessed fall 2000.
2. Impetigo. New Zealand Dermatological Society; 1997–1999. Available at: http://www.dermnet.org.nz/index.html. Accessed fall 2000.

Lice and Mites

1. Scabies. MedicineNet, Inc.; 1996–2000. Available at: http://medicinenet.com. Accessed fall 2000.
2. Scabies. American Academy of Dermatology; 1999. Available at: http://www.aad.org/pamphlets/Scabies.html. Accessed fall 2000.
3. Scabies. New Zealand Dermatological Society; 1997–1999. Available at: http://www.dermnet.org.nz/index.html. Accessed fall 2000.

Warts

1. Warts (common warts). MedicineNet, Inc.; 1996–2000. Available at: http://medicinenet.com. Accessed fall 2000.
2. Warts. American Academy of Dermatology; 1999. Available at: http://www.aad.org/pamphlets/Warts. Accessed fall 2000.
3. What causes warts? American Academy of Family Physicians; 1999. Available at: http://familydoctor.org/handouts/209.html. Accessed fall 2000.
4. Your podiatric physician talks about warts. American Podiatric Medical Association. Available at: http://www.apma.org/topics/Warts.htm. Accessed fall 2000.

Acne

1. Acne vulgaris. New Zealand Dermatological Society; 1997–1999. Available at: http://www.dermnet.org.nz/index.html. Accessed fall 2000.
2. Acne. HealthAnswers.com, Inc.; 2000 Available at: http://healthanswers.com/centers/disease/overview.asp?id5skin1conditions&filename52305.htm. Accessed fall 2000.
3. Acne (pimples). MedicineNet, Inc.; 1996-2000. Available at: http://medicinenet.com. Accessed fall 2000.
4. Questions and answers about acne. The National Institute of Arthritis and Musculoskeletal and Skin Diseases; 1999. Available at: http://www.nih.gov/niams/healthinfo/acne/acne.htm. Accessed fall 2000.

Dermatitis/Eczema

1. Dermatitis. New Zealand Dermatological Society; 1997–1999. Available at: http://www.dermnet.org.nz/index.html. Accessed fall 2000.
2. Pompholyx. New Zealand Dermatological Society; 1997–1999. Available at: http://www.dermnet.org.nz/index.html. Accessed fall 2000.
3. Allergic Contact Rashes. American Academy of Dermatology; 1999. Available at: http://www.aad.org/pamphlets/allergic.html. Accessed fall 2000.
4. Atopic Dermatitis. New Zealand Dermatological Society; 1997–1999. Available at: http://www.dermnet.org.nz/index.html. Accessed fall 2000.

5. Spergel JM, Schneider LC. Atopic dermatitis. Internet Scientific Publications L.L.C.; 1996–2000. Available at: http://www.ispub.com/journals/IJAAI/Vol1N1/AD.html. Accessed fall 2000.
6. Allergic contact dermatitis. New Zealand Dermatological Society; 1997–1999. Available at: http://www.dermnet.org.nz/index.html. Accessed fall 2000.
7. Hand eczema. American Academy of Dermatology; 1999. Available at: http://www.aad.org/pamphlets/hand.html. Accessed fall 2000.
8. Handout on health atopic dermatitis. National Institute of Arthritis and Musculoskeletal and Skin Diseases. Available at: http://www.nih.gov/niams/healthinfo/. Accessed fall 2000.
9. Atopic dermatitis. MedicineNet, Inc.; 1996–2000. Available at: http://medicinenet.com. Accessed fall 2000.
10. Seborrheic dermatitis. American Academy of Dermatology; 1999. Available at: http://www.aad.org/pamphlets/seborrhe.html. Accessed fall 2000.
11. Shaberman BA. The further adventures of eczema boy. *The Washington Post.* 2000. Available at: http://washingtonpost.com/wp-dyn/articles/A19541-2000Jul11.html. Accessed fall 2000.
12. Seborrhoeic dermatitis. New Zealand Dermatological Society; 1997–1999. Available at: http://www.dermnet.org.nz/index.html. Accessed fall 2000.
13. Atopic dermatitis (atopic eczema). National Jewish Medical and Research Center; 1999. Available at: http://www.njc.org/. Accessed fall 2000.

Hives

1. Chronic hives (urticaria): A guide for sufferers. Asthma & Allergy Associates of Florida, P.A.; 1997. Available at:http://www.allergyweb.com/articles/hivespt.html. Accessed fall 2000.
2. Hives. HealthAnswers.com, Inc.; 2000. Available at: http://healthanswers.com/centers/disease/overview.asp?id=allergy&filename=113.htm. Accessed fall 2000.
3. Hives (urticaria): What is it? The Johns Hopkins University; 1996–1999. Available at: http://www.washingtonpost.com/cgibin/gx.cgi/AppLogic+FTContentServer?pagename=health/condition&nextstep=display&disease=10149. Accessed fall 2000.
4. Hives (urticaria) & angioedema. MedicineNet, Inc.; 1996–2000. Available at: http://medicinenet.com. Accessed fall 2000.
5. Urticaria—hives. American Academy of Dermatology; 1999. Available at: http://www.aad.org/pamphlets/Urticaria.html. Accessed fall 2000.

Moles

1. Moles. American Academy of Dermatology; 1999. Available at: http://www.aad.org/pamphlets/Moles.html. Accessed fall 2000.
2. Moles (nevi): What is it? The Johns Hopkins University; 1996–1999. Available at:

http://www.washingtonpost.com/cgi.bin/gx. cgi/AppLogic+FTContentServer? pagename=health/condition&nextstep=display&disease=11074. Accessed fall 2000.

3. Moles. New Zealand Dermatological Society; 1997–1999. Available at: http://www. dermnet. org.nz/index.html. Accessed fall 2000.

4. Freckles. MedicineNet, Inc.; 1996–2000. Available at: http://medicinenet.com. Accessed fall 2000.

5. Seborrheic keratosis. American Academy of Dermatology; 1999. Available at: http://www.aad.org/pamphlets/saborr_kera. html. Accessed fall 2000.

6. Mole patrol. *Washington Post Health*. October 11, 1994.

Psoriasis

1. Psoriasis. MedicineNet, Inc.; 1996–2000. Available at: http://medicinenet.com. Accessed fall 2000.

2. Psoriatic arthritis. MedicineNet, Inc.; 1996–2000. Available at: http://medicinenet. com. Accessed fall 2000.

3. What is psoriasis? National Psoriasis Foundation; 1995, 1991. Available at: http://www.psoriasis. org/ whatis.html. Accessed fall 2000.

4. Psoriasis: Common questions and answers. National Psoriasis Foundation; 1995, 1991. Available at: http://www.psoriasis.org/faq. htmlhttp://www.psoriasis.org/faq.html. Accessed fall 2000.

5. Psoriasis statistics. National Psoriasis Foundation; 1995, 1991. Available at: http://www.psoriasis. org/stat.html. Accessed fall 2000.

6. Question and answers about psoriasis. National Institute of Arthritis and Musculoskeletal and Skin Diseases; 1999. Available at: http://www.nih. gov/niams/ healthinfo/psoriafs.htm. Accessed fall 2000.

7. Psoriasis. American Academy of Dermatology; 1999. Available at: http://www.aad.

org/ pamphlets/Psoriasis.html. Accessed fall 2000.

Skin Cancer

1. Skin cancer information. American Cancer Society; 2000. Available at: http://www2. cancer.org/skinGuide/index_info.html. Accessed fall 2000.

2. What is melanoma? MedicineNet, Inc.; 1996–2000. Available at: http:// medicinenet. com. Accessed fall 2000.

3. Skin cancer. MedicineNet, Inc.; 1996–2000. Available at: http:// medicinenet.com. Accessed fall 2000.

4. Basal cell carcinoma. MedicineNet, Inc.; 1996–2000. Available at: http:// medicinenet. com. Accessed fall 2000.

5. Basal cell carcinoma. New Zealand Dermatological Society; 1997–1999. Available at: http://www.dermnet.org.nz/index.html. Accessed fall 2000.

6. Melanoma. New Zealand Dermatological Society; 1997–1999. Available at: http://www. dermnet.org.nz/index.html. Accessed fall 2000.

7. Squamous cell carcinoma. New Zealand Dermatological Society; 1997–1999. Available at: http://www.dermnet.org.nz/index. html. Accessed fall 2000.

8. Skin cancer. American Academy of Dermatology; 1999. Available at: http://www.aad. org/pamphlets/skincan.html. Accessed fall 2000.

9. What is actinic keratosis? Northeast Dermatology Associates, PA; 1996, 1997. Available at: http://www.nedermatology.com/ skincancer/ak/index.html. Accessed Fall 2000.

10. What you need to know about skin cancer. The Skin Cancer Foundation. Available at: http://www.skincancer.org/home.html. Accessed fall 2000.

11. Huntley A. Malignant melanoma. University of California Davis; 1995, 1998. Available at: http://matrix.ucdavis.edu/tumors/

tradition/introduction.html. Accessed summer 2001.

Burns

1. Burns. MedicineNet, Inc.; 1996–2000. Available at: http://medicinenet.com. Accessed fall 2000.

2. Field T. *Touch Therapy*. London: Churchill Livingstone; 2000:52–58.

3. What are second degree burns? Clinical Reference Systems; 1988. Available at: http://www.brain.com/health_a2z/crs/ burn2.htm. Accessed fall 2000.

Decubitus Ulcers

1. National Pressure Ulcer Advisory Panel frequently asked questions: Pressure ulcer definition and etiology. Available at: http://www. npuap.org/pressureulcerdef. htm. Accessed fall 2000.

2. Pressure sores. Merck & Co., Inc.; 1995–2000. Available at: http://www.merck. com/pubs/mmanual/section10/chapter122/122a.htm. Accessed fall 2000.

3. Rovner S. Treating bedsores with a new approach. *Washington Post Health*. January 31, 1995.

Scar Tissue

1. What's in a scar. American Academy of Dermatology; 1999. Available at: http://www.aad.org/pamphlets/whatsina. html. Accessed fall 2000.

2. Weiss R. Wound-healing gene may soon repair skin. *Washington Post Health*. October 11, 1994.

Ichthyosis

1. Ichthyosis. Merck & Co., Inc.; 1995–2000. Available at: http://www.merck.com/pubs/ mmanual/section10/chapter121/121a.htm. Accessed fall 2000.

Musculoskeletal System Conditions

2

CHAPTER OBJECTIVES

After reading this chapter, you should be able to . . .

- Name three differences between a tender point and a trigger point.
- Name the role of dystrophin in normal muscle function.
- Name three causative factors for muscle spasm.
- Name what feature Paget's disease and osteoporosis have in common.
- Describe the early signs of Lyme disease.
- Name the difference between tendinitis and sprains.

- Name three differences between osteoarthritis and rheumatoid arthritis.
- Name three structures that may be injured in whiplash.
- Name the difference between specific muscle weakness and general muscle weakness.
- Name three muscles and bones that may help to pin or trap the structures damaged with thoracic outlet syndrome.

INTRODUCTION

This chapter discusses disorders and injuries involving muscles, bones, and joint structures: ligaments, tendons, tendinous sheaths, and bursae. Together these structures are the tools that provide humans with shape, strength, and movement. They are composed almost entirely of the material that binds people together and permeates every part of the body: connective tissue.

Injury to any of the connective tissue structures (except bone and sometimes cartilage) can be tricky for many medical professionals to identify. Magnetic resonance imaging (MRI) can be helpful, but its ability to identify soft tissue damage is extremely limited. A thorough clinical examination will still yield the most comprehensive information about injury to muscles, tendons, ligaments, and other connective tissues. Massage therapists, with their in-depth understanding of the musculoskeletal system (particularly the formation of adhesions and scar tissue), are in a unique position to be able to help persons living with these types of injuries.

Bones

Bone Structure

The arrangement of living and nonliving material in bone is fascinating. The collagen matrix on which solid bone is built is arranged as circles within circles. Calcium and phosphorus deposits accumulate on this scaffolding in a similarly circular pattern, leaving holes for a generous blood supply. In addition, most long bones in the body grow in a gently spiraled direction, much like tree trunks. The shaft, or diaphysis, of long bones is hollow, filled with red marrow in youth and yellow marrow in adulthood. All these design features give bone some remarkable properties: terrific resilience, support, and strength combined with a relatively lightweight construction.

The commands to move the rock-like calcium and phosphorus salts around the collagen matrix are carried out by specialized cells. Osteoblasts, or "bone builders," help to lay new deposits, whereas osteoclasts, or "bone clearers," break them down. These cells are located both in the periosteum around the outside of the bone and the endosteum on the inside of the shafts. They can alter the shape of the bones from interior and exterior aspects.

Osteoblasts and osteoclasts perform their duties under the orders of two hormones. Calcitonin, from the thyroid, *lowers* blood calcium levels by telling osteoblasts to pull calcium out of the blood and put it wherever the bones need it most. Parathyroid hormone (PTH) *raises* blood calcium levels by telling the osteoclasts to dismantle calcium deposits and put the valuable mineral back into the bloodstream. There it is available to help with muscle contractions, nervous transmission, blood clotting, and many other functions. Thus, the health and shape of the bones depend not only on a person's physical activity, but also on whatever other chemical demands the body may be making on its calcium banks. This is, in essence, Wolff's law, which states "Every change in the form and the function of a bone, or in its function alone, is followed by certain definite changes in its internal architecture and secondary alterations in its external conformation."[a] In other words, bone is living tissue and will remodel according to the stresses that are placed on it.

Bone Function

The skeleton provides a bony framework, protection for vulnerable organs, and leverage for movement. It also produces new red blood cells and stores calcium and phosphorus for future use. For young people, bone is definitely not a mass of stone-like inert material; in fact, osteoblasts and osteoclasts will easily remodel bone to adapt to whatever stresses are put on it. The younger the body, the higher the percentage of living material that exists within bones. Gradually over years, however, the ratio of inert material to living material shifts; in elderly people bone has little remaining living tissue, and the density of its mineral stores has decreased, hence its brittleness and slowness to heal.

Muscles
Muscle Structure

Muscles are composed of specialized threadlike cells that, with electrical and chemical stimulation, have the power to contract while bearing weight. These cells, or *myofibers*, run the full length of the muscle and are encased in a connective tissue envelope, the *endomysium*. Packets of wrapped myofibers are encased in another connective tissue envelope, the *perimysium*. These bundles are called *fascicles*. Fascicles are bound together by yet another connective tissue membrane, the *epimysium* (Fig. 2-1). Finally, some large muscle groups are further bound by an external connective tissue membrane, which then blends into the subcutaneous layer of the skin, the deep fascia (which is—surprise!—another connective tissue membrane).

Muscle Function

When muscles work they consume fuel and produce both energy (the pulling together of their bony attachments) and wastes. What kinds of wastes are produced depend on how much work is done, how fast and how long it is being done, and what kind of fuel is available to do it. Muscles that work when adequate supplies of oxygen are easily accessible burn very cleanly (*aerobic metabolism*): the waste products they produce are carbon diox-

[a]*Stedman's Medical Dictionary*, 26th ed. Baltimore, Md: Williams & Wilkins; 1995:943.

ide and water. When muscles work without adequate oxygen (*anaerobic metabolism*) a variety of other wastes are produced. Among these is lactic acid, a byproduct of anaerobic combustion that is also a nerve irritant.

This begs the next question: what causes muscle soreness? This issue is the subject of ongoing debate. One factor is probably the accumulation of lactic acid, which irritates nerve endings in overused muscles. Another theory is that some calcium leakage from sarcomeres—segments of myofibrils where chemical reactions take place—may take place. This leakage can then cause microspasms. Soreness may also involve tiny microscopic tears of myofibers. Even with microscopic injuries like these, microscopic pockets of inflammation may also occur. Swelling and tearing stimulate nociceptors (specialized nerve endings designed to transmit messages about tissue damage), which give the brain information about pain and injury.

Massage can influence the processing of chemical residues and minor inflammations in tired muscles by moving fresh, highly oxygenated blood into sore areas while flushing old, toxic, stagnant interstitial fluid out. Imagine a person rinsing an old, dirty, smelly sponge in a stream of clean running water. Every time the sponge is squeezed, dirty, discolored liquid flows out of the sponge. Each time the sponge is released, clean fresh water fills it up again. This is what vigorous, well-applied circulatory massage does for muscles that are sore, tired, and suffused with waste products.

Joints

The joints in the body are organized into three classes: synarthroses ("immovable" joints, such as those between the cranial bones—although even these joints are not *completely* immovable), amphiarthroses ("slightly movable" joints, such as those between the bodies of the vertebrae), and diarthroses ("freely movable" joints). Of these classes of joints, the diarthrotic, or *synovial* joints are by far the most vulnerable to injury. For this reason, it is worth briefly reviewing the structure and function of synovial joints in preparation for a discussion of what happens when they are injured.

Joint Structure

As shown in Figure 2-2, synovial joints are constructed so that no rough surfaces ever have to touch, even in joints that bear an enormous amount of weight, such as knees and

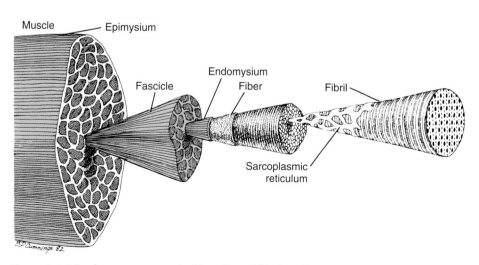

Figure 2-1. Muscles are composed of bundles within bundles, all enveloped by connective tissue membranes

ankles. Articular cartilage, made of densely formed collagen fibers around chondroitin sulfate (very slippery material) and water, cap the ends of bones where they meet. Maintaining the slickness of that cartilage is key to maintaining the health of the joint. Fortunately, each synovial joint has a synovial membrane that produces synovial fluid, creating a generally synovial ("egg-like") environment. As long as the membrane and cartilage stay wet and smooth, the joint stays healthy. It takes only a very small amount of synovial fluid to lubricate the inside of a joint space.

Joint Function

It is a bit redundant to discuss joint function here; this is not a kinesiology text that will define flexion as opposed to extension, or rotation versus circumduction. It is sufficient to say that the function of synovial joints is to allow movement between bones, providing the fulcrum that bones can use for leverage.

Joints, like most other structures in the body, are designed for use. With healthy use, the joint structures stay smooth, slick, and well lubricated. Movement of the joint capsule stimulates the production of synovial fluid, which then circulates through the joint space for the health of all joint components. Lack of movement results in a shortage of synovial fluid; too much movement, especially too much *irritating* movement, can damage articular cartilage or cause the bones of the joint to change shape in such a way that smooth surfaces are made rough, thus opening the door to irreversible arthritis. Other factors that can influence joint health are trauma, calcium metabolism, and nutrition.

Other Connective Tissues

Structures outside the joint capsule (tendons, tendinous sheaths, ligaments, bursae) are also susceptible to damage. Tendons connect muscle to bone and are an early line of defense when a joint undergoes traumatic stress. Depending on the force of the trauma, lig-

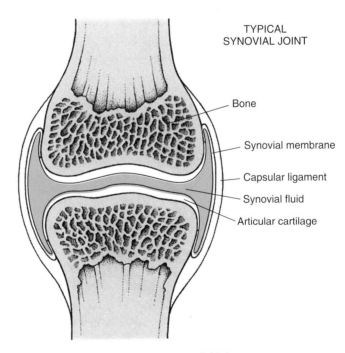

TYPICAL
SYNOVIAL JOINT

Bone

Synovial membrane

Capsular ligament

Synovial fluid

Articular cartilage

Figure 2-2. Synovial joint

aments are also quick to suffer injury: the medial and lateral stabilizers outside the joint capsule and the internal stabilizers are generally damaged before the specialized capsular ligament that comprises the joint capsule itself. Bursae, little fluid-filled sacks that cushion areas where two bones might otherwise knock heads or allow tendons to slide over sharp corners, tend to get irritated with repetitive stress. The body grows new bursae anywhere it needs a little extra protection, and these new bursae can also become irritated and painful.

Connective Tissue Problems in General

Every part of the body is supported by connective tissue. It wraps around muscle cells and neurons as well as supports blood vessels and the tubes of the digestive tract. It is the framework on which bones grow. Connective tissue provides the structure for the functioning cells of most organs. It gives strength and elasticity to most of the body's membranes. Indeed, connective tissue is such a large proportion of the entire human body, it can be said that a person's general health can be determined by the strength, resiliency, and power held in the connective tissues.

What happens when a person's connective tissues become systemically weak? Most people know someone who seems to get injured very easily. Such people can twist an ankle getting out of a car or wrench their back picking up a chair. It seems like pain and injury follow them wherever they go. Very often the culprit in situations like this is a complicated interconnected problem involving long-term stress, poor nutrition, high levels of chronic muscle contraction, elevated cortisol levels in the blood, sleep disorders, and incomplete healing.

The hormone most closely linked to long-term stress is cortisol. This is an important and beneficial chemical that helps to limit inflammation and redirects metabolism away from fast-burning glucose and toward slower-burning proteins. This is a fine mechanism for dealing with the threat of long-term hunger or famine, but what this means for people with elevated cortisol who are *not* suffering from life-threatening food shortages is that cortisol systemically weakens all types of connective tissue, raising the chances for injury and ongoing pain.

When injury occurs, long-term stress, coupled with pain, interferes with the sleep cycles to the point that secretions of somatotropin (growth hormone) are significantly inhibited, as are the neurotransmitters that moderate pain sensation. This makes it difficult to heal from simple injuries and reinforces a pain-stress-sleeplessness cycle that is similar to the pain-spasm-ischemia cycle seen with many muscular problems.

The point of all this is that contrary to how many people view the body, it is not made of a series of interchangeable parts. When a car has a tire that keeps going flat, the owner replaces the tire, and the problem is solved. When a person has an ankle that keeps getting sprained, or a back that is so fragile that he or she cannot pick up a laundry basket, or headaches so severe that they interfere with day-to-day functioning, the answer is not just in the ankle, back, or neck muscles. The answer is in the totality of how mental and emotional states are echoed in the

Connective Tissue Fibers

Connective tissue comes in all shapes and forms in the body. It is difficult to accept that the loose, jiggly deposits of fat in the subcutaneous layer of the skin are technically in the same class of tissue as bones, but it is true. The unifying feature in all types of connective tissue (except blood and lymph) is the presence of particular types of protein fibers. The two that will be examined here are collagen and elastin.

Elastin is a protein fiber that lives up to its name. It is stretchy and has good potential for rebound; in other words, it will snap back to its original size after being stretched out. However, elastin is low in tensile strength; it is relatively easy to break fibers to pieces.

Collagen is another protein fiber, but it is quite different in most qualities from elastin. It has little ability to stretch and poor rebound potential; once collagen has been stretched out, it tends to stay loose rather than go back to its original length. Collagen does have tremendous tensile strength: it takes a great deal of force to stretch collagen, and even more force to physically tear or fray the fibers.

One other property of collagen is that under certain circumstances it can tend to bind things together. If general circulation to an area is impaired, the collagen-based connective tissue membranes that are intended to be slick and slippery for freedom of movement will instead become thick and gluey. Collagen fibers from one structure may even fuse with fibers from a neighboring structure. This can happen at any level within muscle groups or individual muscles: muscle sheaths can stick to each other so that individual muscles can no longer contract independently, fascicles can stick together within muscle bellies, and even individual myofibers can stick together. These sticky places, or *adhesions*, can greatly impair mobility and flexibility while increasing the chances for injury when they are stressed to the point of tearing.

physical body; it is in how eating habits support or do not support healing; and it is in whether the person gets an adequate amount of high-quality sleep. Massage therapists who specialize in helping people with musculoskeletal problems need to address all these issues when clients have recurring, ongoing, or stubborn injuries that do not follow what is usually considered a normal healing process.

The convenient thing about musculoskeletal problems, as far as massage therapists are concerned, is that most are *not* related to an infectious agent; a person cannot catch or spread a sprained ankle. Nor do they usually lead to permanent damage that massage can make worse: increasing circulation does *not* spread tendinitis throughout the body. Skillful, careful, knowledgeably applied massage administered in the appropriate stage of healing can help many musculoskeletal conditions to improve. Sometimes that improvement is just a temporary cessation of pain (which is a noble purpose in itself), but often this work can bring about the lasting changes that make structurally based massage an important factor in the healing process.

Musculoskeletal System Conditions

Muscular Disorders
Fibromyalgia
Myofascial Pain Syndrome
Muscular Dystrophy
Myositis Ossificans
Shin Splints
Spasms, Cramps
Strains

Bone Disorders
Fractures
Osteoporosis
Paget's Disease
Postural Deviations

Joint Disorders
Ankylosing Spondylitis
Dislocations
Gout

Joint Disorders, cont.
Lyme Disease
Osteoarthritis
Patellofemoral Syndrome
Rheumatoid Arthritis
Septic Arthritis
Spondylosis
Sprains
Temporomandibular Joint Disorder

Other Connective Tissue Disorders
Baker Cyst
Bunions
Bursitis
Dupuytren's Contracture
Ganglion Cysts
Hernia
Osgood-Schlatter Disease

Other Connective Tissue Disorders, cont.
Pes Planus
Plantar Fasciitis
Scleroderma
Tendinitis
Tenosynovitis
Torticollis
Whiplash

Neuromuscular Disorders
Carpal Tunnel Syndrome
Herniated Disc
Myasthenia Gravis
Thoracic Outlet Syndrome

Muscular Disorders

FIBRO- MY- ALGIA

simply means muscle pain. Fibromyalgia, fibrositis, myofibrositis, and fibromyositis, are terms that have all been used to put a name to a bewildering set of signs and symptoms that no one has ever completely defined.

Fibromyalgia
Definition: What Is It?

Fibromyalgia is a group of signs and symptoms that involve chronic pain in muscles, tendons, ligaments, and other soft tissues. It is one among a collection of chronic disorders that often go hand-in-hand. FMS is frequently seen with *chronic fatigue syndrome* (Chapter 5), *irritable bowel syndrome* (Chapter 7), *sleep disorders* (insomnia, Chapter 3), and several other chronic conditions.

Demographics: Who Gets It?

FMS affects up to 3% of the U.S. population. Women account for about 85% of all cases, but that number may be misleading because men may be less likely to seek medical intervention for the symptoms that fibromyalgia produces. Fibromyalgia is seen in all ages and economic groups, but its incidence seems to increase with age.

Etiology: What Happens?

This is a very different disorder from most other muscle problems. It is not a viral, bacterial, or fungal infection that causes the problem; it is not usually a direct result of injury, and most researchers do not think it is an autoimmune disorder. Rather, some suggest it is related to sleep disorders, endocrine and neurotransmitter imbalances, and emotional state.

Sleep Disorder   Sleep studies of persons with fibromyalgia reveal that they seldom or never enter the deepest level of sleep, Stage IV sleep. It is in this stage that adults secrete growth hormone: the hormone that stimulates the production of new cells and collagen for healing and recovery. Furthermore, not getting adequate, high-quality sleep reduces serotonin levels. Among other things, serotonin helps to modulate pain sensation. Without adequate secretion of this important neurotransmitter, everything hurts *more*. Thus, a particularly vicious circle develops. A person is under stress and/or experiencing chronic pain. This makes it difficult for the person to sleep. Sleeplessness exacerbates the pain, which further limits the ability to sleep and so on.

Fibromyalgia patients often report getting 8 hours of sleep a night or more, but they also reliably report waking up feeling unrefreshed, as though they'd been working all night long. Studies in which volunteers were deprived of Stage IV sleep showed that the subjects rapidly developed symptoms of fibromyalgia, thus indicating that this is a significant issue in this disorder.[b]

Pain   The origin of the debilitating pain experienced by fibromyalgia patients is one of the most mysterious aspects of the problem. Current studies suggest that the pain is *not* in fact generated in the muscles, as the name implies. Instead, examinations of the cerebrospinal fluid of FMS patients reveal pathologically high levels of two specialized neurotransmitters: *substance P* and *nerve growth factor*. These substances are believed to initiate nerve activity, cause vasodilation, and increase pain sensation. If the excessive secretion of substance P and nerve growth factor are found to be at the center of how fibromyalgia develops, this "muscle-fiber-pain" syndrome may eventually be reclassified as a central nervous system disorder.

Tender Points   Fibromyalgia patients eventually develop tender points that are distributed all over the body (Fig. 2-3) but are concentrated around the neck and shoulders and around the low back. Tender points themselves are not well understood. Histologic studies of affected tissue have yielded no useful information about how these areas develop.

FIBROMYALGIA IN BRIEF

What is it?
Fibromyalgia syndrome (FMS) is a chronic pain syndrome involving the development of a predictable pattern of tender points.

How is it recognized?
FMS is diagnosed when other diseases have been ruled out, and when 11 active tender points are found distributed among all quadrants of the body.

Is massage indicated or contraindicated?
FMS indicates massage. Care must be taken not to overtreat, however, because clients are extremely sensitive to pain and may have accumulations of waste products in the tissues that are difficult to flush out adequately.

---

[b]Nye DA. *Fibromyalgia: A Guide for Patients.* Eau Claire, Wis: Midelfort Clinic; August 13, 1995. Available at: http://Prairie.lakes.com/~roseleaf/fibro/pt-faq.html. Accessed spring 2002.

Signs and Symptoms

The following are some signs and symptoms that characterize FMS:

- Tender points. Nine pairs of these are distributed among all quadrants of the body.
- Widespread pain in shifting locations that is extremely difficult to pin down. The intensity of the pain may vary widely (in other words, patients have good days and bad days). The pain can range from a deep ache to burning and tingling.
- Stiffness after rest.
- Low stamina.
- Sensitivity to cold, especially to damp cold.
- Low pain tolerance.

Diagnosis

No definitive diagnostic test has been developed for FMS. It is often diagnosed when all other diseases with similar signs and symptoms have been ruled out, including Lyme disease, multiple sclerosis, rheumatoid arthritis, lupus, and several others. Obviously, this can be a long and frustrating process.

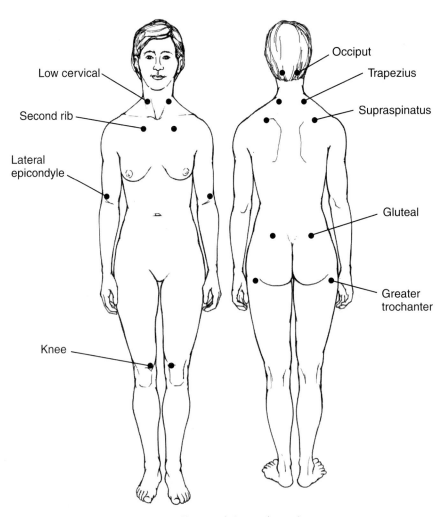

Figure 2-3. Fibromyalgia tender point map

In 1990 the American College of Rheumatology officially defined a set of diagnostic criteria for FMS[c]:

- The patient must report chronic pain for a minimum of 3 months.

- The patient must show at least 11 of 18 mapped tender points to be currently active (that is, they must elicit significant diffuse pain with digital pressure of approximately 4 kg—enough to blanch a thumbnail).

- The active tender points must be widely distributed, with some from each quadrant of the body.

In the palpation of active tender points, many practitioners also look for "control points": areas known *not* to develop tender points. If the patient reports that they, too, are painful, the diagnosis may shift away from fibromyalgia to some other chronic pain problem.

One of the challenges with diagnosing fibromyalgia is in the overlap this condition shows with other disorders. Up to 70% of patients diagnosed with fibromyalgia meet the criteria for a diagnosis of chronic fatigue syndrome. Conversely, about 70% of patients diagnosed with chronic fatigue syndrome meet the criteria for fibromyalgia. Eventually it may be found that these two disorders are simply different manifestations of the same problem. Currently, however, they are approached as two closely related yet etiologically separate problems.

Other conditions that frequently overlap with fibromyalgia include irritable bowel syndrome, hypothyroidism, sleep disorders, *myofascial pain syndrome*, and *temporomandibular joint dysfunction* (this chapter). So much overlap occurs, in fact, that the diagnostic process probably depends on what conditions appear first. In other words, if a person starts with jaw pain, he or she may end up with a diagnosis of temporomandibular joint dysfunction, although the patient's disorder may be systemic. Similarly, if another person first experiences chronic intestinal distress, that patient might never get past a diagnosis of irritable bowel syndrome.

The average fibromyalgia patient spends about 5 years and consults at least five different health care specialists before arriving at a diagnosis. This is a remarkable statistic, considering that this problem is the second most commonly diagnosed musculoskeletal problem in the United States (the first is osteoarthritis).

Complications

While fibromyalgia is not a life-threatening disease, it is often partially or completely debilitating. The pain it causes is "invisible" pain, that is, no recognizable outward signs of a problem are perceptible. The results of imaging tests are negative, and no signs or symptoms of this disorder are readily visible. No single blood test reveals any specific markers for this problem. A person with this syndrome is often discounted as a "faker" or "malingerer" by doctors, employers, and even friends and family. By the time a patient

History of Fibromyalgia Syndrome

The history of the documentation of FMS is a fascinating study of how information that stretches across the globe and over nearly 200 years has been gathered together to create a picture of what is still a very mysterious disorder, but one that is the second most common musculoskeletal diagnosis in the United States today.

1816: Dr. James Balfour first documents a chronic pain syndrome involving sore muscles, stiffness, and fatigue.

1904: Dr. William Gowers of Britain first uses the word "fibrositis," in relation to this disorder. This name implies an inflammatory reaction in muscle or connective tissue fibers.

1940: The word "fibrositis" first finds usage in North American medical texts.

1979: A Canadian group of physicians matches the symptoms of muscle aches to chronic fatigue and sleep disorders.

1981: Research on this condition reveals that it does *not*, after all, involve inflammation of muscle or other tissues. Dr. Muhummad Yunus, an Illinois rheumatologist, coins the term "fibromyalgia" to refer to connective tissue, muscle tissue, and the pain that plagues them both.

1987: The American Medical Association officially recognizes that this disorder, which affects up to 3% of the American population, does indeed exist.

1990: The American College of Rheumatology creates a set of standardized diagnostic criteria for FMS.

1993: The World Health Organization officially recognizes FMS as a disorder.

[c]Gremillion RB. Fibromyalgia. *Physician Sportsmed.* 1998;26(4). Available at: http://www.physsportsmed.com/issues/1998/04apr/grem.htm. Accessed fall 2000.

has reached a definitive diagnosis, the experience with the medical community has often been frustrating and overwhelmingly negative.

Consider what it would be like to live with chronic pain: pain all the time, pain that never stops, pain that no one else can see or understand. When a person lives with pain, and especially when that pain makes it difficult to sleep, he or she may tend to lose perspective about many things. Time ceases to have any real meaning. The person hurts now, has been hurting for a long time, and will always, *always, always* hurt. Ultimately, that pain begins to define the things that such persons can do, what they can eat, where they can go, and in a fundamental way, *who they are*. In other words, persons can become dependent on the experience of pain to tell them that they are alive. Take away that pain, and what is left?

It is not surprising then that *depression* (Chapter 3) is a common and dependable complication of FMS. Depression can exacerbate symptoms as it tends to cause people to isolate themselves from support givers and it disrupts sleep.

Treatment

The prognosis for FMS is that it is a lifelong situation for most people. Treatment focuses on finding ways to *manage* the disorder so that the patient may lead as normal a life as possible.

What seems to work best is a course of therapy that gives the patient control of the healing process. The first priority is to educate the patient as completely as possible about the condition, emphasizing that although he or she may feel incapacitated, this is not a progressive or life-threatening disease.

Next, the responsibility for managing the condition must be put entirely in the patient's hands, through nutrition, sleep, exercise, stretching, and reducing emotional stress. Daily exercise is an important therapy for many fibromyalgia patients. Mild tricyclic antidepressants are often prescribed both to reduce levels of depression and to improve the quality of sleep. Pain-killing drugs are generally avoided, because they interfere with sleep and can be habit-forming.

Massage?

Fibromyalgia patients *live* in pain. Some moments are more severe than others, but a constant, ongoing, uninterrupted body-wide ache is a hallmark of this condition. Their tissues are drowning in irritating chemicals, and they lack the neurotransmitters that block some of the pain transmission. In other words, these people are extremely hypersensitive and very easy to overtreat.

With that consideration, gentle massage is very appropriate for clients with fibromyalgia. Research on massage and fibromyalgia patients shows that massage is effective for reducing reported levels of pain, anxiety, and depression.[d] Massage may be used best to create relaxation and aid with toxic flushing, a little with each session. Fibromyalgia contraindicates the use of ice; any kind of cold can exacerbate symptoms.

It usually takes a long time to become incapacitated by fibromyalgia; it can also take a long time to find ways to cope with this condition. However, if clients can experience being pain-free, even for just a short time after each massage, they will feel more able to take control of their own healing process, which is the most important step toward recovery.

[d]Field T. Touch Therapy. London: Churchill Livingstone, 2000.

CASE HISTORY: FIBROMYALGIA SYNDROME
Kim, Age 48
I'm NOT a hypochondriac! I'm NOT!

Kim was a graphic artist, writer, and creative developer at a children's museum. She was working with the museum at its opening, after just having left an extremely stressful job in another city. It was at this time that she first began to experience new physical symptoms: powerful tingling sensations in her left arm. The sensations felt like an electrical current running up and down her arm. Eventually they spread into her right arm as well. In the beginning, the sensations came and went quickly, but eventually the episodes came in waves, leaving her arms numb and useless for hours at a time.

At first she thought she was having a mini-stroke or even a heart attack, because the initial symptoms were in her left arm. She went to a general practitioner who began to look for signs of stroke or heart attack with an electrocardiogram (EKG), computed tomography (CT) scan, and MRI of her neck and head. When none of these tests were positive, her doctor suggested that she had herniated a disc and recommended that she consult a neurosurgeon.

The neurosurgeon found no signs of a herniated disc and recommended that Kim consult a neurologist to look for signs of multiple sclerosis.

The neurologist found no signs of multiple sclerosis, but felt strongly that Kim was dealing with FMS, and referred her to a rheumatologist.

The rheumatologist confirmed this finding. Kim reported that when her tender points were palpated, "It felt like somebody hit me with a baseball bat."

Kim, like so many other fibromyalgia patients, endured many tests, examinations, and doctor visits before a final diagnosis was made. Because fibromyalgia is an "invisible" condition, she suffered many remarks from friends and co-workers about it all being in her head.

Kim's other symptoms are less dramatic but in many ways just as debilitating as the numbness and tingling in her arms. She has difficulty sleeping and takes a sleeping aid.

She wakes up feeling foggy and extremely stiff. She reports that her pain is worst in the morning, but her neck, shoulders, and sternum hurt "all the time." Her hands and feet are constantly tingling, although this is not as extreme as her initial symptoms.

She has recently developed irritable bowel syndrome with bloating, cramping, gas, and alternating diarrhea and constipation. These symptoms are progressively becoming worse, and although she can control some of them with diet, they still interfere significantly with her life.

Kim also deals with chronic headaches that are probably a result of her fibromyalgia in combination with arthritis in her neck and on-going sinus problems. Her vision has been affected; she reports seeing "specky things." Her balance is inconsistent. She has to keep a finger on the wall as she walks along a hall or she veers off course. Mentally Kim is frustrated (and often amused) by new problems with language. She "flips words" when she's speaking or writing and frequently accidentally substitutes one word for another when she's typing or even listening to other people. For example, she was once attempting to type "try your hand at bartering for products from Nepal," and she typed "try your hand at bartending . . ."

Kim's fibromyalgia is part of a complicated health picture. She is a recovering alcohol and drug abuser and has dealt with depression intermittently for 30 years. She has been treated for post-traumatic stress disorder since leaving her previous job. She has arthritis in her neck, bursitis in her hip, and plantar fasciitis. Her job involves a great deal of sitting, and she feels stiff and painful whenever she stands and moves. Her knees and hips make popping, crackling noises. All these disorders together exacerbate her sleeping problems, which may then exacerbate her fibromyalgia.

Management of Kim's condition is challenging. She takes a course of vitamin and mineral supplements recommended by a fibromyalgia specialist. She recently began taking yoga classes and is excited that they seem to be providing significant relief. She also still spends plenty of time on a full-length massage mat that her mother sent her immediately after finally getting a diagnosis for her problems. She receives chiropractic care for her neck and lots of pet therapy from her two cats. Despite her many obstacles, Kim keeps a positive attitude toward life. She says that although the physical aspects of her condition are taxing, the mental twists and turns it provides are vastly entertaining.

Myofascial Pain Syndrome
Definition: What Is It?

MPS is a situation that develops when muscles undergo injury or trauma, sometimes on a microscopic level, that never goes through a standard healing process. Instead, the injured area gets locked into a repeating pain-spasm cycle.

MYOFASCIAL PAIN SYNDROME IN BRIEF:

What is it?
Myofascial pain syndrome (MPS) is a collection of signs and symptoms that indicate trauma to muscles that leads to a cycle of chronic spasm, ischemia, and pain.

How is it recognized?
MPS is recognized mainly through the development of trigger points in predictable locations in affected muscles. Trigger points are highly painful both locally and in specific patterns of referred pain.

Is massage indicated or contraindicated?
MPS indicates massage, which can "break through" the pain-spasm cycle and help to flush out the irritating metabolic wastes that accumulate around trigger points.

Demographics: Who Gets It?

MPS affects men and women more or less equally; this is one of the features that distinguishes it from another chronic pain syndrome, *fibromyalgia* (this chapter). MPS affects people of all ages, although its prevalence seems to taper off with advancing age. Sedentary people are vulnerable to this condition as well as physically active people.

The incidence of MPS is difficult to estimate. Among one group of patients with chronic pain, 35% of them had active trigger points.[e] However, people with no symptoms can show signs of latent trigger points, which may develop into active MPS with little provocation.

Etiology: What Happens?

This syndrome is marked primarily by the development of trigger points. These are small, sometimes microscopic areas where chronic stress has caused a few muscle fibers to fray. Under normal circumstances, microtrauma would be followed by an inflammatory response, fibroblastic activity, the accumulation of new scar tissue, and the whole incident would be resolved. Instead, a trigger point forms.

A Trigger Point is Born   Consider a stereotypical postal worker. He puts in 8 long hours every day reading illegible zip codes and routing pieces of mail to the correct destinations. He *hates* his job. By 9:30 every morning his shoulders are beginning their day-long journey up to his ears, and his trapezius is doing all the work. Furthermore, his head juts forward and downward so he can read the envelopes. No other muscles can keep it from slumping down onto his chest, so it falls to the trapezius, again, to do the work. It is no great surprise that a few myofibers are traumatized. They do not get the opportunity to relax and exchange waste products for nutrients, and because every myo-fiber in the area is similarly stressed, the blood flow to the area is severely limited.

The combination of mechanical stressors and emotional state has now created an injury. Blood components like histamine and prostaglandins may leak into the area and cause more pain. Any normal muscle's response to injury is to *tighten up*, both as a reaction to pain and as a splinting mechanism against even further injury. The trapezius gets stuck in a pattern of pain, which leads to spasm, which leads to local ischemia, which reinforces the pain, which creates more spasm, ad infinitum. The tiny area where those myofibers first frayed has now become a trigger point.

Histologic studies of trigger points reveal some profound changes in local neuromuscular functioning. Sensory neurons in the area often permanently change into pain sensors. The neuromuscular junction between the motor neurons and their corresponding motor end plates are frequently distorted and suffused in excessive secretions of acetylcholine, the neurotransmitter involved in stimulating muscle contractions.

Satellite Points   Manual pressure on the postal worker's trigger point creates a surprising amount of pain, both locally, and, mysteriously, up over the back of his head, causing headaches. If this situation has been ongoing for a matter of weeks or months, move-

[e]Fomby EW, Mellion MB. Identifying and treating myofascial pain syndrome. *Physician Sportsmed.* 1997;25(2). Available at: http://www.physsportsmed.com/issues/1997/02feb/fomby2.htm. Accessed summer 2000.

ment patterns to compensate for the sore shoulder may redistribute stress throughout the back and neck muscles. The splenius cervicis may experience more stress than it can handle, and *another* trigger point (a *satellite* trigger point) is formed. That satellite point can refer pain to yet another area, around the pectoralis major or minor, for instance. Now a new spot is constantly being told, erroneously, that it is in *pain*. What is the body's reaction to pain? *Tighten up!* That chest muscle may form its own trigger point simply because it has been told that it is hurting, even though no mechanical force is being exerted on it. The cycle goes on, and on, and on.

Trigger points that have not been irritated sometimes go into a latent state. They are not painful nor do they refer pain. Nevertheless, it takes very little stimulus to turn a latent trigger point into an active one. Both latent and active trigger points create palpable "knots" or taut bands that send pain shooting in predictable directions.

It is clear that trigger points form at areas that undergo microscopic amounts of trauma due to postural habits, poor ergonomics, and repetitive motion. These tiny injuries may never be consciously felt, although the trigger points they initiate can be acutely painful. Trigger points can also be a complication of more standard types of injuries, when a person accommodates to the pain and/or limited range of motion that might be the result of an automobile accident, a sports injury, or any other kind of damage.

Unanswered Questions MPS and trigger points have been documented and closely studied since the early 1950s. Still, questions about this condition outnumber answers. Why do trigger points form? Why doesn't the whole inflammatory process turn the affected area to scar tissue? Why doesn't the referred pain pattern from specific trigger points follow nerve pathways, energy meridians, or any other pattern observed (Fig. 2-4)? Finally, why is the location of various trigger points so predictable from one person to the next?

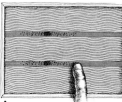

Figure 2-4. Myofascial pain syndrome: trigger points and referred pain patterns

Signs and Symptoms

MPS is recognized by the accumulation of active trigger points. These trigger points have some qualities that make them unique among muscle disorders.

- *Taut bands or nodules.* Trigger points can be palpated in muscle tissue as taut, hypertonic bands of fibers within a mass of muscle that is less tight (Fig. 2-5), or as small nodules that dissipate under static pressure. A muscle flicker or "twitch response" is often seen when a trigger point is palpated.

- *Predictable trigger point map.* Each skeletal muscle in the body has an area or group of areas where trigger points are most likely to form. These areas have been extensively mapped.[f]

- *Referred pain pattern.* Active trigger points are always locally painful under digital pressure, but they often refer pain to other areas in the body as well. Their referred pain patterns are consistent from person to person. However, they do not follow patterns understood in the context of nerve pathways, energy meridians, or other pathways of flow through the body. Referred pain patterns of trigger points have been documented along with the maps of where they occur.

- *Regional pain.* MPS is seldom a whole-body dysfunction (another feature that distinguishes it from fibromyalgia). More often, trigger points flare up in specific regions, often around the neck and shoulders. Jaw muscles are notorious for developing trigger points, which then refer pain all over the face and head. This variety of MPS is often discussed in the context of temporomandibular joint dysfunction.

Taut (palpable) bands in muscle

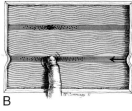

Taut bands

Relaxed muscle fibers

A Local twitch response

Local twitch of band

B

Figure 2-5. Myofascial pain syndrome twitch response

[f]Travell J, Simons DG. *Myofascial Pain and Dysfunction: The Trigger Point Manual.* Baltimore, Md: Williams & Wilkins; 1983.

Other symptoms of MPS are less predictable than trigger point development. Sleep disorders occur occasionally but not consistently. Depression and anxiety are also possible, especially when a person has little success in getting an accurate diagnosis and effective treatment.

Diagnosis

Currently, no specific criteria have been agreed on for a definitive diagnosis of MPS. A diagnosis is usually arrived at after a thorough pain history, physical examination, movement and postural analysis, and palpation of active trigger points.

One complicating factor that interferes with getting a clear picture of this disorder is that *most* people have trigger points. They may be latent (i.e., not actively causing pain), but only a moderate stimulus may cause them to become active. The line between a person with some active trigger points and a person with MPS is vague indeed.

Treatment

Perhaps the best news about MPS is that this is a chronic pain disorder with an excellent prognosis. If it is treated correctly, MPS does not have to be a long-term problem. Finding the correct treatment, of course, is the challenge. Although MPS has much in common with fibromyalgia, the treatment protocols for the two disorders are quite different. Fibromyalgia will not improve if it is treated as MPS; conversely, MPS will not improve if it is treated as fibromyalgia.

A top priority for MPS treatment is to eradicate trigger points. This is accomplished in a number of different ways, including the use of spray and stretch (a topical applica-

WATCH FOR THIS

Fibromyalgia and Myofascial Pain Syndromes

Chronic pain disorders are becoming more and more common as the general population ages. Two such disorders that share some qualities are FMS and MPS. It is certainly possible for these two conditions to occur simultaneously, but they have some differing characteristics that require some different treatment choices.

	FIBROMYALGIA SYNDROME	MYOFASCIAL PAIN SYNDROME
Prevalence	Up to 3% of U.S. population	Unknown
Demographics	85% of diagnosed patients are women	Women and men are equally affected
Prognosis	Life-long problem that can be managed but may never be eradicated	Can be a short-term problem that can be resolved permanently
Primary symptom	"Tender points": predictable areas where a small amount of pressure will yield intense, diffuse pain; tender points are often hypotonic and do not always occur in muscle tissue	"Trigger points": predictable areas within individual muscles where microtrauma has caused an area of hypertonicity; this area may be nodular or appear as a taut band that generates a twitch response; manual pressure on an active trigger point elicits pain locally and also in predictable patterns of referral
Implications for massage	Fibromyalgia patients can benefit from massage, but manual pressure will not "melt" tender points—it will only exacerbate them	Responds well to massage, and sustained static pressure with stretching can be an effective way to break through the "pain-spasm cycle" to eradicate trigger points

tion of an aerosol vapocoolant that temporarily numbs the pain of trigger points while the muscle is stretched), local injections of anesthetics, dry needling, and massage in the form of static pressure along with a passive stretch of the affected fibers. All these approaches work to interrupt the pain-spasm cycle, allowing the tight fibers to relax while the muscle is stretched.

Because MPS often develops out of chronic overuse or poor ergonomics, the patient's movement and work habits are often examined so that perpetuating factors may be eliminated.

Muscle relaxants and nonsteroidal anti-inflammatory drugs (NSAIDs) have not been found to be effective at reducing the pain caused by trigger points.

Massage?

MPS absolutely indicates massage, both for its effectiveness at interrupting the pain-spasm cycle and for its ability to help clean up the debris left behind from chronic muscle tightness. Remember that when muscle cells are working, they cannot exchange nutrients for waste products. Irritating metabolic wastes accumulate in the tissues, perpetuating soreness and fatigue. Massage is an excellent mechanism to help flush the waste away, with the precaution that someone in this condition is easy to overtreat.

Muscular Dystrophy

Definition: What Is It?

Muscular dystrophy is a group of several closely related diseases involving genetic anomalies. These mutated genes lead to the degeneration and wasting away of muscle tissue. It usually begins in the extremities but ultimately can affect the breathing muscles and the heart.

Demographics: Who Gets It?

The two most common varieties of muscular dystrophy (Becker and Duchenne) are X-linked inherited diseases. This means the affected gene is carried by the mother but only passed on to her sons. It *is* possible for a female to have muscular dystrophy, but both her father and mother would have to be positive for the mutated genes, which is a very rare circumstance.

The occurrence of muscular dystrophy varies according to type.

MUSCULAR DYSTROPHY IN BRIEF

What is it?
Muscular dystrophy is a group of related inherited disorders, all of which involve the degeneration and wasting of muscle tissue.

How is it recognized?
Different varieties of muscular dystrophy destroy different areas of skeletal muscles. The age of onset, initial symptoms, and long-term prognosis depend on what kind of genetic problem is present.

Is massage indicated or contraindicated?
The early signs of muscular dystrophy often involve muscles that become tight and constrictive. Physical therapy is often used to prevent or minimize contractures as long as possible; massage can fit in this context as well, as long as the massage therapist is working as part of a health care team.

Etiology: What Happens?

Normal muscles convert fat or glycogen into fuel to do their work of pulling bony attachments together. They do this with the assistance of a special protein, recently identified and named *dystrophin*. Dystrophin is produced by specific genes located close to the periphery of muscle cells, just under the sarcolemma. The most common versions of muscular dystrophy involve a genetic mutation that either prevents the production of dystrophin altogether or allows its production only at subnormal levels.

In the absence of dystrophin to help create energy, muscle cells atrophy and die, to be replaced by fat and connective tissue. Eventually the connective tissue shrinks, pulling bony attachments closer together in a permanent contracture.

Several varieties of muscular dystrophy have been identified, but two are more common than others, and one specifically affects adults; these will be discussed in some detail. Other types of muscular dystrophy are much more rare and will be listed just for identification.

- *Duchenne muscular dystrophy.* This is the most common and most severe variety of the disease. It affects anywhere from 13 to 33 boys out of every 100,000. The genetic anomaly with this condition prevents the production of any dystrophin at all.

- *Becker muscular dystrophy.* This variety of the disease is less common, affecting only 1 to 3 boys out of every 100,000. It is also less severe, because although the production of dystrophin is less than normal, some of this important protein is available to help muscles do their work.

- *Myotonic muscular dystrophy.* This type of muscular dystrophy affects adults more often than children. Its primary symptom is *myotonia:* stiffness or spasm following muscular contraction. This is a progressive disorder, however, which affects many systems. It can cause cataracts, gastrointestinal dysfunction, and heart problems.

- *Other varieties.* Other varieties of muscular dystrophy include *congenital muscular dystrophy* (several rare varieties that are diagnosed at birth or in early infancy), *facioscapulohumeral dystrophy* (a variety that primarily affects the muscles of the face, shoulder, and upper arm), *limb-girdle dystrophy* (this type begins in the shoulders, upper arms, and pelvic area), *Emery-Dreifuss muscular dystrophy* (this shows contractures of the Achilles tendon, elbow, and spine), and *oculopharyngeal muscular dystrophy* (this affects the eyes and pharynx muscles first).

Signs and Symptoms

Signs and symptoms of muscular dystrophy vary according to what type is present, but the two most common varieties (Duchenne and Becker) are very similar in presentation. A toddler might begin to have difficulty in walking or climbing stairs and may complain of leg pain. A waddling gait with an accentuated lumbar curve to compensate for the weakness in the legs will probably develop. Eventually, the child may not put the whole foot down at all, but will walk on tiptoes all the time. The calves may seem to become disproportionately large, in a condition called *pseudohypertrophy,* but in actuality the muscle mass is being replaced with fat and connective tissue.

This condition can progress to affect the spine, joints, heart, and lungs. Most muscular dystrophy patients die at a young age of cardiac or respiratory failure.

Duchenne muscular dystrophy is usually diagnosed between 3 and 5 years of age, and an affected child will probably be in a wheelchair by his or her 12th birthday. Its progression is fairly dependable, and its prognosis is that most patients will not live into their middle 20s.

Becker muscular dystrophy has a similar progression but is usually diagnosed later, has a less severe impact, and has an outlook that may be a great deal brighter, depending on how much dystrophin individual patients may produce.

Muscular dystrophy is occasionally but not always accompanied by mental retardation. Other conditions that accompany these diseases include contractures and *postural deviations* (this chapter) that develop as the skeletal muscles tighten and pull on the spine and rib cage.

Diagnosis

The ability to identify various kinds of muscular dystrophy has taken some giant steps forward in the past 2 decades. The protein dystrophin was isolated and named in 1987. This discovery has made it possible to categorize the different types of muscular dystrophy much more accurately than ever before.

If a child shows signs of some muscular problems, he or she will probably be given a blood test to look for signs of creatine kinase, an enzyme produced by damaged muscles. This is followed by other tests to rule out neurologic problems. Finally, a tissue biopsy specimen may be taken to look for signs of decreased or missing dystrophin.

Treatment

If a positive diagnosis for some variety of muscular dystrophy is made, the family may be encouraged to meet with a genetic counselor to discuss the implications for future children. However, no treatment for a child who already has muscular dystrophy currently exists. Some interventions have been developed to prolong the use of muscles and limbs (massage and physical therapy may be used to minimize the progression of contractures, for instance), and surgery is sometimes recommended to release tight tendons or straighten a distorted spine. Prednisone is a steroidal anti-inflammatory that can preserve function temporarily, but the side effects of long-term use are very serious.

Aside from these interventions, a child with muscular dystrophy is simply aided to be as comfortable and as functional as possible. This usually means learning to use leg braces, a standing walker, and ultimately a wheelchair.

Massage?

This is a disorder of muscle function, but sensation is intact. This makes it a relatively safe condition for massage, as long as the circulatory system is strong and healthy. Massage can be used along with physical therapy to slow the progression of contractures, but it is recommended that massage therapists operate as part of a health care team if they have an opportunity to work with a client who has muscular dystrophy.

Myositis Ossificans

Definition: What Is It?

Myositis ossificans means "muscle inflammation with ossification." This is a bit of a misnomer, because it can happen in any type of soft tissue and it does not always involve inflammation. Its synonym, "heterotopic ossification," is closer to the mark; this describes a malpositioning of some part of the body, specifically bone tissue.

Etiology: What Happens?

In the most common variety of myositis ossificans, an injury occurs that leads to bleeding, usually between fascial sheets where the capillary supply is practically nonexistent. The blood pools between layers of muscles where it quickly coagulates, be-

---

MYOSITIS OSSIFICANS IN BRIEF

What is it?
This is the growth of a calcium deposit in soft tissues. It usually follows trauma that involves significant leakage of blood between fascial sheaths.

How is it recognized?
A radiograph is the best way to see this problem, but it is palpable as a dense mass where, anatomically, no such thing should be.

Is massage indicated or contraindicated?
Massage is always a local contraindication for myositis ossificans, but work around the edges of the area may stimulate the reabsorption of the bone tissue without doing further damage.

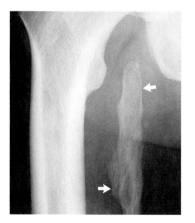

Figure 2-6. Myositis ossificans

coming thick and jelly-like. If the blood is not reabsorbed into the body, the liquid disperses, leaving behind a calcium/iron formation that looks and feels like a bone (Fig. 2-6).

Theories about the calcification process of myositis ossificans vary. Some propose that it is an attempt by the body to "wall off" or separate the injured area. Others suggest that in the original trauma some osteoblasts are released from the damaged periosteum, and they stimulate the deposit of calcium in the soft tissues.

Eventually, the body recognizes that the calcium deposits of myositis ossificans do not belong there, and it will finally begin to break down and reabsorb this bony growth. This can take months or years, but most people experience that the lesion finally just goes away.

Signs and Symptoms

Myositis is identified by a specific bony pattern: within weeks of the injury an outside border of mature bone-like calcium deposits form around an inside area of cellular material. This condition most often affects adolescents and young adults. The muscles most frequently involved are the quadriceps and the brachialis.

Myositis ossificans comes in all shapes and sizes. Radiographs usually show a clearly visible growth adjacent to a long bone. It may be connected to the nearest bone. In the acute stage the area feels bruised; later it will start to feel harder, crusty, and locally very tender. In time, little or no local pain may be present, but a dense, unyielding mass will exist where nothing hard should be.

Treatment

Treatment for myositis ossificans tends to be conservative. It is recommended that patients rest and isolate the injured area in the acute stage to limit further bleeding. In the subacute stage, passive stretching is used to restore range of motion, followed by resistive exercises to restore normal muscle strength.

If a fully mature and calcified mass interferes with muscle or tendon function, it can be surgically removed. This kind of surgery is avoided when possible, however, because eventually the body will finally get around to reabsorbing this deposit of calcium.

Massage?

Myositis ossificans is always a local contraindication. If the injury is acute, it is unwise to risk increasing the bleeding or to impair the healing process by stimulating and stretching the affected tissue. If the leakage has begun to coagulate but has not yet calcified, massage can be instrumental in stimulating reabsorption, but it is still necessary to work just around the edges of the injury; working in the middle of it can aggravate it and lead to more bleeding. If the injury is old, it is *still* a local contraindication; massage may impale soft tissues on the bony growth and cause more internal bleeding. Working within tolerance around the edges, however, can have the benefit of stimulating the body's own mechanisms to reabsorb this old, useless deposit.

Shin Splints

Definition: What Is It?

"Shin splints" is an umbrella term used to describe a variety of lower leg problems. The more technical terms for the injuries that often appear under this heading include acute and chronic exertional compartment syndrome, periostitis, tibial fractures, and medial tibial stress syndrome.

Etiology: What Happens?

Several features make the lower leg susceptible to certain injuries. Before discussing what goes wrong here, let's take a brief look at the construction of the lower leg and foot.

Anatomy Review   Many muscles in the body are almost entirely separate from their attaching bones, touching only at the ends of their tendons. Tibialis anterior and posterior, however, attach to the tibia from beginning to end and almost along the entire length of the muscle bellies. The tibialis anterior fascia actually blends directly into the periosteum along the whole bone (Fig. 2-7). The tibialis posterior attaches to the posterior aspect of the tibia in a similar way; the myofiber sheaths blend directly into the periosteum and interosseus ligament of the tibia and fibula. The soleus muscle also has a long attachment on the medial tibial periosteum.

The musculature of the lower leg is contained in four tough fascial compartments. Each compartment also has its own motor nerve supply. The fascia

<table>
<tr><td>

SHIN SPLINTS IN BRIEF:

What are they?
"Shin splints" refers to a collection of lower leg injuries including muscle tears, periostitis, hairline fractures, and other problems. They are usually brought about by overuse and/or misalignment at the ankle.

How are they recognized?
Pain along the tibia may be superficial or deep, mild or severe. The pattern of pain differs with the specific structures that are injured.

Is massage indicated or contraindicated?
Muscle injuries indicate massage, but it is advised with caution for periostitis or stress fractures, and is contraindicated entirely for acute exertional compartment syndrome.

</td></tr>
</table>

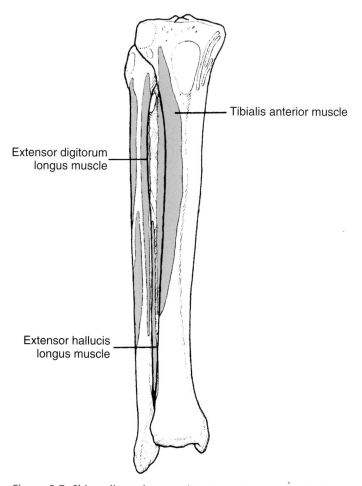

Tibialis anterior muscle

Extensor digitorum longus muscle

Extensor hallucis longus muscle

Figure 2-7. Shin splints: the anterior compartment muscles blend into the periosteum on the tibia

that wraps around groups of muscles in the lower leg is so tough and inelastic that if fluid should build up beyond a certain point, it can interfere with normal lymph and venous drainage. This traps the excess fluid inside the fascial sheath. The pressure this causes can be very painful and can damage muscle tissue and nerves.

The other key piece to lower leg function is the shock-absorbing capacity of the feet. Feet are designed to spread out and rebound with each step. If the foot has inadequate shock absorption—from flat feet (see *pes planus*, this chapter); bad shoes; bad surfaces to walk, run, or jump on; or any combination of these—the tibia and the muscles in the lower leg, especially soleus, tibialis anterior, and tibialis posterior, absorb a disproportionate amount of the shock. They are not designed for this job, however, and ongoing stress causes the periosteum to become irritated, the bone to crack, and the muscles to fray and become inflamed.

Chronic overuse or misalignment may cause the lower leg muscles to suffer some internal micro-tearing along with general inflammation. The periosteum of the injured tibia may also become inflamed. The difficulty with inflammation in this area is that there simply is not room within those fascial sheaths to allow for excess fluid retention. Even a small amount of edema can put pressure on nerve endings and limit blood flow, which in typical vicious-circle fashion, makes it hard for excess fluid to leave the area.

Causes for inflammation in the lower leg include exercising with inadequate foot support or on bad surfaces, unusual amounts of exercise followed by a period of rest (continued gentle movement would help the fluid to keep moving out of the area), suddenly changing an exercise routine, or running mostly uphill, downhill, or on uneven surfaces.

Signs and Symptoms

Pain from shin splints can be mild or severe, and the location varies according to which of the structures has been damaged. It gets worse with whatever actions the affected muscles do: dorsiflexion, inversion, or plantarflexion. Simple muscle injuries are rarely visibly or palpably inflamed. If the tibia is red, hot, and puffy, a more severe injury than just muscle damage to the lower leg is suspected.

Lower Leg Injuries

Muscle strains are the first step in a series of lower leg injuries, all of which may be referred to as "shin splints." The following lists conditions that may fall under this heading and the serious complications that may follow if they are not treated.

- *Tibialis anterior, tibialis posterior injury.* The pain associated with these injuries may be familiar to many people. The ache often runs most of the length of the tibia on the lateral side (for tibialis anterior) or deep in the back of the calf (for tibialis posterior).

- *Medial tibial stress syndrome.* This term refers to a muscular injury on the medial side of the tibia, usually involving the soleus and tibialis anterior.

- *Periostitis.* This is an inflammation of the periosteum, which may happen with damage to the soleus, the anterior tibialis, or posterior tibialis muscles. That seamless connection of membranes begins to rip apart, and the fibers of the muscles pull away from the bone. This condition may sometimes leave the bone feeling bumpy or pitted where scar tissue has knit the connective tissue membranes back together.

- *Stress fractures.* These are small hairline fractures of the tibia. They are extremely painful, and nothing heals them except time. They are frequently the result of "running through the pain." They are best diagnosed by a bone scan, which looks for areas of excessive circulatory activity. Stress fractures of the tibia do not usually show up well on radiographs.

- *Chronic exertional compartment syndrome.* This situation involves the production of excessive fluid in any of the four compartments of the lower leg. The fluid, which is normally increased by up to 20% with exercise, puts mechanical pressure on local nerves, causing pain and inflammation. Symptoms are relieved by rest but recur in a predictable pattern with activity.

- *Acute exertional compartment syndrome.* This is a culmination of a vicious circle of edema which limits blood flow, which limits the exit of excess fluid, which increases edema. Because the fascia on the lower leg is such a tough container, the swelling can actually cause tissue death if it is not resolved naturally or with surgical intervention. Acute exertional compartment syndrome is an emergency situation and should be treated as quickly as possible.

Treatment

The typical approach to mild shin splints is to reduce activity and to alternate applications of heat and cold. If the situation becomes chronic or develops into acute exertional compartment syndrome, steroid injections may be suggested or surgery may be performed to split the fascia and allow room for those compressed blood vessels that were unable to do their jobs. This surgery is followed by physical therapy to limit the accumulation of scar tissue that could bind up the compartments even tighter than before.

Massage?

Shin splints indicate massage as long as the problem is not too advanced. The lower leg muscles are impossible to thoroughly stretch out and clean up with exercise alone, but massage can give them a luxurious inch-by-inch stretching and broadening that cleanses the tissues more efficiently than anything else. In fact, massage is an excellent way to *prevent* shin splints and periostitis from complicating into exertional compartment syndrome.

For really hot, inflamed, painful cases, however, it is necessary to wait until the pain and inflammation has subsided. Obviously, if someone has too much fluid in a closed area, the last thing they need is massage to exacerbate it. What he or she really needs, if the pain is not *much* better in 2 or 3 days, is to see a doctor. Stress fractures and exertional compartment syndrome are serious problems that require medical attention.

Spasms, Cramps

Definition: What Are They?

A spasm is an involuntary contraction of a muscle. Clonic spasms are marked by alternating cycles of contraction and relaxation, whereas tonic spasms are sustained periods of hypertonicity. (*Spasm* is different from *spasticity*, which is discussed in the nervous system conditions, Chapter 3.) The difference between *spasms* and *cramps* is somewhat arbitrary; cramps are strong, painful, and usually short-lived spasms. It can be said that tight, painful paraspinals are in *spasm*, while a charley-horsing gastrocnemius is a *cramp*. The severity of these episodes depends on how much of the muscle is involved. "Spasms" and "cramps" are sometimes used in reference to visceral muscle also (i.e., *spastic constipation*), but the current discussion is restricted to the involuntary contraction of skeletal or so-called voluntary muscle.

Etiology: What Happens?

Four of the most common situations will be addressed here.

- *Nutrition.* Calcium and magnesium deficiencies, in addition to causing all sorts of problems later in life, can also make one prone to cramping, especially in the feet.

- *Ischemia.* When a muscle or part of a muscle is suddenly or gradually deprived of oxygen, it cannot function properly. Rather than becoming loose and weak, it becomes tighter and tighter. This is often a gradual process, but sometimes it is a sudden and violent reaction to an oxygen shortage.

  What causes this oxygen deprivation? Anything that impedes blood flow into the affected areas. Consider a typical tight, painful iliocostalis—one of the paraspinal group of muscles that holds the back erect. Here is a muscle: tight, hard, a little achy, but most of all, overworked. The fibers are shortened and thickened with the effort of keeping the spine upright, and this makes it harder for the supplying capillaries to deliver the goods, namely oxygen. In protest, the iliocostalis draws up even tighter, which further inhibits the influx of oxygen: a vicious circle of ischemia causing spasm, causing pain, which leads to spasm, and so on. Furthermore, muscles that are forced to work without oxygen accumulate the chemical by-products of anaerobic combustion. These metabolic wastes are irritating to nerve fibers, and so they further reinforce the spasm. The whole picture is complicated by the fact that as postural habits develop, the brain comes to interpret these sensations as being normal. The proprioceptors actually reinforce the patterns that cause the problem. This situation can go on for years without any real relief, until the circle of ischemia-spasm-pain is interrupted (Fig. 2-8).

  Pregnancy can be another cause of ischemic cramping. As the fetus lays on the femoral artery (just where it splits off from the abdominal branch), it can interfere with blood flow into the leg, prompting a violent contraction of the gastrocnemius. This is a classic example of an acute cramp or charley horse. Other kinds of circulatory interruptions or nervous system problems can cause them, too. Thus, when making a decision about whether massage is appropriate, it is important to be sure that no underlying pathology (e.g., cardiac weakness) is creating an oxygen deficiency.

- *Exercise-Associated Muscle Cramping.* Amateur and professional athletes often report problems with muscles cramping at or near the end of vigorous workouts. Dehydration, electrolyte imbalance, and hyperthermia may all be contributing factors, but recent research indicates that these cramps may be primarily due to a neurologic abnormality that overexcites muscle spindles (the proprioceptors involved in

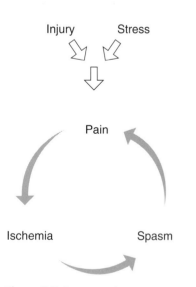

Figure 2-8. Spasm: pain-spasm-ischemia cycle

tightening) while inhibiting the activity of Golgi tendon organs (the propriocep-tors that allow muscles to let go). The target muscles usually cross two joints, and they cramp when they are contracted from a shortened position. Stretching the muscles and manipulating the tendons may stop these cramps, but they tend to recur if the athlete is inadequately warmed up or stretched out before he or she begins to exercise.

- *Splinting.* The last variety of cramps and spasms discussed here is a reflexive reac-tion against injury. Consider acute whiplash. The interspinous and intertransverse ligaments have been severely wrenched, and the body senses a potentially danger-ous instability in the cervical spine. Of course the postural neck muscles contract; as far as they are concerned, they are literally keeping the head from falling off. This kind of spasm is an important protective mechanism. It keeps the injured person from making the kind of movements that could cause further injury. The muscles create an effective splint; the range of motion of affected joints is gener-ally very small. The proprioceptors say, "You can move this far; no further." (For more on this situation see *whiplash*, this chapter.)

Massage?

Ischemic or exercise-related cramps indicate massage, as long as the ischemia is not re-lated to a contraindicated condition. Even when underlying pathology has been ruled out, massage must be used with caution. If a therapist tries to "fluff up" a cramping gas-trocnemius, he or she can damage the fibers. A better strategy is to stretch the tendons and antagonists of the affected muscle to gently but quickly persuade the proprioceptors that they may safely allow the muscle to let go. When the problem has moved out of the acute stage, it is possible to go back and clean up some of the toxic waste left behind, al-ways at the tolerance of the client.

When muscles are splinting an injured area, massage therapists should not interfere with this protective mechanism. If they do, the client will probably get up off the table with his or her newly loosened scalenes, and those muscles will clamp right back down, maybe even tighter than before.

In time, the ligaments surrounding the injured area will be ready to take on some weight-bearing stress, but the muscles may no longer be able to let go spontaneously. *Now* massage can do some real good. By working to soften the hardened muscle tissue, massage can reduce toxicity, improve blood flow, and speed healing. Spasm as a splinting mechanism is to be highly respected. When the injury moves into a subacute stage, massage contributes to a healing process with a minimum of scar tissue, fibrosis, and permanent shortening.

Strains

Definition: What Are They?

Strains are a subject of semantic debate. Some people say that the word "strain" refers only to tendon tears, others insist it refers only to muscle tears. In this text, "strain" refers to an injury to the muscle-tendon unit, with an emphasis on muscles. *Tendinitis,* or inflammation of tendons due to tears, is addressed later.

STRAINS IN BRIEF

What are they?
Strains are injuries to muscles.

How are they recognized?
Pain, stiffness, and occasionally palpable heat and swelling are all signs of muscle strain. Pain may be exacerbated by passive stretching or resisted contraction of the affected muscle.

Is massage indicated or contraindicated?
Muscle strains indicate massage, which can powerfully influ-ence the production of useful scar tissue, reduce adhesions and edema, and re-establish range of motion.

Etiology: What Happens?

Muscle strains and other soft tissue injuries occur from specific trauma, but they appear more often in the context of chronic, cumulative overuse patterns with no specific onset.

When a muscle is injured, the process is essentially similar to tendon and ligament injuries: fibers are torn, the inflammatory process begins, and fibroblasts flood the area with collagen to knit the injury back together. For more details about this process, see the sidebar "Stages of Musculoskeletal Injury" (this chapter).

Signs and Symptoms

Symptoms of muscle strain include mild or intense local pain, stiffness, and pain on resisted movement or passive stretching. Unless it is a *very* bad tear, no palpable heat or swelling will be present. Muscles, unlike tendons and ligaments, are *not* made exclusively of connective tissue, and although this is a good thing in terms of blood supply, an accumulation of excess scar tissue in muscles has different implications than it does in tendons and ligaments:

- *Impaired contractility.* Scar tissue can seriously impede the contractility of uninjured muscle fibers. When the injured muscle tries to contract, it bears the weight not only of its bony insertion, but also the fibers that are disabled by the mass of collagen that binds them up. This significantly increases the chance for repeated injury, more scar tissue, and further weakening of the muscle.

- *Adhesions.* Collagen that is manufactured around an injury does not immediately lay down in alignment with the muscle fibers; it is deposited in haphazard form. Randomly arranged collagen fibers tend to bind up different layers of tissue that are designed to be separate. These areas where one thing gets *stuck* to another are called adhesions. Adhesions can occur virtually wherever layers of connective tissue come in contact with each other. Adhesions may be *within* the muscle, as is frequently seen with the paraspinals, or *between* muscles, when muscle sheaths stick to other muscle sheaths. Hamstrings are a common place to see this phenomenon. Wherever they occur, adhesions limit mobility and increase the chance of injury (Fig. 2-9).

Treatment

The management of muscle injuries has taken some giant steps forward in recent years. Whereas at one time an injured person would be given a prescription for anti-inflammatories and painkillers, it is now recognized that early intervention in the healing process can powerfully affect the long-term quality of the healed tissue.

Although individual specialists approach musculoskeletal injuries with different tactics, some features are consistent:

- *Get a precise diagnosis.* Evaluating muscular injuries requires a thorough patient history and a skilled clinical examination. Other diagnostic procedures (radiographs, bone scans, MRI) may be recommended if the doctor suspects more than a soft tissue injury.

- *Control inflammation.* Inflammation is a valuable tool in dealing with acute injuries, but it can outlive its usefulness and end up causing more harm than good. (See more on *inflammation*, Chapter 5.) RICE therapy (rest, ice, compression, elevation) can help to control this reaction.

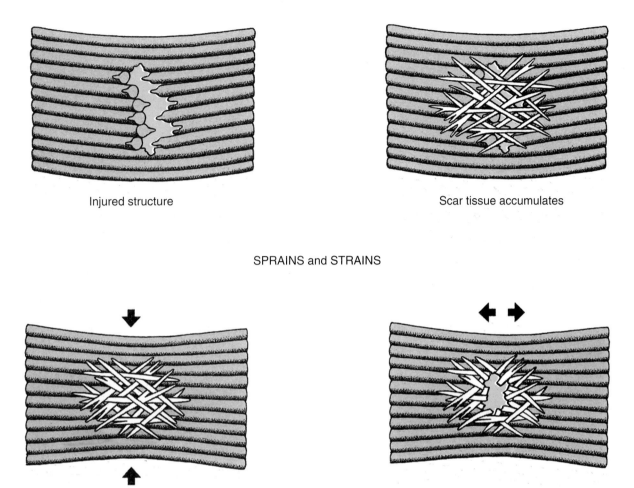

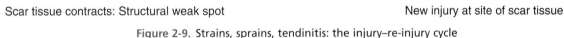

Figure 2-9. Strains, sprains, tendinitis: the injury–re-injury cycle

- *Rehabilitate damaged tissues.* This part of treatment involves exercises that add incremental amounts of weight-bearing stress to the injured muscle to (1) help the scar tissue realign with the original fibers and (2) gradually increase strength and fitness. This may be the most vulnerable time in the process, as athletes who are eager to resume training may try to go too fast and become injured again, and other people may neglect the need to exercise and allow scar tissue to accumulate to inefficient levels.

- *Prevent further injury.* Most chronic muscle injuries are related to controllable factors that can be adjusted to help prevent future problems. These include dealing with muscle imbalances that make one area weaker while another may be tighter, improving technique within specific sports, making sure that equipment is appropriate and in good repair, adjusting training schedules so that changes are incorporated slowly, and taping or bracing vulnerable areas.

Massage?

Skillful, knowledgeable massage can make the difference between a one-time muscle strain that takes a few weeks to resolve and a painful, limiting, chronically recurring condition that makes it impossible to perform an activity the client loves.

Stages of Musculoskeletal Injury
Acute Injuries

The general rule for massage and soft tissue injuries is that massage therapists must *respect the acute stage of injury*. Important things are happening during this time, and therapists ought not to interfere. It is during this stage that the inflammatory reaction begins with the release of chemicals that:

1. Set up edema which limits movement
2. Call in white blood cells to eat up the debris, and
3. Irritate nerve endings so that the person feels pain and takes the injury seriously.

Some types of massage are appropriate with some types of acute injuries, but they are highly specialized and not appropriate for casual experimentation.

How long is an acute injury acute? It depends on the injury, but the most commonly accepted guideline is 48 hours.

Subacute Injuries

This is where massage therapists can be most effective. As they strum over the newly formed scar tissue in an injured tendon or ligament, they are creating an internal environment that is conducive to the best possible healing. The tension and stretch massage creates will help determine the orientation of new collagen fibers. Massage will flush out the irritating chemicals that interfere with the inflow of fresh blood. Massage therapists are instrumental in the rehabilitation of an injured structure so that it will end up looking and behaving as though it never was hurt at all.

Chronic Injuries

In this stage massage therapists can still be major contributors to the healing process, but their effectiveness will be determined by how big, how old, and how accessible the injury is, as well as other variables like the diet and life style of the client. These are the situations in which therapists have to use their most powerful tools: cross fiber friction, ice, stretching, movement recommendations, everything that is at their disposal to rework that gnarled up old scar tissue inside and out.

Once a therapist has a clear picture of what structure or structures have been injured, a variety of bodywork tools may be used. Lymphatic drainage techniques can help to limit edema. Cross fiber and linear friction can influence the way old scar tissue matures and new scar tissue lays down. Passive stretches of healing muscles can also influence the correct alignment of collagen. When massage therapists apply their skills to the proper formation of scar tissue, the reduction of edema, the limiting of adhesions, and the improvement of circulation and mobility, they can help turn an irritating muscle tear into a trivial event.

Bone Disorders

Fractures
Definition: What Are They?

Fractures are any variety of broken bone, from a hairline crack to a complete break with protrusion through the skin.

Fractures come in all shapes and sizes. The basic classes are *complete*, in which the bone is completely broken through, or *incomplete*, in which the bone is only partially broken. Complete fractures may be *open*, in which case the broken fragments of bone protrude through the skin and are susceptible to infection, or *closed*, in which case the damage is entirely internal and involves a minimum of the surrounding soft tissues.

Open or closed complete fractures include *comminuted* fractures (which involve shattering of the broken bone), *impacted* fractures (which are broken bones with one end wedged into the other) (Fig. 2-10), as well as *transverse*, *oblique*, and *spiral* fractures.

Incomplete fractures are always closed. They include *stress* fractures and *compression* fractures. A special variety called a *march* fracture occurs in the metatarsals. *Greenstick* fractures involve bending and partial breakage of the bone.

Mal-union fractures are fractures that heal in a nonanatomic position. Many other types of fractures have been named for the doctors who first described them or the special joints they affect, but they are not discussed here.

Demographics: Who Gets Them?

Approximately 5.6 million people in the United States will experience a broken bone this year. It happens to children often because they engage in the risky behaviors that invite that sort of accident. However, children's bones have a much higher proportion of living cells and flexible cartilage to inert mass than adults' bones do. In fact, bones do not complete their calcification until the end of puberty. Children also have more growth hormone, which allows them a faster and more complete recovery than most adults can hope to attain. Elderly people, while not doing much tree climbing and skateboarding, have bones that are quite a bit more brittle and less resilient than young peoples', and it takes a great deal less stress to cause a fracture for them.

Diagnosis

Big bone breaks are usually obvious: they are painful, they usually follow a specific traumatic event, and they severely limit the function of the affected joints. Some fractures can be difficult to identify without a radiograph or bone scan, particularly if they are accompanied by a great deal of soft-tissue trauma. *Sprained ankles* and *shin splints* (this chapter) are two conditions that frequently hide bone fractures.

Treatment

Most fractures heal well if they are casted to immobilize the bones. Fibroblasts immediately infiltrate the area and build a framework of collagen. These are followed by osteoblasts laying down the framework for bone tissue, which later becomes dense and hard.

Some fractures need more support than a standard cast can offer, especially if the break involves a joint, as in the wrist or ankle. Pins or plates may be introduced to further stabilize the joint, but these carry the risk of introducing infection to the site.

Other fractures, especially those involving the femoral neck or head, may require joint replacement surgery before they heal satisfactorily.

Several grafting procedures have been developed to speed the healing for broken bones. Autologous grafts are insertions of the patient's own bone tissue to provide the scaffolding on which new material may grow. Cadaverous bone has also been used with success, although the replacement process is slower than with an autologous graft. Two other substances are in current use. One is derived from coral, which has a

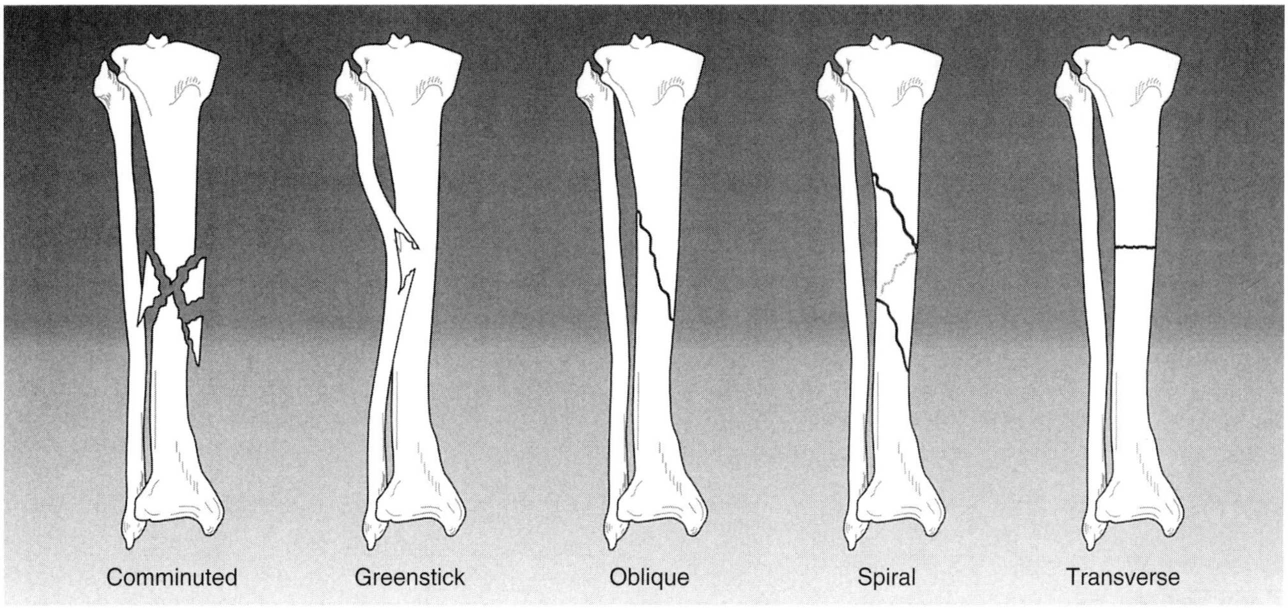

> ### FRACTURES IN BRIEF
>
> **What are they?**
> A fracture is any kind of broken or cracked bone.
>
> **How are they recognized?**
> Most fractures are painful and involve loss of function at the nearest joints, but some may be difficult to diagnose without an x-ray or other imaging techniques.
>
> **Is massage indicated or contraindicated?**
> Acute fractures locally contraindicate massage, but work done on the rest of the body can yield reflexive benefits. Later stages of fracture recovery indicate massage.

| Comminuted | Greenstick | Oblique | Spiral | Transverse |

Figure 2-10. Varieties of fractures

similar growth pattern to human bone; the other is a paste made of cow collagen. All these grafts help bone to heal faster than it would on its own, but none of them are usually strong enough to support the lesion without some kind of fixative device: pins, plates, or screws.

A variety of substances are under investigation that could take the place of various types of bone grafts. These include gels, pastes, and other compounds that may be applied to fractures to provide the framework for the growth of new tissue. Many of these compounds harden quickly to provide strong support for the new growth, and then gradually dissolve and are reabsorbed by the body when the repair is complete.

Massage?

The rules for working with fractures are guided by common sense: acute or unset broken bones obviously contraindicate massage. Casted fractures may result in stasis and edema that can be very much improved by massage, if access is available. Even if access to a broken leg is limited, for instance, reflexive benefits may be gained by working on the other limb. In addition, massage can minimize how movement compensation patterns may affect the rest of the body.

OSTEOPOROSIS IN BRIEF

What is it?
This is loss of bone mass and density brought about by endocrine imbalances and poor metabolism of calcium.

How is it recognized?
Osteoporosis in the early stages is identifiable only by radiographic and bone density tests. In later stages compression or spontaneous fractures of the vertebrae, wrists, or hips may be present. Kyphosis brought about by compression fractures of the vertebrae is a frequent indicator of osteoporosis (see *postural deviations*, this chapter).

Is massage indicated or contraindicated?
Gentle massage is indicated for persons with osteoporosis, with extra caution for the comfort and safety of the client. Massage does not affect the progression of the disease once it is present but may significantly reduce associated pain. Acute *fractures*, however, contraindicate massage (see this chapter).

Osteoporosis
Definition: What Is It?

Osteoporosis means, literally, "porous bones." In this condition calcium is pulled off the bones faster than it is replaced, leaving them thinned, brittle, chalky, and prone to injury.

Demographics: Who Gets It?

This disease affects an estimated 10 million Americans, although it is estimated that up to 18 million more have significant bone thinning but are unaware of their risk. It affects women about 5 times more often than men for several reasons: women have lower bone density to begin with; they bear children—an enormous drain on calcium reserves; and changes in hormone levels have great influence on how well calcium is added to bone mass. Small-boned, thin women get osteoporosis more often than others. Women who are postmenopausal and/or have a history of anorexia are at especially high risk (see *eating disorders*, Chapter 3). White and Asian women are most likely to develop this condition, but African-American and Hispanic women can also have it.

Although a genetic marker for osteoporosis has been identified, other risk factors are major contributors to this disease. Therefore, bone density is determined only about 60% by heredity and 40% by controllable factors such as diet, smoking, exercise, and stress levels. Chronic secretions of cortisol have been shown to be extremely destructive to bone density.[g]

---

[g]Depression, Bone Mass, and Osteoporosis. NIMH, 6/29/01. Available at: http://www.nih.gov/news/pr/June 2001/nimh-29.htm. Accessed winter, 2002.

Etiology: What Happens?

Before the bones are discussed, it is worthwhile to point out a few things about calcium.

Calcium Absorption Calcium requires an acidic environment in the stomach to be absorbed into the body. If calcium enters the body in a form that impedes its contact with hydrochloric acid (i.e., in dairy products or "calcium rich" antacids) the body may not be able to absorb very much of the calcium that is available. Similarly, if natural secretions of hydrochloric acid are reduced, as in older women and men, it becomes even harder to absorb whatever calcium is consumed. Calcium also competes, usually unsuccessfully, with other substances for uptake. Perhaps the most notorious of these is the phosphorus found in carbonated drinks. When a person drinks a lot of soda, the phosphorus blocks out the ability to absorb calcium.

Vitamin D controls how efficiently the body absorbs and retains calcium. The body synthesizes adequate amounts of vitamin D in response to direct sunlight (it takes about 15 minutes of exposure per day), but vitamin D can also be easily supplemented.

Calcium Loss Calcium is constantly lost through sweat and urine. Some substances, specifically meat-based proteins, cause higher levels of calcium to be excreted in urine. Although a person may take in ample supplies of calcium, he or she tends to lose it if a lot of meat is also consumed. This may help to explain why vegetarians have a statistically lower rate of osteoporosis than the general population and why, although the United States is a leading consumer of milk, it also has higher osteoporosis rates than other countries with diets that are lower in animal proteins.

Maintaining Bone Density The shape and density of bones are determined by the activity of osteoclasts and osteoblasts. These cells work to remodel bones according to the commands of calcitonin and parathyroid hormone. If hormones tell the osteoclasts to work faster than the osteoblasts, bone density declines. Osteoclasts pull calcium off bones to respond to immediate needs as they arise.

Bones are *not* the only part of the body that needs calcium. Bones happen to be a convenient storage medium, but calcium is consumed in nearly every chemical reaction that results in muscle contraction and nerve transmission. Calcium is essential to blood clotting and to maintaining the proper pH balance in the blood. These are very important functions, and the body has a strict prioritizing system: chemical reactions that are crucial to moment-to-moment survival are more important than maintaining the density of the vertebrae.

When a person has osteoporosis, it is usually because the body is using the calcium stored in the bones faster than it can be replaced. The bones, especially in the spine and pelvis, get progressively thinner, leaving the person vulnerable to the primary complications of osteoporosis: spinal or hip fractures.

Complications

Complications of osteoporosis center around pathologically weak bones. Thinned vertebrae lead to a loss of height and the characteristic rounded "widow's hump" of kyphosis. Chronic and/or acute back pain appears in this stage as the vertebrae continue to degenerate. People with osteoporosis are also prone to other fractures with little or no cause; these are called *spontaneous* or *pathologic* fractures. Hips, vertebrae, and wrists are particularly vulnerable to breakage. Because older persons are naturally low on both living osteocytes and growth hormone to induce the healing process, it is particularly difficult to recover from any injury of this severity.

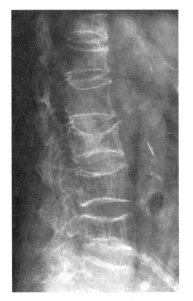

Figure 2-11. Demonstrable bone loss with osteoporosis (compare with Figure 2-12)

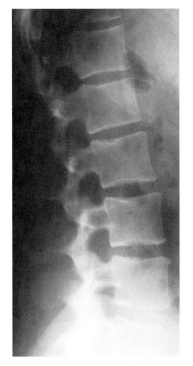

Figure 2-12. Normal spine

Diagnosis

Osteoporosis is a virtually silent disease until it is too late to do anything about it. Even radiographs and bone density tests yield conclusive information only after density loss is between 30 and 40% (Figs. 2-11 and 2-12). In the later stages, however, the disease is often identified by compression fractures in the vertebrae.

One important feature in the diagnosis of osteoporosis, especially in premenopausal women, is to rule out *hyperthyroidism* (see Chapter 8). This condition can cause the release of too much parathyroid hormone, which consequently overstimulates osteoclasts. Hyperthyroidism may be the only type of truly reversible osteoporosis.

Treatment

Once osteoporosis has been identified, a number of treatment options are available to keep it from getting worse. Among these is hormone replacement therapy (HRT). Estrogen influences calcium absorption. Postmenopausal women secrete this hormone only in very small amounts, so replacing it should improve calcium uptake. Unfortunately, estrogen supplements are also associated with breast and uterine cancers, and some research shows that supplementing estrogen is largely ineffective at limiting bone loss in the long run, so HRT is not for everybody. Calcitonin, a synthetic version of the hormone that stimulates osteoblasts, is another treatment option, as are bisphosphates, which inhibit bone breakdown and increase bone density.

Exercise is almost always a part of the osteoporosis treatment strategy. Since bone remodels according to the stresses placed on it, weight-bearing stress ensures that maintaining healthy mass is a high priority. For someone with this condition, gentle weight training or walking is more beneficial than low-impact cardiovascular exercises like swimming or cycling.

Diet also plays an important role in dealing with osteoporosis. Specific vitamins and other substances may improve calcium uptake, even for postmenopausal women, but this book is not the place to discuss them.

Prevention

This is a disease that is easy to prevent, feasible to slow down or halt, and often impossible to reverse. The causes of it are many and varied, but center around one main theme: the time to build up calcium reserves is in youth and early adulthood. The skeleton grows in height until about age 20, but it continues to accumulate *density* until about age 35. After that point it tends to progressively demineralize. Studies show that today many Americans get only half or less of the recommended daily allowance of calcium; this, combined with our dismal rates of getting exercise, does not bode well for future osteoporosis statistics.

Four main steps have been recommended to achieve and maintain optimal bone density and avoid osteoporosis:

1. *Get dietary calcium from easily accessible sources.* These do *not* include dairy products, which interfere with the ability of gastric juice to absorb this important nutrient. Recommended calcium sources include "beans and greens": legumes and green leafy vegetables.

2. *Exercise.* Weight-bearing stress makes it necessary for the body to maintain healthy bone density.

3. *Get Vitamin D.* The recommended daily allowance (RDA) for vitamin D is 200 units, or 5 μg, per day. This can be ingested in supplement form or be naturally synthesized by exposure to sunlight.

4. *Avoid substances and behaviors that pull calcium off bones.* Salt, animal proteins, and alcohol all require calcium to be processed by the body. Cigarette smoking has also been associated with low bone density.

Massage?

In the treatment of clients with osteoporosis, the appropriateness of massage varies from person to person. The only way massage could worsen the situation would be to exert undue mechanical force, which could lead to the possibility of fractures. On the other hand, consider the condition of the muscles of someone with osteoporosis: massage can offer a great deal of symptomatic relief, even if it cannot reverse the degeneration of the bone tissue. In any case, caution is the key with this condition. Massage therapists should not look for miracles; taking someone out of their pain for a few hours is miracle enough.

Paget's Disease

Definition: What Is It?

Paget's disease is a condition in which healthy bone is reabsorbed up to 50 times faster than normal. It is replaced with disorganized fibrous connective tissue, which never completely hardens. This leaves the affected bones weakened and distorted.

Demographics: Who Gets It?

This is one of the most common metabolic bone diseases, second only to *osteoporosis* (this chapter). It affects approximately 3% of persons older than 40 years and 10% of persons older than 80 years in the United States. Men have Paget's disease more often than women, and although African Americans can have it, it is especially prevalent in Whites from Northwestern Europe. It is very rare in Asians.

Etiology: What Happens?

Every day, on a microscopic level, small amounts of calcium in the bones are dissolved into the bloodstream, to be replaced by new supplies. The osteoclasts, which break down bone, and osteoblasts, which build it up, keep each other in balance. In Paget's disease, both the osteoclasts and osteoblasts became hyperactive, and the reshaping process does not function correctly.

This disease typically occurs in two stages. In the vascular stage bone is broken down and replaced— not with high-quality, carefully organized calcium deposits, but with jumbled, chaotic fibrous tissue, supplied by vast numbers of new blood vessels. Then in the sclerotic stage the new material becomes brittle, not strong. This shows in a characteristic mosaic pattern on radiographs. The bones most often affected by this disease are spine, skull, pelvis, femur, and lower leg.

Most people with Paget's disease have it in only one bone, but some have it in two or more. It does not seem to spread from one bone to another, however.

Osteoporosis Statistics[h]

The statistics surrounding osteoporosis are among the most startling of all musculoskeletal diseases. This "silent disease" is responsible for drastic life changes and extraordinary medical costs.

Incidence

Osteoporosis is fully developed in 10 million Americans and is a future threat for approximately 18 million more.

Of people with osteoporosis, 80% are women. Of women older than 50 years of age, half will probably experience an osteoporosis-related fracture. Of men older than 50, 1 in 8 will have a fracture.

Osteoporosis and Fractures

Osteoporosis is directly responsible for 1.5 million broken bones in the United States every year. A rough breakdown of osteoporosis-related fractures is as follows:

- 700,000 vertebral fractures
- 300,000 hip fractures
- 200,000 wrist fractures
- 300,000 other fractures

A woman's risk of hip fracture is equal to her *combined* risk of developing breast, uterine, or ovarian cancer. Women are 2 to 3 times more likely to fracture a hip than men, but men are twice as likely to die of complications related to hip fractures.

Osteoporosis and Medical Costs

The direct costs of treating osteoporosis and related fractures (this is treatment only, not lost work hours or death costs) amounts to $13.8 billion per year or *$38 million per day*, and those costs are rising.

---

[h]Fast facts on osteoporosis. National Institutes of Health Osteoporosis and Related Bone Diseases National Resource Center. Available at: http://www.osteo.org/osteofastfact.html. Accessed fall 2000.

PAGET'S DISEASE:
Sir James Paget was an English surgeon who lived from 1814 to 1899. He was the first to document the bony disorder described here and two types of rare malignancies: extramammary Paget's disease and mammary Paget's disease.

Causes

The cause of Paget's disease is currently unknown, but research is leaning toward the idea of a very slow-acting virus, which may live in the system for years before causing any damage. A genetic component is probable, since Paget's disease often runs in families, but this may simply indicate a susceptibility to the particular virus involved.

Signs and Symptoms

Paget's disease usually has no symptoms until it has become advanced enough to cause visible changes to the affected bones. When it is found early, it is often because a person has a radiograph taken for some other reason and Paget's disease is identified by chance.

Later signs and symptoms of Paget's disease include deep bone pain, palpable heat where the bones are affected, and problems related to a change in bone shape in the affected areas. These can include a loss of hearing and chronic headaches if the skull is affected, pinched nerves and vertebral fractures if the disease is in the spine, and a visible change in bone shape (Fig. 2-13). The long bones of the femur and lower leg may become bowed and distorted.

Complications

Paget's disease has several serious complications brought about by changes in bone size and strength. The most common complication is *fractures* (this chapter) in the affected bones. If the cranial bones begin to put pressure on parts of the central nervous system, deafness or brain damage could result. *Congestive heart failure* (Chapter 4) may occur because the heart must pump blood not only through healthy, normal vessels, but also through whole new networks of vessels in the new, useless fibrous tissue.

Rare cases of Paget's disease may involve a loss of vision as the skull bones interfere with nerves from the eyes, and dental problems as the size of the mandible or maxilla change in relation to the teeth. Approximately 1% of Paget's disease patients develop a rare form of bone cancer.

Diagnosis

This condition is diagnosed primarily by radiograph or bone scan (a test to detect heightened circulation and activity in bone tissue). A blood test to look for alkaline phosphatase (an enzyme produced by overactive osteoblasts) may confirm the diagnosis.

Because this disease has a clear genetic link, family members of Paget's disease patients may be recommended to have blood tests for heightened levels of alkaline phosphatase every few years after they turn 40. This could allow for early diagnosis and more effective treatment of the disease.

Treatment

Treatment of Paget's disease is surprisingly similar to that of osteoporosis; the unwanted breakdown of healthy bone tissue is a feature common to both disorders. Exercise is the first recommendation for patients with Paget's disease to maintain function and healthy bone

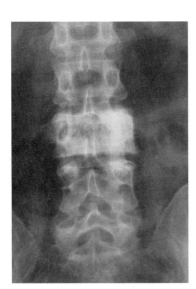

Figure 2-13. Overgrowth of the vertebral body at L3 in this patient with Paget's disease (compare with Figure 2-12)

mass for as long as possible. Aspirin and anti-inflammatories may be suggested for pain relief. Finally calcitonin or bisphosphates may be prescribed to inhibit osteoclast activity.

Massage?

This is a disease involving inflammation, impaired circulation, and weakened bones. All these issues require caution from massage therapists. If a Paget's disease patient is engaging in exercise and physical therapy to maintain bone health, massage could be a useful adjunct to this effort, as long as the client's health care team is informed.

Postural Deviations
Definition: What Are They?

Although it is tempting to think about the spine in terms of a ship's mast, a column, or a tent pole held erect by muscular tension, it is actually much stronger than any of those. The curvatures in the cervical, thoracic, and lumbar regions give the spine 10 times the resistance it would have if it were perfectly straight. Sometimes, though, these natural curvatures are overdeveloped, which reduces resiliency and strength rather than enhancing it. Kyphosis ("humpback"), lordosis ("swayback"), and scoliosis ("S", "C," or "Reverse- C" curves) are the specific postural deviations addressed here (Fig. 2-14).

Etiology: What Happens?

It is sometimes convenient to think about the spine in only two dimensions at a time. In other words, scoliosis would be simply an S-shaped curve from left to right, and lordosis

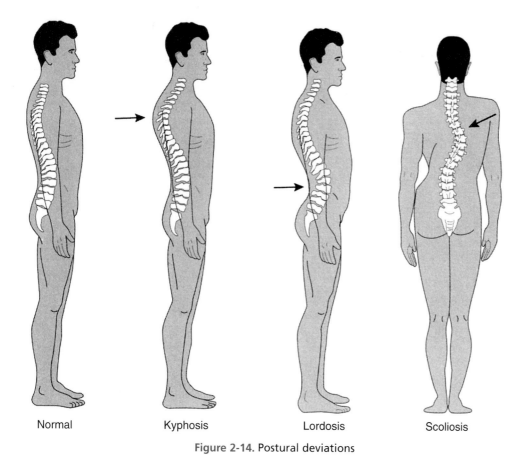

Normal   Kyphosis   Lordosis   Scoliosis

Figure 2-14. Postural deviations

POSTURAL DEVIATIONS IN BRIEF

What are they?
Postural deviations are overdeveloped thoracic or lumbar curves (kyphosis and lordosis) or an S-curve in the spine (scoliosis).

How are they recognized?
Extreme curvatures are easily visible, although radiographs are used to pinpoint exactly where the problems begin and end.

Is massage indicated or contraindicated?
All postural deviations indicate massage as long as other underlying pathologies have been eliminated. Bodywork may not be able to reverse any damage, but it can certainly provide relief for the muscular stress that accompanies spinal changes.

and kyphosis would be exaggerated forward and backward curves. The truth is not nearly so simple. With any imbalance in the stacking of the vertebrae, rotations in one direction or another can complicate the issue. Thus, scoliosis is not merely a left-right aberration, but involves a spiral twisting of the vertebral column as well. Similar lateral imbalances may be observed with most cases of lordosis and kyphosis.

One important thing to remember with postural deviations is the difference between a *functional* problem and a *structural* one. In the early stages of either of these conditions it may be the soft tissues that are pulling the spine out of alignment: a *functional* problem. At this point the condition is probably at its most treatable: muscles, tendons, and ligaments can be exercised, stretched, and manipulated into new holding and movement patterns. Functional deviations can also be brought about by structural problems elsewhere in the body (e.g., unequal leg length). If the soft tissues are left untreated and the bones are constantly pulled in one direction or another, they will eventually change shape to adapt to those stressors. At this point the condition becomes a *structural* dysfunction and is much harder to reverse.

Most cases of postural deviations are idiopathic, that is, of unknown origin. However, a small percentage of structural problems in the spine can be related to congenital or neuromuscular problems like cerebral palsy, polio, spina bifida, or incompletely formed vertebrae. These contributing factors must be addressed before any attempt is made to correct the postural deviations they produce.

Signs and Symptoms

Postural deviations can range from being painfully obvious to quite subtle. A visual examination yields much information about kyphosis and lordosis, and even mild scoliosis may be visible with a forward-bending test. Clients' complaints often include muscular tension and sometimes nerve impairment along with chronic ache and loss of range of motion.

- *Scoliosis* is a problem for approximately 2% of all teenagers. It affects girls 7 times more frequently than boys and almost always involves a bend to the right. It usually appears during the rapid-growth years of late childhood and early adolescence. Mild scoliosis, which is any curve less than 30 to 40° is treated, if at all, with exercise, chiropractic therapy, a corrective brace, and/or electromuscular stimulation to strengthen the muscles of the stretched side of the spine. If the scoliosis appears at more than 40° in childhood, the chances that it will worsen are very great. It typically progresses at 1° every year.

  Complications of scoliosis include neuritis, as misshaped bones press on nerve roots; *spondylosis* (this chapter); and serious heart and lung problems arising from a severely restricted rib cage.

  Surgery for scoliosis involves inserting rods that straighten and fuse the affected vertebrae. This limits spinal mobility but can improve the quality of life for people with advanced scoliosis.

- *Kyphosis* is an overdeveloped thoracic curve. In young people it is very often a result of muscular imbalance and may be treated with physical therapy. Scheuermann's disease is a type of idiopathic kyphosis that affects young men. It is usually painless and is treated with physical therapy and/or braces. Kyphosis in older people may be due to muscular imbalance but could also be a complication of *osteoporosis* or *ankylosing spondylitis* (this chapter). A kyphotic curve of 20 to 40° is considered normal. Surgical intervention is not usually suggested for anything less than a 75° curvature.

- *Lordosis* or swayback is an overpronounced lumbar curve. The architecture and musculature of the low back makes it particularly vulnerable to this kind of imbalance. It can often be much improved by exercise and physical therapy (including massage). Lordosis, although not dangerous in itself, can lead to more serious low back pain (see *herniated disc,* this chapter).

Treatment

Treatment options for different kinds of postural deviations are outlined in the descriptions above.

Massage?

As long as no underlying pathology is contributing to spinal problems, all kinds of postural deviations may indicate massage. In the early stages of these diseases, chronic soft tissue (that is, muscular, tendinous, and ligamentous) stresses pull on the bones and change the architecture of the spine. Caught early enough, many inefficient postural habits can be reversed without permanent damage. Bone is living, adaptable tissue; if left untreated, the vertebrae will eventually remold themselves to permanently imprint a postural pattern.

Massage certainly will not make any of these conditions any worse and could quite possibly offer much relief by simply reducing some of the tension that both causes and accompanies spinal imbalance. If a therapist is very skilled and the circumstances are just right, massage may set the stage for a permanent change in bony alignment.

Joint Disorders

Ankylosing Spondylitis
Definition: What Is It?

AS is a spinal inflammation (*spondylitis*) leading to stiff joints (*ankylosis*). This means really stiff—these joints can become permanently fused. AS is a progressive inflammatory arthritis of the spine caused by an autoimmune reaction. It is sometimes called *rheumatoid spondylitis.*

Demographics: Who Gets It?

AS is an inherited disorder that most often affects men between 16 and 35 years of age. A gene (HLA-B27) has been identified that seems to increase the tendency to develop this disease, but it is not a definitive factor; many people with the AS gene never have symptoms. About 1%, or 2.5 million people, in the United States have some degree of AS; 90% of them are males.

ANKYLOSING SPONDYLITIS:
"Ankyle" comes from the Greek *ankylos*, meaning bent or crooked, and *ankylosis* meaning stiffening of the joints. "Spondylitis" means spinal inflammation. Ankylosing spondylitis: inflammatory stiffening of the spine in a bent position.

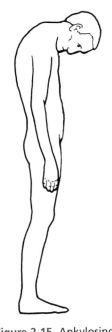

Figure 2-15. Ankylosing spondylitis

Etiology: What Happens?

AS typically begins at the sacroiliac joint on one or both sides. Although it is usually limited to spinal joints, the hips, shoulders, toes, and sternoclavicular joints may also be affected. The affected joints become inflamed in the acute or "flare" stage. When the inflammation subsides, the bony surfaces inside the joint have become damaged. The pattern of inflammation and damage proceeds up the spine, leaving in its wake a trail of injured vertebrae that may eventually fuse in slight or sometimes extreme flexion (Fig. 2-15). If the progression reaches all the way up to the neck, the cervical vertebrae may fuse with the head in a permanently flexed position as well. Fusions may also occur at the vertebral-costal joints, resulting in a locked ribcage and difficulty with breathing.

Signs and Symptoms

AS usually starts as chronic low back pain. Pain is often felt in the buttocks and sometimes all the way down into the heels. This can sometimes lead to a misdiagnosis of herniated disc. The spine and hips feel stiff and immobile; this is usually much worse in the morning or after prolonged immobility.

As with most autoimmune diseases, this condition has acute and subacute stages. During acute episodes a general feeling of illness and a slight fever may be present. The eyes may become dry, red, and uncomfortable. Pain and stiffness gradually spread higher and higher up the spine. The disease is usually limited to the low back but occasionally proceeds up into the neck or other joints in the body.

Complications

Loss of lung capacity is the major complication of this disease. If a person is bent over and the ribs cannot expand, it is very difficult to get an adequate supply of oxygen into the body or to get carbon dioxide out of the body. This results in constant shortness of breath, low stamina, and reduced resistance to chest infections such as pneumonia (from which, depending on posture, recovery can be very difficult).

Spinal fusions and loss of mobility increase the risk of spinal fractures. If the disease makes it all the way up the neck, stiffness at the jaw may make talking and eating difficult.

The inflammatory nature of AS is not restricted to joints around the spine. The inflammation may spread to other organs, including the eyes, lungs, heart, and kidneys.

Diagnosis

AS is diagnosed through observable symptoms, blood tests, and radiographs. It can be difficult to identify in the early stages, because many disorders can cause diffuse back pain and stiffness. It sometimes takes years to confirm a diagnosis of AS. This is especially true when the condition is present in women, for whom the initial symptoms tend to be less predictable.

One feature that can assist in the diagnosis of AS is that it often appears along with other disorders. Particular red flags are chronic prostatitis, iritis (inflammation of the iris of the eyes), *Crohn disease* and *ulcerative colitis* (Chapter 7), and *psoriasis* (Chapter 1). Also, people in the immediate family of an AS patient show statistically higher rates of psoriatic arthritis, Crohn disease, and ulcerative colitis.

Treatment

The first, best option for dealing with AS (which has no known cause and therefore no cure) is exercise. Physical therapy is recommended to develop a series of exercises that will, as much as possible, preserve the suppleness of the spine and the strength of the paraspinals without aggravating the condition. Maintaining correct posture for as long as possible is the primary goal, since the vertebrae tend to fuse in a flexed position.

If exercise alone does not help, painkillers and anti-inflammatories may be prescribed. In very extreme cases surgery may be suggested: an osteotomy is a procedure that cuts through the frozen joints and re-fuses them in a straightened position. If the knees, shoulders, or hips have been impaired, joint replacement surgery may also be suggested.

Massage?

Little is well understood about this disease, and even less is known about how massage might affect it. Because it is an inflammatory condition and because it does spread, massage practitioners must proceed with caution. The massage therapist should always work with this condition in conjunction with a health care team and only when the inflammation is subacute. If the spinal joints are inflamed, the massage therapy appointment should be rescheduled. If a client is in the early stages of this disease, massage may help to preserve precious mobility of the spine. If a client is in a more advanced stage, massage will probably have little effect except pain relief, since the muscles are being stretched over immobile joints.

Dislocations

Definition: What Are They?

When the bones in a joint are separated so that they no longer articulate, the joint is said to be dislocated. It is hard to imagine that happening without damage to most of the surrounding tissues as well: muscles, tendons, blood vessels, and nerves are generally also injured in a traumatic dislocation (Fig. 2-16). Nearby bursae may also become inflamed. Dislocations are most often due to trauma, but some are brought about by congenital weakness of the ligaments. Others are brought about by diseases like rheumatoid arthritis, which may involve degenerated tissue inside joints, raising the risk of having the joint literally fall apart.

Signs and Symptoms

Most of the joints in the body cannot dislocate without *huge* amounts of force. The shoulder, because of the shallowness of the glenoid fossa, and the fingers are the joints most at risk for dislocation (Fig. 2-17). The temporomandibular joint is another common site (see *TMJ Disorders*, this chapter). Symptoms of a newly dislocated joint include swelling, discoloration, loss of function, and, most obviously, a large amount of pain.

DISLOCATIONS IN BRIEF

What are they?
Dislocations are traumatic injuries to joints where the articulating bones are forcefully separated.

How are they recognized?
Acute (new) dislocations are extremely painful. The bones may be visibly separated and the joint may lose all function.

Is massage indicated or contraindicated?
Dislocations indicate massage in the subacute stage, as long as work is conducted within pain tolerance. As the area heals, massage may be useful for managing scar tissue accumulation and muscle spasm around the affected joint.

Complications

Uncomplicated traumatic dislocations are painful and take a long time to heal, but they are not usually serious. Fibrosis and excessive scar tissue of the surrounding soft tissues may develop after prolonged splinting. Occasionally a nerve may be severely damaged by the trauma, but this is the exception rather than the rule.

If, however, the ligaments supporting the damaged joint become stretched, they may lose some of their ability to do their job. The ligaments may even rupture and detach from the bone altogether. When ligaments are permanently damaged, the joint may become unstable and prone to re-injury: "subluxation" if the bones move out of alignment, "spontaneous dislocation" if the bones completely separate. These mishaps are especially common in the shoulder and jaw. The muscles that cross over these unstable joints are likely to be much tighter than is ideal, because the ligaments are not doing their job. This can lead to *myofascial pain syndrome* or *tendinitis* (this chapter). The most serious long-term consequence of ligament laxity is the possibility of developing *osteoarthritis* (this chapter).

Treatment

Acute dislocations require immediate attention. If large joints are not relocated within about 15 minutes, the tissues swell up so much and the muscles contract so tightly that it is difficult to move the joint without a general anesthetic. After the joint is relocated, a radiograph is usually taken to rule out the possibility of a *fracture* (this chapter). The joint is typically splinted for 2 or 3 weeks until the capsular ligament and other supportive ligaments are ready to carry their weight again. Physical therapy is prescribed to strengthen and retrain the muscles surrounding the joint.

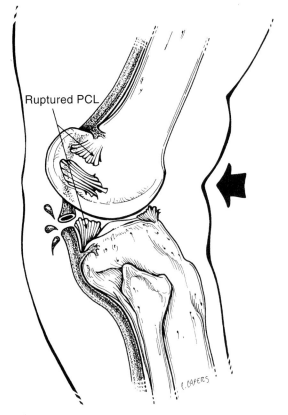

Figure 2-16. Dislocations often involve extensive soft tissue damage

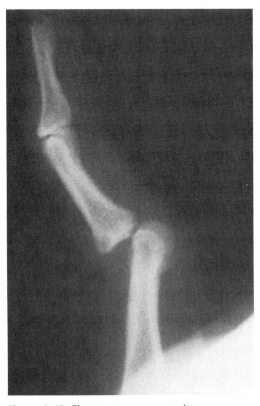

Figure 2-17. Fingers are common sites for dislocations

If the ligaments have ruptured or are simply too lax to support the joint capsule properly, surgery may be recommended. This typically involves shortening and/or reattaching the damaged ligaments to the bone using stitches or staples. Arthroscopic surgery for dislocated shoulders is a technique that may be able to improve joint function without the complications of major surgery. *Thermal capsulorrhaphy* is a type of arthroscopic surgery designed to improve ligament stability. A thermal probe heats up specific areas of the joint capsule. This causes the collagen fibers to shrink, tightening the capsular ligament. This technique is currently used only for shoulders, but it may eventually be applicable to other joints.

An alternative to surgery for chronically lax ligaments is a specialized series of injections of substances called proliferants. They are designed to stimulate the growth of new collagen fibers that, with appropriate stretching and exercise, will lay down in alignment with the original fibers. This procedure can tighten stretched-out ligaments, thus reducing the chance of future injury.

Massage?

Obviously, massage is out of the question for an acute injury of this type. In the subacute stage massage may help untangle the muscular and tendinous scar tissue that is likely to develop as a result of dislocations, as long as the basic rules about working within tolerance, following up with ice, and monitoring results are followed. If a client has an *old* dislocation that occasionally subluxates or even entirely dislocates without trauma, massage does no harm as long as care is taken be sure that he or she is positioned in a way that feels safe and comfortable.

Gout

Definition: What Is It?

Gout is one of the oldest diseases in recorded medical history. In 580 A.D. Alexander of Tralles wrote:

> *Gout sufferers should eat little meat, drink no alcohol and eat the underground stems of calchium (autumn crocus).*[i]

One of the drugs in use today for the treatment of gout is colchicine, a synthetic version of autumn crocus.

Gout has been known as the "disease of kings" because it is associated with rich diets and decadent living. This is witnessed by a list of some of gout's most famous victims: Alexander the Great, Henry VIII of England, Charles V of Spain and his son Phillip II, Dr. Samuel Johnson, Wolfgang von Goethe, and Benjamin Franklin.

Gout is a type of inflammatory arthritis. It has a chemical cause, rather than arising from wear and tear or immune system mistakes.

GOUT IN BRIEF
What is it? Gout is inflammatory arthritis caused by deposits of sodium urate (uric acid) in and around joints, especially in the feet.
How is it recognized? Acute gout causes joints to become red, hot, swollen, shiny, and extremely painful. It usually has a sudden onset.
Is massage indicated or contraindicated? Gout systemically contraindicates massage when it is acute. Gouty joints locally contraindicate massage at all times.

Demographics: Who Gets It?

Gout affects men more than women by a wide margin: 90% of gout sufferers are men, for whom the prime age of disease development is 75 years; 10% are women, and most of those are postmenopausal. The United States has about 1 million gout patients.

[i]DiBacco TV. The pain of gout: Baffling condition left doctors guessing. *Washington Post*. October 11, 1994:Z19.

Etiology: What Happens?

Uric acid is a naturally occurring by-product of protein digestion. Under normal circumstances it is extracted from the blood by the kidneys. If the kidneys are unable to perform this function, either because too much uric acid is present or because they are otherwise impaired, *hyperuricemia* (the state of having higher than normal levels of uric acid in the blood) develops. Hyperuricemia is the primary risk factor for gout.

The transition from hyperuricemia to an acute gouty attack is often precipitated by some specific event: binge eating or drinking, surgery, or a systemic infection. All these things alter fluid levels in the body. When uric acid consolidates, it forms sharp, needle-like crystals that accumulate in and around the foot, grinding on and irritating synovial capsules, bursae, tendons, and other tissues. The foot may be the primary target because of gravity, but it may also have to do with the lower temperature found in extremities that aids in the crystallization process. Typically a person goes to bed feeling fine and then wakes in the night with a foot that is red, throbbing, and painful.

In later stages of the disease, deposits of sodium urate called *tophi* develop inside joints. These tophi progressively erode all the joint structures, leading to a complete loss of function. Tophi also grow along tendons and in subcutaneous tissues. They have been found in myocardium, pericardium, aortic valves, and even the pinna of the ear!

Risk Factors

Uric acid is a waste product from the metabolism of a certain component of nucleic acids called *purines*. A diet that is high in purines tends to produce more uric acid in the body than a diet that is not. Foods that are particularly high in purines include red meat, organ meats, fish, fowl, lentils, alcohol, mushrooms, and some other vegetables (peas, asparagus, and spinach).

Under normal circumstances, uric acid is excreted by the kidneys. Here is where the problems may start.

- *Metabolic gout.* In this situation the kidneys may be functioning normally, but the body is producing too much uric acid for them to keep up. This is the case for someone with a particularly high protein/alcohol intake.

- *Renal gout.* In this case the uric acid load may be normal, but the kidneys are not functioning well. They cannot handle the job of excreting all the uric acid, and so it ends up in the bloodstream and eventually in the feet. This kind of kidney insufficiency may be hereditary or related to other problems such as *diabetes* (Chapter 8) or lead poisoning.

- *Both.* Here the kidneys are compromised *and* the purine intake is high. This is gout waiting to happen.

An elevated level of uric acid (*hyperuricemia*) is clearly connected to gout, but the two things are not always identical. Many people have hyperuricemia without ever having gout. Conversely, some people with gout show normal or even below normal levels of uric acid in the blood.

In addition to a high-purine diet, other risk factors for gout include obesity, sudden weight gain, moderate to high alcohol consumption, high blood pressure, and certain blood disorders that can raise uric acid levels.

Sometimes a person will have just one attack of gout and then never be bothered by it again. Usually, the second attack will come several years later. The third attack will happen after a shorter interval, and the fourth one, shorter still. Each event resolves itself in a few days or weeks. After 10 to 20 years a patient may end up with almost constant acute attacks of this disease, but often by that time the associated problems of this condition may make toe pain the least of his or her worries.

Signs and Symptoms

Acute gouty arthritis has some very predictable patterns. It has a sudden onset and almost always happens in the feet first, especially at the joints of the great toe (Fig. 2-18). It may also appear in the instep, around the Achilles tendon, and in later stages in the knees and elbows.

The acute gouty joint shows all the signs of extreme inflammation The joint may swell up so much that the skin is hot, red, dry, shiny, and exquisitely painful. This phase of inflammation is often accompanied by a moderate fever (up to 101°F or so) and chills.

Complications

The complications of gout are actually complications of having too much uric acid in the bloodstream, which indicates kidneys that are not functioning at adequate levels. Uric acid crystals do not just cause gout, they can also cause *kidney stones* (Chapter 9). If the kidneys become sufficiently clogged by kidney stones, the result is *renal failure* (Chapter 9). Impaired kidneys cannot process adequate fluid. This stresses the rest of the circulatory system, causing *high blood pressure*, the end result of which can be *coronary artery disease* (Chapter 4) or *stroke* (Chapter 3). All these problems—hyperuricemia, kidney insufficiency, gout, high blood pressure, and cardiovascular disease—are closely related.

Diagnosis

Gout is usually easily recognized by its specific pain profile: sudden onset in the feet with long intervals between attacks. However, it sometimes mimics a few other conditions, in-

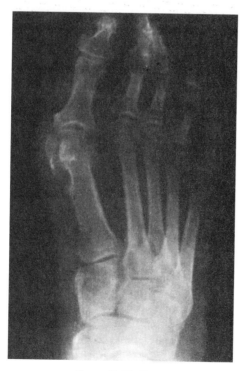

Figure 2-18. Gout

WATCH FOR THIS

Gout and "Pseudogout"

Gout is a variety of arthritis brought about by the accumulation of uric acid crystals in and around joint capsules, especially in the feet. It is a manageable disorder, as long as the person keeps a close watch on uric acid levels. Calcium pyrophosphate dihydrate deposition (CPDD) or *pseudogout* has a very similar presentation, but because it does not involve uric acid or hyperuricemia, it requires a different treatment plan. Massage therapists are not required to be able to tell the difference between gout and pseudogout, but they can certainly counsel clients to explore options if the treatment they receive does not seem to meet their needs.

	GOUT SYNDROME	CPDD ("PSEUDOGOUT")
Prevalence	100:100,000	Unknown
Demographics	90% are men older than 40; women with gout are usually postmenopausal	Women and men are equally affected; most patients are older than 60
Primary symptom	Exquisitely painful inflammation, usually around the great toe, but also in the instep and heel Gout occasionally appears in other joints in later stages, but the foot is usually affected first	Exquisitely painful inflammation, usually at the knee or wrist
Implications for massage	Gout patients usually have some level of hyperuricemia and carry the risk of kidney stones or other urinary system disorders; these need to be ruled out for circulatory massage	This is an idiopathic disease that may be related to other underlying problems; clients with CPDD need to be screened for other contributing factors, but none may be present

cluding *rheumatoid arthritis* and *septic arthritis* (this chapter), psoriatic arthritis, or pseudogout: another chemically based arthritis in which crystals of an entirely different type are deposited in and around joints. The only conclusive diagnosis for gout is an examination of aspirated fluid from an affected joint to look for uric acid crystals.

Treatment

A standard medical approach to gout takes three paths: pain relief (with analgesics *other* than aspirin, which inhibits uric acid excretion); anti-inflammatory drugs, and drugs that modify metabolism and uric acid management. Preventive measures include increasing fluid intake (other than caffeine or alcohol, which act as diuretics), losing weight, and limiting purine-rich foods.

Massage?

Gout is at very least a local contraindication for the affected joints at all times. The last thing this client needs is to have someone grind those little crystals any deeper into the flesh. In its acute stage gout is a systemic contraindication, but it is unlikely that anyone in a full-blown attack would try to keep a massage appointment. Any client who is prone to gout is a good candidate for other circulatory or excretory problems; he should discuss these risks with his health care team before getting massage.

Lyme Disease

Definition: What Is It?

Lyme disease is an infection with the spirochetal bacterium *Borrelia burgdorferi*. This pathogen is spread through the bite of two species of ticks: deer ticks (*Ixodes scapularis*) and Western black-legged ticks (*Ixodes pacificus*). These ticks are very small, especially in the nymph stage when they most frequently affect humans, which can make it difficult to find them on the skin. An engorged deer tick is about 5 mm long (Fig. 2-19).

Demographics: Who Gets It?

Lyme disease has been reported in 48 states and the District of Columbia, but 90% of all cases have been found in the Northeast and Mid-Atlantic states, along with Wisconsin and Minnesota. Smaller concentrations of the disease have been noted in Northwestern California. The nationwide statistics for Lyme disease show an infection rate of 5 of every 100,000 people, but in areas where the disease is endemic, incidence can be as high as 1 to 3% of the population.

Persons most at risk for Lyme disease are those who work or play outside in grassy or wooded areas. Their pets are also at risk for picking up disease-bearing ticks.

Etiology: What Happens?

The life cycle of the deer tick and Western black-legged tick lasts about 2 years. Adult ticks spend fall and winter mating and taking blood meals from warm-blooded hosts. In the spring females detach from their hosts and fall onto the ground to lay eggs. The eggs hatch and the larvae spend summer and fall taking meals from mice, birds, and large mammals, especially white-tailed deer. Dormant in the winter, the larvae molt into the nymph stage the following spring. They climb onto grass or bush stems and wait for a warm-blooded host to brush close by. This is the stage of development during which the animals most often find their way to human hosts. The final molt to the adult tick occurs in the insect's second summer, and the cycle begins again.

Ticks pick up the spiral-shaped bacterium *B. burgdorferi* from the blood of their animal hosts, especially mice. If an infected tick then bites a human, that bacterium may be transmitted to the human host. The bacterial invasion can cause several different reactions, depending on the severity and the stage of the infection.

Signs and Symptoms

Lyme disease moves in stages, with signs and symptoms particular to each.

- *Early localized disease.* This is the first stage of a Lyme disease infection. Ticks are slow feeders, so it may take several days for the bacteria to enter the body and some days after that for symptoms to appear. Early symptoms generally appear between 7 to 30 days after an initial tick bite. They include a circular, red rash (a "bull's eye" rash) that is hot and itchy but not raised from the skin (Fig. 2-20, Color Plate 31) accompanied by high fever, fatigue, night sweats, headache, stiff neck, and swollen lymph nodes.

LYME DISEASE IN BRIEF

What is it?
Lyme disease is a bacterial infection spread by the bites of specific species of ticks. The immune response to the bacteria causes inflammation of large joints, along with neurologic and cardiovascular symptoms.

How is it recognized?
The hallmark early symptom of Lyme disease is a circular "bull's eye" rash at the site of the tick bite. The skin may be red, itchy, and hot, but it is not usually raised or scaly. The rash may be accompanied by fever, fatigue, and joint pain. Later symptoms may include acute intermittent inflammation of one or more large joints, numbness, poor coordination, *Bell's palsy* (Chapter 3), and irregular heart beat.

Is massage indicated or contraindicated?
The inflammation associated with Lyme disease runs in acute and subacute phases. It contraindicates massage during the acute phase. During subacute phases massage may be appropriate to maintain joint function and relieve pain. In this situation it is important to be working as part of a health care team for the maximum benefit and minimum risk to the infected person.

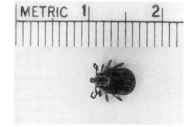

Figure 2-19. Lyme disease: deer tick

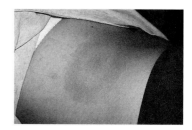

Figure 2-20. Lyme disease: rash (CP 31)

If no rash appears, these early symptoms may be mistaken for flu, mononucleosis, or meningitis.

- *Early disseminated disease.* In this stage the infected person develops systemic symptoms of infection with *B. burgdorferi.* These include cardiovascular symptoms (especially irregular heart beat), neurologic symptoms (chronic headaches, Bell's palsy, numbness, tingling, forgetfulness, and poor coordination), and more general problems including debilitating fatigue.

- *Late disease.* The final outcome of a Lyme disease infection is extreme inflammation of one or more large joints. The knees are the most commonly affected area, but elbows and shoulders are often inflamed as well. Most patients do not have the infection in more than three joints at a time. The inflammation can be extreme enough to damage the joint permanently, especially if it is left untreated.

The tendency for Lyme disease to affect joints is what classifies it as an arthritic condition. In fact, the first cases of Lyme disease ever identified were among a group of children who were all initially misdiagnosed with juvenile rheumatoid arthritis.

History of Lyme Disease

Although this disease was only definitively identified and named in 1982, it has probably been present for much longer.

In the early 20th century doctors made note of red, target-shaped rashes, which were named *Erythema Migrans.* It was noted that people who developed these rashes seemed to have a high incidence of arthritis, but if they were treated with penicillin their chances of developing arthritis were significantly lessened.

Then in 1974 a group of children in Lyme, Connecticut were diagnosed with juvenile rheumatoid arthritis. Parents became suspicious of having such a high concentration of a disease that was not supposed to be in any way communicable. This led to intensive research, during which a scientist named Burgdorfer isolated the spirochete now called *Borrelia burgdorferi.* He found it in highest concentrations in the midgut of deer ticks.

Burgdorfer's discovery in 1982 began a process of surveillance that continues today. The incidence of Lyme disease rises yearly; it currently causes about 12,500 new infections annually.

B. burgdorferi did not make its first appearance with human infections; it probably has been around for ages. As the human population expanded into undeveloped areas, this bacterium suddenly had access to human hosts. It remains to be seen what other kinds of illnesses may be encountered as we continue to expand into previously undeveloped areas.

Diagnosis

The accurate diagnosis of Lyme disease is one of the most contentious issues surrounding this condition. Blood tests that identify antibodies are unreliable—they frequently miss the presence of bacteria, leading to a false-negative test result, or they show the presence of antibodies but cannot distinguish whether the infection is currently active or part of a person's immune system history, leading to a false-positive test result.

This leaves the description of symptoms and the observation of signs as the primary means to make a Lyme disease diagnosis. Unfortunately, up to two-thirds of all patients have no memory of a tick bite, and close to one-half never develop a rash, so doctors must depend on the signs of fever, fatigue, swollen lymph nodes, headache, and so on to make an early diagnosis. All these symptoms can be associated with several other diseases, including mononucleosis, flu, meningitis, and several others.

At this point it is unclear whether Lyme disease is overdiagnosed or underdiagnosed. What is clear is that more accurate diagnostic tests are needed to identify this infection.

Treatment

B. burgdorferi bacteria *do* respond to antibiotics, so the outlook for someone who is diagnosed with Lyme disease in the early stages is often hopeful. Lyme disease seems to require a much longer course of antibiotics than most other bacterial infections, however. It is not unusual for a person to need medication for 6 weeks or more; relapse rates for those who try shorter courses of medication are relatively high.

Lyme disease occasionally becomes a chronic ongoing problem. Patients in this situation may need high doses of antibiotics for 6 to 12 months. Some Lyme disease patients develop chronic symptoms that may last for years and that do not respond to typical antibiotics. Their disease process is much harder to explain or predict. It may turn out that for some of these patients their disease is not Lyme disease alone, but a combination of tick-borne infections.

Prevention

The best protection against Lyme disease is protection from disease-bearing ticks. This means wearing long sleeves and long pants when working or playing in areas where tick infestation is high. Tucking pants into socks or boots may make it harder for ticks to gain access to skin. Wearing light-colored clothing is recommended so that it is easier to find and remove ticks. Using insect repellants can also reduce the risk of tick bites.

Examining the skin after being in a high-risk area is another important preventive measure. Ticks prefer to occupy warm, protected areas like the groin, axilla, backs of knees, and insides of elbows. If a tick is found it should be carefully removed to keep the mouth parts intact, and then the person should report being bitten and take the tick with him or her to the doctor.

Two vaccines have been developed against Lyme disease, but so far they are not recommended for the general public. Persons between 14 and 70 years of age, especially those who spend a good deal of time outdoors, are the target group for these vaccines. They both require a series of injections and do not reach full potential for a year after exposure, but at that point they have shown to be about 90% effective at protecting a person from Lyme disease.

Is It Just Lyme Disease?

Lyme disease is caused by tick-borne bacteria that infect joints and cause debilitating arthritis. Some Lyme disease patients live with pain and progressive inflammation for years despite antibiotics that should provide relief. It has recently been found that some of these patients may have more than Lyme disease alone: deer ticks can carry two other pathogens that affect humans:

- *Ehrlichiosis* is a tick-borne bacterial infection that can easily coexist with Lyme disease. Consequences of an ehrlichiosis infection include low white blood cell and platelet counts. This infection can be cleared with antibiotics from the tetracycline family, but this is a different class of antibiotics than is usually used for Lyme disease alone. Ehrlichiosis is less common than Lyme disease, so some patients may live with this infection for a long time before it is discovered.

- *Babesiosis* is a parasite similar to the protozoan that causes malaria. It can also coexist with Lyme disease. Babesiosis can cause anemia and enlarged spleen. It responds well to quinine *if* it is identified as an infection separate from Lyme disease.

Massage?

The arthritic phase of Lyme disease involves intermittently severe inflammation of joints that is acutely painful. This contraindicates massage when inflammation is acute. At other times, as long as sensation is present and the client is comfortable, a person with Lyme disease may derive significant benefits from massage. Because this disease can affect the nervous and circulatory systems and because treatment for the disease can take a long time to take effect, it is important for massage therapists to operate as part of a client's health care team in this situation, rather than working alone.

Massage therapists who live and work in areas where Lyme disease is especially common should be aware of what deer ticks and Western black-legged ticks look like so that if they should find these parasites during a session, they can counsel clients to receive appropriate medical care.

Osteoarthritis
Definition: What Is It?

Also called *degenerative joint disease*, osteoarthritis is a condition in which synovial joints, especially weight-bearing joints, are irritated and inflamed. This condition is distinguished from other types of arthritis by being directly related to wear and tear of the joint structures.

OSTEOARTHRITIS IN BRIEF

What is it?
This is joint inflammation brought about by wear and tear causing cumulative damage to articular cartilage.

How is it recognized?
Affected joints are stiff, painful, and occasionally palpably inflamed. Osteoarthritis most often affects knees, hips, and distal joints of the fingers.

Is massage indicated or contraindicated?
Arthritis contraindicates massage if it is acutely inflamed. It indicates massage in the subacute stage when bodywork can contribute to muscular relaxation and mobility of the affected joint.

Demographics: Who Gets It?

This is by far the most common type of arthritis in the world. Osteoarthritis affects close to 20 million Americans and is responsible for 7 million doctor visits each year. It is also an occupational hazard for massage therapists, who may get it at the saddle joint of the thumb because it is easy put too much pressure on this joint if good body mechanics are not used.

Etiology: What Happens?

Joints, especially knees and hips, put up with tremendous weight-bearing stress and repetitive movements; their design is a marvel of efficiency and durability. Nevertheless, the environment inside a joint capsule is precarious. Any imbalance can have cumulative destructive impact. Once the path toward arthritis has begun, it may be possible to stop it, but capacity for regeneration is limited at best.

All synovial joints have five features in common: the articulating bones, the cartilage that covers them, a ligamentous joint capsule, a synovial membrane that lines it, and the synovial fluid that serves to lubricate the cartilage. In weight-bearing joints it is important to remember that the articulating layers of cartilage are almost always touching; one layer of cartilage rests directly on top of the other.

Progression

- *Step 1: Cartilage damage.* After years of use or repetitive injury, the cartilage in a knee or hip may begin to flake, just the tiniest bit. If the cartilage on one side of the joint is even slightly roughened, it acts like sandpaper to the cartilage of the opposite side, instead of being smooth for easy, gliding movement. Then the other cartilage gets rough and further damages the first side. Once any cartilage damage inside the joint develops, the downhill slide has begun. The only question is, how far will it go? (Fig. 2-21).

- *Step 2: Bony adaptation.* The cartilaginous surfaces of two articulating bones are now rough instead of smooth. Each time one side moves, the other gets irritated. An inflammatory reaction ensues, releasing enzymes that further damage the cartilage. Since the cartilage is no longer doing its job, the bones (which are living tissue and respond to stresses put on them) begin to adapt. However, bones cannot replace damaged cartilage. Instead of making a new, smooth surface inside the joint capsules, bones have a tendency to thicken at the condyles and make small spurs on the ends, where they sense the most stress. This further limits freedom of movement and increases pain.

- *Step 3: The muscles react.* Any muscles that cross a stiff, painful, and constantly aggravated join tend to tighten up. That is what muscles do when they are in areas of constant pain (see spasms, cramps, this chapter). They may also develop some trigger points in the process, because they will not get to relax as long as that joint is in pain. The tension they cause compresses the joint, making it even more painful, which reinforces the spasm, and so on (see *myofascial pain syndrome*, this chapter).

- *Step 4: Atrophy.* Eventually the person with arthritis will want to stop using the injured joint because it hurts so much. Lack of use leads to atrophy: the wasting away

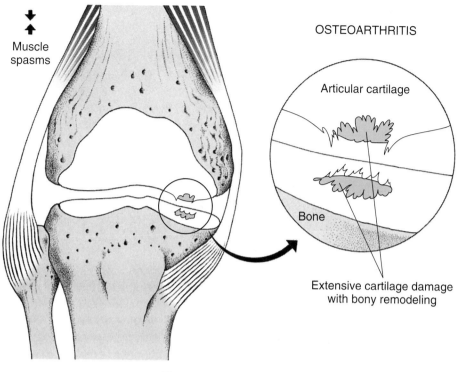

Figure 2-21. Osteoarthritis

of the joint structure and the tissues that surround it. The nearby muscles then get weaker, the synovial membranes stop functioning, and the joint fluid dries up. It could get to the point where even if the person wanted to move again, he or she would not be able to because the muscles and the joint structures have degenerated too far.

Causes

Many changes in the body begin the process of joint degeneration. When the ligaments that surround joints get chronically loose, the joint can become unstable, raising the risk of arthritis (see *dislocations*, this chapter). Repetitive pounding stress, such as running or jumping with inadequate support, can also open the door to problems. Hormonal imbalances and nutritional deficiencies, including inadequate calcium metabolism, may compromise the health of joint structures. Being overweight adds stress to knees and hips. Age itself changes the quality of articular cartilage, making it drier and more prone to injury.

Signs and Symptoms

The symptoms of osteoarthritis all revolve around inflammation of the joint capsule. In the acute stage the joints may be hot, painful, and swollen. More often, arthritis lingers in a chronic stage in which the joints experience ongoing pain and stiffness, especially when they are not warmed up or when they have been overused. Osteoarthritis can be completely debilitating when it occurs at the hip or knee because the pain and limitation are badly exacerbated by walking.

Arthritis Statistics

Arthritis is a term that refers to more than 100 disorders that can cause joints to become swollen, hot, and painful. Some disorders begin and end with joint trouble. Many varieties affect other body systems as well, causing skin problems, vascular inflammation, kidney dysfunction, or other difficulties.

The implications of bodywork for clients who have arthritis are many and far-reaching, especially for varieties that affect more than the musculoskeletal system. Conditions discussed in this text that can involve arthritis as primary or secondary symptoms include the following:

Ankylosing spondylitis	Osteoporosis
Carpal tunnel syndrome	Paget's disease
Crohn's disease	Pseudogout
Fibromyalgia syndrome	Psoriatic arthritis
Gout	Raynaud's syndrome
Lupus	Rheumatoid arthritis
Lyme disease	Scleroderma
Myofascial pain	Septic arthritis
syndrome	Ulcerative colitis
Osteoarthritis	Tendinitis

About 42 million Americans (close to 16%) live with some version of chronic joint inflammation. Arthritis disables more people every year than heart disease and strokes combined. Arthritis treatments cost the U.S. economy approximately $65 billion every year.

The Food and Drug Administration estimates that by 2020 about 60 million Americans will live with chronic arthritis, and 11 million of them will be permanently disabled by it.[j]

[j]Lewis C. Arthritis: Timely treatments for an ageless disease. *FDA Consumer Magazine*. Publication no. (FDA) 00-1313. Available at: http://www.fda.gov/fdac/features/2000/300_arth.html. Accessed fall 2000.

Diagnosis

Osteoarthritis is identified by physical examination and patient history. Tests may be conducted to rule out other conditions, but no blood test absolutely confirms the presence of osteoarthritis. Even radiographs can be misleading. They may be used to back up a diagnosis, but a surprisingly high percentage of people who show osteoarthritis-like bony deformations on a radiograph experience no pain at all. This is because different people are blessed with different thicknesses of cartilage, which does not show up on radiographs. A person with thin cartilage is more likely to feel pain from arthritis than a person with thicker cartilage (see *patellofemoral syndrome*, this chapter).

Treatment

Treatment options for osteoarthritis have improved considerably in recent years. The goals of treatment are to reduce pain and inflammation and to limit or reverse the damage incurred to the joint structures. These goals are accomplished in a number of different ways, depending on how advanced the condition is.

- *NSAIDs.* These are usually the first recourse to deal with arthritis pain. Although some patients do not tolerate the most common NSAIDs well (they can cause stomach irritation), a recently developed variety of painkillers is getting good results. Called *cox-2 inhibitors*, these drugs work to limit the action of the prostaglandin-related enzyme (cyclooxygenase-2) associated with pain and inflammatory response.

- *Exercise.* Arthritis patients are recommended to exercise within pain tolerance to achieve three goals: to improve and maintain healthy range of motion, to increase stamina and lose weight, and to improve the strength of muscles surrounding affected joints.

- *Nutritional supplements.* Glucosamine sulfide and chondroitin sulfide are two substances that may not only limit the progression of arthritis damage, but may be able to reverse it. Research on how (or whether) taking supplements of these naturally occurring connective tissue building blocks helps to repair damaged cartilage is still inconclusive. Although public interest in these supplements is high, they are unregulated by the FDA, and so potency and dosages may vary widely from one brand to another. Still, many people claim to have success with them, and as research continues it may be found that some recovery of damaged cartilage is possible after all.

- *Injections of lubricating fluid.* Another recent development in arthritis treatment has been the injection of lubricants made essentially of hyaluronic acid (the liquid matrix of much of the body's connective tissue) directly into damaged joints. While the patient may have temporary swelling and irritation of the joint after this procedure, this is usually followed by an improvement in the quality and quantity of synovial fluid secreted into the joint capsule.

- *Joint replacement surgery.* A last resort for debilitating osteoarthritis is to replace the surfaces of the affected joint with artificial cartilage. Joint replacement surgery for knees and hips has become a commonplace intervention, and the expected recovery time from such surgery is a matter of weeks.

Massage?

Acute arthritis, like other acute inflammatory conditions, contraindicates massage. However, most osteoarthritis patients seldom experience acute swelling with pain, heat, and redness. Chronic osteoarthritis indicates massage, when goals would be to reduce pain through release of the muscles surrounding the affected joints and to maintain range of motion through gentle stretching and passive movement.

Patellofemoral Syndrome

Definition: What Is It?

PFS is a condition in which the patellar cartilage becomes damaged as it contacts the femoral cartilage. This situation can be a precursor of *osteoarthritis* at the knee (this chapter).

PFS is almost always associated with overuse, although it may be precipitated by a specific injury or trauma. For a long while the term *patellofemoral syndrome* was used interchangeably with *chondromalacia patellae*; it is now recognized that these terms refer to significantly different types of knee problems. More current synonyms for PFS include *anterior knee pain syndrome* and *overutilization syndrome*.

Etiology: What Happens?

If the patellar cartilage is going to wear out, it usually happens in one of two ways. First is by simple overuse. Unfortunately, one person's "I've overused it" is another person's "I barely got started." That's because everyone is born with a different amount of cartilage on the patella. People with "thick cartilage" genes may never get PFS. For people with "thin cartilage" genes, it takes much less use to wear through it and land with a textbook example of overuse PFS.

The other way to wear down patellar cartilage is something that, unlike genetic structure, people have some control over: the alignment of the knee. If the patella is pulled slightly to one side or the other, the wear on the cartilage is uneven and leaves a person vulnerable to cartilage damage. The uneven tracking seen with PFS usually occurs toward the lateral aspect of the knee.

Signs and Symptoms

Symptoms of PFS include pain that is usually felt on the anterior aspect of the knee, stiffness after long immobility, difficulty walking down stairs, and a characteristic crackling, grinding noise on movement.

Diagnosis

PFS can be difficult to diagnose, especially in the early stages before visible damage to the bones has occurred. The problem is that what is often called PFS may actually be an-

---

PATELLOFEMORAL SYNDROME IN BRIEF

What is it?
Patellofemoral syndrome (PFS) is an overuse disorder that can lead to damage of the patellar cartilage.

How is it recognized?
PFS causes pain at the knee, stiffness after immobility, and discomfort in walking down stairs.

Is massage indicated or contraindicated?
PFS indicates massage, as long as the knee is not acutely inflamed. Massage may not be useful to correct this problem, but it will certainly do no harm and can address issues of muscle tightness and imbalance.

other condition, *patellar tendinitis*. This is significant because while PFS is largely unaffected by massage, patellar tendinitis responds beautifully and can have a virtually pain-free resolution, so it is important to have a clear idea of what a client really has. One clue that is sometimes useful is that patellar tendinitis often hurts going *up* stairs (resisted extension of the leg), whereas PFS may hurt more going *down* stairs (the weight of the femur pushing on the patella). However, these two conditions can certainly be present simultaneously. Ultimately, only a doctor using imaging techniques can give an absolutely definitive diagnosis.

Treatment

The long-term prognosis for a person with PFS depends entirely on what he or she does with it. Although damage to the patellar cartilage may set the stage for osteoarthritis in the knee, PFS seldom gets to the point of requiring joint replacement. Nevertheless, this condition is badly irritated by jarring, jouncing, bouncing kinds of exercise. If one kind of activity becomes prohibitive (running and aerobics are not great choices for someone with PFS), it can probably be replaced with something else, like swimming, walking, cycling, or skating. Patients may have to experiment, under a doctor's supervision, to find the exercise activities that work best.

Physical therapy for PFS often includes exercises to strengthen and balance tension in the muscles that cross the knee and that influence knee alignment. The quadriceps, hamstrings, tensor fascia latae, and deep lateral rotators are often addressed in the challenge to improve alignment and stop the progression of damage that PFS can cause.

Massage?

If the knee is inflamed and painful, it is a local contraindication. However, PFS is more often a chronic, low-level irritation that interferes with normal activity, and massage certainly will not make it any worse. Whether massage can be instrumental in *improving* the situation depends on the situation. Massage can address the stiffness and chronic pain experienced in muscle-tendon units that cross the knee joint. If a treatment strategy is developed to retrain the knee extensors to track the patella appropriately over the joint, massage may be a useful part of an effort to slow or stop permanent cartilage damage.

Rheumatoid Arthritis
Definition: What Is It?

RA is an autoimmune condition in which the synovial membranes of various joints are attacked by immune system cells. Unlike most forms of arthritis, RA can also involve inflammation of tissues outside the musculoskeletal system.

Demographics: Who Gets It?

This disease affects 2.1 million (or about 1%) of all Americans. Women are affected about 3 times more frequently than men. Statistics indicate that it is most common among 20- to 40-year-olds, but it can strike anyone, including children and adolescents.

RHEUMATOID ARTHRITIS IN BRIEF

What is it?
Rheumatoid arthritis (RA) is an autoimmune disease in which immune system agents attack synovial membranes, particularly of the joints in the hands and feet. Other structures, such as muscles, tendons, and blood vessels, may also be affected.

How is it recognized?
In the acute phase affected joints are red, swollen, hot, and painful. They often become gnarled and distorted. It tends to affect the body symmetrically, and it is not determined by age.

Is massage indicated or contraindicated?
Only the subacute stage of RA indicates massage. At that point bodywork may be used to re-establish mobility and to reduce the stresses that can trigger another flare.

Etiology: What Happens?

Autoimmune diseases are brought about by a mistake in the vastly complex and usually very effective immune system: normal, healthy tissues are mistakenly identified as threatening invaders and are attacked by immune system agents. Some autoimmune diseases are triggered by pathogens that closely resemble some part of the body's own proteins. A pathogen's protein coat needs to have only five amino acids in the same order as some normal, healthy part of the body to trigger an autoimmune disease response.

In RA an immune system attack is targeted for a specific protein, but that protein *is not* on an invading microbe—it is in the synovial membranes. This leads to all the cardinal signs of inflammation: heat, pain, redness, swelling, and loss of function. In later stages the antibodies may also attack the pericardium, blood vessels, lungs, and fascia.

Several pathogens have been identified that may initiate RA. They include a variety of streptococcus bacterium, *B. burgdorferi* (the same bacterium that causes Lyme disease), and some retroviruses. Contracting and sustaining damage from RA begins with exposure to one of these pathogens. The following is an example of the typical progression of RA:

- A person has a bout with strep throat. The body goes through the usual process of producing T-cells, B-cells, and antibodies and wins the fight; the bacterium is vanquished. Now the person has a regiment of memory cells and antibodies in circulation, looking for any remnants of the invading microorganisms.

- The antibodies get confused. The proteins in the synovial membranes look so much like the proteins in the strep molecules that the immune system raises the alarm and launches a full-scale attack. This is where genetics may play a role; this person's antibodies may actually be programmed to be "auto-antibodies."

- The synovial membrane thickens and swells. Fluid inside the joint capsule begins to accumulate, which causes pressure and pain.

- The inflamed tissues release enzymes that erode cartilage, eventually right down to the bone. This is the process that causes the tell-tale deformation of the joint capsules and gnarled appearance of RA (Fig. 2-22).

- Fibrous scar tissue develops to connect the raw ends of the bones.

- The scar tissue ossifies, and the joint is permanently fused.

Actually, the disease seldom progresses all the way to the final two steps. As serious a condition as RA could be, it rarely fulfills the worst of its promises. After coping with the disease for 10 to 15 years, about 20% of affected people are in remission. Most are able to retain full-time employment. After 15 to 20 years of living with RA only about 10% of affected people are permanently disabled.

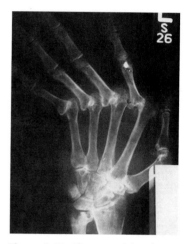

Figure 2-22. Rheumatoid arthritis

Signs and Symptoms

Symptoms of RA vary considerably at the onset of the disease. Many people experience a period of weeks or months with a general feeling of illness: lack of energy, lack of appetite, low-grade fever, and vague muscle pain that gradually becomes sharp, specific joint pain. About 10% experience a sudden onset with joint pain alone. Rheumatic nodules (small, painless bumps that appear around fingers, elbows, and other pressure-bearing areas) are also common indicators of the disease.

In the acute stage the affected joints are red, hot, painful, and stiff, although they improve considerably with moderate amounts of movement and stretching. The joints RA most often attacks are the knuckles in hands and toes. It can also appear in ankles and wrists; knees are less common, and one of the rarest (and most serious) places to get it is in the neck. It generally affects the body bilaterally, although it is sometimes worse on one side than the other.

Like many autoimmune diseases, RA appears in cycles of "flare" followed by periods of remission. Some patients have only a few flares in their life and are never affected again. Moderate cases involve cycles of flare and remission up to several times a year. Severe RA involves chronic inflammation that never fully subsides.

Complications

If someone has RA, it means the immune system is confused about what it should be fighting. Synovial membranes are just one of the types of tissue that may be attacked. Other possibilities include:

* Rheumatic nodules on the sclera (whites) of the eyes.
* Sjögren's syndrome (pathologically dry eyes and mouth).
* Pleuritis, which makes breathing painful and increases vulnerability to lung infection.
* Pericarditis, or inflammation of the pericardial sac around the heart.
* Vasculitis, or inflammation of blood vessels. This complication carries another set of risks: *Raynaud's phenomenon* (this chapter) *skin ulcers* (Chapter 1), bleeding *intestinal ulcers* (Chapter 7). and internal hemorrhaging.

Bursitis (this chapter) and *anemia* (Chapter 4) are also common complications of RA, especially when onset of the disease occurs in childhood.

Advanced structural damage also brings a set of complications. Deformed and bone-damaged joints may dislocate or even collapse, rendering them useless. The tendons that cross over distorted joints sometimes become so stretched that they snap. If the disease is at the C1-C2 joint and the joint collapses, the resultant injury to the spinal column may result in paralysis.

Diagnosis

RA can be difficult to diagnose because its early symptoms are often subtle, they vary greatly from one person to another, and a long list of diseases with similar symptoms must be ruled out before a diagnosis can be conclusive. A sense of urgency exists around a conclusive diagnosis, however, because it has been found that cartilage and bone damage may occur as early as the first or second year of the disease process. If treatment can be administered earlier, this damage can be averted.

RA is typically diagnosed through a description of symptoms, radiographs, and a blood test to check for rheumatoid factor, a substance that is present in most but not all cases. An erythrocyte sedimentation test may be conducted to look for signs of general inflammation, and the blood is also examined for signs of anemia. Even when all signs are positive, the diagnosis is sometimes not considered conclusive until the patient has been under observation for a long while.

Treatment

Once the presence of RA has been confirmed, the goals of treatment are to reduce pain, limit inflammation, halt joint damage, and improve function. Medications that help to achieve these goals are divided into first-line and second-line drugs.

Osteoarthritis Versus Rheumatoid Arthritis

WATCH FOR THIS

Of the 100 conditions that cause painful inflammation of joints, the two most common varieties are osteoarthritis and RA. Osteoarthritis is a wear-and-tear disorder that could possibly be exacerbated by overenthusiastic bodywork but cannot be spread through the body. RA is an autoimmune disorder that *can* spread from joint to joint and should be treated with caution by bodyworkers in the acute or "flare" stage.

It is important for clients to know the source of their joint pain. Massage therapists are not equipped to tell the difference between the two conditions—and of course it is a perfectly reasonable possibility that a client could have both simultaneously. Still, it can be difficult to come to a conclusive diagnosis for joint pain. The following is a brief list of the most common patterns seen with osteoarthritis compared with RA.

	OSTEOARTHRITIS	RHEUMATOID ARTHRITIS
Prevalence	Radiographs show bony deformation in 33 to 90% of people older than 65	Up to 1.5% of the population
Demographics	Most common in people older than 40; men and women are affected equally	Women are affected twice to three times as often as men, although men are more likely to have systemic symptoms; may affect children and adults
Pain patterns	Spine, knees, and hip joints are most frequently affected; distal joints of the fingers and the saddle joint (trapezium-first metacarpal) are also at risk	Joints most commonly affected include the proximal interphalangeal (PIP) joints; the metacarpophalangeal (MCP) joints; and the wrist, elbow, knee, ankle, or matarsolphalangeal (MPT) joints; joints are affected bilaterally
		Pain appears in "flare" and "remission" stages
Other symptoms	None	In early stages and during acute episodes fever, malaise, lack of appetite, and muscle pain may be present; other signs may include rheumatic nodules and the presence of serum rheumatoid factor
Implications for massage	Massage can be useful to maintain range of motion and to relieve pain in muscles that cross over affected joints, as long as inflammation is not acute	During remission, massage can be useful to help maintain joint function
		During acute stages, circulatory massage should be avoided

First-line drugs include NSAIDs to limit inflammation and pain. These are often used along with physical therapy in the hopes that progression can be limited without further intervention.

Second-line drugs attempt to interfere with the disease process. These include steroidal anti-inflammatories and immune suppressant drugs. They often give significant relief but also carry a long list of serious side effects and cannot be used for long-term care.

Until recently RA was treated as conservatively as possible. New research indicates that joint damage occurs much earlier than had been suspected, so many rheumatologists and other specialists now recommend an aggressive course of treatment as soon as the diagnosis is confirmed to limit cumulative joint damage.

Surgery can be a successful option for RA patients if their disease has affected joints that can be treated easily. Joint replacement is sometimes an option, along with surgery to rebuild damaged or ruptured tendons and to remove portions of affected synovial membranes. The synovial membranes grow back, however, so this surgery is a temporary measure.

Massage?

In its acute phase RA is an inflammatory condition caused by agents in the circulatory system. Anything that increases circulation also increases the chance that the disease may spread to other joints in the body. In its subacute phase RA leaves the joints stiff but not inflamed, and the muscles and tendons around them are stressed and tight from chronic pain. RA indicates massage in the subacute stage. Massage can improve mobility and the health of the soft tissues surrounding the joints. In addition to the structural benefits it offers, massage can also be an important part of the keep-healthy-and-stress-free part of prevention strategy. If massage can help to balance the autonomic nervous system, it may also help to reduce the incidence of attack.

SEPTIC ARTHRITIS IN BRIEF

What is it?
Septic arthritis is joint inflammation caused by infection inside the joint capsule.

How is it recognized?
This condition shows the cardinal signs of inflammation: pain, heat, redness, and swelling, although these symptoms may be mild. It is often accompanied by fever.

Is massage indicated or contraindicated?
Massage is contraindicated for septic arthritis until the infection is completely gone from the joint. At that time massage may be useful to help restore function.

Septic Arthritis
Definition: What Is It?

Septic arthritis is a form of arthritis brought about by a bacterial infection. *Neisseria gonorrhea* or *Staphylococcus aureus* are the most common infectious agents.

Demographics: Who Gets It?

Septic arthritis is most common among very young, very old, or immune-suppressed persons. It is unusual for a healthy, middle-aged adult to have this kind of infection.

Etiology: What Happens?

Because no direct blood supply nourishes joints structures, it is not easy for bacteria to get inside a joint. The most common ways for infections to be introduced into a joint capsule are through puncture wounds, contaminated needles (used for intravenous drugs or for steroid injections), or susceptibility brought about by underlying illness, especially gonorrhea, *rheumatoid arthritis* (this chapter), or *diabetes* (Chapter 8).

Once a bacterial colony is established, it will probably thrive in the warm, dark, moist growth medium supplied by synovial capsules. Septic arthritis can become very serious as the bacteria feast on the tissues, filling the joint space with fluid and pus. Permanent damage to the joint may occur if the infection is not treated promptly.

Signs and Symptoms

Symptoms of joint infections include redness, pain, heat, swelling, and mild to high fever, sometimes as high as 104°F, which is quite extreme for adults. Usually just one joint is affected; knees and hips are the most common sites. Surprisingly, the pain generated by septic arthritis is often mild and indistinct when the infection is beginning. This is a problem because studies show that if a person does not receive care within 7 days of contacting an infection, the chances of permanent joint damage are much higher.

Septic arthritis due to gonorrhea has a slightly different pattern. It starts around the sacroiliac joint and progressively moves up the spine much in the manner of *ankylosing spondylitis* (this chapter), but it shares the same inflammatory symptoms as standard septic arthritis.

Diagnosis

Septic arthritis is diagnosed by examining aspirated fluid from an affected joint for signs of bacterial infection. This test may be followed by blood cultures to look for signs of inflammation and an increased white blood cell count. Finally, radiographs or ultrasounds may be used to determine the extent of the infection and the amount of damage.

Treatment

Infected joints are repeatedly aspirated, either with needles or with open shunts. Arthroscopic surgery may be performed to debride or scrape the insides of the synovial capsule to be sure all bacteria are removed. Antibiotic drugs are administered orally, as an injection into the joint, or both. After the infection has subsided, the patient is recommended for physical therapy to prevent, or at least limit, permanent loss of function.

Prognosis

The expected outcome for such limited infections is surprisingly grave. Up to 10% of patients with septic arthritis die of complications from their infections. Thirty percent of patients sustain some lasting damage in the affected joints. Sixty percent of septic arthritis patients can expect to achieve full recovery.

Massage?

Vigorous massage should absolutely not, under any condition, be given to someone with septic arthritis. Range of motion stretches could freely distribute bacteria "hiding" in the corner of a joint. In addition to spreading the infection more thoroughly through the joint capsule, massage could cause the infection to spread to another part of the body. Because this condition often goes hand-in-hand with a high fever, it systemically contraindicates massage until the infection is gone.

Once the possibility of infection is past, however, massage can be beneficial to help restore range of motion and suppleness to the joint and surrounding structures.

Spondylosis

Definition: What Is It?

Spondylosis is the term used to describe osteoarthritis as it happens specifically in the spine. Another term for the same condition is *degenerative joint disease*. In addition to referring to arthritis, the term spondylosis is often used in the context of a narrowing or *stenosis* of the spinal canal.

Etiology: What Happens?

Spondylosis usually occurs in the most mobile parts of the spine: the lumbar and cervical regions. Bony remodeling of the vertebral bodies and joints leads to inflammation and restricted range of motion. Several factors may contribute to the process:

- *Thinning discs.* One contributor to spondylosis is thinned discs that are no longer elastic or resilient. The soft part of the disc calcifies with the aging process, reducing the shock-absorbing capacity between vertebrae.

- *Herniated discs.* Spondylosis is also a frequent complication of *herniated discs* (this chapter). Damaged discs, like thinning ones, cannot easily absorb shock and bear

SPONDYLOSIS IN BRIEF

What is it?
Spondylosis is osteoarthritis of the spine.

How is it recognized?
It is identifiable on a radiograph, which shows a characteristic thickening of the affected vertebral bodies, facets, and ligamentum flava. Pain is present only if pressure is exerted on nerve roots, which also causes numbness, paresthesia, and specific muscle weakness. Otherwise, the only sign of spondylosis may be slow, progressive loss of range of motion in the spine.

Is massage indicated or contraindicated?
Spondylosis indicates massage with caution. Muscle splinting to protect against movement that may be dangerous is often a feature of this condition; massage therapists should not interfere with this mechanism.

weight. This puts extra stress on the vertebrae, which according to Wolff's law, adapt by becoming thickened and distorted.

• *Chronic misalignment.* Misalignment signals bones that *should* be touching to thicken in a peculiar pattern that is exclusive to spondylosis. The bony growths, called *osteophytes*, can also grow inside joint capsules or in the intervertebral foramen, where they put pressure on the nerve roots that live there (Fig. 2-23). Eventually, arthritic vertebrae may fuse together completely (Fig. 2-24).

Signs and Symptoms

Sometimes spondylosis has no symptoms whatever. If the bony changes are *not* pressing on nerve roots but growing somewhere that impedes movement, the main symptom is a slowly progressive, painless, but irreversible stiffening in the spine.

When the osteophytes *do* press on nerve roots, the symptoms include shooting pain, tingling, pins and needles, numbness, and muscle weakness only in those muscles supplied by the affected nerve. One distinguishing feature of nerve pressure from osteophytes is that the pain is absolutely consistent; if the bone spurs are in a place to create pain when a person is in a certain position or posture, that pain is predictable and will probably get worse over time.

Pain from lumbar spondylosis has a pattern all its own. Patients with arthritis in the low back often feel pain in the low back and legs that is consistently aggravated by standing and walking, and usually relieved by sitting or forward bending. This pattern helps to distinguish lumbar spondylosis from disc or other problems that can cause pain from the back into the legs.

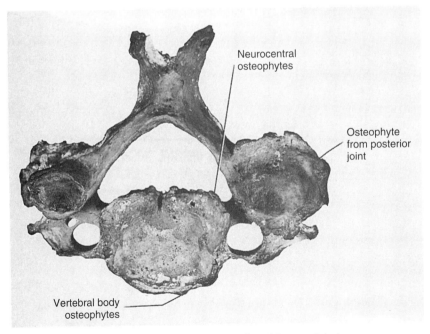

Neurocentral osteophytes

Osteophyte from posterior joint

Vertebral body osteophytes

Figure 2-23. Osteophytic growths with spondylosis

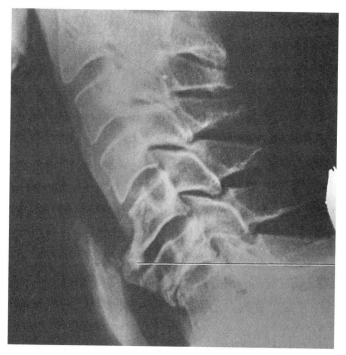

Figure 2-24. Fusion of vertebral bodies with spondylosis

Complications

Spondylosis itself is a slowly progressing arthritis that mostly affects middle-aged and elderly people who have accumulated the kind of wear and tear in their spine that would make them vulnerable to this kind of condition. What makes spondylosis more dangerous is the seriousness of the complications that can arise from it:

- *Spreading problems in the spine.* This is not a progressive disease that travels through the blood. However, if two vertebrae become fused through bony remodeling, that puts much more stress on the joints above and below the fusion to provide mobility. Those joints can then become unstable, develop arthritis, and experience the same bony remodeling that created the first problem. The stress of hypermobility may also cause disc problems. Herniated discs can be both a *predisposing factor* and a *complication* of spondylosis.

- *Nerve pain.* This is the consequence of having osteophytes grow where they can put pressure on nerve roots in the foramina.

- *Secondary spasm.* This accompanies nerve pain. Muscle spasm may be confined to the paraspinals, where it exacerbates the problem by compressing the affected joints, or it may follow the path of referred pain. Muscles may also go into spasm to protect the spine from movement that would otherwise be excruciatingly painful.

- *Blood vessel pressure.* Osteophytes in the neck are sometimes situated to press on the vertebral arteries as they go up the transverse foramina. If the head is turned or bent in a certain position, the patient may feel dizzy, have headaches, or have double vision from impaired blood flow into the head.

- *Spinal cord pressure.* This is an extremely serious complication of spondylosis in the neck. In 5 to 10% of patients with spondylosis symptoms, osteophytes may grow in

Spondylo-Tongue Twisters

The terminology used in the discussion of arthritis and stenosis in the spine can be puzzling. Here is a brief summary of some of the most confusing terms:

- *Spondylosis.* A general term for any degenerative condition of the vertebrae. This comes from the Greek root *spondylo-* for "vertebra."

- *Spondylolysis.* A specific defect in vertebrae, usually in the lumbar spine, which impairs the weight-bearing capacity of the bone. The word roots are *spondylo-* and *lysis*, or "loosening."

- *Spondylolisthesis.* An anterior displacement of the body of a lumbar vertebra onto its inferior vertebra or onto the sacrum. This is a combination of *spondylo-* and *olisthesis*, Greek for "a slipping and falling."

a place to put pressure not on the nerve roots, but in the spinal cord itself. This is felt as progressive weakening down the body, possible loss of bladder and bowel control, and even paralysis. Surgery for this condition involves creating a larger foramen for the spinal cord to pass through and permanently fusing the involved vertebrae.

Diagnosis

The characteristic thickening or hypertrophy of the vertebral bodies that accompanies spondylosis is easily identified on a radiograph. The facet joints in the lumbar spine tend to become distorted in a predictable pattern, and the ligamentum flava—the ligament that lines the spinal canal—often thickens and buckles with spondylosis.

Radiographs of 25 to 50% of all people older than 50 years of age show signs of spondylosis. Radiographs of 75% of people older than 75 years are positive for spondylosis—and most people never experience arthritic pain![k] Therefore, if a mature person complains of low back or neck pain, a radiograph is likely to indicate spondylosis, although the pain may actually be from something completely different (e.g., an injured disc or inflamed spinal ligaments).

Treatment

Treatment for spondylosis depends on which (if any) complications present themselves. Anti-inflammatories are the usual first recourse. Movement and exercise can limit progression once the damage has begun.

If symptoms get worse, a variety of surgeries can create more space for nerve roots or the spinal cord. These often involve spinal fusions, however, and they work best for younger patients who have not been having arthritic symptoms for a long time or in more than one joint.

Massage?

Massage for spondylosis is appropriate with caution. When the joints are acutely inflamed, the surrounding muscles tend to splint them against painful movement. This splinting mechanism is important and must be respected by massage therapists. For this reason, and because of the other serious complications of spondylosis, in this situation it is highly recommended to work with a primary caregiver who has a complete set of radiographs for the patient.

Sprains
Definition: What Are They?

Sprains are tears to ligaments, the connective tissue strapping tape that links bone to bone throughout the body.

[k]Cervical spondylosis. NYU Department of Neurosurgery. Available at: http://mcns10.med.nyu.edu/spine/spine_surgery_p5.html. Accessed fall 2000.

Etiology: What Happens?

Sprains, strains, and tendinitis are all injuries to structures that are composed largely of connective tissue fibers arranged in linear patterns. They have much in common in the way of symptoms, healing mechanisms, and treatment protocols. Thus, much of the information presented here is applicable to all three conditions. Their differences will be emphasized, as well as guidelines for how they may be seen in the same light.

Anatomy Review Linearly arranged structures like muscles, tendons, and ligaments are injured when some of their fibers are ripped. The severity of the injury depends on what percentage of the fibers are affected. First-degree injuries involve just a few fibers. Second-degree injuries are much worse. Third-degree injuries are ruptures (i.e., the entire structure has been ripped through and no longer attaches to the bone).

The process of repairing muscle, tendon, or ligament tears involves laying down new collagen fibers *not* in alignment with the injured structure, but in whichever way the fibroblasts happen to deposit them (see *inflammation*, Chapter 5). The perfect combination of movement, stretching, and weight-bearing stress in the subacute phase of recovery helps to reorient the fibers in alignment with the injured structure. If this happens in the best possible way, the new scar tissue actually becomes part of the muscle fascia, tendon, or ligament. If a new injury is immobilized, however, the scar tissue becomes dense and contracted, pulling on all the uninjured fibers nearby and significantly hampering the weight-bearing capacity of the ligament.

> ### SPRAINS IN BRIEF
>
> **What are they?**
> Sprains are injured ligaments. Injuries can range from a few traumatized fibers to a complete rupture.
>
> **How are they recognized?**
> In the acute stage pain, redness, heat, swelling, and loss of joint function are evident. In the subacute stage these symptoms are abated, although perhaps not entirely absent. Passive stretching of the affected ligament is painful until all inflammation has subsided.
>
> **Is massage indicated or contraindicated?**
> Subacute sprains indicate massage. Bodywork can influence the healthy development of scar tissue and reduce swelling and damage due to edematous ischemia. Therapists must take care to rule out bone fractures or other injuries that sprains may temporarily mask.

Distinguishing Features

What makes sprains unique? A few things distinguish sprains from strains and tendinitis, which are discussed in other sections.

- *Sprains are injured ligaments, not muscles or tendons.* Ligaments are the connectors that hold the bones together. Structurally they are a little different from tendons; the dense linear arrangement of collagen fibers affords little stretch and almost no rebound. If a ligament is stressed enough to become injured, it tends to tear before it stretches. If it *does* get stretched, it will not rebound to its original length and will not stabilize the joint as well as it did before the injury. This ligament laxity is also seen with chronic injury–re-injury situations.

- *Sprains are more serious than strains and tendinitis.* Because tendons and muscles tend to be more elastic and less densely arranged than ligaments, they will stretch before a ligament does. The "lines of defense" in joint injuries are muscles, tendons, ligaments, and joint capsule; thus, a sprain is one step away from a *dislocation* (this chapter). Furthermore, ligaments do not have the same rich blood supply as muscles and are denser than tendons. This means they do not have the same access to circulation, which makes them slower to heal than muscles or tendons.

- *Sprains tend to swell.* With a few exceptions, acute sprains swell much more than muscle strains or tendinitis; this is one way to differentiate between injuries.

Swelling is a protective measure that recruits the body's healing resources and limits movement, which prevents further injury. Ligaments are sometimes contiguous with the joint capsules of the joints they cross over, so an injury to them sometimes signals the joint to swell. Ligaments that are *not* attached to joint capsules swell much less than those that are.

Signs and Symptoms, Acute Stage

Acute sprains show the usual signs of inflammation: pain, heat, redness, and swelling, with the added bonus of *loss of function* because the rapid swelling splints the unstable joint and makes it extremely painful to move. Sprains in any stage of inflammation are especially painful with passive stretches of the structure.

Sprains can happen at almost any synovial joint, but the anterior talofibular ligament of the ankle is the most commonly sprained ligament in the body. Ligaments overlying the sacroiliac joint are also very commonly injured, as are various ligaments around the knees and fingers.

Signs and Symptoms, Subacute Stage

In the subacute stage, signs of inflammation may still be present but have subsided somewhat, and the joint begins to regain some function. The physiologic processes are no longer geared toward blood clotting and damage control; they shift toward clearing out debris and rebuilding torn fibers. The amount of time that passes between acute and subacute stages varies with the severity of the injury, but the 24 to 48 hour rule is usually dependable. Nevertheless, some injuries can waver back and forth between acute and subacute, especially in response to certain kinds of activity or massage.

Complications

Injured ligaments can occasionally lead to more serious problems. Sprains are such a common injury that it is important for massage therapists to be familiar with all their repercussions.

- *Masking symptoms.* An acute sprain may mask the symptoms of a bone fracture, especially in the foot. It is important for a client to have a radiograph taken to rule out fractures before a massage therapist begins work on a sprained ankle.

- *Repeated injury.* Internal scar tissue (scar tissue that accumulates within a specific structure) that never remodels just lies there in a big, gummy mass. It can interfere with the function of undamaged fibers. It can weaken the integrity of the whole structure, which, along with the increase in ligament laxity, makes repeated injury a very common complication of sprains. This pattern is also present with strains and tendinitis.

- *Ligament laxity.* In addition to having torn some fibers, a ligament that has been injured is often looser than an uninjured ligament. This is because it has been asked to stretch further than it could go, and ligaments have almost no rebound capability. When a joint becomes unstable because of loose, lax ligaments, excessive movement of the bones becomes possible. The bones may rock around and knock together, causing *osteoarthritis* (this chapter) and a host of other problems.

Treatment

A long time ago, the recommendations for sprains included hot soaks and total immobilization. Clearly, both these strategies were counterproductive: heat increases edema and the accumulation of scar tissue, while immobilization prevents the fibers from becoming aligned with the injured structure.

These days *RICE therapy* (rest, ice, compression, elevation) is considered the norm, with an emphasis on moving the joint within range of pain tolerance as soon as possible. The potential benefits are clear: ice keeps edema at bay, limiting further tissue damage from ischemia; compression does the same; and elevation also encourages lymph flow *out* of an already impacted area. Introducing movement is exactly what bodies are designed to do to help form scar tissue that strengthens rather than weakens an injured ligament.

If exercise is overdone, more tearing happens and more scar tissue is produced. If too little exercise is done, the scar tissue glues itself in its original random arrangement and binds up the undamaged ligament fibers as well, increasing the risk of future injury. If it's done *just right*, exercise and stretching "teach" the new collagen fibers which way to lie, and the fibers remodel themselves according to the stresses put on them. Interestingly, the issue of when exactly to introduce movement and weight-bearing stress is still not settled; different ligaments seem to have different needs. Most evidence points toward early mobilization as an important part of the rehabilitation of most ligament sprains.

Massage?

Massage is *great* for sprains. It can reduce adhesions and influence the direction of new collagen fibers in the healing process. It can address edema and toxic accumulations from secondary muscle spasm. Massage also helps with stiffness from the temporary loss of joint function. Most massage must be done *after* the acute stage has subsided. Modalities for dealing with acute sprains are effective, but it is a highly technical field and not for casual experimentation.

Temporomandibular Joint Disorders

Definition: What Are They?

The term temporomandibular joint disorders can mean a multitude of problems in and around the jaw. This collection of signs and symptoms is usually associated with malocclusion (a dysfunctional bite), bruxism (teeth grinding), and loose ligaments surrounding the jaw that cause excessive movement between the bones, damage to the internal cartilage, and possible dislocation of the joint (see *dislocations*, this chapter). TMJ disorders are also referred to as TMD, for **t**emporo**m**andibular joint **d**isorders."

Demographics: Who Gets It?

It is difficult to pin down exact numbers of people who live with distortions in the jaw. Some estimates suggest that up to

TEMPOROMANDIBULAR JOINT DISORDERS IN BRIEF

What are they?
Temporomandibular joint (TMJ) disorders arise when constant strain, stress, and malocclusion of the jaw lead to pain and loss of function of the TMJ.

How is it recognized?
Symptoms of TMJ disorder include head, neck, and shoulder pain; ear pain; mouth pain; clicking or locking in the jaw; and loss of range of motion in the jaw.

Is massage indicated or contraindicated?
Massage can be useful for TMJ problems if intervention is begun before bony deformation begins. However, this condition can be difficult to diagnose, so it is important to be working with other medical professionals in these situations.

20% of the U.S. population has some degree of TMJ disorders, but only a small fraction may ever seek help. Of those who do, women outnumber men by about 3 to 1.

Etiology: What Happens?

When chronic misalignment, trauma, or muscle tension affects the highly specialized joints at the jaw, a person may find it difficult to open or close the mouth without pain. Chewing and swallowing become problematic, and pain in the jaw can reverberate systemically throughout the body. The construction of the jaw is so intricate, it is easy for structures to become injured or improperly balanced.

Anatomy Review   The TMJ is like no other joint in the body. Far from being a simple hinge joint, the TMJ moves up, down, forward, back, and side to side. The jaw is unusually mobile, as the shape of the joint actually stretches with the position of the mouth (Fig. 2-25). A fibrocartilage disc cushions the two bones (the temporal bone and the condyle of the mandible) but, like the menisci in the knee, this disc is sometimes pulled awry or injured, which can lead to problems in the joint. Lastly, a muscle involved in this joint, the lateral pterygoid that attaches directly to the fibrocartilage disc, is an unusual structure: it does not relax by order of the central nervous system. Instead, it constantly pulls on the disc, acting as a kind of spring. This constant tension makes the lateral pterygoid especially prone to trigger points, which can both mimic and precipitate TMJ syndrome.

Causes

The American Dental Association estimates that 44 to 99% of TMJ problems are precipitated by some kind of trauma. This may be direct impact to the face or head or indi-

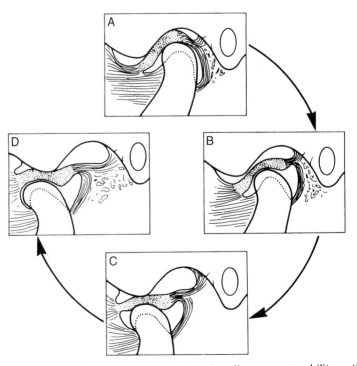

Figure 2-25. The temporomandibular joint allows great mobility as the jaw moves forward

rect repercussions of trauma elsewhere in the body. For instance, a childhood fall could set up imbalances in the spine, which would culminate in neck and jaw problems.[l]

TMJ disorder may also be a frequent consequence of car wrecks. A whole scenario of the progression of "jaw-lash" has been developed to explain the whiplash-like results seen after this kind of acceleration-deceleration accident (see *whiplash*, this chapter).

Precipitating trauma aside, this is often a "circular" disorder. That is, the things that cause TMJ problems can also be the symptoms. This is true of teeth grinding, muscle tightness, and *osteoarthritis* (this chapter). RA occasionally strikes here, but osteoarthritis is a far more frequent cause for TMJ problems. Other factors include misalignment of the bite and congenital malformations of the bones. Some sources suggest that TMJ syndrome is entirely a muscular disorder, but this is contradicted when the problems progress to arthritis and bony adaptation. Travell points out that when the jaw flexors, especially the lateral pterygoid, are overengaged, the constant pulling mechanically displaces the internal disc, thus starting the downward slide toward arthritis. In other words, *myofascial pain syndrome* (this chapter) that is linked to painful trigger points is both a cause and a complication of this disorder. According to her findings, about 70% of the people who complain of TMJ disorder symptoms show some disc displacement.[m]

It is impossible to ignore the emotional component of TMJ disorders. If one looks at the body as a physical expression of the emotional state, it is easy to see how closely chronic emotional stress and chronic jaw stress are linked together. Regardless of whether a precipitating injury occurred, people who persistently clench their teeth are setting themselves up for jaw problems in the future.

Signs and Symptoms

The signs and symptoms of TMJ disorders are as follows:

- *Jaw, neck, and shoulder pain.* This can be from actual deterioration of bony structures inside the capsule (arthritis), or it can be local and referred pain generated by tight, trigger-point laden muscles.

- *Limited range of motion.* Deformation or displacement of the cartilage inside the joint can make it difficult or impossible to open the mouth all the way.

- *Popping in the jaw.* This is usually attributed to having the disc or bone out of alignment, which then interferes in jaw opening. A similar "clicking" sensation is sometimes felt by people with knee problems involving the discs there.

- *Locking of the joint.* Again, this is a result of having the fibrocartilage disc interfere with normal joint movement.

- *Grinding teeth (bruxism).* Like many things about this disorder, this symptom is also a possible cause of the problem. A chronically shortened set of jaw flexors leads to clenching and grinding of teeth, especially during sleep, when the joint should be as relaxed as possible.

- *Ear pain.* Because of the location of the joint, pressure may be exerted directly on the eustachian tubes. Symptoms in this case include a feeling of stuffiness in the ears and loss of hearing.

---

[l]Shankland WE, II. Causes of TMJ. American Academy of Face, Head and Neck Pain. Available at: http://www.netset.com/~docws/page4.html. Accessed winter 1998.
[m]Travell J, Simons DG. *Myofascial Pain and Dysfunction: The Trigger Point Manual.* Baltimore, Md: Williams & Wilkins; 1983:176.

- *Headaches.* A total of 2000 lb/square inch of pressure are placed at the second molar when the teeth are clenched. It is no surprise that the cranial bones would be affected if this happens all night long. Headaches can also be related to trigger points of muscles in spasm and to cervical subluxation.

- *Chronic misalignment of cervical vertebrae.* This is probably a result of the muscular hypertonicity that is generated by this problem. As pain refers from the jaw to the neck and shoulders, the muscles there tighten up and pull asymmetrically on the neck bones. No matter how often the neck is adjusted, or how brilliantly the neck muscles are massaged, this pain-spasm cycle will not abate until the jaw situation is addressed.

Diagnosis

Many conditions present signs and symptoms similar to TMJ disorder but will not respond to the most advanced kinds of interventions. Therefore, it is important to differentiate between true TMJ disorder, which involves bony or cartilaginous deformation inside the joint capsule, and the other diseases and conditions that can cause head, neck, and shoulder pain.

First among these differential diagnoses is MPS. More than any other condition, this one is both a precursor and a complication of TMJ disorder. Jaw surgery will not resolve trigger points, but resolving trigger points could eliminate the need for future jaw surgery. It is important to remember though, that true TMJ disorder can (and probably will) be present simultaneously with MPS. Other conditions that cause head, neck, and shoulder pain include:

- *Sprain* of the ligament that attaches the stylomandibular joint to the base of the skull can cause pain in the jaw and head. This is also called *Ernest syndrome.*

- *Trigeminal neuralgia,* also called *Tic Douloureux* is an extremely painful result of damage to the trigeminal nerve (See Chapter 3).

- *Occipital neuralgia* is damage to the greater or lesser occipital nerves.

- *Osteomyelitis* is a complication of dental surgery in which tissue death occurs at the site of extracted teeth, which causes pain in the face.

Some diagnostic tools that identify TMJ disorder include MRI, which can show whether the internal cartilage is chipped or subluxated; radiographs of the jaw and head; and electromography, which shows muscle function around the joint. A trained clinician can also feel a subluxation when fingers are inserted in the ear of the patient during chewing.

Treatment

Treatment for TMJ disorder is divided into surgical and nonsurgical options. In most cases nonsurgical options are tried first. These include applying heat to painful areas, physical therapy, ultrasound and massage for jaw muscles, anti-inflammatory medications, and local anesthetics. Special splints that reduce bone-to-bone pressure may be prescribed, although some specialists are concerned that poorly fitted splints make matters worse. Proliferant injections to tighten the ligaments that surround the jaw may also be effective. If these noninvasive techniques are successful, the TMJ disorder may be averted before permanent bony distortion or cartilage damage inside the joint occurs.

In some situations the onset of symptoms may be very fast (e.g., a car wreck or a fall). If such a patient has been severely debilitated, or if noninvasive techniques have been unsuccessful and other problems have been ruled out, surgery may be considered. Several different surgeries have been developed. These range from an outpatient procedure in which scar tissue and adhesions are dissolved by injecting special substances into the joint, to arthroscopic surgery to manipulate the cartilage, to full prosthetic joint replacement.

Massage?

Massage can be especially useful in the early teeth-clenching stages of TMJ problems not only by addressing the jaw flexors, but also by helping to increase the client's awareness of this habit. It is surprising how often people grit their teeth without realizing it; the proprioceptors can adapt to assume that this is *normal*, even if it is not *optimal*. Of course, in addition to helping reduce excessive muscle tone, massage can also deal with some of the referred pain patterns that can be such a problem with this condition.

Other Connective Tissue Disorders

Baker Cysts

Definition: What Are They?

Baker cysts are posterior extensions of the joint capsule of the knee.

Etiology: What Happens?

Baker cysts form when the joint capsule at the knee develops a pouch at the posterior aspect. A structural weak spot of the joint capsule, called the popliteal recess, is the most common site for these extensions. Baker cysts are relatively common in children, in whom they usually spontaneously resolve within a few months. When they occur in adults, it is usually connected to general joint inflammation: osteoarthritis, RA, or meniscus tears.

Baker cysts are not usually dangerous. The only risks they pose is that a cyst could become big enough to press on nerves or impair blood flow through the lesser saphenous vein in the back of the leg. If that is the case, clients may experience some numbness, which contraindicates massage, or they could be at risk for forming blood clots, another contraindication.

Signs and Symptoms

Baker cysts themselves are generally asymptomatic, but the affected knee is often painful from the underlying cause of inflammation. The cysts usually extend into the medial side

---

BAKER CYSTS IN BRIEF

What are they?
Baker cysts are fluid-filled extensions of the synovial membrane at the knee. They protrude into the popliteal fossa, usually on the medial side.

How are they recognized?
Baker cysts are usually painless sacs that are palpable deep to the superficial fascia in the popliteal fossa. They may cause pain or a feeling of tightness in the knee in flexion.

Is massage indicated or contraindicated?
Massage is locally contraindicated in the popliteal fossa anyway, especially if a Baker cyst is present. In addition, if any signs of circulatory disruption (coldness, clamminess, edema) are palpable distal to the cyst, that whole area is a contraindication, and the client needs to be cleared of the possibility of thrombosis.

of the popliteal fossa and may protrude down the leg, deep to the gastrocnemius (Fig. 2-26). Patients with Baker cysts often report a feeling of tightness or fullness when the knee is in flexion.

Baker cysts occasionally spontaneously rupture, the symptoms of which mimic *thrombophlebitis* (see Chapter 4), deep acute pain in the calf with temporary edema from the leaking fluid.

Treatment

Most Baker cysts are first treated with ice and NSAIDs in the hopes that they might spontaneously resolve. If this is unsuccessful, they may be aspirated followed by cortisone shots to resolve joint inflammation. This is often an impermanent solution, however, as they may easily come back.

Surgery to remove the cyst is another possibility, although even in this case another cyst may form if the area is irritated again. Baker cysts are resolved most successfully when the underlying cause for joint inflammation is effectively identified and treated.

Massage?

It is possible, although unlikely, that massage could rupture a Baker cyst, but a therapist would have to be working much deeper in the popliteal fossa than good sense allows. Because of the possibility of pressure on the lesser saphenous vein, Baker cysts are considered local contraindications for massage. Therapists should watch for signs of fluid accumulation and poor blood return below the knee: coldness, clamminess, and edema that is more pronounced on the cysted side than the uncysted side (Fig. 2-27). These are all

BAKER CYSTS
Dr. William Baker was a British surgeon who lived from 1839 to 1896. He was the first to note and document the odd, usually painless swellings some people have in the popliteal fossa.

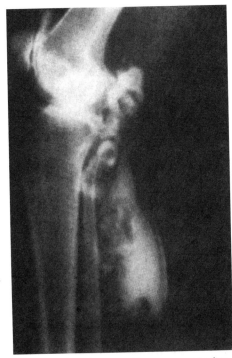

Figure 2-26. Baker cyst: the mass posterior to the femoral condyle is probably the original cyst; the mass in the gastrocnemius is where it may have leaked its fluid.

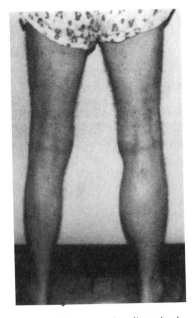

Figure 2-27. Note the disparity in size and color between the two calves.

signs that the cyst is big enough to cause a problem. If this is the case, it and everything distal to it is considered a local contraindication. The client should be advised to visit a doctor to rule out the possibility of thrombophlebitis.

Bunions

Definition: What Are They?

Bunions are also known as *hallux valgus*, which means, "laterally deviated big toe." The first phalanx of the great toe is distorted toward the lateral aspect of the foot. The joint capsule stretches, and callus grows over the protrusion. A smaller version of the same problem sometimes appears at the base of the little toe; this is called "tailor's bunion."

Demographics: Who gets them?

Bunions occur approximately 10 times more often in women than in men. Anyone can get them, but the condition is linked to a habit of wearing high-heeled, narrow-toed shoes. A genetic weakness in the toe joints may predispose some people to bunions regardless of footwear, but anyone can get bunions.

Etiology: What Happens?

Bunions begin with a bony misalignment in which the proximal phalanx of the great toe is laterally deviated. This misalignment may be the result of an overarched foot, which places excessive pressure on the medial aspect of the foot. Bunions also arise when feet are forced into pointed-toe shoes, shoes that are too small, and shoes with high heels. A history of other joint problems in the feet (i.e., osteoarthritis or RA) may also precipitate bunions.

The distortion of the metacarpal-phalangeal joint in itself can cause erosion and irritation, but the acute pain of bunions is more often related to a variety of *bursitis* (this chapter). Bursae spontaneously generate in places subject to a lot of wear and tear. The bump formed by a bunion is a natural spot for that protective impulse. If that new bursa should get irritated and inflamed, it becomes a case of friction bursitis, which can be extremely painful and even debilitating. Ultimately, if this badly misaligned weight-bearing joint is not somehow corrected or supported in a way that limits erosion of the joint structures, the patient can also develop bone spurs and/or degenerative joint disease, which can make it chronically painful to do anything, including walking.

Signs and Symptoms

Bunions look like an enormous lump on the medial side of the metatarsal-phalangeal joint of the great toe. If the bunion is not irritated, a simple protrusion, often covered with a thick layer of callus will be obvious (Fig. 2-28). If the bursa happens to be inflamed, the area will be red, hot, and painful.

Treatment

The first steps in treating a bunion are to remove whatever irritants are causing it or making it worse. This usually means switching footgear or cutting holes in shoes to make

---

BUNIONS IN BRIEF

What are they?
A bunion is a protrusion at the metatarsal-phalangeal joint of the great toe that occurs when the toe is laterally deviated.

How are they recognized?
Bunions are recognizable by the large bump on the medial aspect of the foot. When they are inflamed they are red, hot, and possibly edematous.

Is massage indicated or contraindicated?
The point of a bunion locally contraindicates massage, especially when it is inflamed. Massage elsewhere on the foot or body is very much appropriate within pain tolerance to help with compensation patterns that occur when it is difficult to walk.

BUNIONS:
This term comes from an Old French word, *buigne*, which means a bump on the head. Its synonym, "hallux valgus," comes from the Latin for "big toe turned outward."

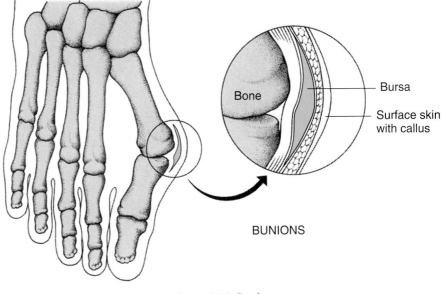

Figure 2-28. Bunion

room for the protrusion. Other noninvasive techniques include the use of massage and ultrasound to reduce internal adhesions and inflammation. Elevating the heel to an appropriate height can diminish pain, and a corticosteroid injection can reduce inflammation. If damage has developed inside the joint and if the bunion is causing enough pain to limit the patient's activity, surgery may be recommended to realign and fuse the joint. This can eradicate the bunion but it can also eradicate any movement at the joint, so surgery is considered a last-ditch option.

Massage?

Acutely inflamed bunions locally contraindicate massage; massage elsewhere on the body is perfectly safe. If no acute inflammation is present, massage is appropriate, although the bump itself is still a local contraindication because of the risk of irritating a bursa or osteophyte. Massage does *not* make bunions go away. Therapists do not have access to genetic patterning or to the inner workings of the affected joint. The best massage can do is work with the compensation patterns that ripple through a body when it is forced to move differently because of foot pain. This can mean concentrating on the intrinsic muscles of the affected foot, and it can mean working with the extrinsic muscles for gross movement everywhere else on the body.

Bursitis

Definition: What Is It?

Bursae are small closed sacks made of connective tissue. They are lined with synovial membrane and are filled with synovial fluid. Bursitis is inflammation of the bursae: these fluid-filled sacks, when irritated, generate excess fluid, which causes pain and limits mobility. Most bursae are very small, but the ones that protect the knee and shoulder can be quite large.

Bursitis comes in all shapes and forms, some of which have descriptive names such as *housemaid's knee* and *student's elbow*, which occurs on the point of the olecranon (Fig. 2-29). *Weaver's bottom* is bursitis on the ischial tuberosity. Trochanteric, or hip bur-

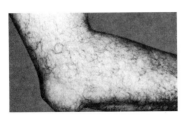

Figure 2-29. Bursitis: student's elbow

sitis, is another common variety. The most common type of bursitis, at the pad between the humerus and the acromion, is called subacromial bursitis, but could be labeled *"jack hammerer's shoulder."*

Etiology: What Happens?

Imagine stretching a rubber band over the sharp edge of a table. Now imagine moving it back and forth for several minutes. It would not be long before that rubber band would fray and then break. If a small water balloon is inserted between the rubber band and the edge of the table, the rubber band (i.e., tendon) has freedom to move without the friction caused by the table (i.e., bone). The water balloon (i.e., bursa) has protected it from damage. Bursae serve to ease the movement of tendons over bony angles (Fig. 2-30). They also cushion the bones where they would otherwise bang against each other. Bursae pad people's sharpest corners: they are on elbows, knees, heels, ischial tuberosities, and between layers of fascia. Bursae can grow anywhere the body experiences extra wear and tear around a joint.

Without bursae to protect them, several tendons would fray and rupture in short order. Some bones that are not meant to touch *would* touch, with great force. Sharp corners, like elbows or hallux valgus (*bunions,* this chapter), would have no protection.

Causes

culpable (n)

Repetitive stress is usually the culprit behind bursitis. Performing the same movement or rubbing the same spot over and over, day after day, sooner or later irritates that fluid-filled sack. Then the inflammatory process tries to pack a tangerine's worth of fluid into a sack the size of a grape, which *hurts.* In response to the pain, the muscles that surround the joint go into spasm, splinting the injury. This drastically limits the range of motion of the affected joint. Sometimes the muscles can actually aggravate and prolong an attack of bursitis by compressing the joint and the bursa at the same time.

Bursitis often occurs in concert with other inflammatory conditions. It tends to accompany general area inflammation, so if a person has shoulder tendinitis, bursitis is often present as well. (Unfortunately, it is hard to treat the tendinitis if the bursitis is in the way.) It also attends *rheumatoid arthritis* (this chapter) and some chronic infections, especially syphilis and *tuberculosis* (Chapter 6).

BURSITIS IN BRIEF

What is it?
A bursa is a fluid filled-sack that acts as a protective cushion at points of recurring pressure, eases the movement of tendons and ligaments moving over bones, and cushions points of contact between bones. Bursitis is the inflammation of a bursa.

How is it recognized?
Acute bursitis is painful and is aggravated by both passive and active motion. Muscles that tighten around the affected joint may severely limit range of motion. It may be hot or edematous if the bursa is superficial enough to be palpated.

Is massage indicated or contraindicated?
Acute noninfectious bursitis locally contraindicates massage. Massage elsewhere on the body during an acute phase, and directly on the muscles of the affected joint (within pain limits) in a subacute phase, is perfectly appropriate.

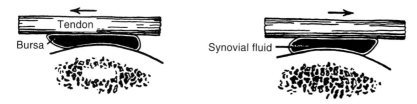

Figure 2-30. Bursae allow tendons to move freely over bony prominences

Signs and Symptoms

The symptoms of bursitis include pain on *any* kind of movement, passive or active, along with heat, edema, and extremely limited range of motion because of the muscular splinting reaction to pain. If the affected bursae are deep, no heat or edema may be palpable, but the pain and limitation of movement may still be present.

Diagnosis

Bursitis is not usually caused by an infectious agent, and bursae do not show up on radiographs. Therefore, its diagnosis largely depends on ruling out anything else it could be, which includes tendinitis, arthritis, ligament sprains, and any other problems specific to the joint or area being affected.

Treatment

Opinions vary about the duration of the average bursitis episode. Some orthopedists predict several weeks; others suggest it usually clears up in about 2 weeks. For some people bursitis can last much longer: untreated bursitis can become a chronic situation that lasts several months or even years. Obviously, a great deal depends on which bursae are inflamed and the precipitating factors. Treatment strategies range from NSAIDs, to warm moist applications (cold is too intense for this inflammation; the muscles seize up and make it worse), to aspiration of excess fluid, to corticosteroid injections. One or two injections generally clear away even chronic inflammation, and since the chemical is being injected into a closed cavity, one does not have to deal with the same side affects that a systemic dose of steroids involves.

As a last resort, some doctors suggest the possibility of a *bursectomy* to simply remove a badly inflamed bursa. However, the only way to be sure that the bursitis is permanently cured is to get rid of the aggravating factors that caused it. No matter how often or how effectively bursitis is treated, if the stimulus that irritated the bursa to begin with is not removed, no treatment will be permanently successful. Even removing the bursa may eventually backfire, because the body can grow new ones! What does removing the irritating stimulus mean? It means learning some new movement patterns that do not put so much stress in just one spot. It means strengthening the muscles that surround the affected joint. It means finding a different way to do a job or possibly even finding a new line of work.

Massage?

This is a local contraindication, especially in an acute phase. It is tempting to try to release the muscles around an inflamed bursa. This temptation must be resisted. Although the muscles are likely to be tight, working to loosen them does not solve any problems until the inflammation itself has subsided. Bursitis usually does not involve a pathogen that can spread, so massage is certainly appropriate for the rest of the body. (If the bursitis *is* caused by an infectious agent, it systemically contraindicates massage until the infection has subsided.)

In the subacute stage, a skilled massage therapist can address the muscles that cross over the affected joint and may well have some success at decompressing the bones that are re-irritating the affected bursa. As with any condition that involves prolonged pain and immobility, it is a good idea to look for compensation patterns that may cause pain.

Dupuytren's Contracture

Definition: What Is It?

This condition, also called *palmar fasciitis*, is an idiopathic thickening and shrinking of the palmar fascia that limits the movement of the fingers. Usually the ring and little fingers are most severely affected, although the index and middle fingers may also be bent (Fig. 2-31).

Demographics: Who Gets It?

This condition strikes mostly middle-aged white men. It shows some statistical links to alcoholism and epilepsy, but no direct connections have been established. About 10% of Dupuytren contracture patients have other family members with the same condition.

Etiology: What Happens?

No one knows exactly *why* the palmar fascia shrinks in this condition, although some think it may have to do with repetitive trauma. Proliferations of type III collagen fibers have been identified both in the fascia on the palm and in the fingers.

Signs and Symptoms

Dupuytren's contracture may be mildly painful in early stages but usually becomes painless. It is sometimes progressive. The pattern is unpredictable and varies greatly from person to person. Some people only experience the growth of tough, fibrous bumps on their hands, whereas others end up with severely bent, strangulated, unusable fingers. Dupuytren's contracture is bilateral in almost 50% of all cases.

Treatment

If this condition is left untreated, the connective tissue simply strangles the muscles and nerves until the affected fingers eventually lose all function. If it is caught before too much atrophy occurs, corticosteroid injections to reduce fascial build-up can be an effective treatment. Injections of collagenase, an enzyme that dissolves collagen, is another treatment option.

Surgical intervention is generally not recommended until fingers become bent and too stiff to move. At that point, surgery involves making several zig-zag cuts in the palm to release the fascia, followed by skin grafts, physical therapy, and massage to limit the growth of scar tissue. Even when surgery is successful, Dupuytren's contracture recurs in about one-third of all cases.

Massage?

Dupuytren's contracture does not stem from nerve injury, and sensation is present in the hand, at least before the progression has damaged nerves. Therefore, massage is appropriate. The connective tissue involved with Dupuytren's contracture is particularly tough and strong. Although massage certainly will not make the condition any worse, it may not make it better either. Massage is a good preventive measure for contractures, but if this condition is already present it may not be possible to reverse it.

DUPUYTREN'S CONTRACTURE IN BRIEF

What is it?
Dupuytren's contracture is an idiopathic shrinking and thickening of the fascia on the palm of the hand.

How is it recognized?
This is a painless condition that usually affects the ring and little fingers, pulling them into permanent flexion.

Is massage indicated or contraindicated?
Dupuytren's contracture indicates massage as long as sensation is present, although massage may do little to reverse the process if it has gone too far.

DUPUYTREN'S CONTRACTURE
Baron Guillaume Dupuytren (1777-1835) was a French surgeon and pathologist who documented this condition and other specific diseases and conditions. He also put his stamp on several surgical procedures, including Dupuytren's suture, Dupuytren's amputation, and Dupuytren's tourniquet.

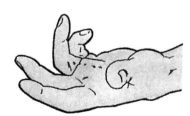

Figure 2-31. Dupuytren's contracture

Massage is sometimes recommended along with physical therapy and exercise to help minimize the growth of scar tissue in postsurgical situations.

Ganglion Cysts

Definition: What Are They?

bolsa

Ganglion cysts are small connective tissue pouches filled with fluid. They grow on joint capsules or tendinous sheaths. They usually appear on the wrist, the hand, or the top of the foot.

Etiology: What Happens?

Although some ganglion cysts seem to be a response to a direct trauma, the vast majority of them simply appear without an identifiable reason. A ganglion cyst is essentially a synovial pouch that forms as an extension of a joint capsule or tenosynovial sheath; in this sense they are very similar to *Baker cysts* (this chapter).

Ganglion cysts are not inherently dangerous, but when they appear on the distal phalanges of the fingers they can interfere with normal fingernail growth. They may also interfere with joint capsule function at the distal interphalangeal joint.

Signs and Symptoms

Ganglion cysts may be too small to notice or they may grow to the size of a small tennis ball, obstructing joint function and getting in the way of a normal range of motion. Most ganglion cysts are not usually painful, except that they have a habit of growing in places where they can be easily irritated: on the fingers and around the wrists (Fig. 2-32). This can put them in a state of chronic irritation and can make it difficult for them to heal and subside.

When a cyst grows on the flexor tendon of a finger, movement of that finger may become limited and painful. Some cysts around the wrist or ankle joints may become large enough to limit the normal range of motion for those joints. The majority of ganglion cysts are not acutely painful.

Treatment

Generally the treatment for ganglion cysts is to leave them alone. It may take a while, but they usually resolve themselves without interference. They may be aspirated to relieve internal pressure, but they grow back about half the time. The traditional "home remedy" for ganglion cysts used to be to smash them with a Bible. *aplastar* *sin embargo* Patients are not recommended to use this option, however, as smashing a ganglion cyst with a book or any other heavy object may rupture the cyst and will probably also cause a great deal of other soft tissue damage as well.

Cysts may be surgically excised if they are big enough to be a significant problem. They often grow back, but are usually not as large as the original cyst.

Massage?

Ganglion cysts are a local contraindication. Massage certainly cannot make ganglion cysts bigger, worse, or more painful, *unless* they are overstimulated. Massage cannot make

---

GANGLION CYSTS
"Ganglion" comes from the Greek word for swelling, or knot. It is used to describe the small fluid-filled sacs that can develop around hand and feet joints, but the term is also used in reference to the nervous system where clusters of nerve cell bodies are also referred to as ganglia.

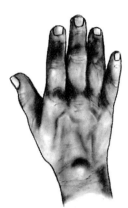

Figure 2-32. Ganglion cyst

them go away either, so massage therapists should leave them alone. If however, a client has a mysterious bump on the wrist, foot, or anywhere else, it is important to get a diagnosis before working anywhere in the area.

Hernia

Definition: What Is It?

"Hernia" means hole. Specifically in this case it means "hole through which contents that are supposed to be contained are protruding." Muscles may herniate through fascial walls; vertebral discs may herniate; the brain may even herniate through the cranium. This section discusses the most common types of hernias, which occur in various places around the abdomen.

Etiology: What Happens?

Hernias can be caused by a number of different factors, from congenital weakness of the muscular wall, to childbirth, to abnormal straining that increases intra-abdominal pressure. They can go undetected for a long time if they have a slow onset and the hole is large enough that the intestine is not impaired in any way. Most hernias are *reducible*, which means that the contents can easily be put back where they belong manually. Generally, though, they will worsen, bulging more and more often, and perhaps a bigger and bigger hole may develop. Therefore, once a hernia has been identified, surgery to tighten up or close the hole is recommended sooner rather than later. Where a hernia is most likely to happen and what it feels like depends a lot on gender and what makes the abdominal contents push against the walls.

> ### HERNIA IN BRIEF
>
> **What is it?**
> A hernia is a hole or rip in the abdominal wall or the inguinal ring through which the small intestines may protrude.
>
> **How is it recognized?**
> Abdominal hernias usually show some bulging and mild to severe pain, depending on whether a portion of the small intestine is trapped.
>
> **Is massage indicated or contraindicated?**
> Untreated hernias locally contraindicate massage. If the hernia is accompanied by fever or other signs of infection, it systemically contraindicates massage. Recent hernia surgeries fall under the category of *post-operative situations* (Chapter 11). Massage is acceptable for sites of old hernia surgeries with no complications.

Signs and Symptoms

The signs and symptoms of hernias depend on what part of the abdominal wall has been compromised.

- *Epigastric hernia.* This is a bulging above the stomach. In this condition the linea alba is split, and a portion of the omentum pushes through. The symptoms, besides a visible lump protruding above the belly button, may include a feeling of tenderness or heaviness in the area, but seldom extreme pain. This hernia happens with women and men, but it is more common in men.

- *Paraumbilical hernia.* This is another split of the linea alba, this time right at the navel. It is sometimes a complication of childbirth. The symptoms are the same as the epigastric type, but the bulge is lower. This type of hernia is almost always experienced by women.

- *Femoral hernia.* This is the female equivalent to the inguinal hernia. In this case the abdominal contents protrude through the femoral ring just below the inguinal ligament. Femoral hernias usually happen only in women, and they can be hard to detect. They can be very dangerous, however, because the hole around the intestine is usually quite small, which increases the chance of strangulation or obstruction of the intestine.

- *Inguinal hernia.* This is the most common variety of hernia. Inguinal hernias are holes in the abdominal wall at the inguinal ring. This opening for the spermatic

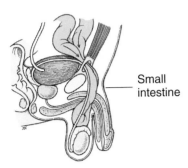

Figure 2-33. Inguinal hernia

cord to enter the abdomen is a structurally weak spot. A sudden change in internal abdominal pressure, like coughing, sneezing, or heavy lifting, may force a section of small intestine right through at this point (Fig. 2-33).

Complications

The seriousness of a hernia is determined by how big it is. Paradoxically, the bigger the better, at least for the short term. Small holes, as seen with femoral hernias, have a much greater danger of trapping the intestine in such a way that it cannot function. Either it becomes obstructed, in which case the patient experiences abdominal pain, nausea, and vomiting, or it becomes strangulated, cut off from its blood supply. In this case the area rapidly becomes red, enlarged, and extremely painful. If no medical intervention is taken, the strangulated loop of intestine will become infected and possibly necrotic.

Treatment

Surgery is frequently recommended even for mild hernias, because they tend to get worse as time passes. Sewing up a small stretch of abdominal fascia is much easier than repairing a big rip. The standard surgical technique involves inserting a small piece of mesh at the site of the tear. This helps to distribute the force of abdominal pressure more evenly than do stitches or staples alone, reducing the risk of subsequent hernias at the surgery site.

If a person does not need immediate surgery, a special corset or truss may be recommended to prevent sudden changes in abdominal pressure. Nevertheless, these are considered to be only a temporary measure, not a solution to the problem.

Massage?

If a client has been diagnosed with a hernia but has not had surgery, that part of the body locally contraindicates any kind of deep massage. Vigorously stretching the fascia around an already weakened area could have disastrous results. If, on the other hand, a client has had surgery, the guidelines for postoperative cautions are followed. If his or her hernia surgery is ancient history, and no pain is present, massage does not pose a danger in any way.

Osgood-Schlatter Disease
Definition: What Is It?

OSD is a condition involving irritation and inflammation at the site of the quadriceps insertion on the tibial tuberosity. It occurs when the quadriceps muscles are vigorously used in combination with rapid growth of the leg bones.

Demographics: Who Gets It?

OSD is a condition that is practically exclusive to adolescent athletes. It is especially common among people who participate in sports that involve running, jumping, and making fast, tight turns. Soccer, basketball, figure skating, and dancing are all sports with a high incidence of athletes in whom OSD develops.

OSD occurs in both boys and girls, although it is more common in boys. The average age of onset for boys is 11 to 18 years of age; for girls it can occur a little earlier, between 10 and 16 years of age.

Incidence of OSD in the United States is unknown. Some experts estimate that it affects between 16 and 20% of young athletes to some extent.

Etiology: What Happens?

When children enter their teen years, they begin a time of rapid bone growth, especially in their femurs and tibias: the bones that eventually determine how tall a person will be. Most of the time the muscles, fascia, and other connective tissues in the legs can easily keep up with the accelerated growth rate during this time, but when the quadriceps muscles are particularly taxed through demanding athletics, the combination of stresses can cause the insertion of this powerful muscle group to become irritated and inflamed.

OSD involves acute inflammation of the quadriceps insertion at the tibial tuberosity. The tendon can pull away from the bone, causing a variety of *tendinitis* (this chapter), or in extreme cases the tibia itself can become damaged and even develop an avulsion: a forceful separation of a part of the bone from chronic tendinous tension. Even if the tibia does not break, it is common for OSD patients to develop a large, permanent bump at the tibial tuberosity; this is where the bone adapts to the constant pull of the quadriceps insertion (Fig. 2-34). OSD is usually unilateral, but a small number of athletes may develop inflammation at both knees.

The severity of OSD varies greatly from one person to the next; one person may have to be careful about not overstressing the knee, while another athlete may have to quit the team altogether. It is generally a self-limiting condition, which means when the connective tissue growth "catches up" to the bone growth, the pain and irritation finally subside. Unfortunately, this can take anywhere from several months to 2 years.

Signs and Symptoms

OSD is easy to identify because the people susceptible to it are such an unambiguous group: athletic teens. In acute stages of OSD the knee is hot, swollen, and painful, just distal to the patella at the tibial tuberosity. Any activity that stresses or stretches the quadriceps aggravates symptoms.

When OSD is not acute, pain and inflammation are resolved, but the characteristic bump of the remodeled tibia is permanent. A person who had OSD as a child may never be comfortable kneeling because of tibial distortion.

Treatment

Treatment for OSD focuses on reducing pain and limiting damage to the quadriceps attachment at the tibia. Mild cases can be managed by heating the knee with hot packs before athletic events and icing them afterward. NSAIDs may be suggested to help with pain and inflammation, and doctors or physical therapists may recommend that stretches designed to reduce tension in the quadriceps be performed several times a day.

OSGOOD-SCHLATTER DISEASE IN BRIEF

What is it?
Osgood-Schlatter disease (OSD) is the result of chronic or traumatic irritation at the insertion of the quadriceps tendon in combination with adolescent growth spurts.

How is it recognized?
When OSD disease is acute, the tibial tuberosity is hot, swollen, and painful. The bone may grow a large protuberance at the site of the tendinous insertion.

Is massage indicated or contraindicated?
An acute flair of OSD locally contraindicates circulatory massage, which could exacerbate inflammation. Techniques for reducing lymphatic retention and work elsewhere on the body are certainly appropriate. A client with a history of OSD but no current inflammation at the knee may benefit from the pain relief and reduction in quadriceps muscle tone that massage can provide.

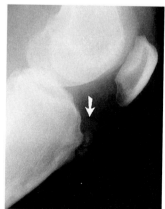

Figure 2-34. Osgood-Schlatter disease: a protuberance on the tibia is visible, and the blurry area indicated by the arrow shows where inflammatory edema has accumulated

More severe cases may require that the athlete suspend his or her activity until the pain and inflammation have been gone for several weeks. In the meantime, the knee may be supported with a brace or cast. This period is followed by aggressive quadriceps exercise to strengthen the muscles and reduce the chance of a recurrence when the athlete becomes active again.

In rare cases, the knee may require surgery to remove bits of the tibia that may have been pulled off and suspended in the tibial tendon.

Massage?

In its acute stages OSD locally contraindicates circulatory massage, which only exacerbates inflammation. Other techniques that may reduce edema can be appropriate, as is work anywhere other than the affected knee.

When the knee is not acutely painful, massage may be useful in reducing quadriceps tension that pulls on the tibial tendon. Massage is unlikely to resolve or reverse a case of OSD, but it may help to deal with the pain it causes and speed up recovery so that a teen athlete may more quickly and safely resume activity.

Pes Planus

Definition: What Is It?

This is the medical term for feet that lack the medial arch between the calcaneus and the great toe, the lateral arch between the calcaneus and the little toe, and the transverse arch that stretches across the ball of the foot. In other words, pes planus means *flat feet*.

Etiology: What Happens?

Pes planus may develop because of a congenital problem in the shape of the foot bones or the strength of the foot ligaments. Occasionally it can be caused by trauma leading to the rupture of the posterior tibialis tendon. It may arise from the unending battle between the deep flexors and everters, combined with footwear that offers little or no support to the intertarsal ligaments that are supposed to hold up the arches (Fig. 2-35). Interestingly, these factors may also lead to the exact opposite of flat feet, jammed arches, or *pes cavus*.

PES PLANUS IN BRIEF

What is it?
This is the medical term for flat feet.

How is it recognized?
Flat feet lack well-defined arches. Pronation of the ankle may also be present.

Is massage indicated or contraindicated?
Pes planus indicates massage. In some cases the health of intrinsic foot muscles and ligaments can be improved to the point where alignment in the foot is also improved. In cases where the ligaments are lax through genetic or other problems, massage may not correct the situation but it will not make it worse.

Complications

Whichever direction the tarsal bones go— to the floor or to the roof—if they lack mobility, a critical feature of foot architecture is missing: shock absorption. Each time the foot hits the ground, thousands of pounds of downward pressure should be softly distributed through the tarsal bones, which flatten out and then rebound in preparation for the next step. If the arches are somehow compromised and the bones lose their rebound capacity, all that force reverberates through the rest of the skeleton. This is how flat feet or jammed arches can lead to arthritis in the feet, heel spurs, *plantar fasciitis* (this chapter), knee problems, hip problems, back problems, and even headaches. This is the biggest idea that should echo throughout good anatomy training: *everything in the body is connected to everything else.* Pes planus is an excellent example of how an "insignificant" problem in one place can create *very* significant problems elsewhere. These problems can be hard to track down and correct unless a therapist knows where to look.

Treatment

Unless they lead to serious arthritis or plantar fasciitis, flat feet often do not hurt in the feet as much as cause dysfunction in other places in the body. When this is the case, the feet may never be treated at all. If it is known that the alignment of the feet is a problem, highly supportive shoes, perhaps with orthotic inserts, may be recommended. Physical therapy to strengthen the peroneus longus and tibialis posterior muscles may also be suggested. Rarely, surgery may be performed to repair injured tendons that can contribute to flat feet, to reshape foot bones, or to fuse foot joints for reduced pain and improved stability.

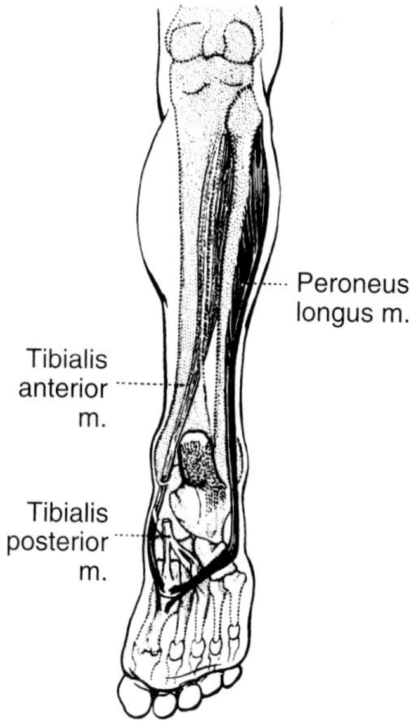

Massage?

Pes planus indicates massage. If the problems are congenital, massage will not have much lasting effect, but even temporary relief from pain is better than nothing. Furthermore, massage can ameliorate some of the distant effects of flat feet (e.g., knee strain or hip rotation).

If flat feet are related to muscular or ligamentous stresses, massage may have some success at equalizing the tensions between antagonistic muscles and stimulating circulation to the ligaments. Deep, specific massage tips the scales, drawing lots of fresh blood to ligaments that otherwise would not get it.

Figure 2-35. The "stirrup" of lower leg muscles that support the medial arch of the foot

Plantar Fasciitis

Definition: What Is It?

This is a condition involving pain and inflammation of the plantar fascia, which stretches from the calcaneus to the metatarsals on the plantar surface of the foot.

Demographics: Who Gets It?

This is a common problem; 95% of all heel pain is diagnosed as plantar fasciitis. Up to 2 million cases are reported per year, and that includes only people who seek treatment. It affects men and women equally. Although children *can* get it, adults are far more susceptible because their plantar fascia has generally lost some of its youthful elasticity.

Two populations seem to be at highest risk for developing plantar fasciitis: runners (some estimates suggest that up to 10% of all runners experience plantar fasciitis at some time), and non-athletes who may be overweight, especially if a sudden change is made that puts unusual stress on the foot.

PLANTAR FASCIITIS IN BRIEF

What is it?
Plantar fasciitis is pain and inflammation caused by injury to the plantar fascia of the foot.

How is it recognized?
Plantar fasciitis is acutely painful after prolonged immobility. Then the pain recedes but comes back with extended use. It feels sharp and bruise-like, usually at the anterior calcaneus or deep in the arch, but the pain can appear almost anywhere the plantar fascia goes.

Is massage indicated or contraindicated?
Plantar fasciitis indicates massage. It can help release tension in deep calf muscles that put strain on the plantar fascia; it can also help to affect the development of scar tissue at the site of the tear.

Etiology: What Happens?

When the plantar fascia is overused or stressed by misalignment, its fibers tend to fray. This is essentially the same as a tendon or ligament tear (Fig. 2-36). Radiographs very frequently show that a bone spur has developed at the attachment to the calcaneus. It was once assumed that these bone spurs caused the pain of plantar fasciitis. It is now clear that

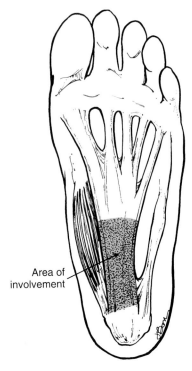

Figure 2-36. Plantar fasciitis

Area of involvement

the chronic irritation of injured fascia stimulates the growth of bone spurs, not that bone spurs cause fascial irritation.

The pain that accompanies plantar fasciitis occurs when the foot has been immobile for several hours and is then used. The fibers of the fascia begin to knit together during rest and are re-torn each time the foot goes into even gentle weight-bearing dorsiflexion.

Causes

Causes of plantar fasciitis are varied, but most boil down to overuse or alignment stresses. Being overweight can predispose someone to plantar fasciitis, as can wearing shoes without good arch and lateral support. Flat or pronated feet are associated with this problem. Very tight calf muscles are also contributing factors, especially for runners. Plantar fasciitis may occur as a secondary complication to an underlying disorder such as *gout* or *rheumatoid arthritis* (this chapter).

Signs and Symptoms

Plantar fasciitis follows a distinctive pattern that makes it easy to identify: it is acutely painful for the first few steps every morning. Then the pain subsides or disappears altogether, but becomes a problem again with prolonged standing, walking, or running. A sharp "bruised" feeling either just anterior to the calcaneus on the plantar surface or deep in the arch of the foot often marks this disorder.

Treatment

The most important thing to do for plantar fasciitis is to remove the tensions that cause the plantar fascia to be re-injured every morning when the foot first hits the floor. This can be accomplished in a number of ways: heating up and massaging the foot and lower leg before getting out of bed can make the tissue more flexible. Shoe inserts can be helpful to keep the foot from going into deep dorsiflexion; these should be in *all* shoes, including bedroom slippers. Someone with plantar fasciitis should *never* go barefoot until the fascia can stretch without tearing. Another helpful device is a night splint that holds the foot in a slightly dorsiflexed position. This allows the plantar fascia fibers to knit back together in a way that will not be stressed and re-torn so easily.

NSAIDs and topical anti-inflammatories, ice, stretching, and deep massage to the calf muscles and the site of the tear are frequently prescribed for plantar fasciitis. Corticosteroid injections are sometime given to reduce inflammation if other interventions are unsuccessful, but steroids may weaken the collagen fibers and increase the risk of plantar fascia rupture, so they are used only sparingly. As a last-ditch option surgery may be performed to sever the plantar fascia altogether. This may eradicate pain but it also creates more instability in the foot, which can lead to problems in the rest of the body.

No single treatment is universally effective; each patient must experiment with the treatments that meet his or her own needs. It takes patience to overcome this stubborn injury; even the most successful treatment options often take up to 12 weeks to resolve injuries completely.

Massage?

Plantar fasciitis can respond well to bodywork. Massage is often suggested both to decrease tension in the deep calf muscles and to have an organizing influence on the growth of scar tissue on the plantar fascia itself.

Scleroderma

Definition: What Is It?

Scleroderma is a chronic autoimmune dysfunction in which abnormal proteins called *autoantibodies* attack and damage small arteries. This stimulates the production of excessive amounts of collagen in the skin, hence the name: *sclero* (from Greek for "hard") *–derma* (from Greek for "skin").

Demographics: Who Gets It?

Like many autoimmune diseases, scleroderma affects women more often than men; in this case the ratio is about 4 to 1. It is a relatively rare disease, affecting approximately 300,000 people in the United States. The majority of scleroderma patients are women between 35 and 54 years of age. It is rare in children and elderly people.

Etiology: What Happens?

Scleroderma is the result of an overactive immune system that launches attacks against normal tissue. In this case the tissue under attack is the lining of arterioles. Damage to these small blood vessels causes local edema and the stimulation of nearby fibroblasts to spin out huge amounts of collagen, the basis for scar tissue. Eventually the edema subsides, but the scar tissue deposits remain hard and unyielding for years. Scleroderma takes two forms: localized or systemic.

- *Localized scleroderma.* When scleroderma is localized, the areas of blood vessel damage are usually limited to the skin of the hands and face. The initial edema may last for several weeks or months, the thickening of the skin may accumulate over a course of about 3 years, and then the symptoms will gradually stabilize or even reverse.

- *Systemic scleroderma.* When scleroderma is a systemic problem, blood vessel damage occurs in the skin as with localized scleroderma but also in other organs and systems. Tissues most at risk are in the digestive tract, the heart and circulatory systems, the kidneys, lungs, and various parts of the musculoskeletal system, especially synovial membranes in joints and around tendons. When systemic scleroderma attacks the lungs, kidneys, or heart, the prognosis becomes much more serious. This disease can be fatal.

Causes

The cause of scleroderma is unknown, but several contributing factors have been identified. One of the most interesting features of this disease is that a large number of patients have accumulated "chimeric cells" in their sclerotic deposits. These are cells that contain genes not only of the patient but of someone else as well: they are usually leftover fetal cells, from pregnancies that may date from many years previously. Somehow these fetal cells, which traveled from child to mother during gestation, manage to survive in the mother, where they may stimulate an autoimmune attack many years later. When scleroderma occurs in children, men, or in women who have never had a child,

---

SCLERODERMA IN BRIEF

What is it?
Scleroderma is a chronic autoimmune disorder involving damage to small blood vessels that leads to abnormal accumulations of scar tissue in the skin. Internal organs may also be affected.

How is it recognized?
Scleroderma can have many varied symptoms, depending on which tissues are involved. The most common outward signs are edema followed by hardening and thickening of the skin, usually of the hands and face.

Is massage indicated or contraindicated?
Scleroderma may indicate massage if circulatory and kidney damage is not advanced. Clients whose systems are not capable of keeping up with the changes circulatory massage brings about may benefit from bodywork with less mechanical impact.

it is postulated that the chimeric cells may be maternal cells that traveled into the patient during gestation.

The presence of chimeric cells alone does not seem to be the only stimulus for the autoimmune activity associated with scleroderma. However, when these cells are present and a person experiences other kinds of triggers, the chance for the disease to develop is much higher. Other triggers for scleroderma involve exposure to specific chemicals, including vinyl chloride, epoxy resins, uranium, and aromatic hydrocarbons.

Signs and Symptoms

Scleroderma can produce a huge variety of symptoms, depending on which blood vessels are under attack. The term "CREST syndrome" has been coined as a mnemonic for the most common scleroderma symptoms:

C: Calcinosis refers to the accumulation of calcium deposits in the skin.
R: *Raynaud's phenomenon* is a result of impaired circulation and vascular spasm in the hands (See Chapter 3).
E: Esophageal dysmobility refers to sluggishness of the digestive tract and chronic gastric reflux.
S: Sclerodactyly is "hardening of the fingers," a result of the accumulation of scar tissue in the hands (Fig. 2-37, Color Plate 32).
T: Telangiectasia is a reddish discoloration of the skin caused by permanently stretched and damaged capillaries.

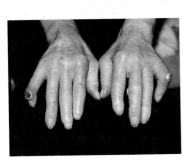

Figure 2-37. Scleroderma (CP 32)

Other symptoms of systemic scleroderma include skin ulcers where circulation prevents normal nutrition for healthy cells, changes in pigmentation, and hair loss. Muscles may become weak while tendons and tendinous sheaths become swollen. Lungs may accumulate edema where blood vessels are under attack. Heart pain, arrhythmia, and heart failure may develop as the heart tries to push blood through a system that cannot accommodate it. Kidneys, working under high blood pressure and damaged arterioles, may go into renal failure. *Trigeminal neuralgia* (Chapter 3) and Sjögren's syndrome (pathologically dry mucous membranes) may also be a part of the scleroderma picture.

Treatment

Scleroderma is typically treated by symptom. Calcium channel blockers may be recommended for Raynaud's phenomenon, diuretics for kidney function, antacids for gastric reflux, and NSAIDs for muscle and joint pain. Physical or occupational therapies are often used to maintain flexibility in the hands. Patients are usually advised to avoid smoking, cold conditions, and spicy foods to minimize symptoms.

As more research is conducted on the presence of chimeric cells in many scleroderma patients, medications may be developed to help the body recognize these "non-self" entities more efficiently and eradicate them before they can trigger significant damage.

Massage?

Scleroderma is a disease that presents very differently in each client. One person may have some stiffness and coldness in the hands, while another may be undergoing dialysis because the kidneys are failing. The decision about massage in the context of scleroderma must be made based on the client's circulatory health and resiliency. It is inappropriate to try to mechanically push fluid through a system where the blood vessels are either inflamed or severely scarred. Bodywork that does not challenge fluid flow, however, may be beneficial.

Tendinitis

Definition: What Is It?

Tendinitis involves injury and inflammation in tendinous tissues. The injury process has much in common with strains and sprains, and in fact these injuries may sometimes be difficult to delineate from each other.

Etiology: What Happens?

Tendinitis can occur anywhere in the tendon, but tears happen most frequently at the tenoperiosteal junction or the musculotendinous junction. These areas mark the shift of one tissue type into another. Although the transition may be gradual, this is still a weak point in the structure that is vulnerable to injury.

Signs and Symptoms

The symptoms of tendinitis are very similar to muscle strains although they may be more intense. The acute stage may show some heat and swelling, depending on which tendons are affected. Most tendon swelling is not visible, with a few exceptions, particularly in the Achilles tendon and the posterior tibialis tendon at the medial ankle, both of which may swell significantly with injury.

In all stages of tendinitis stiffness and pain are present on resistive movements and in stretching. It is easier to get a bad tendon tear than it is to get a bad muscle tear; muscles are much more elastic than tendons. This condition will have a more distinct acute and subacute stage than muscle strains.

Treatment

The quality of the healing of a torn tendon depends largely on what happens during the subacute and maturation phase of scar tissue development. Although the initial collagen fibers generated by the inflammatory response lie down randomly during the subacute phase of healing, weight-bearing stress and stretching will cause them to rearrange in alignment with the direction of force once the initial inflammation has subsided. A more in-depth discussion of the stages of injury is covered in *inflammation* (Chapter 5).

If an injured tendon gets too little stress during its maturation phase, the scar tissue fibers do not realign and the tendon will be permanently weakened and prone to developing adhesions to nearby structures. If the injured tendon gets *too much* use during this time it can rip again, go back into an acutely inflamed state, and accumulate excessive scar tissue. The challenge for the injured person and the health care team is to figure out how much is just the right amount of weight-bearing stress for the maximum benefit to injured tendons.

As with muscle and ligament tears, standard medical approaches to this kind of injury often focus on symptom abatement rather than scar tissue management. Unfortunately, this can create a stubborn, serious problem out of a potentially very minor one, as the un-

---

TENDINITIS IN BRIEF

What is it?
Tendinitis is inflammation of a tendon, usually due to injury at the tenoperiosteal or musculotendinous junction.

How is it recognized?
Pain and stiffness are usually present, and in acute stages palpable heat and swelling will occur. Pain is exacerbated by resisted exercise of the injured muscle-tendon unit.

Is massage indicated or contraindicated?
Tendinitis indicates massage. In the acute stage, lymph drainage techniques may help to limit and resolve inflammation. In the subacute stage, massage may influence the production of useful scar tissue, reduce adhesions and edema, and reestablish range of motion.

Tendinitis? Tendinosis? Is There a Difference?

Inflammation is not the only cause of tendon pain and weakness. A related disorder, *tendinosis*, has been labeled to describe tendons that have sustained significant damage but are no longer inflamed. Tendons with tendinosis may have significant accumulations of disorganized scar tissue and a reduction in weight-bearing strength, but the inflammatory process is no longer at work—that is, until the structure is re-injured.

Massage is frequently suggested for athletes and other patients with tendinosis to stimulate circulation and improve nutrition in the avascular connective tissue structures, as well as to help stretch and mobilize the muscles involved with the damaged tissues.

Massage and Orthopedic Injuries

Injuries of muscles, tendons, and ligaments are among the most common complaints clients may have and are among the most satisfying things massage therapists can treat. Cross fiber friction, linear friction, proprioceptive neuromuscular facilitation (PFN), lymph drainage, and dozens of other modalities have been developed to help create a healing process that is efficient and long-lasting.

The purpose of this text is to provide information about the appropriateness of massage in the context of many diseases and disorders, but *not* to give specific guidelines about exactly what modalities to use when and in what circumstances. That judgment must be made by the individual therapist, depending on his or her own bodywork skills and the needs of the client. For this reason, many orthopedic injuries are not specifically addressed in the body of the text, since they fit into the broader headings of strains, sprains, and tendinitis.

Nonetheless, it is useful to make a list of some of the most common orthopedic injuries and some reference to where they may fit in the context of massage.

Soft tissue injuries can often be identified with carefully isolated resisted contractions or passive stretches, but it must be remembered that injuries seldom happen in a vacuum: they often appear in combination with other damage. This is why it is important to accompany a massage therapist's informed opinion with a thorough diagnosis conducted by a medical professional.

resolved scar tissue weakens rather than strengthens the tendon. Fortunately, recent advancements in the understanding of how scar tissue develops have begun spreading into more mainstream applications, so the "take these painkillers and don't move it for 2 weeks" kinds of treatment strategies for soft tissue injuries are becoming less common.

Massage?

Tendinitis definitely indicates massage. Again, this condition is more serious than a simple muscle tear, and the acute phase must be respected to allow the body to begin the process of cleaning up debris and laying down new fibers in peace. Practitioners familiar with lymph drainage techniques may be able to limit the accumulation of edema and minimize scar tissue. In the subacute stage massage is valuable not only for the mechanical action it can have on badly placed collagen fibers, but for the circulatory turnover it stimulates in the area of avascular tendons.

Sprains, strains, and tendinitis all respond best to mechanical types of massage in a subacute phase as soon as the acute symptoms have passed. This is when direct manipulation can have the most profound influence over the quality of healing. The sooner it is treated, the more complete resolution a client is likely to have. Even years-old injuries respond well to massage if the circumstances are right. It may not be possible to completely reverse 10-year-old tendinitis, but for a client who has been living with pain and limitation, any improvement is better than nothing.

Tenosynovitis

Definition: What Is It?

Tenosynovitis is a situation in which tendons that pass through a synovial sheath become irritated and inflamed.

Etiology: What Happens?

Some tendons have to pass through very narrow, crowded passageways or around sharp corners to get to their bony attachments. Without any lubrication those tendons and their neighbors would soon be worn to a frazzle. They *do* have lubrication that is provided by special sheaths made of connective tissue and lined with synovial membrane: tenosynovial sheaths. As the tendon or group of tendons pass through the sheath, synovial fluid is secreted to provide lubrication and ease of movement (Fig. 2-38).

Repetitive stress, percussive movement, or constant twisting can cause the tendons inside tenosynovial sheaths to become irritated. The sheath may become inflamed and then shrink around the tendons in such a way that it inhibits

TENOSYNOVITIS IN BRIEF

What is it?
Tenosynovitis is the inflammation of a tendon and/or its surrounding tenosynovial sheath. It can happen wherever a tendon passes through a sheath but is especially common in the wrist and hand.

How is it recognized?
Pain, heat, and stiffness mark the acute stage of tenosynovitis. In the subacute stage only be stiffness and pain may be present. The tendon may feel or sound gritty as it moves through the sheath. It is difficult to bend the fingers with tenosynovitis and even harder to straighten them.

Is massage indicated or contraindicated?
Tenosynovitis contraindicates massage in the acute stage of inflammation and indicates massage when the swelling has subsided.

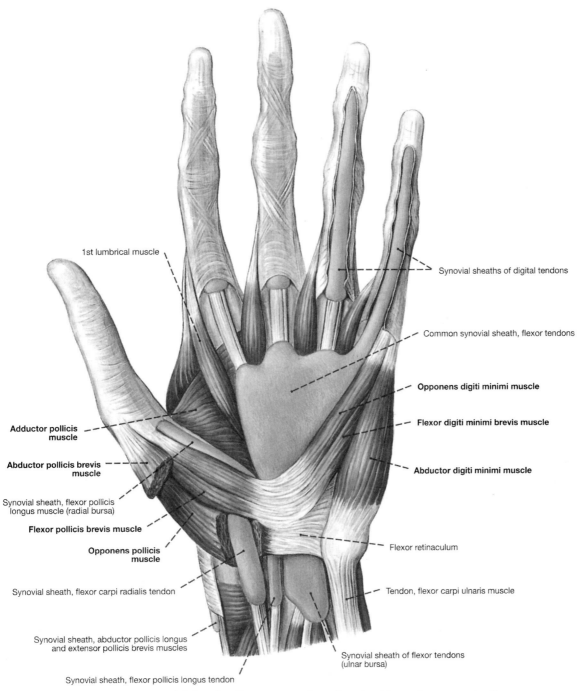

1st lumbrical muscle

Synovial sheaths of digital tendons

Common synovial sheath, flexor tendons

Opponens digiti minimi muscle

Flexor digiti minimi brevis muscle

Abductor digiti minimi muscle

Adductor pollicis muscle

Abductor pollicis brevis muscle

Synovial sheath, flexor pollicis longus muscle (radial bursa)

Flexor pollicis brevis muscle

Opponens pollicis muscle

Synovial sheath, flexor carpi radialis tendon

Synovial sheath, abductor pollicis longus and extensor pollicis brevis muscles

Synovial sheath, flexor pollicis longus tendon

Flexor retinaculum

Tendon, flexor carpi ulnaris muscle

Synovial sheath of flexor tendons (ulnar bursa)

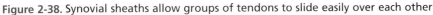

Figure 2-38. Synovial sheaths allow groups of tendons to slide easily over each other

freedom of movement. A cycle of stiffness followed by irritating movement, which creates more stiffness, pain, and inflammation, may develop.

Causes

Tenosynovitis is usually caused by trauma, repetitive movement, or excessive exercise. It can happen anywhere synovial sheaths protect tendons: the wrist, the ankle, the long head of the biceps, or near the thumb where it has a special name: *De Quervain's tenosynovitis.*

Occasionally it can be caused by a local infection that inflames the synovium, but it is usually brought about by mechanical stress. Tenosynovitis also occurs as a complication of other inflammatory wrist problems like *rheumatoid arthritis* or *fractures* (this chapter).

Signs and Symptoms

Symptoms of tenosynovitis are predictable: local pain, sometimes with swelling and heat. In the case of "trigger finger" it maybe difficult to bend the joint, and *unbending* it is even harder (excessive force must be applied to slide the tendon through its sheath, and the joint usually extends with a sudden "pop"). A grinding noise or gritty feeling called crepitus occurs when the affected joint is moved. Movement of the tendon through the sheath tends to exacerbate the problem, but lack of movement decreases the production of synovial fluid. It can be a very frustrating condition because nothing seems to make it better.

Treatment

If the synovium is inflamed because of infection, the obvious course is to treat it with antibiotics. Non-infectious tenosynovitis is typically treated with anti-inflammatory drugs, then injected with steroids, and failing that, the synovium is surgically split.

Massage?

This is an inflammatory condition, and even worse, the inflammation is confined to a very small, crowded space. This makes it counter-productive to work when the condition is hot and painful, since all massage will do is make it hotter and more swollen. During the acute phase tenosynovitis locally contraindicates massage.

When inflammation is not acute, however, massage can help to reduce inflammation, flush out toxins, and create very specific movements of structures against each other to prevent the accumulation of scar tissue and/or adhesions. Massage may not be able to solve the problem of irritation inside the synovial sheath, but it can improve the nutrition and freedom of movement available to the affected structures.

Torticollis
Definition: What Is It?

Torticollis ("wryneck") is an umbrella term for any condition that causes the head to be pulled to one side. A unilateral spasm of a neck muscle or muscles causes the head to become stuck in flexion and rotation.

Etiology: What Happens?

Torticollis can be a simple matter of having "slept funny" so that the neck is stiff and painful all day, or it could be a symptom of a more serious underlying problem.

- *Congenital torticollis.* In this situation a genetic abnormality results in the development of only one sternocleidomastoid

---

TORTICOLLIS IN BRIEF

What is it?
Torticollis is a unilateral spasm of neck muscles. It can be caused by a variety of factors, including mild musculoskeletal injury, congenital abnormalities, or central nervous system problems.

How is it recognized?
Flexion and rotation of the head are the main symptoms. The spasm may be constant or intermittent. Torticollis may also cause pain in the neck, shoulders, and back.

Is massage indicated or contraindicated?
This depends on the cause of the problem. Simple wryneck from trigger points, cervical misalignment, ligament sprain, or trauma may be appropriate for massage if no acute inflammation is present. Spasmodic torticollis patients may benefit from pain relief offered by massage, but work should be done in cooperation with the patient's health care team. If symptoms do not improve, or if signs of systemic infection are present, a more thorough diagnosis should be sought.

muscle. Because so many other muscles can rotate and flex the head, this problem may be overcome by physical therapy (Fig. 2-39).

- *Infant torticollis.* In the late stages of pregnancy the fetus may lie with the head twisted to one side. This can create a shortened or weakened sternocleidomastoid as well as cranial bone distortion. This condition is usually successfully treated with exercise and special helmets designed to reshape the cranial bones.

- *Spasmodic torticollis.* This condition is the most common type of *focal dystonia* (abnormal muscle contraction related to a central nervous system disturbance). The spasms may be tonic (sustained contractions), clonic (tremors), or both. Spasmodic torticollis affects adults, creating chronic pain in the neck, back, and shoulder. It has a slow onset that peaks within 2 to 5 years. Occasionally it spontaneously resolves but may occur again in later years.

- *Wryneck.* This is a simple stiff neck, often caused by irritation of the intertransverse ligament at C_7. A cervical misalignment may also create the problem, which will not be relieved until both the muscles and the bony alignment have been addressed. Trigger points and spasm in the splenius cervicis are another possible cause. Short-lived cases of wryneck may be brought about by sleeping in a bad position or some other event or trauma that might cause irritation in the neck muscles.

- *Other.* Torticollis can, on rare occasions, be the earliest presenting sign of a more serious condition. Cases have been documented in which it was the first symptom of bone cancer in the spine (the tumor may affect the motor and/or sensory neurons), bone infections, and even a serious infection of the adenoids (i.e., lymph nodes in the neck that can get so filled with pus that they irritate and cause spasm in the nearby muscles).

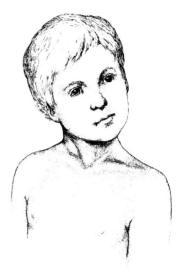

Figure 2-39. Torticollis

TORTICOLLIS
This comes from the Latin *tortus*, "twisted," and *collum*, "neck." Torticollis is a general term for a twisted neck, which its synonym, "wryneck," implies.

Signs and Symptoms

Symptoms of torticollis vary according to the predisposing causes. For specific information, refer to the types of torticollis described above.

Treatment

Treatment for torticollis depends on the underlying cause. Congenital or infantile situations call for exercise to strengthen the auxiliary muscles. For spasmodic torticollis, special drugs or even surgery to limit the spasms may be recommended. Wryneck from subluxated vertebrae can be addressed by bony manipulation. Specific frictions to the lesion may resolve wryneck caused by ligament irritation; if the scar tissue is very old and difficult to access, corticosteroid injections to limit inflammation and reduce scar tissue may be helpful. Torticollis related only to muscle spasm and trigger points responds well to massage.

Massage?

Chiropractic treatment or manipulation *with* massage for uncomplicated wryneck is a powerful combination, because both

Common Tendon Injuries

Rotator Cuff Tears
These can affect any combination of the rotator cuff muscles of the shoulder. One of the trickiest things about rotator cuff tears is that they can refer pain down the arm or even into the wrist and hand. This can make it difficult to make a clear diagnosis. Rotator cuff injuries can involve chronic tendinosis (damage to tissues without acute inflammation) or acute tendinitis. They often respond well to friction and rehabilitative exercise.

Patellar Tendinitis
This is obviously an injury to the quadriceps attachment somewhere around the patella or distally in the patellar tendon on the way to the tibia. Several things make patellar tendinitis difficult to pin down: the quadriceps are so strong that they often will not be painful with resisted contractions unless they are already fatigued; the patellar tendon is large and thick and it can be difficult to pin down exactly where the lesion has developed; and this injury is frequently misdiagnosed as PFS (this chapter). The latter can be problematic because PFS implies damage *inside* the joint capsule, whereas this condition really involves irritation *outside* the joint.

Common Tendon Injuries—
continued

Patellar tendinitis often arises in conjunction with muscular imbalances and overuse. It responds well to massage, both at the site of injury and generally around the lower extremity as the injured person works to create better balance.

Epicondylitis

This is a term that has been used to refer to irritation of either the extensors or flexors of the forearm. "Golfer's elbow" refers to flexor problems, and "tennis elbow" refers to extensor injuries. These injuries respond very well to friction and carefully gauged exercise but *will not* improve if the massage is applied to the wrong area. The greatest challenge with both flexor and extensor injuries is isolating the damaged structure and the exact site of injury.

Common Ligament Injuries

Ankle Sprains

Most ankle injuries involve rolling outward and stressing structures on the lateral side of the foot. The most commonly injured ligament in the body is the anterior talofibular ligament, which is almost always a part of lateral ankle sprains.

Ligaments are not contractile structures, so they are not isolated by muscle contractions and are not rehabilitated by exercise. Rather, friction, stretching, and gradually increasing weight-bearing stress are the interventions that work best for most ankle sprains.

If a ligament ruptures, it will be unable to stabilize its joint. This situation may require surgery to reattach the ligament and restore its ability to function.

Cruciate Ligament Sprains or Ruptures

The anterior and posterior cruciate ligaments (ACL and PCL) inside the knee joint capsule are responsible for most of the anterior-posterior stability of this massive weight-bearing joint. When they are injured, the whole joint becomes unstable and susceptible to further injury.

Cruciate ligament sprains break the pattern of most orthopedic injuries: they do not benefit from immediate mobilization and are not accessible for friction or other hands-on therapies. Instead, these injuries often require arthroscopic surgery to repair the damage, followed by physical therapy to limit scar tissue and restore function. Massage can be useful in the postsurgical recovery period but will have no access to an untreated cruciate ligament injury.

the hard and soft tissues receive the attention they need. Nevertheless, torticollis can be an early symptom of some other more serious problems, so if the client is not improving or if he or she is showing any other signs of infection, a more complete diagnosis is necessary.

Whiplash
Definition: What Is It?

Whiplash or cervical acceleration-deceleration (CAD) is a broad term used to refer to a mixture of injuries, including sprains, strains, and joint trauma. Bone fractures, herniated discs, and concussion are commonly seen along with these soft tissue injuries and so are often addressed simultaneously. Whiplash injuries are usually, but not always, associated with car accidents in which the head "whips" backward and forward in rapid succession (Fig. 2-40).

Etiology: What Happens?

The nature of damage incurred by whiplash accidents depends on many variables, including the direction of impact, the speed with which the vehicles were moving, the relative weight of the vehicles involved, whether the individual was wearing a seatbelt, the position of the individual's head, and whether the individual was aware of the impending impact and had time to brace. Analysis of rear-impact accidents shows that the initial movement of the head is into extension, as the momentum of the car seat forces the thorax forward while the head initially stays stable. Then energy is magnified by the leverage of the neck to increase the forward-moving acceleration of the head. At an impact of 20 mph the maximum acceleration of the head has been measured at 12 G![n]

Accidents of this nature put the cervical muscles (especially the sternocleidomastoid, scalenes, and splenius cervicis) at risk (see *strains*, this chapter). Spinal ligaments may also be damaged (see *sprains*, this chapter). Two ligaments that massage cannot touch are also frequently traumatized: the anterior and the posterior longitudinal ligaments. However, the supraspinous and the intertransverse ligaments are commonly injured ligaments that *are* accessible. Other structures that may be injured with CAD include the esophagus and larynx; spinal discs that may herniate or rupture; vertebrae that can come out of alignment or fracture; the TMJ; the spinal cord, which may get stretched and then become edematous; and the brain, which can become bruised and damaged in concussion.

[n]Mahar R. Musculotendinous injuries of the neck. Summer, 1987. Available at: http://www.theberries.ns.ca/Archives/Whiplash.html. Accessed fall 2000.

Signs and Symptoms

A great deal of crossover exists between what may be considered a symptom of whiplash and what is a complication, or resulting disorder. The following list includes both:

- *Ligament sprains.* The supraspinous and intertransverse ligaments that connect the vertebrae to each other are very vulnerable to injury in a whiplash type of accident. These ligaments can refer pain up over the head, into the chest, and down the arms. It is important to know about these structures because referred pain from ligaments can often be misdiagnosed as pain from nerve damage.

  Ligament sprains often take a long time to heal and tend to accumulate a great amount of excess scar tissue. They may be the most common cause of lasting pain and dysfunction when a whiplash injury occurs.

- *Misaligned cervical vertebrae.* This is generally shown clearly on a radiograph. Vertebrae may be displaced to the front, back, side, or rotated one way or another. In some very extreme cases fractures may occur. Left untreated or incompletely treated, misaligned vertebrae with lax ligaments and lack of structural support may develop *spondylosis* (this chapter).

- *Herniated disc.* This is not inevitable, but it frequently happens that the neck ligaments are so stressed in a trauma of this force that the annulus cracks too, allowing the nucleus pulposus to seep into spaces where it does not belong. Car wrecks

WHIPLASH IN BRIEF:

What is it?
Whiplash is an umbrella term referring to a collection of soft tissue injuries that may occur with cervical acceleration/deceleration. These injuries include sprained ligaments, strained muscles, damaged cartilage and joint capsules, and TMJ problems. Although whiplash technically refers to soft tissue injury, damage to other structures including vertebrae, discs, and the central nervous system frequently occurs at the same time.

How is it recognized?
Symptoms of whiplash vary according to the nature of the injuries. Pain at the neck and referring into the shoulders and arms along with chronic headaches are the primary indicators.

Is massage indicated or contraindicated?
An acute whiplash injury contraindicates circulatory or mechanically based massage. In the subacute and mature phases of scar tissue formation, however, massage along with chiropractic treatment or manipulation can contribute greatly to a positive resolution of the problem.

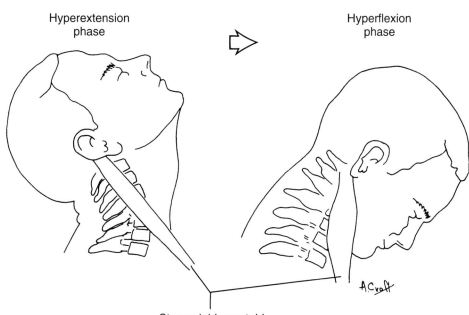

Hyperextension phase

Hyperflexion phase

Sternocleidomastoid

Figure 2-40. Cervical acceleration-deceleration whiplash

Common Joint Injuries

Meniscus Tears

The menisci are mobile pieces of cartilage that help track the femur on top of the tibia. Occasionally they can crack, tear, fragment, or otherwise sustain damage. This situation requires surgery to remove loose bits of cartilage before joint surfaces become rough and arthritic. Because they are inside the joint capsule, massage therapists have no access to meniscus injuries. Massage can be beneficial in the postsurgical recovery period, however.

Acromial Clavicular (AC) Joint

The gliding joint where the clavicle meets the acromion of the scapula is a vulnerable spot because it is subject to bumps, falls, and other trauma. When the joint is inflamed, movement at the shoulder is limited and painful. AC joint problems often respond well to friction followed by ice to limit inflammation.

Frozen Shoulder (Adhesive Capsulitis)

This disorder involves the synovial joint capsule at the glenohumeral joint. Often precipitated by some other inflammatory problem (bursitis or tendinitis), the joint capsule gradually adheres to the articulating bones, causing pain, inflammation, and loss of range of motion. The onset is usually gradual. It will often spontaneously resolve without intervention, although it may leave a permanent loss of range of motion at the joint. Physical therapy is often recommended for persons with frozen shoulder to minimize and reverse the adhesive process; massage can fit into this context as well.

and other major traumas of this type are the easiest way to cause a herniation in the cervical region (this chapter).

- *Spasm.* In the acute stage the paraspinals and other neck muscles go into spasm to "splint" or give extra support to the stretched neck ligaments. This reaction has a tendency to outlive its usefulness. Spasm of neck muscles also significantly limits range of motion and blood flow to nearby connective tissues.

- *Trigger points.* Traumatized muscles often develop trigger points, that is, localized tight areas that refer pain, often into the head, causing chronic headaches.

- *Neurological symptoms.* These can include dizziness, blurred vision, abnormal smell or taste, tinnitus (ringing in the ears), or loss of hearing. These signs indicate cranial trauma: the brain has been bruised and may have some internal bleeding. This is usually the result of a specific blow (e.g., hitting the head on the steering wheel), but postconcussion syndrome can also happen without direct impact.

- *TMJ disorders.* Direct impact of the jaw on a steering wheel or dashboard can obviously damage the TMJ, but some research suggests that the joint can be traumatized just by the rapid acceleration/deceleration that accompanies whiplash injuries. TMJ disorders (this chapter) often go unaddressed until the more critical, acute aspects of whiplash have passed.

- *Headaches.* These arise for a variety of reasons, including but not limited to referred pain and trigger points from spasmed muscles in the neck, sprained ligaments that refer pain up over the head, cranial bones that may be out of alignment, stress and its autonomic action on blood flow and muscle tightness in the neck and head, TMJ problems, and concussion (see Chapter 3).

Diagnosis

Some assumptions can be made about which precise structures have been injured based on whether the car wreck was a direct head-on or a rear-end collision. However, these assumptions do not hold true if the collision occurred at any kind of angle or if the patient's head was turned in any direction at the moment of impact.

Techniques that are currently available to measure the extent of injury (e.g., MRI, radiographs, CT scans, nerve conduction velocity tests) are extremely valuable for evaluating one particular type of whiplash damage: direct, mechanical nerve pressure. Pressure on a nerve causes "radicular pain," that is, pain that radiates directly along the distribution of the affected nerve. Care must be taken, however, to delineate between what these tests show and what patients report. MRIs or radiographs frequently show signs that actually do not create symptoms for the patient.

Unfortunately, much of the pain associated with whiplash injuries is *not* radicular pain, but referred pain brought about by trauma to connective tissue and muscle tissue that feed into the same nerve root as the associated spinal nerve. This type of damage is much harder to quantify. It is best evaluated with good palpation skills that reveal information about localized tenderness, muscle spasm, and trigger point activity.

Treatment

Neck collars are used for acute whiplash patients to take the stress off their wrenched ligaments and to try to reduce muscle spasm. The sooner the injured structures are put back to use, the less scar tissue accumulates. Therefore, collars are strictly for short-term use, as this kind of immobilization can create more long-term problems than benefits.

Further treatment for whiplash depends on the type and severity of the specific injuries. It has been noted that a majority of whiplash patients recover completely within 1 year, but anywhere from 5 to 20% may have long-lasting pain. It is difficult to assess whether this disability is from unresolved injury, psychological stress associated with long-term injury, or other factors. The fact that much of the pain generated by whiplash injuries is difficult to measure makes this a condition that is easy to take advantage of by patients willing to "work the system" for financial gain, and easy to discount by health care professionals and insurers who become frustrated with patients' slow recovery.

Massage?

The acute stage of this injury contraindicates mechanical massage. This is an important phase of healing that massage therapists must not disrupt. Gentle reflexive work with the intention of balancing the autonomic nervous system rather than making changes in the tissue may ameliorate the emotional trauma and shock such an injury often incurs. As long as it does not disrupt the cellular activity at the site of the injury, this type of work is a fine idea.

If it has been established that no other serious disorder (such as a herniated disc or spinal fracture) is present, chiropractic treatment or manipulation alone can be sufficient to undo the damage done to the cervical vertebrae in a whiplash injury. If muscle spasm is not addressed, bony adjustments are difficult to perform and probably will not hold for long because the muscles will simply pull the bones out of alignment again. Furthermore, in the absence of the circulation that can be stimulated by massage, the injured ligaments have little access to nutrition. They tend to accumulate masses of scar tissue that bind to other ligaments and other muscles sheaths, thus turning a temporary loss of range of motion into a permanent one.

CASE HISTORY: WHIPLASH
Client X: The Sneezer

A massage therapist met with a first-time client approximately 1 year after the client had been involved in a car accident. The client was still in considerable pain. He was diagnosed with whiplash and was seeking massage under prescription from his doctor.

The therapist worked slowly and carefully and was encouraged by the client to go deeper into his neck muscles, all the way down to the transverse processes of the neck vertebrae. He felt better after the massage; his muscles were looser and he had an improved range of motion.

Several hours later, the client sneezed. The force of the motion wrenched his neck and re-injured the tissues so that he was in greater pain, more spasm, and had much less range of motion than he had *before* his massage. He returned for another session, but it was ineffective at reducing his pain and dysfunction. He never sought massage again.

What is the moral here? It is utterly unclear whether the first massage put the client at risk of re-injuring himself just by sneezing. The therapist followed all the rules of good sense, worked under medical supervision, and let the client guide her into how much pressure felt comfortable to receive. Yet, it is necessary to entertain the possibility that the massage somehow *did* put the client at risk, even though the therapist was well-informed and made what seemed to be the right decisions. The point is that no two people will go through the same kind of healing process, and no two people will respond to massage the same way. Massage therapists must weigh the benefits and risks of their work on a case-by-case basis. It is impossible to rely only on books and rules to make decisions about whether to give massage.

Chiropractic or manipulative therapy *with* massage can yield good results, blending the best of soft tissue work (to prevent or reduce muscle spasm, scar tissue accumulation, adhesions, fibrosis, and ischemia) with the best of bony alignment. It is not unusual for someone to emerge from whiplash recovery consisting of this kind of care in better shape than before they began.

Neuromuscular Disorders

CARPAL TUNNEL SYNDROME IN BRIEF

What is it?
Carpal tunnel syndrome (CTS) is irritation of the median nerve as it passes under the transverse carpal ligament into the wrist. It can have several causes.

How is it recognized?
CTS can cause pain, tingling, numbness, and weakness in the part of the hand supplied by the median nerve. Pain may also radiate proximally up the forearm.

Is massage indicated or contraindicated?
Depending on the underlying factors, some CTS cases may respond well to massage. The massage therapist should work on or around the wrist and stop immediately if any symptoms are elicited. A medical diagnosis is necessary to know which type of CTS is present.

Carpal Tunnel Syndrome
Definition: What Is It?

CTS is a set of signs and symptoms brought about by the entrapment of the median nerve between the carpal bones of the wrist and the transverse carpal ligament that holds down the flexor tendons (Fig. 2-41). The median nerve supplies sensation to the thumb, forefinger, middle finger, and half of the ring finger (Fig. 2-42) If it is caught or squeezed in any way, it can create symptoms in the part of the hand the nerve supplies.

Demographics: Who Gets It?

It is estimated that CTS affects up to 1% of the U.S. population and up to 10% of people older than 40 years of age. Up to 1 million surgeries for this condition are performed every year.

As the physical demands of many occupations have changed over the past few decades, many jobs have become more specialized. Fewer movements are needed to accomplish assigned tasks, but those movements may be performed several thousand times a day. This is true for persons who have manufacturing jobs and for persons working on computers, cash registers, and assembly lines. The National Institute for Occupational Safety and Health reports that the incidence of CTS in job-related settings increased by 300% between 1982 and 1992.[°]

CTS is an occupational hazard for massage practitioners and anyone else who performs repetitive movements for several hours every day: people who work with keyboards, string musicians, bakers, and check-out clerks. Women with CTS outnumber men by about 3 to 1; this may be because their carpal tunnels are smaller to begin with, and thus less irritation can cause symptoms.

Etiology: What Happens?

Pressure on the median nerve may arise from several sources. To develop a treatment strategy (and to assess the appropriateness of massage), the aggravating factors must be

---

[°]NIOSH facts: Carpal tunnel syndrome. National Institute of Occupational Safety and Health. June, 1997. Document no. 705001. Available at: http://www.cdc.gov/niosh/ctsfs.html. Accessed fall 2000.

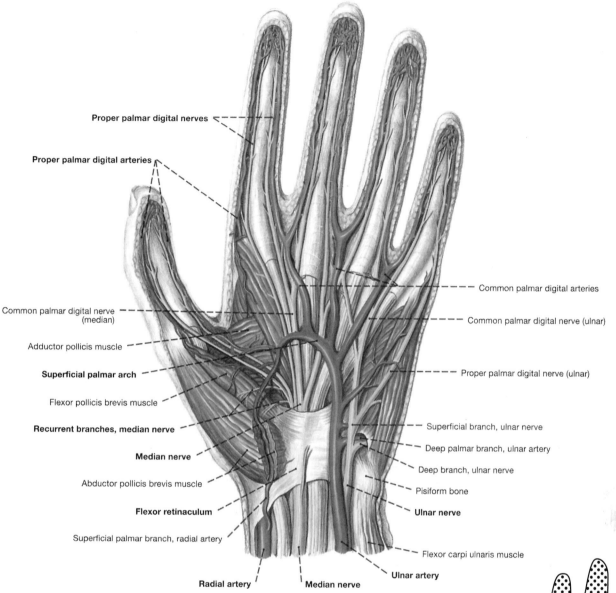

Proper palmar digital nerves

Proper palmar digital arteries

Common palmar digital nerve (median)

Adductor pollicis muscle

Superficial palmar arch

Flexor pollicis brevis muscle

Recurrent branches, median nerve

Median nerve

Abductor pollicis brevis muscle

Flexor retinaculum

Superficial palmar branch, radial artery

Radial artery   **Median nerve**

Common palmar digital arteries

Common palmar digital nerve (ulnar)

Proper palmar digital nerve (ulnar)

Superficial branch, ulnar nerve

Deep palmar branch, ulnar artery

Deep branch, ulnar nerve

Pisiform bone

Ulnar nerve

Flexor carpi ulnaris muscle

Ulnar artery

Figure 2-41. The carpal tunnel is formed by the transverse carpal ligament (flexor retinaculum) and the carpal bones

determined. The following are some possible causes and their basic medical treatment strategies:

- *Edema.* Fluid retention, which is common for overweight people as well as menopausal and pregnant women, creates extra pressure in an area where there's no room to spare. The wrist is particularly susceptible because of its normal gravitational position; it is easy for fluid to pool here. CTS due to edema is usually bilateral and is quite common. It is most often treated with diuretics or other methods designed to help get rid of excess fluid.

- *Subluxation.* Sometimes the carpal bones, especially the capitate bone in the center of the distal row of carpal bones, subluxate toward the palmar side. This can put mechanical pressure on the median nerve which cannot be relieved by diuretics, anti-inflammatories, or any other drugs. This type of CTS is almost always

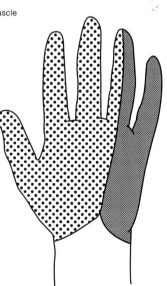

Figure 2-42. Carpal tunnel syndrome affects the thumb, index finger, middle finger, and half of the ring finger

unilateral. Manipulation is the treatment of choice, although the bones often move back into place without intervention. Waiting for that to happen can be something of a gamble, however, because the longer the irritation goes on, the higher the chances of sustaining nerve damage, and the less likely it is that the problem will spontaneously resolve.

- *Fibrotic build-up.* This is the most common variety of CTS. The human body simply was not designed to perform the same movements for 8 hours a day, 5 days a week. In an attempt to keep up with demands, the body tends to *hypertrophy*, or grow bigger and thicker wherever it is used most. This is true of muscles and bones, and it also happens with the tendons and synovial sheaths at the wrist. If they thicken because of overuse, they can press on anything soft trying to get through tiny "tunnel" formed by the carpal bones, namely, the median nerve. The transverse carpal ligament may also swell with chronic irritation, adding to the pressure on the median nerve.

  Treatment of this situation often begins with a wrist splint: the goal is to keep the carpal tunnel in a neutral position (in which it is as open as possible) and to require less work from the supportive tissues. Steroidal or nonsteroidal anti-inflammatory drugs may be prescribed. Corticosteroid injections into the wrist may also be recommended to reduce inflammation and melt excess connective tissue. If the ligaments surrounding the wrist have become loose enough to allow nearby structures to become irritated, proliferant injections may be recommended to tighten them.

  Treatment for CTS due to fibrotic build-up culminates with surgery: the transverse carpal ligament is split, and some of the accumulated connective tissue is scraped away. Innovations in endoscopic surgery techniques allow surgeons to use tiny incisions and pencil-thin cameras to cut through the transverse ligament from the inside of the carpal tunnel without opening the rest of the tissues of the hand. This allows for a much shorter recovery time and a reduced risk of fresh scar tissue accumulation that would lead to a recurrence of symptoms.

CTS is one of several conditions brought about by repetitive stress (i.e., repetitive stress injuries [RSIs]). The physical stress of repeating the same movements hour after hour, day after day is one part of this picture, but nutritional deficiencies, poor alignment, fatigue, and the resulting risk for trauma and accidents are also contributing factors.

Signs and Symptoms

Depending on the source and severity of the problem, CTS can manifest as tingling, pins and needles, burning, shooting pains, intermittent numbness, and weakness as innervation to the hand muscles is interrupted. The thenar pad may flatten out as the thumb muscles atrophy from lack of nerve stimulation. It is often worse at night when a person may sleep on the arm or turn the wrist into awkward positions. It can be painful enough to wake someone out of a deep sleep. Logically it should not, but often it does involve pain going proximally *up* the forearm from the wrist. (Nerves generally only refer distally.) If pressure is taken off the nerve promptly, no long-term symptoms may persist. The worst-case scenario involves permanent damage to the median nerve, resulting in some loss of muscle function and sensation in the hand.

Diagnosis

CTS is generally diagnosed by the description of symptoms and two simple tests. *Tinel's test* involves tapping on the wrist while the hand is extended. *Phalen's maneuver* involves holding the wrist in flexion for 2 minutes or more to see if symptoms occur in this position. These are often followed by a nerve conduction test that measures the speed of nerve impulses passing through the wrist into the hand. Unfortunately, nerve conduction tests can be inaccurate up to 20% of the time.

Doctors also look for underlying conditions that can contribute to nerve pain in the hands, specifically hypothyroidism, diabetes, pregnancy, and obesity. Any of these factors may cause pain and irritation of the median nerve but they will not be relieved with standard CTS interventions. It is important to get a very solid diagnosis before attempting to treat this problem because several other disorders can cause similar problems.

Many factors can cause pain or reduced sensation in the wrist and hand. The possibilities include but are not limited to the following:

- *Neck injuries.* Herniated discs and irritated neck ligaments refer pain distally. The worse the irritation, the further the pain refers.

- *Shoulder injuries.* Some rotator cuff tendons also refer pain down the arm. The worse the injury, the further it refers. Again, *really* bad shoulder injuries can actually cause pain in the wrist and hand.

- *Thoracic outlet syndrome.* Nerve and vascular entrapment at the pectoralis minor and/or scalenes can create pain in the wrist.

- *Other wrist injuries.* These can include osteoarthritis, rheumatoid arthritis, tendinitis, and ligament sprains, all of which can cause pain in the wrist and hand, and none of which are affected by any standard treatments for CTS.

The difficult thing about CTS is that injuries often run in combinations. In other words, wrist and hand pain can be caused by any blending of real CTS factors and factors that mimic CTS, but which do not respond to typical CTS remedies or interventions.

Treatment

The treatment options for CTS depend entirely on the causes. Treatments may range from vitamin therapy to bony manipulation to surgery. (For more details, review *causes* in this section.)

Various kinds of CTS and other nerve impairment problems often respond well to acupuncture. The National Institute of Health has conducted studies that come to the conclusion that acupuncture is a useful adjunct treatment for this and other nerve conduction disorders.[p] If a client is not getting relief through other noninvasive methods and is reluctant to consider surgery, acupuncture may be a viable alternative.

Massage?

The appropriateness of massage absolutely depends on which kind of CTS the client has, and that determination is not a massage therapist's job. So what can a responsible therapist do? He or she can work conservatively, check with the client's health care team, and monitor results. Edematous CTS responds well to massage that focuses on draining the forearm. Fibrotic CTS may improve with massage, depending on the thickness and location of the fibrosis. CTS due to a subluxation *may* respond to massage and traction, but wrist adjustments are *not* in the scope of practice of massage.

If work on or around the wrist creates any symptoms, work must stop immediately! If, on the other hand, a client experiences some improvement, the therapist may be on the

[p]Packer-Tursman J. Treatment of choice. Special to The Washington Post. October 17, 2000:Z35. Available at: http://www.washingtonpost.com/wp-dyn/articles/A21028-2000Oct17.html. Accessed fall 2000.

right track. One should proceed slowly, have a clear image of what needs to be accomplished, and work with a doctor for a definitive diagnosis.

Herniated Disc

Definition: What Is It?

A herniated disc is an intervertebral disc in which the soft nucleus pulposus or the annulus fibrosis extend beyond their normal borders. If the disc puts pressure on the spinal cord or spinal nerve roots, pain will be present. If the bulge does not interfere with nerve tissue, no symptoms may be present.

Etiology: What Happens?

A typical intervertebral disc is a complex package. It has an outer wrapping of very tough, hard material called the *annulus fibrosis* that envelopes a soft, gelatinous center called the *nucleus pulposus*. Ideally, the shape of the nucleus should be roughly spherical, with the harder annulus layers forming flat surfaces above and below the ball. This combination of textures gives the disc the advantages of strength and resiliency, which it needs to do its job of separating and cushioning the vertebrae (Fig. 2-43). The spine is capable of bearing a great deal of weight, partly thanks to this arrangement of the discs.

The outer ring of annulus fibrosis is an arrangement of concentric circles of collagen fibers. These fibers are arranged in such a way that the tighter they are pulled, the stronger they become. On the other hand, the closer the vertebrae, the looser (and weaker) the collagen fibers. This has great implications for the nucleus pulposus, which relies on a very tight, solid exterior wall for support.

The annulus fibrosis is very strong, but studies show that it starts to degenerate at about 25 years. It can sustain multitudes of micro-traumas, but they all contribute to setting the stage for future trouble. At the same time, the nucleus pulposus tends to shrink and dry with age. By the time most people are in their 50s, the nuclei of their discs are no longer soft and

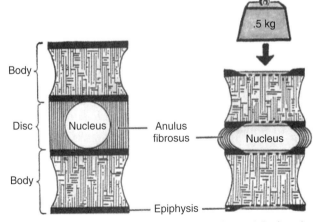

Figure 2-43. Intervertebral discs increase the weight-bearing capacity of the spine

gelatinous; they have hardened and thinned. This process begins in the neck where the discs are thinner, but eventually also affects the more massive lumbar discs.

When the nucleus pulposus protrudes through a hole or crack in the annulus (the hernia), it can press on nerve tissue and cause very severe problems. This scenario is generally the case for people younger than 45 to 50 years of age. For older people the annulus itself may crack and exert pressure on nerve tissue. Of course, if these protrusions do not press on nerve roots or the spinal cord, no symptoms may develop.

Causes

Causes of disc injury may vary according to the general health of the connective tissues of the person involved. For some people it takes a major trauma like a car accident to damage the tissues enough to cause pain. For people with weak, loose intervertebral ligaments, the spine is less stable and the risk of disc damage from ordinary everyday activity is higher. The classic scenario for this kind of disc damage is an incident that involves simultaneous lifting and twisting.

Progression

When an intervertebral disc is injured and puts pressure on nerve tissue, it is often because of a certain sequence of events on top of a lifetime of normal wear and tear. Here is a typical example of how a lumbar disc may herniate:

- A person bends over to pick up something heavy (e.g., a basket full of laundry). Going into trunk flexion flattens the anterior portion of the nucleus and opens up a posterior space while stretching the posterior fibers of the annulus.

- The person jerks into an erect posture, possibly twisting at the same time, while carrying a heavy load. Suddenly coming back into extension, especially while carrying something heavy, quickly redistributes the nucleus and shoots it into that posterior space with great force.

- The protruding section of nucleus presses against the weakest part of the posterior annulus and breaks through, which then puts pressure on nerve roots. Or, the force of the motion, combined with the brittleness of the annulus, causes the annulus to crack and put pressure on nerve tissue.

Many variations may develop on this theme. Discs that cause pain usually bulge posterolaterally, because that is the path of least resistance in the tight space they inhabit, but they can also go to the left or the right side (Fig. 2-44). A "mushroom" disc may bulge in both directions. Occasionally a disc bulges directly posteriorly, which puts pressure on the spinal cord if it is in the neck or the cauda equina in the lumbar spine. This is a very serious situation that can lead to permanent damage. However, the protrusion is usually on nerve roots rather than the spinal cord, and the amount of herniated material is very small. It dries up and takes pressure off the nerve roots within a few days or weeks. This leaves the disc permanently thinned but does not necessarily lead to long-lasting problems.

L4 and L5 herniations are the most common with the kind of lifting or lifting-and-twisting injury that has been described here. Cervical herniations are a common problem for car crash survivors; the action of a *whiplash* (this chapter) can be very similar to the injury described above. Thoracic herniations are possible but rarer since the ribs make the thoracic spine much more stable than its cervical and lumbar counterparts.

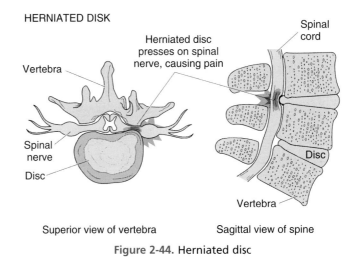

Figure 2-44. Herniated disc

It will not make a great deal of difference to the applicability of massage to specific cases, but it is useful to be able to recognize the terminology for different types of disc problems that may turn up in a diagnosis.

- *Bulge.* This refers to a situation in which the entire disc protrudes beyond the normal boundaries of the vertebral body.

- *Protrusion.* In this case the nucleus pulposus extends out of the annulus at a specific location. If it protrudes posterolaterally, it will tend to put pressure on nerve roots. If it protrudes straight back, it could put pressure on the spinal cord or cauda equina.

- *Extrusion.* This is a protrusion of a small piece of the nucleus with a narrow connection back to the body of the nucleus. In some cases the protrusion can separate from the nucleus altogether.

- *Rupture.* The nucleus pulposus has burst and leaked its entire contents into the surrounding area. Ruptures are less painful than other disc problems, because the pressure has been removed from the nerve tissue.

Signs and Symptoms

Discs have no direct nerve or blood supply, so the only symptoms they elicit are from the pressure that they put on surrounding ligaments and nerve fibers. The pressure can come and go as the patient's position and alignment shifts; thus, the symptoms may be intermittent. This is very important: it is appropriate to work with a herniated disc client when their symptoms are abated, but it is *not* appropriate to work when the affected disc is irritated and painful. Symptoms of an acute situation include:

- *Local and radicular pain.* Pain is felt locally from inflammation and ligament irritation as well as along the dermatome for the affected nerve roots. A dermatome chart is a critical piece of equipment for a massage therapist working with this population.

- *Specific muscle weakness.* It is important to clarify the difference between *general* weakness, which occurs after a period of disuse or injury to whole muscle areas, and *specific* weakness, which occurs fairly quickly and *only in the muscles supplied by the affected nerve.*

- *Paresthesia.* Tingling or "pins and needles." It happens along the affected dermatomes.

- *Reduced sensation.* This is sensation that is impaired but not completely absent. Reduced sensation is also a common symptom of ligament damage (which may frequently accompany disc damage).

- *Numbness.* Total numbness is one distinguishing factor between disc problems and ligament injuries. A disc protrusion can completely cut off sensation to areas within a particular dermatome.

Diagnosis

A definitive diagnosis is important for herniated discs because many of the signs and symptoms listed above may be caused by other disorders entirely. Many neurologists agree that herniated discs account for less than 2% of all neck and back pain.

Treatment

The best resolution for a herniated disc is for the bulging nucleus pulposus to be reabsorbed into the center of the disc and for the annulus to close down behind it. Chiropractors and osteopathic physicians work to correct bony alignment to create a maximum of space for the nucleus to retreat. Medical doctors recommend strict bed rest for the same reason. Traction may be used if warranted. Physical therapy and special classes on correct posture and body mechanics are often recommended to people recovering from disc problems. Drugs prescribed for herniated discs (muscle relaxants and painkillers) are intended to deal with the tendency for muscles to seize up in response to this kind of trauma. If nothing else is working, cortisone is sometimes injected into the area. This powerful anti-inflammatory helps only about half the time and is often considered the last resort before surgery.

If bed rest does not help and the protrusion does not run its course of drying up and disintegrating, it may be necessary to consider other kinds of intervention. One option is called *chemonucleolysis.* This procedure involves injecting a preparation of papain, an enzyme from papayas that dissolves proteins (it is also used in meat tenderizer) into the disc. This material reduces the size of the protrusion, takes pressure off the nerve tissue, and so restores the patient to a pain-free state without major surgery. *Transcutaneous diskectomies,* the removal of disc material through a tiny incision, are sometimes also possible. Open surgery is generally recommended, however, when the disc is putting pressure directly on the spinal cord. In this procedure a portion of the posterior arch of the vertebra is cut, and the protruding part of the disc is removed, along with the rest of the nucleus pulposus. Another surgical option is to fuse the affected vertebrae together. This certainly increases stability at the spot, but may lead to hypermobility at the joints above and below the fusion as they compensate for the loss of motion at the fused joint. Hypermobility then increases the risk of future herniations at the joints above and below the site of the original problem.

Massage?

Most people with herniated discs have good days and bad days. They should not receive massage on bad days. On good days, the therapist should work with the intention of creating space for the retreat of the bulging tissue. Referred pain and muscle spasms always accompany this condition. Compensation patterns that develop with chronic back pain also demand attention.

It is especially important not to work alone with a herniated disc. Muscle spasm can serve an important protective function for newly damaged discs, and releasing it too soon may put a client in danger (see *spasms*, *cramps*, this chapter). Working with another professional who can handle the bony and/or medical end of it will help the client get better faster and more completely than her or she would have by working with either professional alone.

WATCH FOR THIS

Is It Really a Herniated Disc?

Herniated discs are generally diagnosed through a combination of radiographs, CT scans, myelograms, and MRIs. It is important to arrive at a clear diagnosis, because similar symptoms may be exhibited by three other conditions that require vastly different treatment: *spondylosis* (this chapter), ligament *sprains* (this chapter), and, infrequently, bone tumors.

Spondylosis may lead to osteophytes that can put direct pressure on nerve tissue.

Irritated spinal ligaments running between spinous or transverse processes can refer pain along the same dermatomes as the nearby discs. Ligament sprains do *not* cause total numbness or specific muscle weakness, however, and they respond well to specific types of massage (see *sprains*, this chapter).

Bone tumors, by far the least common of these options, may involve growths in the spine that put mechanical pressure on nerve roots in much the same way as bulging discs.

Individuals seeking a definitive diagnosis for their back, neck, arm, and/or leg pain may be frustrated by the fact that spondylosis, herniated discs, and irritated spinal ligaments may all exist simultaneously and in any combination. The following are some basic guidelines for sorting out the most common sources of pain.

FEATURES	HERNIATED DISC	SPONDYLOSIS	LIGAMENT IRRITATION
Best diagnostic tool	MRI to see soft tissue distortion	Radiograph or CT scan for bony definition	A skilled clinical exam to identify areas of injury
When the person coughs or sneezes . . .	Symptoms are elicited	Symptoms do not change	Symptoms do not change
Factors that make it worse	Sitting for long periods, flexion of the spine	Extension of the spine	Standing, twisting movements
Pattern of weakness	Specific muscle weakness in the muscles supplied by the affected nerve root	Specific muscle weakness in the muscles supplied by the affected nerve root	General muscle weakness may gradually appear if the situation is present for a prolonged period
Pattern of pain	Shooting electrical pain along dermatome, numbness, reduced sensation, paresthesia; may be intermittent as the disc changes shape and size	Same symptoms as with a herniated disc are dependably elicited when the spine is in a position that lets osteophytes press on nerve tissue	Pain (usually not electrical) along dermatome, reduced sensation, paresthesia

Myasthenia Gravis
Definition: What Is It?

In 1890 a German doctor named Welhelm Erb documented several patients with a "grave muscular weakness." This was the first written reference to what is now called myasthenia gravis. MG is an autoimmune disease that involves the degeneration or destruction of specific receptor sites at neuromuscular junctions. It is a progressive disease but is usually manageable with the right kinds of intervention.

Demographics: Who Gets It?

Although MG has been diagnosed in babies as young as 1 and in adults as old as 80, it is seen most often in women in their 20s and men in their 50s. It affects approximately 14 of every 100,00 people, and anywhere from 24,000 to 36,000 Americans live with this condition.

Etiology: What Happens?

MG is one of the best-understood autoimmune diseases. In learning about this condition, we have come to a much clearer understanding of the chemistry of muscular contractions. Before we examine the disease process, however, it will be worthwhile to review how nerves normally work with muscles.

Anatomy Review: The Neuromuscular Junction   Every motor neuron contacts its muscle cell at a specialized area on the cell membrane called the motor end plate. At this junction, a chemical called *acetylcholine* is released from the motor neuron. Acetylcholine moves across the synaptic cleft onto specialized receptor sites within the motor end plate. This depolarizes the muscle cell membrane, allowing sodium ions to move into the cell, and calcium and potassium to move out. This process initiates muscular contraction. Acetylcholine, a neurotransmitter associated with increased excitability, is a key player in the lightning-fast cascade of events that translates electrical stimulation into chemical reactions and muscle contraction.

Autoimmune Response: Two Theories   Two theories have developed about the origins of the autoimmune reactions that lead to MG. One states that B-cells trained in the thymus are inappropriately sensitized against acetylcholine receptor sites on motor end plates. This causes the production of antibodies that attack the sites, reducing their efficiency or blocking them altogether. The fact that the thymus gland of people with MG is abnormal up to 90% of the time points to this possibility. Thymic abnormalities usually involve hypertrophic thymuses or the growth of benign tumors ("thymomas") that are easily removed.

Another theory behind the development of MG is that the immune system simply misinterprets the target tissue, in this case, acetylcholine receptor sites, as "non-self." This kind of autoimmune mistake is usually made after exposure to some pathogen with a protein coat pattern similar to the target tissue. Some evidence has been found that exposure to the *herpes simplex* (Chapter 1) virus can lead to MG.

In either case, molecular studies of affected motor endplates reveals that acetylcholine receptors are impaired or completely disabled in MG patients. This means that the muscle cell cannot be stimulated by its motor neuron.

MYASTHENIA GRAVIS IN BRIEF

What is it?
Myasthenia gravis (MG) is a neuromuscular disorder in which an autoimmune attack is launched against acetylcholine receptors at the neuromuscular junction. This makes it difficult to stimulate a muscle to contract, leading to fatigue and weakness.

What does it look like?
MG can develop at any age, but is most common in women in their 20s and in men in their 50s. It often begins with weakness in facial muscles and in the muscles used in speaking, eating, and swallowing. MG is a progressive disease but is usually treatable with medical intervention.

Is massage indicated or contraindicated?
Massage can be appropriate for persons with MG, because this disease does not affect sensation. Massage may not affect acetylcholine uptake in any positive way but it will not make it worse. Care must be taken to respect the side effects that accompany medications used to treat MG.

Signs and Symptoms

Most people with MG report weakness and fatigability in affected muscles. The process begins most often around the eyes or lower face. Early signs include a flattened smile, droopy eyelids ("ptosis"), and difficulty with eating, swallowing, and speaking.

Symptoms tend to fluctuate during the day, being worst early in the morning and late at night. Repetitive activity, emotional stress, overexertion, exposure to heat, and some medications can make symptoms much worse.

The typical MG patient experiences degeneration of muscle function for 2 or 3 years after diagnosis. Symptoms then tend to level off, sometimes even going into complete remission. However, MG is a progressive disease, and without intervention it can move from the muscles of the face and head to the muscles of the arms and legs, and ultimately to the muscles that control respiration. This is the final stage of the disease, although it is rarely seen now that effective treatments for this condition have been developed.

Treatment

Before the 1970s the prognosis for MG was indeterminate at best. About one-third of people died of the disease, about one-third experienced permanent damage and loss of motor function, and about a third experienced spontaneous remission with no lasting effects. When the relationship between acetylcholine and muscle contractions was finally unraveled, it opened new possibilities for treatment.

Treatment of MG usually has a double intention: to boost nerve transmission and to suppress immune system activity at neuromuscular junctions. Medications include drugs that limit the normal destruction of acetylcholine by local enzymes (this allows the acetylcholine more time and opportunities to bind with whatever receptor sites are functioning) and steroids that suppress immune system activity. Surgery is occasionally recommended to remove an abnormal thymus gland. In the event of an MG crisis (a sudden onset that threatens the patient's ability to breathe), plasmapheresis may be used to remove antibodies from the blood. This is an invasive procedure with only short-term benefits, so it is usually used in only extreme circumstances.

Massage?

MG is a disorder that involves motor loss but no sensory loss. It is exacerbated by stress, repetitive motion, and overexertion. Massage could be appropriate for MG patients, bearing in mind that excessive heat can also aggravate symptoms, and that these clients may be taking immunosuppressive medications that put them at increased risk for susceptibility to other people's infections.

Thoracic Outlet Syndrome
Definition: What Is It?

TOS is neurovascular entrapment. The nerves of the brachial plexus or the blood vessels running to or from the arm (or some combination of both) are impinged or impaired at the thoracic outlet (the area behind the clavicle between the insertions of the trapezius and sternocleidomastoid).

Etiology: What Happens?

The brachial plexus, that tangled network of spinal nerves that supplies the arm with sensation and motor control, is composed of spinal nerves C5 to T1. These nerves interconnect as they travel a complicated path to get to their final destinations in the arm. They go from intervertebral foramina through the anterior and medial scalenes, between the clavicle and the first rib, under the pectoralis minor, and around the humerus. If some part of the plexus is somehow compressed along the way, the client feels it somewhere along the distance of that nerve. The nerve roots C8 and T1, both of which contribute to the ulnar and median nerves, are most at risk for compression with TOS.

Pinched nerves are only one part of TOS. This is a neuro*vascular* entrapment, and the vessels at risk are the subclavian vein and the axillary artery, which is the distal portion of the subclavian artery. These vessels, although not being vulnerable to osteophytes and herniated discs like the nerves, are equally at the mercy of the compression that can happen when muscles in small spaces get too tight (Fig. 2-45).

Contributing Factors

Symptoms of TOS can be caused by any factor that impinges brachial plexus nerves or blood vessels to and from the arm, anywhere from the neck to the shoulder. Although postural habits and bony growth patterns can make a person susceptible to TOS, it often seems to be precipitated by a specific traumatic event such as a hyperextension injury (see *whiplash*, this chapter) or a repetitive stress situation similar to the factors seen with CTS.

THORACIC OUTLET SYNDROME IN BRIEF

What is it?
Thoracic outlet syndrome (TOS) is a collection of signs and symptoms brought about by occlusion of nerves and blood supply to the arm.

How is it recognized?
Depending on what structures are compressed, TOS shows shooting pains, weakness, numbness, and paresthesia ("pins and needles") along with a feeling of fullness and possible discoloration of the affected arm from impaired circulation.

Is massage indicated or contraindicated?
This depends on the source of the problem. TOS from muscle tightness indicates massage. TOS symptoms due to muscle degeneration or some other disorder such as *spondylosis* or *herniated disc* (this chapter) will not respond well to massage.

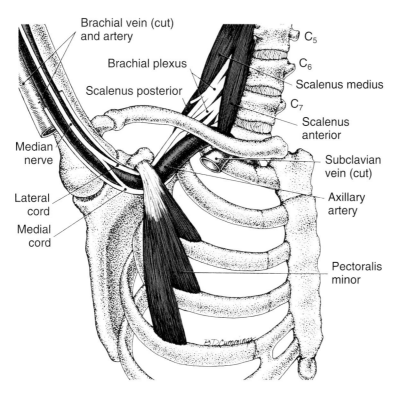

Figure 2-45. Thoracic outlet syndrome

Although TOS is only diagnosed when that impingement occurs at the thoracic outlet, other factors can contribute to identical symptoms. Treating this condition successfully means finding out exactly where that interference is happening. Some possibilities include the following:

- *Cervical misalignment.* This could be a subluxation, but would more likely be a rotation *with* subluxation of any combination of lower cervical vertebrae. Which nerves are affected (and therefore the location of the symptoms) depends on what level or levels of spinal nerves are being compressed.

- *Cervical ribs.* In about 1% of the population, the transverse processes of the cervical vertebrae grow longer than normal, extending into territory where they do not belong. On a radiograph they look like little ribs sticking out into the soft tissues of the neck. They are usually unilateral, and C_7 is the vertebra that grows them most frequently.

- *Bone spurs.* Imagine growing a bone spur that intrudes right into the nerve root at C_6 (or any other cervical nerve root). Symptoms would be very similar to those of classic TOS (see *spondylosis*, this chapter).

- *Rib misalignment.* The joints that join the ribs to the spine are full synovial joints called *zygapophyseal joints.* Like the intervertebral joints, the rib joints sometimes subluxate. When this happens to the first rib, two different spots could cause problems: directly under the anterior scalene, and between the coracoid process and the ribs. In both of those locations, the brachial plexus nerves can easily be caught between a bone (the first rib) and a hard place (a tight muscle or another bone).

- *Tight muscles.* The anterior and medial scalenes as well as the pectoralis minor are the muscles most immediately involved with TOS. Microscopic studies of the scalenes of TOS patients show that the muscles are often bound up with large amounts of scar tissue. This can make the muscles tight and unyielding, putting mechanical pressure on the nerve roots.

- *Atrophied muscles.* Many cases of TOS may be related to muscle atrophy as an outcome of chronic muscle tightness. The pectoralis minor, in a constant battle with the rhomboids and levator scapulae, is especially prone to this phenomenon, particularly for people with a "caved in" kind of posture. Eventually the pectoralis minor becomes shrunken and fibrotic, while its antagonists on the back, especially the rhomboids, become stretched out and hypotonic. If muscles that support the shoulder girdle are abnormally underdeveloped, the clavicle and scapula may collapse onto the ribs, compressing and irritating brachial plexus nerves and the subclavian vein.

Signs and Symptoms

Symptoms of TOS include shooting pains, numbness, reduced sensation, weakness, tingling, and pins and needles. Added to these are the vascular symptoms of a feeling of "fullness" when blood return from a vein is blocked, or coldness and weakness when blood flow to the axillary artery is impaired. A difference in coloration of the affected arm may also be noticeable. Symptoms tend to be worse at night, when the patient lifts the affected arm over the head, or when the patient is tired from other activities.

Diagnosis

Several tests for TOS have been developed. Unfortunately, none of them is always accurate for every patient, so a diagnosis is usually based on a physical examination combined with a description of symptoms from the patient. The challenge then is to locate exactly where the impingement is taking place.

In the Wright hyperabduction test, the hand is placed over the head and the head is turned toward the affected side. If this exacerbates symptoms or reduces the strength of the pulse of the affected side, impingement to the axillary artery and lower brachial plexus nerves is suspected.

In Adson's test the head is extended and rotated toward the affected side. The client takes a deep breath. If the radial pulse on the affected side diminishes or even completely disappears, a diagnosis is made.

TOS that is due to muscle atrophy may show best when a client lies on the affected side and the pulse is diminished from axillary artery compression.

Nerve velocity conduction tests and electromyograms (tests that measure electrical activity during muscle action) are sometimes used, but they are often inconclusive. Radiographs, MRIs, and other imaging techniques may be used to look for bone spurs, cervical ribs, or other mechanical obstructions but yield little information about chronic muscle tightness or atrophy.

Confusing Signs

Many things cause pain in the shoulders, arms, wrists, and hands. Some of these problems are often missed by standard diagnosis, simply because most soft tissue injuries do not appear on most medical tests. This is unfortunate, because it makes it hard for people to receive an accurate diagnosis for their most common and treatable problems. The following are a few causes of pain in the shoulder, arm, wrist, or hand that can be hard to pin down in an accurate diagnosis:

Arthritis in shoulders, elbows, or wrists
Cervical rib pressing on the brachial plexus
CTS
Costal misalignment
Elbow tendinitis
Herniated disc
Injured cervical ligaments
Rotator cuff tendinitis
Shoulder bursitis
Spondylosis
Tight scalenes, pectoralis minor
Vertebral misalignment
Wrist tendinitis or sprain

Treatment

TOS treatment depends on its cause, which is why an accurate diagnosis is important. Different strategies are more appropriate for spondylosis than for tight scalenes, for instance. TOS due to muscle atrophy or tightness responds best to strengthening exercises and stretching. A small percentage of TOS patients are good candidates for surgery, which has the goal of releasing pressure on the affected nerves. This can mean removing a cervical rib, resectioning of the first rib, or both.

Massage?

If TOS is not from muscular spasm or weakness, massage will not make much lasting difference. If it *is* related to muscular problems, it can respond very well to massage. The client should also learn some specific stretches and exercises for pectoralis minor, its antagonists, and the scalenes to make the massage have lasting impact.

Chapter Review Questions: Musculoskeletal Conditions

1. What is the relationship between fibromyalgia and sleep disorders?

2. Name three differences between tender points and trigger points.

3. What is the most common variety of arthritis?

4. Why are herniated discs in the thoracic spine rare?

5. Why are women more prone than men to osteoporosis?

6. Describe how pes planus can lead to headaches.

7. What kind of muscle spasm is an important part of the healing process?

8. Name three structures that may be damaged in a whiplash injury.

9. In which stage of healing do soft tissue injuries generally contraindicate circulatory massage? Why?

10. What does RICE stand for?

11. List the lines of defense against a joint injury.

12. Define "specific weakness."

13. Describe the pain-spasm-ischemia cycle.

14. Describe the differences between strains, sprains, and tendinitis.

15. Describe the relationship between stress and chronic injury.

Bibliography, Musculoskeletal System Conditions

General References, Musculoskeletal System

1. de Dominico G, Wood E. *Beard's Massage.* Philadelphia, Pa: WB Saunders; 1997.
2. Damjanou I. *Pathology for the Health-Related Professions.* Philadelphia, Pa: WB Saunders; 1996.
3. Travell J, Simons DG. *Myofascial Pain and Dysfunction: The Trigger Point Manual.* Baltimore, Md: Williams & Wilkins; 1983.
4. Clemente CD. *Anatomy: A Regional Atlas of the Human Body.* 3rd ed. Baltimore, Md: Urban & Schwarzenburg; 1987.
5. Tortora GJ, Anagnostakos NP. *Principles of Anatomy and Physiology.* 6th ed. New York NY: Harper & Row; 1990.
6. *Taber's Cyclopedic Dictionary.* 14th ed. Philadelphia, Pa: FA Davis; 1981.
7. *Stedman's Medical Dictionary.* 26th ed. Baltimore, Md: Williams & Wilkins; 1995.
8. Memmler RL, Wood DL. *The Human Body in Health and Disease.* 5th ed. Philadelphia, Pa: JB Lippincott; 1983.
9. Juhan D. *Job's Body: A Handbook for Bodywork.* Barrytown, NY: Station Hill Press; 1987.
10. Mulvihill ML. *Human Diseases: A Systemic Approach.* 2nd ed. Norwalk, Conn: Appleton & Lange; 1987.
11. Kunz JRM, Finkel AJ, eds. *The American Medical Association Family Medical Guide.* New York, NY: Random House; 1987.
12. Marieb EM. *Human Anatomy and Physiology.* Redwood City, Calif: Benjamin/Cummings; 1989.

13. Benjamin B, Borden G. Listen to Your Pain: *The Active Person's Guide to Understanding, Identifying and Treating Pain and Injury.* New York, NY: Penguin Books; 1984.

14. Kapandji IA. The Physiology of the Joints: Annotated Diagrams of the Mechanics of the Human Joints. Volume One: Upper Limb. 5th ed. New York, NY: Longman Group Limited, Churchill Livingstone; 1982. (reprinted 1986).

15. Kapandji IA. The Physiology of the Joints: Annotated Diagrams of the Mechanics of the Human Joints. Volume Two: Lower Limb. 2nd ed. New York, NY: Longman Group Limited, Churchill Livingstone; 1970. (reprinted 1985).

16. Kapandji IA. The Physiology of the Joints: Annotated Diagrams of the Mechanics of the Human Joints. Volume Three: The Trunk and Vertebral Column. New York, NY: Longman Group Limited, Churchill Livingstone; 1974. (reprinted 1985).

Fibromyalgia Syndrome

1. Slavkin, H. DDS. Chronic disabling diseases and disorders: The challenges of fibromyalgia. Insights on Human Health, National Institute of Dental Research. Available at: http://www.talkaboutsleep. com/related/fms_challenges.htm. ©2001. Talk About Sleep, Inc. Accessed spring 2002.

2. FMS: Fibromyalgia syndrome. Excerpted from Starlanyl DJ. *The Fibromyalgia Advocate.* ©2001. Available at: http://www.sover. net/~devstar/ fmsdef.htm. Accessed spring 2002.

3. Fibromyalgia: Coping with the pain. Mayo Foundation for Medical Education and Research; 2000. Available at: http://www. mayohealth.org/mayo/9710/htm/ fibromya.htm. Accessed fall 2000.

4. Gremillion RB. Fibromyalgia. *Physician Sportsmed.* 1998;26(4). Available at: http:// www.physsportsmed.com/issues/1998/ 04apr/grem.htm. Accessed fall 2000.

5. Fibromyalgia basics: Symptoms, treatment and research. Fibromyalgia Network. Available at: http://www.fmnetnews. com/pages/basics.html. Accessed fall 2000.

6. Fibromyalgia (fibrositis). MedicineNet, Inc.; 1996–2000. Available at: http:// medicinenet.com. Accessed fall 2000.

7. Nye D. A physician's guide to fibromyalgia syndrome. http://www.med1.de/50773. Accessed summer 2000.

8. Nye D. Fibromyalgia—A physician's guide. Available at http://pages.prodigy.net/ turnip/ drnye1.htm Accessed summer 2000.

9. The American Fibromyalgia Syndrome Association, Inc. Update Volume 5, Issue 1. Available at : http://www.afsafund. org/ updates.htm. Accessed summer 2000.

10. Nye D. A patient's frequently asked questions about fibromyalgia. Available at: http://www.muhealth.org/~fibro/ fram_fpt.html Accessed summer 2000.

11. Field T. *Touch Therapy.* London: Churchill Livingstone. 2000.

12. Mann S. Cognitive/somatic pain management with fibromyalgia and chronic myofascial pain. *Massage Ther J.* 1995;34(4):35–45.

Myofascial Pain Syndrome

1. Fomby EW, Mellion MB. Identifying and treating myofascial pain syndrome. *Physician Sportsmed.* 1997;25(2). Available at: http://www.physsportsmed.com/issues/1997/ 02feb/fomby2.htm Accessed summer 2000.

2. Starlanyl D. Fibromyalgia/myofascial pain syndrome handout # 1. Available at: http://www.pendulum.org/related/FMS/ fm-pain.htm Accessed summer 2000.

3. Starlanyl D. Fibromyalgia syndrome or myofascial pain syndrome? Available at: http://www.sover.net/~devstar/ Accessed spring 2002.

4. SPA-Treatment of myofascial pain syndrome requires team effort. Specialty Physicians Alliance; 2000. Available at: http://www.spa-ortho.com/library/ gen2.htm Accessed summer 2000.

Muscular Dystrophy

1. Muscular dystrophy: What is it? 1996–1999 Available at: http://www. washington post.com/cgi-bin/gx.cgi/ AppLogic+ FTContentServer?pagename =health/condition &nextstep=display &disease=10383. Accessed fall 2000.

2. Facts about Duchenne and Becker muscular dystrophies (DMD BMD). Muscular Dystrophy Association. Available at: http://www.mdausa. org/publications/fa-dmdbmd-treat.html. Accessed fall 2000.

3. Emery AEH. The muscular dystrophies. *Br Med J.* 1998. Available at: http://www.bmj. com/ cgi/content/full/317/ 7164/991. Accessed fall 2000.

Myositis Ossificans

1. Takle TE, D'Alessandro DM, D'Alessandro MP. Virtual pediatric patients case 3— An adolescent with leg pain. Author(s) and University of Iowa; 1992–2000. Available at: http://www.vh.org//Providers/ Simulations/VirtualPedsPatients/Case03/ Case03.html. Accessed fall 2000.

2. Myositis ossificans. www.Bonetumor.org. Available at: http://www.bonetumor.org/ page177.html. Accessed fall 2000.

Shin Splints

1. Hutchinson MR, Cahoon S, Atkins T. Chronic leg pain: Putting the diagnostic pieces together. *Physician Sportsmed.* 1998;26(7). Available at: http://www. physsportsmed.com/issues/1998/ 07jul/ hutch.htm. Accessed fall 2000.

2. Edwards P, Myerson MS. Exertional compartment syndrome of the leg: Steps for expedient return to activity. *Physician Sportsmed.* 1996;24(4). Available at : http://www. physsportsmed.com/issues/ apr_96/edwards.htm. Accessed fall 2000.

3. Shin splints. MedicineNet, Inc.; 1996–2000. Available at: http:// medicinenet.com. Accessed fall 2000.

Spasms, Cramps

1. Schwellnus MP. Skeletal muscle cramps during exercise. *Physician Sportsmed.* 1999;27(12). Available at: http://www. physsportsmed.com/ issues/1999/11_99/ schwellnus.htm. Accessed fall 2000.

Strains

1. Kannus P. Immobilization or early mobilization after an acute soft-tissue injury? *Physician Sportsmed.* 2000;28(3). Available at: http://www.physsportsmed.com/ issues/2000/03_00/kannus.htm. Accessed fall 2000.

2. O'Connor FG, Howard TM, Fieseler CM, Nirschl RP. Managing overuse injuries: A systematic approach. Physician Sportsmed. 1997;25(5). Available at: http://www. physsportsmed.com/issues/1997/ 05may/ oconnor.htm. Accessed fall 2000.

Fractures

1. Farley D. New ways to heal broken bones. *FDA Consumer Magazine.* 1996; April. Available at: http://www.fda.gov/fdac/ features/396_bone. html. Accessed fall 2000.

2. Orthopedic Surgery.com? Surgery-Biz.;1999–2000. Available at: http://www. surgerybiz.com/1199surg/1199surgstory01. cfm. Accessed fall 2000.

Osteoporosis

1. Slavkin HC. Building a better mousetrap: Toward an understanding of osteoporosis. Available at: http://www.nidcr.nih. gov/ slavkin/ slav1199.asp. Accessed fall 2000.

2. Fast facts on osteoporosis. National Institutes of Health Osteoporosis and Related Bone Diseases National Resource Center. Available at: http://www. osteo.org/osteo-fastfact.html. Accessed fall 2000.

3. Low-dose estrogen spares bones, enhances hormone replacement therapy. National Institute of Arthritis and Musculoskeletal and Skin Diseases; 1999. Available at: http://www.nih.gov/niams/news/spotlight/ lowdose.htm. Accessed fall 2000.

4. Preventing and reversing osteoporosis. Physicians Committee for Responsible Medicine. Available at: http://www.pcrm.org/issues/ Nutrition_Curriculum/nutr_curr_7.html. Accessed fall 2000.

5. Preventive medicine and nutrition: Calcium and strong bones: protecting your bones. Physicians Committee for Responsible Medicine. Available at: http://www. pcrm.org/ health/Preventive_Medicine/ strong_bones.html. Accessed spring 2002.

6. Matsen F, III, ed. Osteoporosis. University of Washington Orthopaedics Arthritis Source; 2000. University of Washington. Available at: http://www.orthop. washington.edu/bonejointozzzzzzz1_2. html. Accessed fall 2000.

7. Depression, Bone Mass, and Osteoporosis NIMH, 6/29/01. Available at: http://www.nih.gov/news/pr/jun2001/nimh–29.htm. Accessed winter 2002.
8. Brown D. Simple genetic test may identify increased risk of osteoporosis. *Washington Post*. January 20, 1994:A3.

Paget's Disease

1. Matsen F, III, ed. Paget's disease. University of Washington Orthopaedics Arthritis Source; 2000 University of Washington. Available at: http://www.orthop. washington.edu/bonejoint/yzzzzzzz1_2. html. Accessed fall 2000.
2. Information for patients about Paget's disease of bone. National Institutes of Health Osteoporosis and Related Bone Diseases National Resource Center. Available at: http://www. osteo.org/pdisbone. html. Accessed fall 2000.
3. Paget's disease of the bone. The Johns Hopkins University; 1996–1999. Available at: http://www.washingtonpost.com/cgi-bin/gx.cgi/ AppLogic+FTContentServer? pagename=health/condition&nextstep= display&disease=9565. Accessed fall 2000.
4. Kurtsweil P. Help for people with Paget's disease. *FDA Consumer Magazine*. 1996;October. Available at: http://www.fda.gov/fdac/features/ 896_pag.html. Accessed fall 2000.
5. Paget's disease. HealthAnswers.com, Inc.; 2000. Available at: http://healthanswers. com/centers/ body/overview.asp?id=bone +muscle+joint&filename=1667.htm. Accessed fall 2000.

Postural Deviations

1. Clay JH. Scoliosis: Information & treatment. James H. Clay; 1996–1999. Available at: http://www.danke.com/Orthodoc/ scoliosis.html. Accessed fall 2000.
2. Kyphosis—Questions and answers. Orthospine; 1998–1999. Available at: http://www. orthospine.com/hottopics/qa_kyphosis. htm. Accessed fall 2000.
3. Scoliosis In children and adolescents. MedicineNet, Inc.; 1996–2000. Available at: http://medicinenet.com. Accessed fall 2000.
4. In depth review of scoliosis: Introduction. Scoliosis Research Society. Available at: http://www.srs.org/htm/library/review/ review00.htm. Accessed fall 2000.
5. Odom JA, Jr. Spinal deformities: Benefits of early screening and treatment. Joel R. Cooper; 1995. Available at: http:// medicalreporter.health.org/tmr0795/ scoliosis0795.html. Accessed fall 2000.

Ankylosing Spondylitis

1. Adult spine surgery service frequently asked questions: Ankylosing spondylitis surgery. Milton S. Hershey Medical Center; 2000. Available at: http://www.collmed. psu.edu/ortho/ spine/FAQs_AS.html. Accessed fall 2000.
2. Ankylosing spondylitis. MedicineNet, Inc.; 1996–2000. Available at: http://www. MedicineNet.com. Accessed fall 2000.

3. Ankylosing spondylitis. Adapted from the pamphlet originally prepared for the Arthritis Foundation by Frank C. Arnett, MD, Professor of Internal Medicine, University of Texas Medical School at Houston. Available at: http://www.orthop.washington.edu/arthritis/ankspond/ankspond_print.html. Accessed fall 2000.
4. Matsen F, III. Ankylosing spondylitis. University of Washington; 2000. Available at: http://www.orthop.washington.edu/Bone%20and%20Joint%20Sources/azzzzzzz1_1. html Accessed fall 2000.

Dislocations

1. Thermal Capsulorrhaphy Effective. American Academy of Orthopaedic Surgeons Academy News. 3/2/01. Available at: http://www.aaos.org/wordhtml/2001news/ a02-6.htm. Accessed spring 02.
2. Dorman TA, Ravin TA. *Diagnosis and Injection Techniques in Orthopedic Medicine*. Baltimore, Md: Williams & Wilkins.

Gout

1. Flieger K. Getting to know gout. U.S. Food and Drug Administration. Available at: http://www.seekwellness.com/gout/ getting_to_know_gout.htm. Accessed fall 2000.
2. Gout and hyperuricemia. MedicineNet, Inc.; 1996–2000. Available at: http://www. MedicineNet.com. Accessed fall 2000.
3. Questions and answers about gout. National Institute of Arthritis and Musculoskeletal and Skin Diseases. Available at: http://www.nih.gov/ niams/ healthinfo/ gout.htm. Accessed fall 2000.
4. Calcium pyrophosphate dihydrate crystal deposition disease (CPPD) (pseudo gout). Arthritis Foundation; 2000. Available at: http://www. arthritis.org/answers/ diseasecenter/cppd.asp. Accessed fall 2000.
5. Matsen F, III. Pseudogout. University of Washington; 2000. Available at: http://www.orthop.washington.edu/ bonejoint/pzzzzzzz1_2.html. Accessed fall 2000.
6. DiBacco TV. The pain of gout: Baffling condition left doctors guessing. *Washington Post*. October 11, 1994:Z19.

Lyme Disease

1. Lyme disease: Introduction. Division of Vector-Borne Infectious Diseases, National Centers for Disease Control and Prevention. Available at: http://www. cdc.gov/nci-dod/dvbid/lymeinfo.htm. Accessed fall 2000.
2. Lyme disease: Natural history. Division of Vector-Borne Infectious Diseases, National Centers for Disease Control and Prevention. Available at: http://www. cdc.gov/ ncidod/dvbid/ Lymehistory.htm. Accessed fall 2000.
3. Lyme disease diagnosis. Division of Vector-Borne Infectious Diseases, National Centers for Disease Control and Prevention. Available at: http://www.cdc.gov/ncidod/

dvbid/Lymediagnosis.htm. Accessed fall 2000.
4. Lyme disease: Epidemiology. Division of Vector-Borne Infectious Diseases, National Centers for Disease Control and Prevention. Available at: http://www. cdc.gov/ ncidod/dvbid/ lymeepi.htm. Accessed fall 2000.
5. Lyme disease: Vaccine. Division of Vector-Borne Infectious Diseases, National Centers for Disease Control and Prevention. Available at: http://www.cdc.gov/ncidod/ dvbid/lymevaccine.htm. Accessed fall 2000.
6. Lyme disease: The bacterium. Division of Vector-Borne Infectious Diseases, National Centers for Disease Control and Prevention. Available at: http://www. cdc.gov/ ncidod/dvbid/Bburgdorferi.htm.htm. Accessed fall 2000.
7. Lyme disease. Arthritis Foundation; 2000. ©2000 Arth. Found. Available at: http://www.arthritis.org/ readarthritistoday/2000_03_04_101_lyme. asp. Accessed fall 2000.
8. Diagnosis of lyme disease. National Institute of Allergy and Infectious Diseases. Available at: http://www.niaid.nih.gov/ dmid/lymediag.htm. Accessed fall 2000.
9. Phalen KF. Lyme disease: A ticking bomb. *The Washington Post*. 2000. Available at: http://www.washingtonpost.com/ac2/ wp-dyn/A41547-2000Oct10? language = printer. Accessed fall 2000.
10. Lyme disease. MedicineNet, Inc.; 1996–2000. Available at: http://www. MedicineNet.com. Accessed fall 2000.
11. Basic information. International Lyme and Associated Diseases Society. Available at: http://www.ilads.org/ axioms.htm. Accessed spring 2002.
12. Campbell CA. Lesser-known cousins to Lyme grab attention. *Newark Star Ledger*. 1994-2000. Available at: http://www2.lymenet.org/domino/news.nsf/UID/ Ledger20-Jun-2000. Accessed fall 2000.

Osteoarthritis

1. Osteoarthritis (OA). Arthritis Foundation; 2000. Available at: http://www.arthritis.org/ Answers/DiseaseCenter/oa.asp. Accessed fall 2000.
2. Dunkin MA. On the front lines of arthritis research. Arthritis Foundation; 2000. Available at: http://www.arthritis.org/ ReadArthritisToday/ 2000_03_04_MA_ ACR.asp. Accessed fall 2000.
3. Lewis C. Arthritis: Timely treatments for an ageless disease. Food and Drug Administration Publication No. (FDA) 00-1313. Available at: http://www.fda.gov/fdac/ features/2000/300_arth.html. Accessed fall 2000.
4. Thumb arthritis. Southeastern Hand Center. Available at: http://www.handsurgery. com/arthritis.html. Accessed fall 2000.
5. Osteoarthritis. American College of Rheumatology; 2000. Available at: http://www.rheumatology.org/patients/ factsheet/oa.html. Accessed fall 2000.

6. Kelly GS. The role of glucosamine sulfate and chondroitin sulfates in the treatment of degenerative joint disease. *Alt Med Rev.* 1998;3(1). Available at: http://www.thorne.com/altmedrev/.fulltext/3/1/27.html. Accessed fall 2000.

Patellofemoral Syndrome

1. Post WR. Patellofemoral pain: Let the physical exam define treatment. *Physician Sportsmed.* 1998;26(1). Available at: http://www.physsportsmed.com/issues/1998/01jan/post.htm. Accessed fall 2000.
2. Patellofemoral Syndrome. MedicineNet, Inc.; 1996–2000. Available at: http://www.MedicineNet.com. Accessed fall 2000.

Rheumatoid Arthritis

1. Rheumatoid arthritis. American College of Rheumatology; 2000. Available at: http://www.rheumatology.org/patients/factsheet/ra.html. Accessed fall 2000.
2. Focus on. . . Rheumatoid arthritis. Medical Sciences Bulletin; 1996–1999. Available at: http://pharminfo.com/pubs/msb/rheumart.html. Accessed fall 2000.
3. Rheumatoid arthritis (RA). Arthritis Foundation; 2000. Available at: http://www.arthritis.org/Answers/DiseaseCenter/ra.asp. Accessed fall 2000.
4. Handout on health—Rheumatoid arthritis. PharmInfoNet. Available at: www.niams.nih.gov/hi/topics/arthritis/rahandout.htm. Accessed spring 2002.
5. Rheumatoid arthritis. MedicineNet, Inc.; 1996–2000. Available at: http://www.MedicineNet.com. Accessed fall 2000.
6. Mayeaux EJ. 2000 Revised ARA criteria for the classification of rheumatoid arthritis. Louisiana State University Medical Center. Available at: http://lib-sh.lsumc.edu/fammed/intern/ra.html. Accessed spring 2002.

Septic Arthritis

1. Toyoshima H, Toth PP, Graber MA. Rheumatology: Septic arthritis. In: *University of Iowa Family Practice Handbook.* 3rd ed. University of Iowa: 1992-2000. Available at: http://www.vh.org/Providers/ClinRef/FPHandbook/Chapter06/05-6.html Accessed fall 2000.
2. Pommering TL, Wroble RR. Septic arthritis of the shoulder: Treating an atypical case. *Physician Sportsmed.* 1996;24(5). Available at: http://www.physsportsmed.com/issues/may_96/pomm.htm. Accessed fall 2000.

Spondylosis

1. Cervical spondylosis. NYU Department of Neurosurgery. Available at: http://mcns10.med.nyu.edu/spine/spine_surgery_p5.html. Accessed fall 2000.
2. Lumbar stenosis (spondylosis). NYU Department of Neurosurgery. Available at: http://mcns10.med.nyu.edu/spine/spine_surgery_p3.html. Accessed fall 2000.

3. Weiss R. Back pain and MRIs: Vivid diagnostic images are a mixed blessing. *Washington Post Health.* July 19, 1997:Z7.

Sprains

1. Lai M. "It's just a sprain": Understanding the consequences of ankle injuries. Available at: http://www.hcs.harvard.edu/~hsr/hsr/winter97/sprain.html. Accessed fall 2000.
2. Kannus P. Immobilization or early mobilization after an acute soft-tissue injury? *Physician Sportsmed.* 2000;28(3). Available at: http://www.physsportsmed.com/issues/2000/03_00/kannus.htm. Accessed fall 2000.
3. O'Connor FG, Howard TM, Fieseler CM, Nirschl RP. Managing overuse injuries: A systematic approach. *Physician Sportsmed.* 1997;25(5). Available at: http://www.physsportsmed.com/issues/1997/05may/oconnor.htm. Accessed fall 2000.
4. Bassewitz HL, Shapiro MS. Persistent pain after ankle sprain: Targeting the causes. Physician Sportsmed. 1997;25(12). Available at: http://www.physsportsmed.com/issues/1997/12dec/shapiro.htm. Accessed fall 2000.

Temporomandibular Joint Disorders

1. Temporomandibular joint disorder. MedicineNet, Inc.; 1996–2000. Available at: http://medicinenet.com. Accessed fall 2000.
2. Temporomandibular joint (TMJ) pain-dysfunction syndrome. In: Buttaravoli, Stair, eds. *Common Simple Emergencies.* Longwood Information. Available at: http://www.clark.net/pub/ electra/cse0401.html. Accessed fall 2000.
3. Goldman KE. What is temporomandibular joint disease? Kim E. Goldman; 1995–2000. Available at: http://www.calweb.com/~goldman/tmj.html. Accessed fall 2000.
4. What is TMD? And do you have it? American Academy of Head Neck and Facial Pain. The Q Group; 1997. Available at: http://www.aahnfp.org/self-help.html. Accessed fall 2000.
5. Shankland WE, II. Causes of TMJ. American Academy of Face, Head and Neck Pain. Available at: http://www.netset.com/~docws/ page4.html. Accessed winter 1998.

Baker Cysts

1. Baker's cysts (popliteal cyst). MedicineNet, Inc.; 1996–2000. Available at: http://medicinenet.com. Accessed fall 2000.
2. Baker's cyst/popliteal cyst. C.R. Wheeless; 1996. Available at: http://www.medmedia.com/o2/219.htm. Accessed fall 2000.
3. Yu WD, Shapiro MS. Cysts and other masses about the knee: Identifying and treating common and rare lesions. Physician Sportsmed. 1999;27(7). Available at: http://www.physsportsmed.com/issues/1999/07_99/yu.htm. Accessed fall 2000.
4. Benjamin B. Understanding Baker's cyst. *Massage Ther J* 1993;32(3).

Bunions

1. Bunions. MedicineNet, Inc.; 1996–2000. Available at: http://medicinenet.com. Accessed fall 2000.
2. Bunions. Don't crowd your toes. Mayo Clinic Health Oasis; 2000 Mayo Foundation for Medical Education and Research. Available at: http://www.mayohealth.org/mayo/0004/htm/bunions.htm. Accessed fall 2000.
3. Bunion/Hallux Valgus. University of Washington, Harborview Medical Center, Department of Orthopaedics; 2000. Available at: http://www.orthop.washington.edu/ankle/Bunions.htm. Accessed fall 2000.
4. Positano R, Waller J. Are other treatments for bunions as helpful as surgery? *Washington Post Health.* August 24, 1993.

Bursitis

1. Hip bursitis. A simple shot often helps. Mayo Clinic Health Oasis; 2000. Mayo Foundation for Medical Education and Research. Available at: http://www.mayohealth.org/mayo/9709/ htm/bursitis.htm. Accessed fall 2000.
2. Bursitis: Common problem, simple care. Mayo Clinic Health Oasis; 2000. Mayo Foundation for Medical Education and Research. Available at: http://www.mayohealth.org/mayo/9506/htm/bursitis.htm. Accessed fall 2000.

Dupuytren Contracture

1. Dupuytren's contracture: C.R. Wheeless; 1996. Available at: http://www.medmedia.com/ o2/192.htm. Accessed fall 2000.
2. Eaton C. Dupuytren's contracture. FISH. Available at: http://www.eatonhand.com/hw/hw009.htm. Accessed fall 2000.
3. Dupuytren's syndrome, Dupuytren's disease and contractures of the palm and fingers. The Center for Orthopaedics & Sports Medicine; 1999. Available at: http://www.arthroscopy. com/sp04012.htm. Accessed fall 2000.

Ganglion Cyst

1. Ganglion cysts. MedicineNet, Inc.; 1996–2000. Available at: http://medicinenet.com. Accessed fall 2000.
2. Ganglions. Southeastern Hand Center. Available at: http://www.handsurgery.com/ganglions.html. Accessed spring 2002.
3. Ganglion cyst. Manus; 2000. Available at: http://www.indianahandcenter.com/med_gang.html. Accessed fall 2000.

Hernia

1. Hernia. MedicineNet, Inc.; 1996–2000. Available at: http://medicinenet.com. Accessed fall 2000.

Osgood Schlatter Disease

1. Meisterling RC, Wall EJ, Meisterling MR. Coping with Osgood Schlatter disease. Physician Sportsmed. 1998;26(3). Available at: http://www.physsportsmed.com/issues/

1998/03mar/wall_pa.htm. Accessed fall 2000.

2. American Academy of Family Physicians. Osgood-Schlatter disease: A cause of knee pain in children. In: *Iowa Health Book: Family Practice.* University of Iowa; 1992–2000. Available at: http://www.vh.org/Patients/IHB/FamilyPractice/AFP/June1995/Knee.html . Accessed fall 2000.

3. Osgood-Schlatter disease. InteliHealth Inc.; 1996–2000. Available at: http://www.intelihealth.com/IH/ihtIH/WSIHW000/9339/24676.html. Accessed fall 2000.

4. Wall EJ. Osgood-Schlatter disease: A practical treatment for a self-limiting condition. Physician Sportsmed. 1998;26(3). Available at: http://www.physsportsmed.com/issues/1998/ 03mar/wall.htm. Accessed fall 2000.

Pes Planus

1. The five minute orthopaedic consultant. Ahn, Nicholas: Flat foot. Department of Orthopaedic Surgery. Johns Hopkins Bayview Medical Center. Available at: http://jhbmc. bayview.jhu.edu/Ortho/consultant/5mcf.html#FlatFoot. Accessed fall 2000.

2. Flat feet. Angsko; 1996. Available at: http://www.footcaredirect.com/flatfeet.html. Accessed fall 2000.

Plantar Fasciitis

1. Plantar fasciitis. Angsko; 1996. Available at: http://www.footcaredirect.com/heel.html. Accessed fall 2000.

2. Petrizzi MJ, Petrizzi MG, Roos RJ. Making a tension night splint for plantar fasciitis. *Physician Sportsmed.* 1998;26(6). Available at: http://www.physsportsmed.com/issues/1998/ 06jun/petrizzi.htm. Accessed fall 2000.

3. Orthoses face off in heel pain treatment. *Physician Sportsmed.* 1997;25(2). Available at: http://www.physsportsmed.com/issues/1997/ 02feb/nb_heel.htm. Accessed fall 2000.

4. Roberts WO. Plantar fascia injection. *Physician Sportsmed.* 1999;27(9). Available at: http://www.physsportsmed.com/issues/1999/09_99/roberts.htm. Accessed fall 2000.

5. Plantar fasciitis. The Center for Orthopaedics & Sports Medicine; 1999. Available at: http://www.arthroscopy.com/sp09001.htm. Accessed fall 2000.

6. Roberts S. Plantar fasciitis, heel spurs, heel pain. Scott Roberts; 1996–2000. Available at: http://heelspurs.com/_intro.html#vs. Accessed fall 2000.

Scleroderma

1. Scleroderma. American College of Rheumatology; 2000. Available at: http://www.rheumatology.org/patients/factsheet/scler.html. Accessed fall 2000.

2. Scleroderma. InteliHealth Inc.; 1996–2000. http://www.intelihealth.com/IH/ihtIH/WSIHW000/9339/10646.html. Accessed fall 2000.

3. Zweiman B. Scleroderma. American Academy of Allergy, Asthma and Immunology; 1997–1999. Available at: http://www.aaaai.org/ aadmc/inthenews/news/ 1999archive/scleroderma.html. Accessed fall 2000.

4. Fetal cells found in skin lesions of women with scleroderma. The National Institute of Arthritis and Musculoskeletal and Skin Diseases. Available at: http://www.nih.gov/niams/news/fetalfin.htm. Accessed fall 2000.

5. Scleroderma: Early diagnosis is important. Mayo Foundation for Medical Education and Research; 2000. Available at: http://www.mayohealth.org/mayo/9705/htm/sclero.htm. Accessed fall 2000.

6. Scleroderma fact sheet. Scleroderma Foundation; 2000. Available at: http://www.scleroderma.org/fact.html. Accessed fall 2000.

7. Lehman TJA. Scleroderma. Available at: http://www.goldscout.com/sclero.html. Accessed fall 2000.

Tendinitis

1. O'Connor FG, Howard TM, Fieseler CM, Nirschl RP. Managing overuse syndromes: A systemic approach. *Physician Sportsmed.* 1997;25(5). Available at: http://www.physsportsmed.com/issues/1997/05may/oconnor.htm. Accessed fall 2000.

2. Cook JL, Khan KM, Maffulli N, Purdam C. Overuse tendinosis, not tendinitis part 2: Applying the new approach to patellar tendinopathy. *Physician Sportsmed.* 2000;28(6). Available at: http://www.physsportsmed.com/issues/ 2000/06_00/khan.htm. Accessed fall 2000.

3. Thornton JS. Pain relief for acute soft-tissue injuries. *Physician Sportsmed.* 1997;25(10). Available at: http://www.physsportsmed.com/issues/ 1997/10oct/thornton.htm. Accessed fall 2000.

Tenosynovitis

1. What is De Quervain's stenosing tenosynovitis? Available at: http://www.indianahandcenter.com/med_deq.html. Accessed fall 2000.

Torticollis

1. Dystonia. MedicineNet, Inc.; 1996–2000. Available at: http://medicinenet.com. Accessed fall 2000.

2. CSMC pediatrics/medical genetics: Management of plagiocephaly and torticollis. Cedars Sinai Medical Center Department of Pediatrics. Available at: http://www.csmc.edu/pediatrics/ refguide/helmet/helmet.html. Accessed fall 2000.

3. 9.02 Torticollis (Wryneck). Common simple emergencies. Longwood Information LLC. Available at: http://www.ncemi.org/cse/ cse0902.htm. Accessed fall 2000.

4. Ross M, Dufel S. Torticollis. Emedicine. Available at: http://www.emedicine.com/

cgi-bin/ foxweb.exe/showsection@/em/ ga?book=emerg&topicid=597

5. The dystonias fact sheet. National Institute of Neurological Disorders and Stroke. Available at: http://www.ninds.nih.gov/health_and_medical/pubs/dystonias.htm. Accessed fall 2000.

Whiplash

1. Hachinski V. Whiplash. American Medical Association; 1995–2000. Available at: http://archneur.ama-assn.org/issues/v57n4/rfull/ ncn90000.html. Accessed fall 2000.

2. Mahar R. Musculotendinous injuries of the neck. Available at: http://www.theberries.ns.ca/ Archives/Whiplash.html. Accessed fall 2000.

3. Carette S. Whiplash injury and chronic neck pain. *N Engl J Med.* 1994;330(15). Available at: http://www.nejm.org/content/1994/0330/ 0015/1083.asp. Accessed fall 2000.

4. Eccles R, Jr. The failure of standard orthopedic and neurologic tests. Part I. Dynamic Chiropractic; 2000. Available at: http://www.chiroweb.com/archives/13/18/30.html. Accessed fall 2000.

5. Eccles R, Jr. The failure of standard orthopedic and neurologic tests. Part II. Dynamic Chiropractic; 2000. Available at: Accessed fall 2000.

Carpal Tunnel Syndrome

1. Carpal tunnel syndrome & tarsal tunnel syndrome. MedicineNet, Inc.; 1996–2000. Available at: http://medicinenet.com. Accessed fall 2000.

2. Carpal tunnel syndrome. InteliHealth Inc.; 1996–2000. Available at: http://www.intelihealth.com/IH/ihtIH/WSIHW000/9339/9485.html. Accessed fall 2000.

3. NIOSH facts: Carpal tunnel syndrome. National Institute of Occupational Safety and Health. Document #705001. Available at: http://www.cdc.gov/niosh/ctsfs.html. Accessed fall 2000.

4. Carpal tunnel syndrome. Medical Multimedia Group. Available at: http://www.sechrest.com/mmg/reflib/ctd/cts/cts.html. Accessed fall 2000.

5. Packer-Tursman J. Treatment of choice. *Special to The Washington Post.* October 17, 2000:Z35 . Available at: http://www.washingtonpost. com/wp-dyn/articles/A21028-2000Oct17.html. Accessed fall 2000.

6. Stroud R. Minimally invasive surgical techniques of the hand and upper extremities. *Orthop Technol Rev.* 2000;2(8). Available at: http://orthopedictechreview.com/issues/sep00/pg18.htm. Accessed fall 2000.

Herniated Disc

1. Cervical disc disease. NYU Department of Neurosurgery. Available at: http://mcns10. med. nyu.edu/spine/ spine_surgery_p4.html. Accessed winter 2001.

2. Lumbar disc disease. NYU Department of Neurosurgery. Available at: http://mcns10.

med.nyu.edu/spine/spine_surgery_p2.html. Accessed winter 2001.

3. El-Khoury G. Diagnosis of disc disease. The University of Iowa; 1992–2001. Available at: http://www.vh.org/Providers/ Textbooks/DiagnosisDiskDisease/ DiagnosisDiskDisease.html. Accessed winter 2001.

4. Humphrys SC, Eck JC. Clinical evaluation and treatment options for herniated lumbar disc. American Academy of Family Physicians; 1999. Available at: http://www.aafp. org/afp/990201ap/575.html. Accessed winter 2001.

5. Murphy D. Is it safe to adjust the cervical spine in the presence of a herniated disc? Dynamic Chiropractice; 2000. Available at: http://www. chiroweb.com/archives/ 18/13/17.html. Accessed winter 2001.

6. Aptaker RL. Neck pain: Part 1: Narrowing the differential. *Physician Sportsmed.* 1996;24(10). Available at: http://www. physsportsmed.com/issues/nov_96/ aptaker2.htm. Accessed winter 2001.

Myasthenia Gravis

1. About myasthenia gravis (MG). Muscular Dystrophy Association. Available at: http://www.mdausa.org/publications/ fa-mg.html. Accessed fall 2000.

2. Myasthenia gravis, description, disorder and autoimmune involvement. Available at: http://www.macalester.edu/~psych/ whathap/UBNRP/Gravis/real_mg_ directory.html#menu. Accessed fall 2000.

3. Howard JF. Myasthenia gravis–A summary. Author and Myasthenia Gravis Foundation of America; 1997. Available at: http://www. myasthenia.org/information/summary.htm. Accessed fall 2000.

4. Myasthenia gravis. MedicineNet; 1996–2000. Available at: http:// medicinenet.com. Accessed fall 2000.

Thoracic Outlet Syndrome

1. Sanders RJ. Thoracic outlet syndrome. Available at: http://www. healthlinkusa.com/308_getpage.asp?http:// www.ecentral.com/members/rsanders/. Accessed fall 2000.

2. A patient's guide to cumulative trauma disorders: Thoracic outlet syndrome. Medical Multimedia Group. Available at: http://www.medicalmultimediagroup.com/ pated/ctd/tos.html. Accessed spring 2002.

3. Thoracic outlet syndrome. C.R. Wheeless; 1996. Available at: http://www.medmedia. com/o13/62.htm. Accessed fall 2000.

Nervous System Conditions

3

CHAPTER OBJECTIVES

After reading this chapter, you should be able to . . .

- Name three diseases that could be confused with multiple sclerosis.
- Name the neurotransmitter that is in short supply in Parkinson's disease.
- Name the causative agent of herpes zoster.
- Name three variations of depression.
- Name three variations of anxiety disorders.

- Name two types of stroke.
- Name which nerve is involved in Bell's palsy.
- Name three complications of spinal cord injury.
- Name two signs that a headache could be a medical emergency.
- Name what feature multiple sclerosis and Guillain-Barré syndrome have in common.

INTRODUCTION

By the time most massage therapists finish their training, they probably know more about the nervous system than they ever suspected existed and probably still feel like rank amateurs on the subject. That feeling is common to most people who study this topic. Fortunately, only a passing familiarity with the structure and function of this system is needed to make educated decisions about massage and most nervous system disorders. Most of the conditions considered here affect the peripheral nerves rather than the central nervous system. Thus, this introductory discussion focuses mainly on the structure and function of the parts of the nervous system massage therapists can touch—which, not coincidentally, are also the parts of the system that are most vulnerable to injury.

Function

What are nerves? Nerves are bundles of individual neurons: single-celled fibers capable of transmitting electrical impulses from one place to another. At their most basic level, their function is to transmit information from the body to the brain (sensation) and signals from the brain back to the body (motor control). Interconnected neurons in the brain also provide the potential for consciousness, creativity, memory, and other fascinating abilities, but these are beyond the scope of what massage therapists are qualified to deal with and therefore are not discussed here.

Structure

Peripheral nerves are composed of bundles of long filaments (neurons) that run from the spinal cord to wherever in the body they supply sensation or motor control. Each neuron is a single living cell. It is a bit boggling to realize that the neuron running from the low back to the skin of the great toe is all one unbroken microscopic fiber, but that is the case. Neurons have three parts: the dendrite (which carries impulses *toward* the cell body), the cell body, and the axon (which carries impulses *away* from the cell body). Sensory neurons therefore have exceptionally long dendrites to carry information toward the cell body in the dorsal root ganglia; they have short little axons to continue carrying their impulses into the spinal cord. Motor neurons have tiny dendrites and cell bodies in the spinal canal, and very long axons to carry messages out to their terminating sites in the muscles and glands. Motor and sensory neurons communicate via synapses in the spinal cord, usually by way of some combinations of central, or association, neurons. At the same time that an immediate response is generated at the spinal cord level, the information also travels up the spine into the brain. This immediate reaction is called the reflex arc (Fig. 3-1).

Most neurons in the peripheral and central nervous system have a waxy insulating coating called myelin. This layer of material speeds nerve conduction along the fiber and prevents the jumping of electrical impulses from one fiber to another. In the peripheral nervous system, neurons have another protective feature called *neurilemma*; this is an outer covering of special cells that can help to regenerate damaged tissue (Fig. 3-2).

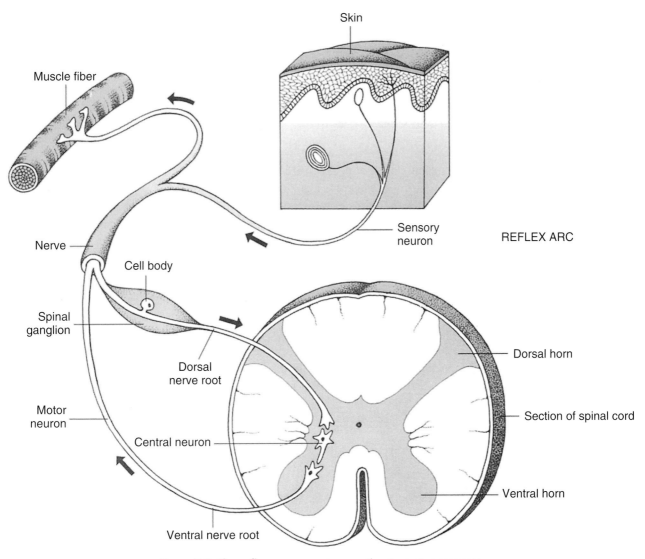

Figure 3-1. The reflex arc connects sensation to motor response

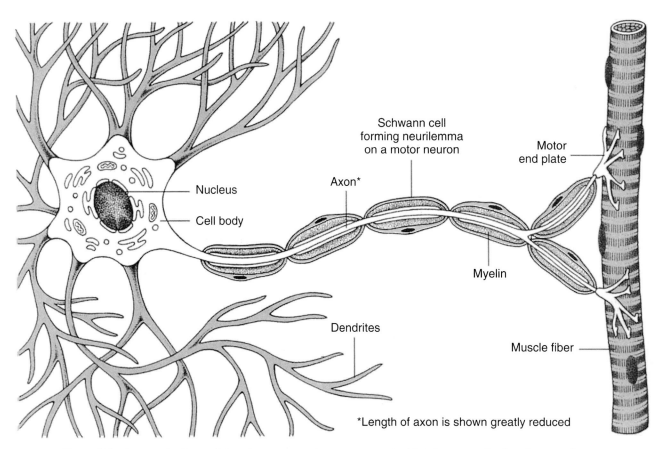

Figure 3-2. Neurons in the peripheral nervous system are covered with Schwann cells, forming neurilemma

Peripheral nerves typically run close to the bone where they are protected from most injuries. They are vulnerable in a few places, however. These spots are *endangerments* for massage therapists, who could potentially cause injury to delicate tissues at these points (self-defense classes call them *targets*). For specific information on nerve endangerments, see Appendix 3.

It is a convenient analogy to think about nerves as bundles of electrical wires. The similarities are obvious. Here are thousands of filaments carrying electrical impulses, each one wrapped by an insulating layer of myelin, and they are bundled together for efficiency. The analogy stops, however, when one considers the effect of external pressure on nerve fiber transmission. In *Job's Body*, Deane Juhan points out that a piece of electrical cable with a truck parked on continues to carry its electrical messages, but a sciatic nerve squeezed by a tight piriformis will have a drastically reduced flow of energy through it.[a] Nerves function with a combination of electrical and fluid flow; fluid flow is severely limited by external pressure. Consider the implications of pressure on a femoral nerve that is hugged by a psoas in spasm, or the brachial plexus nerves running through a tangled maze of scalenes, and pectoralis minor muscles.

General Neurological Problems

Most of the nervous system disorders that massage can affect involve some kind of mechanical pinching or distortion of peripheral nerves as they wend their ways from the

---

[a]Juhan D. *Job's Body: A Handbook for Bodywork*. Barrytown, NY: Station Hill Press; 1987.

spinal cord to their destinations in the body. Peripheral nerve damage has a generally good prognosis because of the regenerative properties provided by the neurilemma.

Other neurologic problems involve the brain or spinal cord, which have very limited ability to regenerate and which massage obviously cannot directly access. Even when the spinal cord has been injured, overlapping patterns of innervation created by the twists and turns of the plexi often allow at least partial use of what would otherwise be a totally lost limb. This is a remarkable advantage that begins to explain the benefits of the confusing routes that nerves take through the plexi. The best plan, when faced with a client who has sustained central nervous system damage, is to address the *symptoms* of these disorders as well as possible, looking for sensation where it is present, and to create as hospitable an internal environment as possible.

Organic and mechanical problems with the central and peripheral nervous systems are one class of neurologic problems that massage therapists may encounter. Psychiatric disorders, which can also be classified as neurologic problems, are another situation altogether. Many people have a bewildering array of mental or psychological qualities that set them apart from the arbitrary standards called "normal." Some of these people seek massage as a way to deal with some of the difficulties that their "abnormalities" create.

Massage therapists can thus be put in the precarious position of deciding whether their work is an appropriate part of someone's healing (or even just coping) process. Sometimes the answer will clearly be "no" (e.g., with someone who is obviously in need of psychological counseling instead of or in addition to massage). At other times it will be less clear, and it will be necessary to seek out the opinion of other professionals. Mental health patients who are taking heavy, long-term doses of medication are in a particularly vulnerable position regarding massage. Although massage is usually a good thing, it can change the internal chemistry of the body and brain significantly. When massage elicits a parasympathetic response, the types of neurotransmitters and hormones circulating in the body may shift radically away from "flight or fight" chemicals to substances that allow for relaxation and even sleepiness. If a client is taking medication to achieve equilibrium, it is inappropriate for a well-meaning but ignorant massage therapist to throw the client off balance. The client's medical and health care team must always be consulted before massage is given.

Disorders of the nervous system can produce a bewildering variety of startling and sometimes intimidating symptoms. In working with these patients, as with all others, massage therapists must remember that their prime objective must always be, "Do no harm."

Nervous System Conditions

Chronic Degenerative Disorders
Alzheimer's Disease
Amyotrophic Lateral Sclerosis
Multiple Sclerosis
Parkinson's Disease
Peripheral Neuropathy
Tremor

Infectious Disorders
Encephalitis
Herpes Zoster
Meningitis
Polio
Post Polio Syndrome

Psychiatric Disorders
Anxiety Disorders
Chemical Dependancy
Depression
Eating Disorders

Nervous System Injuries
Bell's Palsy
Cerebral Palsy
Reflex Sympathetic Dystrophy
Spinal Cord Injury
Stroke
Trigeminal Neuralgia

Other Nervous System Disorders
Guillain-Barré Syndrome

Headaches
Seizure Disorders
Sleep Disorders

Chronic Degenerative Disorders

Alzheimer's Disease

Definition: What Is It?

Alzheimer's disease is a progressive degenerative disorder of the brain causing memory loss, personality changes, and eventually death. The precise causes of the disorder are not fully understood, but it is now known that although most people can look forward to a certain degree of memory loss as they age, the severe dementia associated with Alzheimer's is not normal and not an inevitable fate for every person.

Demographics: Who Gets It?

Alzheimer's disease affects about 5% of the U.S. population, or about 4 million people. It affects about half of all people living in nursing homes, and costs approximately $24 to $48 million per year in direct medical expenses.

The incidence of Alzheimer's disease increases with age. Whereas only 1% of people younger than 75 years of age are significantly affected, more than 25% of those older than 85 have severe dementia. Most cases of Alzheimer's disease are diagnosed around age 80. Because baby boomers will soon be entering the at-risk age group, it is estimated that by 2050 this disease will disable approximately14 million people.[b]

Alzheimer's affects more women than men, but this may be related to the fact that women generally live longer than men, rather than a gender-based predisposition.

Etiology: What Happens?

Alzheimer's disease is named for a German doctor, Alois Alzheimer, who in 1906 first documented the trademark lesions in the brain seen with this disease. He performed an autopsy on a female patient who died in a mental institution in her mid-50s. He noted two specific changes in her brain tissue: plaques and tangles. These observations have become the primary postmortem diagnostic features of this disease and have become the focus of the leading edge of research today.

Features of Alzheimer's Disease

Plaques   Sticky deposits of a certain type of naturally occurring cellular protein called beta amyloid have been noted on brain tissue of people with Alzheimer's disease. Beta amyloid is a protein produced by many cells throughout the body, and it occurs in different lengths and qualities, depending on where it is found. In the brain it seems to be particularly adhesive. When it accumulates in sufficient amounts, the deposits appear to

[b]What is Alzheimer's disease? Meditopia!; 1996. Available at: http://www.meditopia.com/alzwhat.html. Accessed winter 2001.

stimulate an inflammatory response in the brain that kills not only the cells affected by beta amyloid plaques, but nearby unaffected cells as well.

Neurofibrillary Tangles   Another Alzheimer's-related protein is called tau. This substance helps to physically support long fibers in the central nervous system that allow cells to communicate. The tau proteins in Alzheimer's patients degenerate, and the long fibers collapse and become twisted and tangled together. Eventually the cells, which are incapable of transmitting messages to each other, shrink and die.

Low Neurotransmitters   The presence of beta amyloid plaques and tau-related tangles means that fewer brain cells function at normal levels. With the loss of neural tissue, levels of neurotransmitters in the brains of Alzheimer's patients become pathologically low. This makes it difficult for the functioning nerve cells that remain to communicate with each other. Consequently, the Alzheimer's patient loses both access to memories and the ability to process new information.

Genetics   Although having Alzheimer's disease in the family only marginally increases a person's chance of developing it, some specific genetic markers have been found that can identify a higher-risk population. The genes involved probably determine how effectively a person can clear off beta amyloid plaques. Genetic research has yielded especially clear markers for people susceptible to an early onset of the disease.

The majority of the information about how Alzheimer's develops has been gathered in the past 10 years. As the understanding of this disease progresses, it will probably be found that its causes are multi-faceted, involving issues as complex as genetics, exposure to environmental toxins, high cholesterol levels, low estrogen levels (in women), and possibly some other variables that have yet to be explored.

Signs and Symptoms

Stage 1   The first stage of Alzheimer's disease is a gradual loss of memory and/or cognitive function. Patients may have difficulty performing complex tasks like balancing a checkbook or cooking dinner. Holding a job may become an unrealistic expectation. The patient may lose interest in favorite activities, and a decrease in judgment may lead to inappropriate choices, like wearing a bathrobe to the store.

These early signs can be alarming for many individuals, who foresee a bleak future in the grips of this disease. Depression, which has some similar symptoms to Alzheimer's, may complicate the whole mental health picture. Stage 1 Alzheimer's generally lasts for about 2 to 4 years.

Stage 2   Later signs may involve a deterioration of language skills: it becomes harder to remember specific names or words when they are needed, and patients may have increasing difficulty in expressing themselves. The ability to recognize people begins to fade, and the patient may experience disorientation (easily getting lost or wandering away from familiar territory), confusion, and anxiety. Daily tasks like brushing teeth or getting dressed become prohibitively difficult. This stage of the disease usually lasts from 2 to 8 years.

Stage 3   As the disease progresses, Alzheimer's patients become unable to remember anything or to process new information. Patients may still respond to touch, sound, and eye contact, but they are unable to bathe or dress themselves. Eventually they lose bowel and bladder control and are bedridden. Most Alzheimer's patients eventually die of infection, as in *pneumonia* (see Chapter 6), or complications due to falls (see *pulmonary embolism*, Chapter 4).

Diagnosis

Diagnosis of Alzheimer's disease is problematic because the presence of plaques and tangles can only be confirmed posthumously. This disease is now diagnosed through a variety of tests to rule out other causes of dementia, in combination with mental status examinations. It is important to try to come to an accurate diagnosis of Alzheimer's for two reasons. First, because the earlier treatment is introduced, the longer memory may be preserved. Second, dementia and loss of memory can sometimes be indicators of diseases *other* than Alzheimer's, some of which can be reversible.

As our ability to gather information about living brains develops, it may become easier to diagnose Alzheimer's. One possibility is a refined examination of cerebrospinal fluid, which could show increased levels of tau (because it is breaking off its normal support system of long central nervous system fibers) and reduced levels of beta amyloid (because it is adhering to nerve cells). Other new technologies may allow physicians to observe interactions of brain chemicals at a molecular level in living patients. In other words, it may become possible to observe exactly how and when neurotransmitters are being produced and how they are stimulating connections in neural tissue.

Differential Diagnosis

Alzheimer's is only one of several diseases that can cause dementia and memory loss. Some conditions involve permanent brain damage, but others may be only temporary problems if they are treated appropriately.

Causes of permanent memory loss other than Alzheimer's include the following:

- *Vascular dementia.* This is caused by a narrowing of the arteries to the brain, usually associated with advanced cardiovascular disease.

- *Stroke and transient ischemic attack (TIA).* These events cause brain tissue to die because of an interruption in blood supply. These issues are more fully discussed elsewhere in this chapter.

- *Parkinson's disease.* This disease involves the degeneration of certain motor centers in the brain but also often involves dementia. Parkinson's disease is also discussed in this chapter.

- *Lewy body dementia.* Lewy bodies are protein deposits similar to beta amyloid plaques that lead to dementia. This disease has features in common with both Alzheimer's and Parkinson's disease.

- *Huntington's disease.* This is another progressive degenerative central nervous system disease involving the destruction of nerve cells and resulting changes in personality and intellect. Huntington's is a genetic disease.

- *Creutzfeldt-Jakob disease.* This is a type of dementia that affects young and middle-aged people. It is associated with eating meat that is contaminated with bovine spongiform encephalitis (mad cow disease).

Other conditions can cause memory loss that is recoverable. Naturally, it is important to consider these possibilities before deciding that a patient has irreversible Alzheimer's disease. Some examples of things important to test for include:

- Chronic high blood pressure

- Depression

- Diabetes

- Hypothyroidism

- Side effects to medication

- Vitamin B_{12} deficiency

Treatment

Treatment options are perhaps the most exciting part of the tremendous advances being made in Alzheimer's research. As a better understanding of this disease is achieved, methods to slow or even prevent it are being developed at an astounding pace.

Current treatment options often revolve around the deficit of neurotransmitters in the brain that make it difficult for nerves to communicate. Cholinesterase inhibitors are often prescribed to prevent the re-uptake of acetylcholine, an essential neurotransmitter that is often in short supply for Alzheimer's patients. These drugs effectively improve memory, at least in the short term. Other medications may be prescribed to address some of the behavioral and mood distortions seen with Alzheimer's.

Medications directed at the prevention or reversal of beta amyloid plaques may be developed in the future; some of these are already being used successfully in mice. Other promising options include the use of some non-steroidal anti-inflammatory drugs (NSAIDs) that seem to limit the reaction to plaques that causes cell damage. Observations that postmenopausal women who supplement estrogen have a lower risk of Alzheimer's disease, and that some antioxidants seem to limit the progression of the disease, may also point the way to effective future treatments.

Massage?

Alzheimer's disease patients, even in advanced stages of the disease when language is difficult or impossible, still respond positively to touch. Research done on the effects of massage with Alzheimer's patients shows that although bodywork does not slow or reverse the disease, it improves the quality of life for patients to the extent that they become measurably less disruptive, show better sense of orientation, and have more positive social interactions in nursing home settings.

Two cautions must be kept in mind when working with Alzheimer's patients. One is that most of these clients are elderly, and consequently may have a number of other complicated disorders that may contraindicate various kinds of bodywork. The other is that when a client cannot communicate clearly, it becomes the responsibility of the massage therapist to interpret nonverbal signals about how the bodywork is being accepted. Alzheimer's clients generally respond well to massage, but if they become anxious and frightened for unknowable reasons, the therapist must be sensitive to the client's mental and emotional state.

Amyotrophic Lateral Sclerosis
Definition: What Is It?

Also known as *Lou Gehrig's disease*, this is a progressive condition that destroys motor neurons in the spinal cord, leading to the atrophy of voluntary muscles.

Demographics: Who Gets It?

Three types of ALS have been identified: sporadic, which accounts for 90 to 95% of the cases in the United States; familial, which shows a genetic link for 5 to 10% of U.S. cases; and the Mariana Island variety, which is endemic to a specific population in the Western Pacific islands.

AMYOTROPHIC LATERAL SCLEROSIS IN BRIEF

What is it?
Amyotrophic lateral sclerosis (ALS) is a progressive disease that begins in the central nervous system. It involves the degeneration of motor neurons and the subsequent atrophy of voluntary muscles.

How is it recognized?
Symptoms of ALS include weakness, fatigue, and muscle spasms. It appears most frequently in patients between 40 and 70 years of age.

Is massage indicated or contraindicated?
ALS indicates massage, with caution, when a massage therapist works as part of a health care team.

ALS usually affects people between 40 and 70 years of age; the average age at diagnosis is 55. Familial ALS tends to have a younger onset than the sporadic type. Between 4000 and 5000 new cases of ALS are diagnosed in the United States every year; approximately 30,000 people in this country are living with this disease right now. Men get it only slightly more often than do women. One of the most interesting features about this disease is that it has a virtually identical incidence among all nations and races. Two populations carry a higher-than-normal risk in the United States—electrical utility workers and airline pilots.

Etiology: What Happens?

The cause or causes of ALS is unknown. When the disease develops, it leads to the degeneration of motor neurons in the spinal cord, which leads to the progressive and irreversible atrophy of voluntary muscle.

Several possible causative factors have been identified, including some features that are strikingly similar to *Alzheimer's disease* (this chapter): tangled neural fibers and deposits of abnormal proteins on clumps of cells. ALS interrupts only motor function, however, and does not affect intellect or memory.

Other possible causes of ALS include imbalances in neurotransmitters that can lead to cell death, a genetic susceptibility to damage from free radicals (this has been reliably established in the case of familial ALS), and exposure to environmental toxins such as lead, agricultural chemicals, and selenium. It is important to point out, however, that these theories are simply observations; causative factors for ALS have not been defined.

Signs and Symptoms

ALS presents different early symptoms in different people. The most common pattern is stiffness, weakness, and awkwardness in one body part, which slowly spreads to other parts of the body. About one-third of ALS patients have their first symptoms in the legs; another third begin with changes in hand and arm function; and the final third begin with "thick speech" and difficulty with swallowing. Fasciculations, or visible muscle twitching, may be present. One side of the body is typically affected more than the other, but the stiffness eventually spreads and moves proximally up the limbs, eventually affecting the trunk muscles for breathing.

ALS does not affect sensory neurons or intellectual capacity.

Diagnosis

No single test can identify ALS. It is typically diagnosed through patient history, physical examination, nerve conduction studies, and electromyographs, all of which show loss of muscle function caused by lack of nerve stimulation. Tests are also conducted to differentiate ALS from other conditions that have some similar symptoms, for instance *muscular dystrophy* (see Chapter 2), *hyperthyroidism* (Chapter 8), *multiple sclerosis*, *post polio syndrome*, and *peripheral neuropathy* (all in this chapter).

Treatment

Up until very recently, treatment for ALS has been strictly palliative, that is, aimed at managing the severity of the symptoms only. Some of these options include moderate exercise and physical and occupational therapy to maintain muscle strength as long as possible. Heat and whirlpools are used to control muscle spasms, and speech therapy helps with difficulties in swallowing and speech. Assistive devices such as leg braces, arm braces, or wheelchairs can improve a patient's ability to function. In advanced cases swallowing may be so difficult that the insertion of a stomach tube (gastrostomy) may be recommended. Since this disease does not impede cognitive or emotional processes, psychological therapy for ALS patients and their families is an important part of the treatment plan.

Drug treatment of ALS has traditionally been used only to help combat general fatigue or secondary infections, but drugs have now been developed that slow the progression of the disease and keep motor nerves active for longer. They are not a cure for ALS, but they may significantly prolong the lives of people affected by this disease.

Prognosis

Once diagnosed, this disease, which has no known cure, usually results in death within 2 to 10 years. Death is usually due to complications of paralysis, particularly systemic infections such as *pneumonia* (Chapter 6) or *kidney infection* (Chapter 9). One-half of all ALS patients die within 3 years of diagnosis; 90% die within 6 years. Some ALS patients, however, have survived for decades. How? No one knows.

Massage?

This disease is not blood- or lymph-borne, it does not involve sensory paralysis, and it is not contagious. It is treated with heat, exercise, and physical therapy. Therefore, *within limits*, and in the absence of other contraindicating circumstances, massage may also be appropriate. Massage therapists who work with ALS patients should do it as part of a health care team and keep careful notes on their work to make available to others.

Multiple Sclerosis

Definition: What Is It?

This condition is characterized by the inflammation and then gradual degeneration of myelin sheaths in the spinal cord and brain. It is thought to be an autoimmune disease, but the triggering pathogen has not yet been identified.

Demographics: Who Gets It?

MS affects Whites about twice as often as any other ethnic group. Its highest incidence is among people who live far from the equator (either north or south), or who did so before they were 15 years old.

MS is generally diagnosed in patients between 20 and 40 years of age. Young women are diagnosed up to twice as often as young men, but when it is diagnosed among older patients, the female-male distribution is about the same.

Between 300,000 and 350,000 Americans live with MS; about 9,000 new cases are diagnosed every year.

Etiology: What Happens?

The word *sclerosis* means hardened scar or plaque. In MS myelin is attacked, and in the inflammatory process it is replaced with scar tissue. As the myelin is replaced, the electrical impulses meant to tie the whole system together literally short circuit. This results

---

MULTIPLE SCLEROSIS IN BRIEF

What is it?
Multiple sclerosis (MS) is an idiopathic disease that involves the destruction of myelin sheaths around both motor and sensory neurons in the central nervous system.

How is it recognized?
MS has many symptoms, depending on the nature of the damage. These can include fatigue, eye pain, spasticity, tremors, and a progressive loss of vision, sensation, and motor control.

Is massage indicated or contraindicated?
Subacute stages of MS, when the client is in remission, indicate massage. Circulatory or other vigorous types of bodywork should be avoided during periods of flare.

in motor and sensory paralysis instead of coordinated movement and feeling. The signs and symptoms of the disease, like so many disorders of the central nervous system, depend entirely on where and how much nerve tissue has been damaged.

MS, like many autoimmune diseases, often works in cycles of inflammatory "flares" followed by periods of remission. During flares the myelin is under attack and is replaced by scar tissue. During remission inflammation subsides, and some regeneration of myelin may occur. In this way MS patients may lose some neurologic function during flares but regain some or all of it during remission.

Causes

Currently, the leading theories behind MS point to immune system attacks against some component of myelin sheaths in the central nervous system. This leads to an inflammatory response that destroys the protective myelin sheath and may eventually attack the nerve tissue itself. Most autoimmune diseases have some specific pathogenic trigger that begins the immune system mistake, leading to tissue damage. No specific trigger has been identified for MS.

It also seems clear that a genetic predisposition raises the risk of developing MS, but this seems to be a relatively small factor. The population-wide risk of developing MS is less than 0.1%; people with a first-degree relative who has the disease have a 1 to 3% risk. Identical twins carry a 30% risk of developing the disease if their twin has it.

This collection of information indicates that MS is probably an autoimmune disease to which some people are genetically predisposed, but that requires some kind of environmental trigger to initiate the disease process. The fact that in a few isolated cases the incidence of MS among a local population is much higher than the statistical norm supports the influence of environmental factors that are not yet understood.

Signs and Symptoms

This disease is sometimes called *The Great Imitator* because its initial symptoms can look like a variety of other diseases, depending on what area of nerve tissue has been affected. The order with which symptoms appear also varies greatly from one person to the next. Some of the most dependable signs and symptoms include:

- *Weakness.* The onset of this problem may be gradual or sudden. It comes about because the loss of myelin makes nerve transmission slow.
- *Spasm.* This can take the form of chronic muscle stiffness or of active acute cramping. (See *Spasms, cramps,* Chapter 2).
- *Changes in sensation:* MS patients often report numbness or paresthesia ("pins and needles") in various parts of the body. These sensations may last for hours or days.
- *Optic neuritis.* Attacks on the myelin of the optic nerve result in extreme eye pain, coupled with progressive loss of function. Vision may be minimally impaired (e.g., color distortions) or it may be fully lost until the episode has past. Most MS patients recover full or close to full vision when they go into remission.
- *Urologic dysfunction.* MS patients may find it difficult to urinate or they may experience incontinence.
- *Sexual dysfunction.* Difficulty in maintaining an erection for men, or in having an orgasm for women are sometimes early signs of this disease.
- *Difficulty walking.* This problem can be a product of several different factors including muscle stiffness, numbness, and loss of coordination.

- *Loss of cognitive function.* A frequently overlooked issue for many MS patients is a change in mental ability. Short-term memory and the ability to learn and perform complex tasks are often challenged. A majority of MS patients have limited loss of cognitive function but can compensate. A smaller percentage experience severe changes in cognitive skills.

- *Depression.* This is a complication of many chronic progressive diseases, especially in situations as unpredictable as those created by MS. Up to 70% of MS patients live with depression, which can exacerbate symptoms.

- *Lhermitte's sign.* In this neurologic test, electrical sensations run down the spine when the neck is in flexion.

- *Digestive disturbances.* Many MS patients experience severe digestive disturbances (nausea, diarrhea, constipation) that vary greatly from day to day.

- *Fatigue.* Perhaps the most common symptom for all MS patients is debilitating fatigue, which is particularly exacerbated by heat. The fatigue may be a result of slower or impaired nerve transmission (this requires fewer muscle fibers to work harder), muscle spasm, and other factors.

Progression

The progression of this disease is highly unpredictable. It has a few characteristic patterns, but some patients move from one pattern type to others within their disease process. Some of the basic patterns are as follow:

- *Relapse/remitting (R/R).* Definite periods of flare are followed by long periods of remission. It may be years between episodes.

- *Primary progressive (PP).* Patients show a steady decline in function; episodes of flare are frequent.

- *Benign MS.* The patient has only one flare in his or her lifetime.

- *Malignant MS.* This is a rapidly progressive form of the disease with little respite (if any) between flares.

Other presentations of MS are combinations of R/R or PP patterns.

Diagnosis

No single test can definitively diagnose MS. The disease is identified through a description of symptoms, a family health history, a spinal tap to look for raised antibody levels and myelin fragments, and magnetic resonance imaging (MRI) scans that can reveal central nervous system lesions. (The lesions shown in MRI scans may be from sources other than MS, however, so they are not considered factors for a definitive diagnosis). Nerve conduction tests to measure the speed of electrical impulses through nerves may also be conducted.

Several conditions can produce MS-like symptoms. Part of a thorough diagnosis is ruling out the following conditions:

- Lyme disease

- Herniated or ruptured disk

- Human immunodeficiency virus/acquired immune deficiency syndrome (HIV/AIDS)

- Lupus

- Scleroderma

- Central nervous system tumors
- Vascular problems in the brain
- Fibromyalgia
- Complications of encephalitis
- B_{12} or folic acid deficiency

The process of coming to a conclusive diagnosis of MS is so challenging that conditions are often labeled as "possible MS" and "probable MS" before tests results are conclusive.

Treatment

Until recently, standard treatment options for MS included symptomatic treatment (e.g., for fatigue or muscle pain) with doses of steroidal anti-inflammatories to quell the severity of flares. Steroids can reduce symptoms in the short run but have not been shown to have long-lasting benefits. In addition, their side effects can be severe. Therefore, they are usually used only as a temporary measure.

A new class of drugs called beta interferon has been developed to work specifically to limit immune system activity. Initial studies find that these drugs can shorten the duration of periods of flare and prolong periods between episodes. They are cumulatively toxic to the heart and liver, however, and must be used extremely sparingly.

Research into MS treatment is now examining the possibility of transplanting myelin-producing cells into MS patients. This may become the standard treatment option until the understanding of the exact causes of the disease yield enough information to stop the myelin damage before it starts.

Other interventions for people living with MS include mild exercise and physical or occupational therapy designed to maintain strength and function for as long as possible. Eating well and getting adequate amounts of high-quality sleep are important for maintaining health and prolonging remissions. Stress management techniques, including massage, are often recommended for the same reasons.

Prognosis

Although not much is understood about the cause of this disease, many statistics have been collected about how it affects the people who have it. Until recently, up to 50% of all MS patients had some level of disability within 10 years of the onset of their disease; 66% of all MS patients could expect to be in a wheelchair at 30 years after their diagnosis. Those statistics may change as beta-interferon–based medicines slow the progression of the disease.

MS is not a terminal disease in itself. People who have MS generally have a life span about 6 years shorter than average. People who die prematurely of this disease are usually immobile, and they fall prey to an opportunistic disease such as a *kidney infection*, *urinary tract infection* (Chapter 9), or *pneumonia* (Chapter 6).

Massage?

This disease usually has acute and subacute periods; it indicates massage in the subacute stages. However, care *must* be taken not to overstimulate the client, which can result in painful and uncontrolled muscle spasms. Symptoms may also be exacerbated by heat, so therapists must avoid allowing their clients' core temperature to rise by working in an overly warm environment.

Every client with MS presents symptoms and problems differently. If sensation is present, massage can be useful as an agent against stress (which seems to trigger relapses), depression, and spasticity. Massage also helps to maintain the health and mobility of the tissues. In areas where sensation is not present, non-mechanical types of work (i.e., very light effleurage and energy work) is more appropriate.

MULTIPLE SCLEROSIS
Tricia, 36 Years Old
"It takes all the courage I can muster just to stand up in the morning."

Everyone has problems. Everyone gets in their own world so much. Now I look at someone with a disability and I wonder if they have it. You start to watch people walk and wonder if they've got it.

One and a half years ago we had just moved into a new house and my youngest child had just started school. For the first time in 15 years I was looking forward to having some time, to getting on with my life.

Then there was a pain in my left heel that felt like a stone bruise. We were just back from a long vacation, so I thought it was from too much walking. Two weeks later there was a lack of sensation in my foot and it traveled up my leg to my knee. It began affecting my right leg too. Then there was numbness and tingling in my left hand. It felt like I had just had a shot of Novocain—it was that kind of tingling.

Try walking on the balls of your feet for a whole day. Then you'll get an idea of how hard it was. I couldn't put my heels down because there would be a sharp tingling "funny bone" feeling. My walking was so labored, I got to the point where I would rather shimmy on my chest like an army guy to get from room to room. I wasn't crying, I wasn't upset, it was just easier to crawl.

At the same time as feeling stressed about not knowing what was happening to me, I put off going to the doctor. I finally went to my OB for my headaches. He gave me migraine medication, but it didn't work.

He sent me to a neurologist who checked me out and watched me walk. Then while I was sitting there he went out into the hall with another doctor and they started speaking in medical jargon that I couldn't understand; it made me really nervous. When he came back he asked me, "Will you come in for a spinal tap?"

"Why?"

"There are some things we want to check out."

"What do you think I have?"

"I think you have MS."

"Excuse me?"

I never *dreamed* it would be something like this.

They started me on IV steroids. The next morning I got up after a bad night, and for the first time in 2 months I could walk normally. I was so excited, I woke my family and called my mom on the phone. But by the end of that morning I was already beginning to feel tired. My condition deteriorated in spite of the steroids. By the end of the week I couldn't even get up off the couch to let the home care nurse in.

My neurologist finally sent me to the University Hospital. There they did lots of other tests, more spinal taps, and an MRI. The MRI showed tiny spots in my brain, but nothing like what they were expecting. The spinal taps all came back negative.

They had me talking to teams of doctors. I talked to neurologists, immune specialists, nutritionists, and psychiatrists. The head of the department was prepared to tell my family I had chronic progressive MS, which meant I could be dead in a matter of weeks. I finally decided that I needed to be home, I needed to be with my family, so I checked out even though they didn't want me to.

I continued physical therapy at a local clinic. At first they would have me sit in a warm pool with jets of water after I exercised, and I would go home feeling so drained and worn out, it was awful. Finally they adjusted that part of it and I did better.

Today I still don't have much sensation below my knees. It takes all the courage I can muster to just to stand up in the morning. I never know what kind of day I'll have, whether I'll be able to walk without a cane, whether I'll be tied to the house because my digestive system is unpredictable. I have terrible headaches that begin on the lower half of one side of my face and go up into my ear. I have days when I can't eat at all. I've had episodes of dizziness and double vision. I'm not on steroids now, but I take an anti-depressant for the headaches. We're still struggling to find the right dose. My greatest fear, even more than being in a wheelchair, is that I will lose bladder or bowel control, or go blind.

But my doctor says my scenario is good. It's been a year and a half without any exacerbations and he says I'm in remission. The only thing that's worse are my headaches, which are more painful and happen more often.

MULTIPLE SCLEROSIS—continued
Tricia, 36 Years Old
"It takes all the courage I can muster just to stand up in the morning."

I think everything depends on your attitude. A major thing for me is to feel needed. If I have a purpose, I feel better. My aunt has MS, and she practically runs her family business. It's just amazing to see her get up and go. She says there are some days that if she didn't have that business to go to, she wouldn't be able to get out of bed. I have a chance now to see what other people have to deal with, and some of them are so much worse off than I am, because of physical problems, but other kinds of problems too. I have five wonderful children and a husband who loves me. My doctor thought I was going to die, and here I am in remission. I just feel so lucky to be here.

PARKINSON'S DISEASE IN BRIEF

What is it?
Parkinson's disease is a degenerative disease of the substantia nigra cells in the brain. These cells produce the neurotransmitter dopamine, which helps the basal ganglia to maintain balance, posture, and coordination.

How is it recognized?
Early symptoms of Parkinson's include general stiffness and fatigue; resting tremor of the hand, foot, or head; stiffness; and poor balance. Later symptoms include a shuffling gait, a "mask-like" appearance to the face, and a monotone voice.

Is massage indicated or contraindicated?
Parkinson's disease indicates massage with caution. Care must be taken for the physical safety of these clients who cannot move freely or smoothly.

PARKINSON'S DISEASE

Dr. James Parkinson (1755–1824) was a British physician who first documented this chronic degenerative nervous system disorder.

Parkinson's Disease
Definition: What Is It?

Parkinson's disease, first discussed by the British physician James Parkinson in 1817 as the "shaking palsy," is a movement disorder involving the progressive degeneration of nerve tissue and a reduction in neurotransmitter production in the central nervous system.

Demographics: Who Gets It?

Parkinson's disease affects about 1 person out of every 1000 of the population overall, but its incidence rises considerably with age. It occurs at a rate of approximately 1–2:100 in persons older than 50. Men with Parkinson's disease outnumber women by about 3:2.

Approximately 500,000 people with Parkinson's live in the United States today; about 50,000 new cases are diagnosed each year.

Etiology: What Happens?

Parkinson's disease is one of a variety of conditions classified as "movement disorders." It involves changes in central nervous system structures that cause them to work inefficiently. To discuss this condition thoroughly, it is necessary to review some of the inner workings of the brain.

Anatomy Review

Voluntary muscle control is managed in two areas of the brain: the basal ganglia and the cerebellum. The basal ganglia are found at the lower edges of the cerebrum. They are little pockets of gray matter embedded in white matter that work with the cerebellum to provide learned reflexes, motor control, and coordination. ("Coordination" here means the balance in action between prime movers and their antagonistic muscles.)

Healthy basal ganglia cells are supplied with a vital neurotransmitter, dopamine, by another nearby structure, the *substantia nigra* (also known as "black stuff"). In Parkinson's disease, the substantia nigra cells die, depriving the basal ganglia of dopamine. Without dopamine, the basal ganglia cannot maintain the careful balance between agonists and antagonists in the body; thus, coordination degenerates and controlled movement becomes very difficult.

For Parkinson's symptoms to appear, the substantia nigra must be about 60% lost. This loss of tissue results in an 80% loss of dopamine production in the area of the basal ganglia. New imaging techniques that can track chemical reactions in the brain may allow diagnoses of Parkinson's disease before the damage has reached this advanced stage.

Causes

No one really knows what causes the substantia nigra to degenerate in the majority of Parkinson's disease cases. Environmental agents may be found to be one cause; a statistical rise in patients younger than 50 years of age substantiates that theory. In some families a genetic connection is clear, and research has identified specific sites of genetic abnormality for those individuals with familial Parkinson's. A small percentage of cases can be traced to specific other issues: carbon monoxide poisoning may be one factor, as is heavy metal poisoning and exposure to pesticides. It can also follow repeated head trauma (*pugilistic parkinsonism* is a diagnosis given to affected boxers), neurovascular disease, and exposure to certain drugs. The drug-induced form is reversible.

Whatever the root cause, research is focusing on the process of *apoptosis* (cellular "suicide") that occurs in the substantia nigra. One theory holds that immune system agents create a surplus of chemical messengers in the substantia nigra that carry instructions for cells to self-destruct. A similar problem with apoptosis of specific nervous system cells has been seen in other neurodegenerative diseases like *amyotrophic lateral sclerosis* and *Alzheimer's disease* (this chapter).

Signs and Symptoms

Symptoms of Parkinson's disease can be divided into primary and secondary problems. Primary symptoms arise from the disease itself, whereas secondary symptoms are direct results of primary symptoms.

Primary Symptoms

- *Nonspecific achiness, weakness, and fatigue.* Parkinson's disease has a slow onset and is most common in elderly people. Therefore, these early symptoms are often missed, either because they are too subtle to be seen or because of an assumption that a certain amount of fatigue and stiffness is just a natural part of growing older.

- *Resting tremor.* This phenomenon is present in about 75% of all Parkinson's patients and is often one of the first noticeable symptoms. A rhythmic shaking or "pill rolling" action of the hand is often seen. Tremor may also affect the foot, head, and neck. This tremor is most noticeable when the patient is at rest but not sleeping. It often disappears entirely when the patient is engaged in some other activity.

- *Bradykinesia.* This means difficulty in initiating or sustaining movement. It can take a long time to begin a voluntary movement of the arm or leg, and the limb's movement may be halting and interrupted midstream. Parkinson's patients sometimes report feeling "rooted to the floor" when they can visualize moving a leg, but it does not happen without sustained effort.

- *Rigidity.* Gradually the muscles, particularly the flexor muscles, of Parkinson's patients become permanently hypertonic. This can give rise to a characteristically stooped posture as the trunk flexors contract more strongly than the paraspinals.

This is particularly visible when Parkinson's accompanies *osteoporosis* (Chapter 2), as it often does. Rigidity also makes it difficult to bend or straighten arms and legs and can cause a particular "mask-like" appearance to the face as the facial muscles lose flexibility and ease of movement (Fig. 3-3). This also accounts for a reduced rate of eye blinking and increased drooling and difficulty with eating and swallowing.

The rigidity that accompanies Parkinson's is not the same thing as spasticity, which implies a different kind of nerve damage. (See *spinal cord injury*, this chapter.) Rigidity indicates massage (with caution), whereas spasticity generally does not.

- *Poor postural reflexes.* Disruption in the activity of basal ganglia cells results in uncoordinated movement and poor balance. Parkinson's patients are particularly susceptible to falling.

Secondary Symptoms

- *Shuffling gait.* Difficulty in bending arms and legs make walking a special challenge for Parkinson's patients. Often the ability to swing the arm is noticeably diminished on one side. The patient takes small steps and may then have to stumble forward to avoid falling. This chasing after the center of gravity is called a *festinating gait.*

- *Changes in speech.* Parkinson's patients experience progressive rigidity of the muscles in the larynx that control vocalization. Their speech gradually becomes monotone and expressionless and progresses toward constant whispering. Muscular changes in the mouth and throat also create problems with swallowing and drooling, particularly while laying down.

- *Changes in handwriting.* The loss of coordination in fine motor muscles changes the ability of a Parkinson's patient to write by hand. "Micrographia" or progressively shrinking, cramped handwriting is one of the later symptoms of this disease.

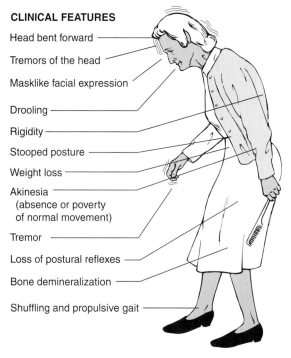

CLINICAL FEATURES

Head bent forward
Tremors of the head
Masklike facial expression
Drooling
Rigidity
Stooped posture
Weight loss
Akinesia
(absence or poverty
of normal movement)
Tremor
Loss of postural reflexes
Bone demineralization
Shuffling and propulsive gait

Figure 3-3. Clinical features of Parkinson's disease

- *Sleep disorders.* Parkinson's patients experience a variety of sleep disorders, from a complete reversal of normal sleeping schedules to sleeplessness, because it is difficult or impossible for them to move in bed.

- *Depression.* The progressive nature of this condition makes anxiety and depression a very predictable part of the disease process. Depression can also be related to insomnia or it can be a side effect of medication. Sometimes the symptoms of depression can outweigh the symptoms of the disease, and treatment for depression can lessen Parkinson's symptoms as well.

- *Mental degeneration.* This is a subject of some controversy. Some sources suggest that advanced Parkinson's patients experience memory loss and deterioration of thought processes. Others suggest that mental problems are side effects of Parkinson's medication and not necessarily a part of the disease itself.

Treatment

In Parkinson's disease a dopamine deficiency develops in the basal ganglia of the brain. A synthetic precursor of dopamine called *levodopa (L-dopa)* can cross the blood–brain barrier, but it is usually a temporary solution. Patients seem to build up a resistance to the drug, and it has a number of troubling side effects including hallucinations and dementia. Some dopamine agonists can be substituted when it becomes necessary, or L-dopa can be prescribed with other drugs that serve to mediate side effects.

Other drug therapies include substances that slow the metabolism of dopamine, so that whatever is available stays for a longer time, and substances that stimulate dopamine receptors in the basal ganglia, so that uptake of the neurotransmitter happens more easily. None of these is a permanent solution, however. Physicians working with Parkinson's patients must monitor their medications carefully and make frequent adjustments.

New discoveries about the pathology of neural tissue have yielded several other treatment options for Parkinson's patients whose conditions do not respond to medication. One of them is deep brain stimulation, in which an electrode is inserted in the thalamus. The patient can activate the thalamus by passing a magnet over a pacemaker-like device that is implanted in the chest. Stimulating the thalamus in this way causes an immediate cessation in tremors. Other surgical options include alterations to the thalamus and other midbrain structures to try to modulate motor dysfunction. As neurosurgery advances, these surgeries are becoming safer and more dependable, but they are still considered a viable option only when medications are no longer effective. Stem cell implantation, the insertion of cellular "blanks" that will grow into healthy substantia nigra cells, holds some promise for the future of Parkinson's disease treatment.

Physical, speech, and occupational therapies are often used to maintain the health and general functioning levels of Parkinson's patients for as long as possible. Psychotherapy and support groups are recommended to cope with the effects of depression.

Massage?

Parkinson's patients experience progressive stiffness and rigidity of voluntary muscles. Massage, given by a therapist as part of a health care team, can be a valuable tool not only to maintain flexibility and range of motion, but also to reduce anxiety and depression. It is important to work in cooperation with a client's primary physician, because massage may affect the need for anti-depressive medication. In addition, clients with Parkinson's disease do not have the freedom of movement that most other people do, and they may have great difficulty in getting on and off tables safely. Some massage therapists solve this problem by doing their work with these clients on the floor.

Peripheral Neuropathy

Definition: What Is It?

Peripheral neuropathy is not a disease in itself, but a symptom or a complication of other underlying conditions. Peripheral nerves, either singly or in groups, are damaged through lack of circulation, chemical imbalance, trauma, or other factors.

Etiology: What Happens?

Most cases of peripheral neuropathy are complications of long-standing bouts with *diabetes* (Chapter 8) or *alcoholism* (see *chemical dependency*, this chapter). More rarely this condition develops because of certain vitamin deficiencies (especially B_{12}) or exposure to toxic substances. The toxins in question include arsenic, mercury, lead, and the organophosphates in insecticides.

Peripheral neuropathy can be associated with various cancers, *HIV/AIDS*, *lupus*, (Chapter 5), *rheumatoid arthritis*, *scleroderma* (Chapter 2), and other diseases that cause vasculitis or inflammation of blood vessels.

Mechanical pressure on nerves can also cause peripheral neuropathy. Examples of this kind of problem include *carpal tunnel syndrome* and *herniated disc* (Chapter 2), *trigeminal neuralgia* (this chapter), and any kind of trauma or tumors that might result in nerve pressure. Inflammation of a single nerve, as seen in trigeminal neuralgia, is referred to as *mononeuropathy*. If several nerves are involved, as seen with lupus, it is called *polyneuropathy*.

Signs and Symptoms

Most cases of peripheral neuropathy begin very subtly and slowly. Damage to sensory neurons produces burning pain or tingling in the hands and feet, which gradually spreads proximally into the limbs and finally the trunk. Extreme sensitivity to touch can follow, but that is eventually replaced by a far more dangerous symptom: numbness. Numbness is dangerous because if a person cannot feel something— a toe, for instance— the person cannot tell if it has been injured or infected. Secondary ulcers and infections are common complications of numbness with any disease.

Damage to motor neurons causes weakness and possibly limited or uncontrolled movement. Specific muscle weakening and atrophy are also part of advanced peripheral neuropathy.

Treatment

Treatment of peripheral neuropathy depends on the underlying pathology causing the nerve damage. Over-the-counter pain relievers are the first resort. Topical ointments with pepper sometimes offer some relief. Chronic pain is often treated with tricyclic antidepressants (which can interfere with pain perception) or anti-seizure medications (which can help ameliorate sharp, jabbing types of pain). Other therapies include TENS

PERIPHERAL NEUROPATHY IN BRIEF

What is it?
Peripheral neuropathy is damage to peripheral nerves, usually of the hands and feet, often as a result of some other underlying condition such as alcoholism, diabetes, or lupus.

How is it recognized?
Sensory damage, motor damage, or both may be present. Symptoms include burning or tingling pain beginning distally and slowly moving proximally, loss of movement or control of movement, hyperesthesia, and eventual numbness.

Is massage indicated or contraindicated?
Peripheral neuropathy contraindicates massage when numbness interferes with the client's ability to give accurate feedback. In other cases, therapists will need to make case-by-case judgments about whether massage fits in the context of the underlying factors.

units (electrical stimulators that interrupt pain transmission), biofeedback, acupuncture, relaxation techniques, and massage to improve circulation in the affected extremities.

The good news is if the disease is interrupted early, the peripheral nerves may be able to regenerate and the patient may regain full function. If it is left untreated, peripheral neuropathy can become a chronically painful long-term condition.

Massage?

If a client has undiagnosed tingling or numbness, he or she needs to see a physician; it could be any number of things, peripheral neuropathy included. If a client is numb or has reduced sensation, these are contraindications too, since the client is unable to give informed feedback about comfort levels. Clients with nerve damage are likely to be hypersensitive; massage may exacerbate or soothe this symptom.

Massage therapists must make case-by case decisions for clients with peripheral neuropathy to balance the possible benefits (soothing irritable nerves, improving circulation) with the possible risks (further irritating irritable nerves, damaging numb tissue).

Tremor

Definition: What Is It?

This condition refers to involuntary twitching, which can be a symptom of a number of different types of central nervous system problems. The key characteristics of tremor disorders are that the movements are rhythmic oscillations of antagonistic muscle groups, and the movement occurs in a fixed plane.

Etiology: What Happens?

Tremors can occur in a variety of ways. The most common versions are discussed below. They are generally classified as *resting tremor* (the oscillations occur when the patient is at rest), *postural tremor* (the oscillations occur when the patient attempts to hold a limb against gravity, i.e., holding an arm out in front of him), and *active* or *activity-specific tremor* (the oscillations occur when the patient attempts to use the hands or whatever part of the body is affected).

Tremors may be further classified by whether they are *physiologic* (exacerbated by stress, fear, or underlying problems such as alcohol withdrawal, *hyperthyroidism* [Chapter 8], or drug reactions) or *pathologic* (either idiopathic or caused by some other disease). A third class of tremor has been labeled *psychogenic*, referring to tremors brought about by mental or emotional imbalances. These tremors disappear when the patient is distracted by other stimuli.

It is important to understand why a person may be experiencing tremors, because treatment options for this disorder vary according to cause and classification. Some of the most common tremor types are listed below:

- *Essential tremor* is an idiopathic chronic tremor that is not secondary to any other pathology. Three to 4 million people in the United States have essential tremor, which is slowly progressive but not usually debilitating. Onset can occur as early as adolescence, but essential tremor most often appears at about 45 years of age. It is often an inherited disorder.

TREMOR IN BRIEF

What is it?
Tremor is rhythmic, involuntary muscle movement. It can be a primary disorder (unrelated to other problems) or it can be a symptom of other neurologic diseases.

How is it recognized?
Tremor is identified through uncontrolled fine or gross motor movements.

Is massage indicated or contraindicated?
Tremor may indicate massage as long as no contraindicating conditions are contributing factors.

CHOREA
This word, which is a synonym for tremor, comes from the Greek *choreia*, a "choral dance." It has the same root as the word "chorus," which gives some insight into what those Greek choruses were doing during all those tragedies.

Some medications can treat essential tremor, and moderate alcohol consumption can relieve symptoms. Too much alcohol, however, makes it worse.

- *Huntington's disease* is a hereditary degeneration of nerve tissue in the cerebrum. Symptoms do not usually appear until adulthood, when tremors and progressive dementia become irreversible. The average age of onset is between 35 and 50 years. It affects approximately 5 of every 1 million people in the United States.

    Huntington's disease is diagnosed by computed tomography (CT) scan, MRI, and DNA marker studies.

- *St. Vitus' dance*, or chorea minor, is a rare disorder. This is a problem that begins in childhood or occasionally during pregnancy. There is no known cure, but the prognosis is not so bleak; it usually passes without serious incident, although sedation during convulsive episodes may be recommended.

- *Parkinson's disease* is another central nervous system disorder involving involuntary movement, but it is discussed elsewhere in this chapter.

- *Other factors* that can cause tremor include *alcohol withdrawal*, *peripheral neuropathy* (this chapter), and damage to the cerebellum.

Massage?

If a client has episodes of uncontrolled muscular contraction and the condition has not been diagnosed, it is important to get medical clearance before performing massage. It may be that massage can help to reconnect these patients with their bodies in a way that is beneficial, but it is vital to work as part of a health care team.

Infectious Disorders

ENCEPHALITIS IN BRIEF

What is it?
Encephalitis is inflammation of the brain usually brought about by a viral infection.

How is it recognized?
Signs and symptoms of encephalitis include fever, headache, confusion, and personality and memory changes. In rare cases, encephalitis may cause permanent neurologic damage or even death.

Is massage indicated or contraindicated?
Acute encephalitis contraindicates massage. If encephalitis is part of a client's history but there are no signs of present infection or neurologic damage, massage is acceptable.

Encephalitis
Definition: What Is It?

Encephalitis is a central nervous system infection usually caused by a variety of different viruses.

Demographics: Who Gets It?

Until recently, many different types of encephalitis were considered to be "endemic" to certain areas, that is, specifically limited to geographical regions. As more people travel to different places, however, strains of virus that had previously been restricted to certain areas are being found all over the world.

Encephalitis infections are relatively rare. Even with a recent introduction of a previously unknown strain in the United States, national incidence stays between 150 and 3000 cases per year.

Etiology: What Happens?

Most cases of encephalitis are transmitted by mosquitoes. The virus usually affects other animals first; wild and domestic birds and horses are common hosts. Mosquitoes bite an infected animal and pick up the virus, and then bite a human, introducing the virus into the human's bloodstream.

Encephalitis infections affect the brain and sometimes the spinal cord. Very often infections are mild and do not lead to long-lasting damage. Occasionally, and especially if the patient is very young or very old, encephalitis infections can cause permanent neurologic damage or even death.

Encephalitis is usually brought about by a viral infection, but occasionally it is from something more exotic like a paramecium carried by the tsetse fly. Inflammation of the brain can also be a complication of other diseases, notably *HIV/AIDS* (Chapter 5).

Signs and Symptoms

Symptoms of encephalitis can range from being so mild they are never even identified to very, very severe. How the disease presents itself depends on the virus involved and the age and general health of the patient. Infants, the elderly, and AIDS patients are most vulnerable to the very extreme forms of the disease, whereas others only rarely experience any lasting damage from the inflammation.

The mild end of the symptomatic scale includes a sudden onset of fever with headaches, drowsiness, irritability, and disordered thought processes. In more severe cases the drowsiness can progress to stupor and then coma. The patient may also experience double vision, confused sensation, impaired speech or hearing, convulsions, and partial or full paralysis. Changes in personality, intellect, and memory may develop, depending on which parts of the brain are affected.

Diagnosis

The presenting symptoms for any central nervous system disturbance are so varied and individualized it is difficult to make a conclusive diagnosis without a full range of intrusive testing. For encephalitis this means a spinal tap to look for signs of inflammation in the cerebral spinal fluid, along with a CT or MRI scan to look for signs of inflammation. This is much better than how it was done long ago, when a biopsy of brain tissue was required to make a diagnosis!

Treatment

Viruses do not respond to antibiotic therapy, which is designed to disable bacteria only. Encephalitis is treated with anti-viral medications to slow viral activity, along with steroids to limit inflammation, and sedatives to moderate convulsions.

Prognosis

The prognosis for encephalitis depends on the vulnerability of the patient, the virulence of the pathogen, and how early treatment is administered. Very often healthy people can emerge from a short-term infection with no lasting damage. Nevertheless, prolonged inflammation in the central nervous system may cause permanent damage to structures that have little or no capacity to heal. Thus, permanent paralysis or cognitive changes may be the result of a serious bout with this disease.

West Nile Encephalitis: Watching a Virus Take Hold

In August 1999, six residents of Queens, New York, checked into local hospitals with high fevers in combination with debilitating headaches. Five of them also developed alarming neurologic symptoms: weakness, paralysis, and even coma.

Initial tests suggested an outbreak of Saint Louis encephalitis (SLE), a mosquito-borne viral infection. However, patients showed a different pattern than usually seen with SLE; several of them were much sicker than medical professionals expected. Within days several more people in the area were reporting similar symptoms.

At the same time, a few miles to the north of where most of the encephalitis patients were, birds in the Bronx zoo were dying at a startling rate. Crows all over the city were showing an alarming mortality rate. Horses in nearby suburbs were also falling to a mysterious brain fever.

It took some time, but epidemiologists finally put the phenomena together and realized that the viruses attacking humans were the same as those attacking the birds and horses. It was firmly established that the infectious agent was one never before seen in the United States. West Nile encephalitis virus was being transmitted from horses and birds to humans by common mosquitoes.

By the time the first frost killed the mosquito population, a total of 56 confirmed cases were identified among humans, with 7 deaths. The people who died of encephalitis were all older than 68 years of age.

It has never been firmly established exactly how the West Nile virus got to New York. One of the patients had been to Africa the previous June and might have been infected then, or it is possible that one of the birds in the Bronx zoo carried the virus into the United States. Aggressive mosquito abatement programs limited the spread of the disease.

The appearance of the West Nile virus in the United States provides an unprecedented opportunity to observe how an infectious agent spreads through a new environment. By the end of 2000, 83 human cases had been reported, with a total of 9 deaths. In summer of 2001 the first human cases were confirmed outside the New York City area: two people in rural Florida tested positive for the infection.

This virus has some other unusual features. Although epidemics of this disease have been recorded in Africa, the Middle East, and parts of Europe since 1950, it has never been associated with a high mortality rate among people or animals—until now. This raises the possibility that the virus found in New York in 1999 is a new, more virulent strain of the West Nile virus. Furthermore, concurrent with the New York outbreak, another epidemic of a West Nile-type of virus was happening in Volgograd, Russia. This outbreak, however, had a much higher incidence (84 cases in a city of about 2 million) and a much higher mortality rate (40 deaths or nearly 48%).

How does this bode for the future? It is difficult to say. This virus carries several challenges, including how to develop ways of predicting high-risk areas for outbreaks of the disease, creating measurably useful mosquito abatement programs, and setting up a wide-ranging surveillance program to carefully monitor the geographical progress of the disease.

Massage?

Major signs of an encephalitis infection, especially headache, fever, and irritability, *systemically contraindicates massage.* If, on the other hand, encephalitis shows up on a medical history as a long ago infection, and the client has no permanent damage, massage should be just fine.

Herpes Zoster
Definition: What Is It?

Also known as *shingles*, this condition is a viral infection of the nervous system. In this case the targeted tissues are the dendrites at the end of sensory neurons. Imagine growing painful, fluid-filled blisters on all the nerve endings of a specific dermatome. That is fair idea of what a bad case of shingles feels like. Shingles affects about 300,000 people in the United States every year. It seldom affects the same person twice, unless that person is severely immunocompromised.

Etiology: What Happens?

The virus at fault here is the chickenpox virus, *varicella zoster virus.* When a person is exposed to chickenpox in childhood, the normal course of events is to go through the disease process, have painful itchy blisters, let them fade away, and then go back to business as usual. The difference with chickenpox is that although a full complement of anti-chickenpox antibodies are present, the virus is never fully expelled from the body. Instead, it goes into a dormant state in the dorsal root ganglia (the meeting point for all the sensory neurons in each dermatome). Then later in life the virus may reactivate.

Sometimes the immune response quells future attacks before any symptoms appear. However, if the virus awakens when the immune system is below par for some other reason—stress, old age, other diseases—a person might get chickenpox again, but adults are much more likely to get shingles.

Causes

It is hard to predict what causes a reactivation of the varicella zoster virus. Contributing factors include the ones listed above: stress, old age, impaired immunity because of other diseases (shingles is notorious for accompanying advanced *tuberculosis* or *pneumonia* [Chapter 6]), or having had an initial infection before 18 months of age. Shingles occasionally occurs after severe trauma or as a drug reaction. Of course, if an adult has never been exposed to chickenpox, that person is vulnerable if they have contact with the varicella zoster virus.

Although the fluid in zoster blisters is filled with virus, shingles is not particularly contagious, unless people come in contact with it while their own immune systems are depressed or if they have never been exposed to the virus. In this case, an adult may get either shingles or chickenpox, but shingles is more likely.

Signs and Symptoms

Pain is the biggest symptom of this disease. Pain is present for 1 to 3 days before the blisters appear. Pain is present for the 2 to 3 weeks in which blisters develop, erupt, and scab over. Pain is often present for months after the lesions have healed and the skin is intact again.

The blisters may grow along the entire dermatome of the host dorsal root ganglion, but more often they appear along an isolated stretch. It is nearly always a unilateral attack. (Fig. 3-4), Color Plate 33). Sensory nerves that supply the trunk and buttocks are the most frequently affected, although the trigeminal nerve may also be attacked.

Complications

The most common complication of herpes zoster is secondary bacterial infection of the blisters. Other complications involve a viral attack on the trigeminal nerve, which can lead to eye damage, hearing loss, and temporary or permanent facial paralysis. *Post herpetic neuralgia* is a complication in which the pain generated by the viral attack outlives the infection by weeks or months.

> ## HERPES ZOSTER IN BRIEF
>
> ### What is it?
> Herpes zoster, or shingles, is a viral infection of sensory neurons from the same virus that causes chickenpox.
>
> ### How is it recognized?
> Shingles creates rashes and extremely painful blisters unilaterally along the affected dermatomes. The trunk or buttocks are the most common areas, but it occasionally affects the trigeminal nerve.
>
> ### Is massage indicated or contraindicated?
> This is an extraordinarily painful condition and contraindicates massage in the acute stage. After the blisters have healed and the pain has subsided, massage is appropriate.

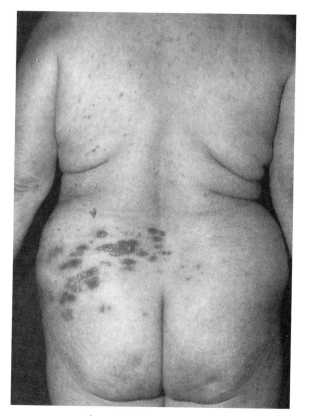

Figure 3-4. Herpes zoster

Herpes zoster occasionally leads to secondary viral and bacterial infections. Pneumonia, encephalitis, and meningitis are all possible complications of this disease.

Treatment

Herpes zoster is treated mainly palliatively. Acyclovir, the antiviral medication used for herpes simplex, has some success with herpes zoster; it is believed to shorten any possible bouts with post herpetic neuralgia. Beyond that, soothing lotion, steroids for anti-inflammatory action, and painkillers are the interventions used most often.

Massage?

Herpes zoster is the kind of disease that is very kind to massage practitioners: during an acute outbreak of this condition the *last* thing clients want is someone to *touch* them. Occasionally very mild outbreaks may occur, which may only locally contraindicate massage, according to the tolerance of the client. After the infection has passed and the lesions have completely healed, massage is perfectly appropriate.

Meningitis
Definition: What Is It?

Meningitis is "meninges" + "itis": an inflammation of the meninges, specifically the pia mater and arachnoid layers of connective tissue membrane that surround the brain and spinal cord.

Demographics: Who Gets It?

More than 70% of meningitis infections are in children younger than 5 years of age. Most dangerous cases of meningitis are among people whose resistance is low: immunosuppressed people, babies, and the elderly. An estimated 17,500 people in the United States have meningitis each year.

Etiology: What Happens?

Meningitis is usually caused by bacterial or viral infection. It is important to know the causative factor for this condition because the severity and treatment options vary according to the pathogen.

- *Bacterial meningitis.* This infection is usually due to an invasion of *Streptococcus pneumoniae* or *Neisseria meningitides* bacteria. Bacterial meningitis tends to be more severe than viral infections, and the risk of long-term central nervous system damage, specifically hearing loss or mental retardation, is much higher. It does respond to antibiotics, as long as the correct ones are administered early in the disease process.

- *Viral meningitis.* The viruses that can cause meningitis are many and varied and include a number of enteroviruses (usually associated with intestinal infections), her-

---

MENINGITIS IN BRIEF

What is it?
Meningitis is an infection of the meninges, specifically the pia mater and the arachnoid layers.

How is it recognized?
Symptoms of acute meningitis include very high fever, rash, photophobia, headache, and stiff neck. Symptoms are not always consistent, however, and may appear in different combinations for different people.

Is massage indicated or contraindicated?
Meningitis, a contagious and inflammatory disease, strictly contraindicates massage in the acute phase. It is perfectly fine for people who have recovered from meningitis with no lasting damage to receive massage.

pes, Coxsackie virus, and others. Viral meningitis tends to be less severe than bacterial meningitis and seldom causes permanent damage.

Signs and Symptoms

The symptoms of an acute meningitis infection include very high fever and chills, a deep red or purple rash, extreme headache, irritability, aversion to bright light, and a stiff, rigid neck. The neck is held tightly because any movement or stretching of the swollen meninges is excruciatingly painful. Drowsiness and slurred speech may be present. More extreme infections cause nausea, vomiting, delirium, and even convulsions or coma.

A bacterial meningitis infection incubates from 2 to 10 days. It takes up to 3 weeks for viral infections to develop. Symptoms generally peak and then recede over a period of 2 to 3 weeks.

Diagnosis

Meningitis is diagnosed through a spinal tap that examines the cerebrospinal fluid for pus, fragments of pathogens, and reduced glucose levels (the infectious agents consume the glucose that would normally be available to the central nervous system).

Treatment

If the pathogen is identified as a bacterium, large doses of antibiotics are administered immediately to forestall the possibility of central nervous system damage. Viral meningitis is generally treated with supportive therapy: rest, fluids, and good nutrition while the patient's immune system fights back.

Most people emerge from meningitis infections with no lasting damage.

Communicability

Meningitis can be contagious. Its mode of transmission is much like the common cold. An infected person sneezes or coughs and covers the mouth. He or she then touches some surface (e.g., a doorknob), thereby spreading the infection to that surface. Uninfected persons then touch the doorknob and thereby contaminate their hand. They then touch their eyes or mouth and have now been exposed to the pathogen. Meningitis brought about by the intestinal enterovirus family can also be spread by oral-fecal contact, which is an issue when it occurs in young children or in day care settings.

Some parts of the world experience epidemics of meningitis. The "meningeal belt" of sub-Saharan Africa has seasonal outbreaks of the severe bacterial version of this disease.

Not all the people exposed to meningitis-causing pathogens contract the disease. A high percentage of exposed people experience no symptoms or symptoms of a cold or mild flu. Only approximately 1 of every 1000 people exposed to meningitis develop the disease.

Prevention

In the United States the *Haemophilus influenzae* (HiB) vaccine is probably the most effective prevention against children getting meningitis. Before this vaccine was available, *H. influenzae* was the most common causative agent of bacterial meningitis infections. Vaccines against two of the three types of meningococcus bacteria have been developed, but they are generally recommended only for people planning to travel to places where epidemics are in progress.

Massage?

Meningitis contraindicates massage in the acute stage. These people do not just need bed rest—they may need hospital care. Clients who have recovered from meningitis with no lasting effects are perfectly appropriate candidates for massage.

POLIO IN BRIEF

What is it?
Polio is a viral infection, first of the intestines and then (for about 1% of exposed people) the anterior horn cells of the spinal cord.

How is it recognized?
The destruction of motor neurons leads to degeneration, atrophy, and finally paralysis of skeletal muscles.

Is massage indicated or contraindicated?
The polio virus does not affect sensation or cognition. Therefore, massage is very appropriate for polio survivors, as long as acute phase of the infection has passed.

POLIO

This is from the Greek word for "gray." Polio denotes damage to the gray matter of the central nervous system. Poliomyelitis indicates damage and inflammation in the gray matter, specifically in the spinal cord (*myelos* means "marrow").

Polio
Definition: What Is It?

Poliomyelitis or *infantile paralysis*, as it used to be known, is a viral disease. Most viruses have a target tissue, or a "favorite food," so to speak. Herpes zoster targets sensory neuron dendrites; most cold viruses attack mucous membranes. HIV goes after helper T-cells. The polio virus targets intestinal mucosa first and anterior horn nerve cells later.

Etiology: What Happens?

The polio virus usually enters the body through the mouth; contaminated water is the usual medium. It gets past the acidic environment of the stomach and sets up an infection in the intestine. New virus is released in fecal matter, possibly to contaminate water elsewhere.

For 99% of people exposed to the polio virus, this is the end of the story. Symptoms resemble a severe flu: headache, deep muscular ache, and high fever. These are followed by an intestinal infection, a bout with diarrhea, and then the infection is over. However, in about 1% of people who are infected, the virus travels into the central nervous system, where it targets and destroys nerve cells in the anterior horns of the spinal cord. This impedes motor messages leaving the spinal cord, which in turn leads to rapid deterioration and atrophy of muscles and motor paralysis.

A few facets of polio are worth examining. First, when people are exposed to this virus in infancy, they seldom become seriously ill. The later the exposure, the more dangerous this virus can be. So although this disease has been identified from as far back as 3,000-year-old Egyptian carvings, it did not really become a public menace until sanitation services were set up in heavily populated areas. Although these measures reduced the rates of cholera, typhoid, and a host of other infectious diseases, they also prevented middle and upper class infants from exposure to the polio virus. Then, when they were exposed at later ages, the disease took a heavier toll. For many years polio was considered a disease of the upper classes.

Second, as stated above, a polio infection usually resolves itself in a short bout of flu-like symptoms. It only infects the spinal cords of about 1% of the people who are exposed to it. That does not sound like much, but it means that if 10,000 children go swimming in a contaminated lake, 100 of them will experience some level of paralysis.

The paralysis caused by polio is motor only; sensation is still present. Because the motor nerves tend to overlap each other in the extremities, some muscle fibers may still function, even though a whole level of motor neurons may have been damaged. Another way to describe it is to consider the dermatomes for the quadriceps. Even if all the impulses to the motor neurons in L2 have been eliminated, other motor neurons to the same muscle group are supplied by L3 (Fig. 3-5). Furthermore, anterior horn cells that survive the initial attack can create new nerve connections to help re-establish motor control during recovery. Unfortunately, these cells can become overtaxed later in life, giving rise to *post polio syndrome* (this chapter).

The most serious form of this disease, *bulbar polio*, attacks not only the anterior horn cells of the spinal column, but the nuclei of some cranial nerves as well. Patients with this kind of damage risk death due to respiratory or heart failure. It was these patients, mostly children, who were confined to the "iron lungs" that were a big part of the American medical landscape in the 1930s and 1940s.

Treatment

Moist heat applications, physical therapy, and massage have been used to treat polio survivors once the initial infection has subsided. Together hydrotherapy and massage can help to limit contractures and to keep functioning muscle fibers healthy and well nourished.

Prevention

Polio is stunningly easy to prevent. Two inexpensive, stable, easy to administer vaccines are effective against this disease. The Salk vaccine injects weakened polio virus into the bloodstream, causing the recipient to create a set of antibodies against it. This vaccine, although protecting the patient, does not eliminate the possibility of that person's transmitting the disease to someone else. People who handle the diapers of infants who have received the oral vaccine need to be aware that live virus may be in the fecal matter. Immune-suppressed persons should avoid contact with infants who are undergoing this treatment.

The Sabin vaccine, an oral medication, introduces weakened viruses into the digestive system, where they attract antibodies exactly where the virus first tends to reside. The advantages of the Sabin vaccine are that this approach prevents the patient from being a carrier of the disease and from creating an internal immune response. Because it is given orally rather than hypodermically, it can be administered by anyone.

State health departments vary in how they recommend polio vaccines be administered. Many of them now recommend giving both the oral and injected vaccines, providing the best of both worlds to their patients.

Massage?

Massage therapists in the United States are *extremely* unlikely to encounter an acute case of polio in practice. Polio survivors experience only a motor paralysis; sensation is still intact. Massage can be performed for these clients with good possibility of benefit and little risk of danger.

Post Polio Syndrome
Definition: What Is It?

PPS is a progressive muscular weakness that develops anywhere from 10 to 40 years after an initial infection with the polio virus.

Polio: Almost Extinct

The statistics on polio are extremely promising. In 1988, the Global Poliomyelitis Eradication Initiative combined efforts with the World Health Organization (WHO), UNICEF, Rotary International, and the Centers for Disease Control in the largest public health effort ever coordinated for the eradication of a disease.

Thorough coverage with the appropriate vaccines is vital, however. A small outbreak on the island of Hispaniola between December and January of 2000–2001 was the result of a mutated virus derived from incompletely administered oral vaccines. Twenty-one children between 2 and 12 years of age were infected, and two died. Outside of this incident, however, acute polio has not been seen in the Americas since 1991. The last reported case in Europe was in 1998.

Countries with little or no incidence of polio infection are still vulnerable to invasion with the virus, especially along borders with countries where the virus is still active. Therefore, it is recommended that even "safe" countries maintain their vaccination schedules until the globe is free of the polio virus. It is expected that with vaccination programs in place, polio in the wild will be extinct by 2002.

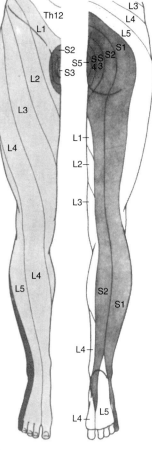

Figure 3-5. Dermatome patterns in the leg muscles allow multiple nerves to supply muscle groups; this way, if one nerve root is damaged, the muscle group will still be useable

POST POLIO SYNDROME IN BRIEF

What is it?

Post polio syndrome (PPS) is a group of signs and symptoms common to polio survivors, particularly those who experienced significant loss of function in the acute stage of the disease.

How is it recognized?

Symptoms of PPS include a sudden onset of fatigue, achiness, and weakness. Breathing and sleeping difficulties may also occur.

Is massage indicated or contraindicated?

PPS indicates massage.

Demographics: Who Gets It?

It is estimated that approximately 300,000 polio survivors live in the United States. Of them, about 25% have some symptoms of PPS, although polio survivors are also more than usually prone to arthritis, tendinitis, and other orthopedic problems that mimic PPS.

Etiology: What Happens?

PPS is not a resurgence of the original polio infection. Instead, it seems to be the result of normal aging combined with the loss of some percentage of anterior horn cells from the initial polio attack. The surviving cells, in spite of or because of whatever new synapses they were able to make in the recovery process, may be severely overtaxed. PPS may be the result of overstressed motor neurons.

Signs and Symptoms

Now that polio is little more than a memory for most people, an unexpected phenomenon is being found among its survivors. Some people who had polio as children, especially those who experienced significant loss of function, have found that as they reach middle age they have a sudden and sometimes extreme onset of fatigue, achiness, and weakness, not always in just the muscles originally affected. Breathing difficulties, sleep disturbances, and trouble swallowing may also develop. These symptoms usually begin many years after the original infection. They tend to run in cycles in which function is progressively lost, followed by periods of stability, and then more loss of function.

Diagnosis

One interesting phenomenon that has developed along with PPS is the discovery that many people who were treated for polio in the 1940s and 1950s may have been misdiagnosed. Several other neurologic problems can present similarly to polio, but survivors of these diseases who develop muscular pain and weakness in middle age will *not* be experiencing post polio syndrome, and so they need to pursue other treatment options.

PPS is diagnosed by looking for a confirmed prior episode of paralytic polio, along with an electromyogram to look for changes to anterior horn nerves. Other diseases, like *amyotrophic lateral sclerosis* (this chapter) must also be ruled out.

Treatment

PPS does not mean the polio virus has become reactivated; it is not a new infection. It is treated as a problem that may be fixed by reducing muscular and neurologic stress: adjusted braces, a change in activity levels, and exercise programs that encourage the use of muscles *not* supplied by the damaged nerves. People with PPS need to avoid excessive use of their affected muscles, since exercise to these damaged tissues can cause permanent damage to the working fibers.

Massage?

PPS indicates massage, which reduces muscle tone, improves local nutrition, and generally decreases strain on the nervous system.

Psychiatric Disorders

Anxiety Disorders

Definition: What Are They?

Anxiety disorders are a collection of distinct psychiatric disorders that all have to do with irrational fears and extensive efforts to avoid or control them. Anxiety disorders range from being mild to being completely debilitating.

Demographics: Who Gets Them?

Statistics for specific types of anxiety disorders will be discussed individually, but overall it is estimated that up to 19 million people in the United States have some type of anxiety disorder. Many anxiety disorders are more common in women than in men, but men are more likely to seek treatment for disorders that make it hard to function in public settings. These disorders take a huge toll on a person's ability to complete school or hold a job. Consequently, a disproportionately high percentage of people with anxiety disorders never earn a high school diploma and are in the lowest end of socioeconomic ranking.

Etiology: What Happens?

"*Am I safe?*" At this moment every person who is alive and awake is asking this question at some level of consciousness. The answer for people with anxiety disorders is, "*Probably not.*"

Each type of anxiety disorder has its own etiology, but some group generalizations can be made. These disorders involve neurotransmitter imbalances in the brain, although which parts of the brain vary by individual problem. The areas most frequently affected are parts of the limbic system: the area of the brain that stores memory and compares it to current experience to gauge an appropriate sympathetic or parasympathetic response. Many people with anxiety disorders tend to interpret incoming stimuli as potentially threatening and consequently live in a constant sympathetic state. Other parts of the brain that are frequently affected are the basal ganglia (the site that initiates much muscular activity) and the frontal lobes (the area associated with judgment and decision-making).

The neurotransmitters that are most frequently disturbed by anxiety disorders include norepinephrine (chemically related to epinephrine), gamma-aminobutyric acid (GABA), and serotonin.

Some types of anxiety disorders can always be linked to a specific trigger. Posttraumatic stress disorder, for instance, is initiated by some traumatic incident. Other types can occasionally but not always be traced to an initial event. A genetic link appears to be a factor in some types of anxiety disorders, but the specific genetic mutation has not been found. This blend of genetics, life-changing events, and neurotransmitter imbalances produces emotions and behaviors that can completely debilitate a person, making it impossible to go to school, to maintain relationships, or to hold a job. The risk of depression and suicide with several anxiety disorders is many times higher than it is with the general population.

ANXIETY DISORDERS IN BRIEF

What are they?

Anxiety disorders are a group of mental disorders that have to do with exaggerated, irrational fears and the attempts to control those fears. Some anxiety disorders come and go, some are chronic progressive problems, and others reach a peak and then sometimes recede or remain stable. All anxiety disorders begin as emotional responses that create inappropriate sympathetic reactions.

How are they recognized?

Although triggers for individual cases may vary, many anxiety disorders involve sympathetic reactions in the body, including fast heart rate, sweating, dizziness, faintness, nausea, and other symptoms. In addition, some disorders bring about feelings of impending death, a sense of physical detachment, unwelcome or frightening thoughts, and other reactions.

Is massage indicated or contraindicated?

If the stimulus of bodywork is perceived as something safe and welcome, then massage can have a useful place in dealing with a variety of anxiety disorders.

Types of Anxiety Disorders

Dozens of distinct anxiety disorders have been documented, each with a specific list of criteria for diagnosis. What follows is a list of some of the most common ones, along with brief descriptions.

- *General anxiety disorder (GAD).* This disorder affects about 4 million people in the United States. Women with GAD outnumber men by approximately 2 to 1. This disorder involves chronic, exaggerated, consuming worry and the constant anticipation of disaster. It does not cause the person to avoid stressful situations, but he or she lives in a constant state of anxiety that makes it difficult to accomplish many tasks. It appears earlier and develops more slowly than other anxiety disorders.

  GAD is diagnosed when symptoms persist for 6 months or longer. Physical symptoms included insomnia, fatigue, muscle tension, and headaches. More than half of all GAD patients also deal with depression, substance abuse, and other anxiety disorders.

- *Panic disorder.* Panic disorder is characterized by the sudden onset (often with no identifiable trigger) of very extreme sympathetic symptoms: a pounding heart, chest pain, sweatiness, dizziness, faintness, and alternating flushing and chilling. Hyperventilation causes numbness and tingling in the lips and extremities. A feeling of being smothered, of impending doom, and the nearness of death usually lasts for about 10 minutes but may persist for many hours.

  Panic disorder affects about 2.4 million Americans, with women again outnumbering men by about 2 to 1. It is complicated by worrying about having another attack—fear of fear. When it causes a person to avoid situations in which panic attacks have happened before or may happen in the future, it can cause another anxiety disorder, agoraphobia, or fear of open places. Gradually a person's perceived "safety zone" shrinks to the point where he or she becomes reluctant to leave the immediate environment. About one-third of all panic disorder patients develop agoraphobia.

  People with panic disorder are 4 times more likely than the general population to abuse alcohol or drugs and 18 times more likely to commit suicide, although this rarely happens *during* a panic attack. Panic disorder patients also have high rates of depression, *migraine headache* (this chapter), and *irritable bowel syndrome* (see Chapter 7).

  Panic disorder is one of the most successfully treated of all anxiety disorders, but treatment is most successful if it is initiated before the onset of agoraphobia.

- *Posttraumatic stress disorder (PTSD).* Traditionally associated with soldiers returning from the horrors of war, PTSD has also been known as "shell shock." It affects about 5.2 million Americans, most of them men.

  PTSD is a disorder involving persistent visceral memories of a specific ordeal, which could be combat, physical or sexual abuse, rape, assault, torture, natural disaster, or any other life-threatening event. Sometimes a PTSD patient was a witness to an attack or threat to someone else. Memories of the event are relived in nightmares and waking flashbacks. Patients often becomes withdrawn, irritable, and occasionally aggressive as these memories intrude more and more frequently into their lives. Some PTSD patients find that their symptoms subside with time and eventually no longer affect them, but others find that without treatment this is a life-long problem.

Symptoms of PTSD usually appear within 3 months of the triggering event, but some patients are not affected until many years later. People with PTSD tend to be hypervigilant, always on the lookout against the possibility of a repeated attack or trauma. Studies of the brain activity of PTSD patients show some differences in brain chemicals depending on whether the trauma was impersonal, like a hurricane or flood, or a personal attack, like a rape or kidnapping. Survivors of impersonal experiences generally have less severe symptoms, although the severity of the stressor does not necessarily correspond to the severity of the symptoms.

- *Obsessive-compulsive disorder (OCD).* OCD is a combination of intrusive, uncontrollable, unwelcome thoughts *(obsessions)* along with highly developed rituals designed to try to quell or control those thoughts *(compulsions)*. About 3.3 million Americans have it, and the ratio of men to women is about even. Unlike many other anxiety disorders, OCD can come and go throughout a lifetime and is not always progressive.

   Some of the most common obsessions experienced by OCD patients include fear of contamination by dirt, germs, or sexual activity; fear of violence or catastrophic accidents; fear of committing violent or sexual acts; and fears surrounding disorder or asymmetry. The rituals used to battle these fears include repeated hand-washing (often to the point of damaging the skin); refusing to touch other people or contaminated surfaces; repeatedly checking locks, stoves, irons, or other appliances; counting telephone poles; carefully and symmetrically arranging clothes, food, or other items; and persistently repeating words, phrases, or prayers. Although many people occasionally engage in some of these behaviors, OCD patients often devote hours everyday to the rituals that are designed to keep them safe.

- Phobias: social and specific
  - *Social phobia*

    Social phobia is also called *social anxiety disorder*. It involves intense, irrational fears of being judged negatively by others or of being publicly embarrassed. It can involve specific situations, like speaking or performing in public, or it can involve any social setting. Physical symptoms include blushing, sweating, trembling, and nausea, but many social phobia patients display no outward signs of their disorder.

    Whereas many people may feel shy or nervous among strangers, patients with social phobia are significantly distressed and even disabled by their fear, which can interfere with work, school, or relationships.

    Social phobia affects some 5.3 million people in the United States. Women with social phobia outnumber men, but men are generally more likely to seek treatment. About 16% of all social phobia patients are alcoholics. They are 4 times more likely to have depression and have a higher than normal risk for suicide.

  - *Specific phobias*

    A phobia is an intense, irrational fear of something that poses little or no real danger. Some common phobias include fear of closed-in places, heights, flying, elevators, tunnels, and bridges. Untreated phobias can severely restrict a person's ability to hold a certain kind of job, live in a certain kind of building, or perform mundane tasks such as grocery shopping.

    About 6.3 million people have specific phobias. Women outnumber men. Persons with this disorder often respond better to controlled desensitization and relaxation techniques than they do to medication.

Signs and Symptoms

Signs and symptoms of anxiety disorders vary according to type. Although they usually involve irrational fears and inappropriate sympathetic nervous system responses, they present differently by each variety and in each patient. The *Diagnostic and Statistical Manual of Mental Disorders*[c] has extensively documented signs, symptoms, and diagnostic criteria for each of the individual anxiety disorders, but brief descriptions of their signs and symptoms have been included in the descriptions above.

Treatment

Most anxiety disorders are treated with a combination of medication and psychotherapy. Some varieties respond better to psychotherapy and the development of coping skills alone, while others also require chemical intervention to re-establish neurotransmitter balance in the central nervous system. Most patients with anxiety disorders can find some combination of therapies that successfully treats their problem—if they seek treatment. Sadly, many patients are incorrectly diagnosed or never seek treatment at all.

Medications to treat anxiety disorders fall in three classes: antidepressants, anti-anxiety drugs, and beta-blockers. Antidepressants include selective serotonin reuptake inhibitors (SSRIs), tricyclics, and monoamine oxidase inhibitors (MAOIs). Anti-anxiety medications include benzodiazepines: tranquilizers that influence levels of the neurotransmitter GABA. These can be effective drugs, especially since they can produce results in a short period. Unfortunately they can also be highly addictive and react dangerously with alcohol. Therefore, they are not appropriate for long-term treatment or for anxiety patients who are also chemically dependent on alcohol or other drugs (which is a high percentage of this population). Beta-blockers are usually prescribed for high blood pressure patients to decrease the force of heart contractions. They can also help to ameliorate some of the heart-pounding discomfort of panic attacks and social phobias, but they are strictly palliative—they do nothing to fix the problem, they simply quell some of the symptoms.

Psychotherapeutic techniques used for anxiety disorders vary from supported resistance to compulsive behaviors for OCD patients, to controlled exposure to frightening stimuli for people with specific phobias, to various forms of behavioral-cognitive therapies to help patients learn ways to cope with and often overcome the irrational fears that limit their lives.

Massage?

Relaxation techniques, breathing exercises, and biofeedback are often taught to anxiety disorder patients as coping mechanisms; it seems reasonable that massage and bodywork would fit under this heading as well. It is important to remember, however, that massage therapy is a fine choice for an anxiety disorder patient *as long as the stimulus is perceived as safe and nurturing.* Although a therapist's intent may be completely benign and supportive, the survivor of touch abuse or other types of trauma may not be able to interpret it as such.

Some people with issues and phobias about touch may specifically seek out massage as a way to experience positive touch in their lives. It is a privilege to work with these clients, but massage therapists must be especially vigilant about maintaining clear and careful boundaries around these relationships, so that no one—neither the therapist nor the client—feels taken advantage of or abused.

[c]Diagnostic and Statistical Manual of Mental Disorders-IV TR 2000. Washington, DC: *American Psychiatric Press; 2000.*

Chemical Dependency

Definition: What Is It?

Here is a controversial topic! While definitions for chemical use, abuse, and dependence are relatively clear, the whole issue is clouded by value judgments imposed on whether a substance is legal. A person may become addicted to nasal decongestants or to cocaine, but decongestants are not generally considered a substance abuse problem, whereas cocaine certainly is a problem.

This section focuses on the prevalent attitudes about which substances are prone to abuse and dependence, but the general rules about addiction and recovery are the same regardless of the substance being discussed.

Alcoholism is a form of chemical dependency that, because of its prevalence in the culture and the profound effects it has on virtually every system of the body, is discussed here as a specific subset of chemical dependency.

The issue of chemical dependence falls into three categories: use, abuse, and dependence or addiction.

- *Use.* "Use" is easy to identify; if a person ingests a substance specifically to change mood or physical experience, that could be called substance use.

- *Abuse.* Abuse is harder to define, especially when the substances under question are examined without the qualifiers of "legal" and "illegal." After all, are caffeine or sugar inherently less damaging than an illegal substance like cannabis? What is more "abusive"—smoking a cigarette or eating a cheese Danish?

  The official definition of substance abuse is simply the use of a substance in a way that is potentially harmful to the user or to other people. Abuse is identified when use of the product interferes with a person's ability to function normally, when the user's behavior becomes unacceptable to those around him or her, and when the person continues to use the substance despite the recurring problems it causes.

- *Dependence.* The line between *abuse* and *dependency* is sometimes blurry. Most experts agree that abuse becomes dependency when the user develops a progressive tolerance, and so must use more of the substance to achieve the same effects, and when signs of physical and psychological addiction develop, which lead to a need to avoid the unpleasant effects of withdrawal.

CHEMICAL DEPENDENCY IN BRIEF

What is it?
Chemical dependency is the use of material in methods or dosages that result in damage to the user and people whom the user contacts. The issue of chemical dependency covers the use of both legal and illegal substances.

How is it recognized?
Specific symptoms of chemical dependency are determined by what substances are being consumed. Generally speaking, the symptoms of dependence include a craving for the substance in question, an inability to voluntarily limit use, unpleasant or dangerous withdrawal symptoms, and increasing tolerance of the substance's effects.

Is massage indicated or contraindicated?
People who are recovering from chemical dependency can benefit from massage, as long as no contraindicating conditions have developed as part of the abuse. Massage is contraindicated for people who are intoxicated at the time of their appointment.

Demographics: Who Becomes Chemically Dependent or Alcoholic?

Statistics on chemical dependency are difficult to gather, especially since many people never get medical treatment, and they may move back and forth between being a substance user and being free from use.

The National Institute of Mental Health estimates that up to 17% of people 18 years of age or older have experienced some kind of substance abuse, although not all of them become dependent.[d] The National Institute on Alcohol Abuse and Alcoholism projects that 4% of all adult women and 11% of all adult men meet the criteria for alcoholism or other types of chemical dependency.[e]

Dependency is more common in men than in women. The peak years for dependency among adults are 18 to 29 years of age. The lowest rates of chemical dependency are found among adults older than 65 years.

Etiology: What Happens with Chemical Dependency?

The process of developing dependence on a particular substance depends on the chemical make-up of that product and the susceptibility of the user. Many of the most common addictive drugs available today work in the central nervous system by changing the rate at which dopamine, the neurotransmitter produced in the substantia nigra, is reabsorbed at key synapses. Dopamine in certain parts of the brain can trigger pleasure responses, but if it lingers too long, the receptors become desensitized. In other words, it takes more dopamine—and more drug—to produce the same pleasurable results.

Etiology: What Happens With Alcoholism?

Alcohol slows activity of the brain and nervous system. While it is technically a depressant, the loss of inhibitions felt by the drinker can give the impression that alcohol is a stimulant. The effect of alcohol on specific organ systems is discussed in more detail in the *complications* section of this article.

Risk Factors

Several risk factors contribute to a person's susceptibility to chemical dependency.

- *Genetic predisposition.* The rate of drug abuse and alcoholism is demonstrably greater in the families of other addicts than in the general population. This is partly an environmental and availability issue, but studies have shown that even children who are not raised with their chemically dependent parents have a higher than normal incidence of addiction themselves.

- *Other mental illness.* The presence of *depression* and/or *anxiety disorders* (this chapter) raises the risk of a person becoming a substance abuser, as he or she may attempt to self-medicate to cope with problems.

- *Environmental factors.* These include availability of the substance in question, peer pressure, self-esteem, a history of physical or sexual abuse, being a child in the household of a substance abuser, and other stressors that may make drug use look like a reasonable choice to the person at risk.

- *Age.* The younger persons are when they begin to use an addictive substance, the more likely they are to develop a long-term dependency.

- *Medical reasons.* A patient's need for medication sometimes outlives the problem that required the initial prescription. Addiction to painkillers and sleeping pills are examples of this phenomenon.

[d]Nationwide Trends 13567. National Institute of Drug Abuse (NIDA), US Department of Health and Human Services, National Institutes of Health. 3/00. Available at: http://165.112.78.61/Infofax/nation-trends.html. Accessed winter 2001.
[e]National Institute of Alcohol Abuse and Alcoholism. Alcohol alert. 2000;48. Available at: http://silk.nih.gov/silk/niaaa1/publication/aa48.htm. Accessed winter 2001.

Types of Addiction

Once a person has become dependent on a substance, two things happen: it takes more and more of the substance to achieve the desired affects, and to *stop* using the substance can create physical responses that are daunting to contemplate. Addiction is defined in two categories: psychological addiction and physical addiction. Most addicts have a combination of these two phenomena.

- *Psychological addiction.* This is a dependency on the pleasurable or satisfying sensations that some substance provides. In other words, addicts just like the way they feel when they are "using."

- *Physical addiction.* This is a dependency arising from the need to avoid withdrawal symptoms, which can involve hallucinations, nausea and vomiting, seizures, and general physical pain.

A few issues are important to bear in mind in any discussion of chemical dependency. One is that even easy-to-get, over-the-counter drugs can change body chemistry and make it very hard to cope without them. Nasal decongestants are an excellent example. Why should a body's antihistamines do any work if some externally supplied nasal decongestant will do it for them? The difficulty lies in how long it takes to convince the body that no more decongestants will be consumed. The same kinds of dependency can develop with the use of sleeping pills, muscle relaxants, and some kinds of painkillers.

The other thing to remember is that the body builds up chemical tolerances to most kinds of drugs. That is, it takes more and more decongestant to clear up that stuffy nose, more sleeping pills, more painkillers, more caffeine, and so on. The higher the doses a person needs to feel satisfied, the harder it is to shake the dependency.

Signs and Symptoms of Chemical Dependency and Alcoholism

Symptoms of chemical dependency vary according to the substance, but four main features are consistent: the person feels a persistent craving for the substance, the person is unable to voluntarily control the use of the substance, the person develops an increasing tolerance to the effects of the substance and so must consume more to achieve the same results, and cessation of use creates unpleasant and alarming withdrawal symptoms.

In addition to these signs, the addict or alcoholic may also devote a significant amount of time to the process of using and then recovering from substance use. The person may neglect responsibilities to family, job, friends, and other relationships because of the distraction of substance abuse. The addict often denies that the substance use seriously impedes or endangers his or her life: "I'm not dead yet, so that proves I'm okay."

Complications of Chemical Dependency

Complications depend on the substance in question. They can range from paranoid delusions, to coma, or even death. Some of the worst effects of drug use are not limited to the users, however. People close to substance abusers also suffer tremendously. Drug-related violent crime, car accidents, industrial accidents, impaired judgment leading to the spread of HIV, and high rates of child abuse are other complications of chemical dependency that affect many people beyond the user.

Complications of Alcoholism

Alcohol use affects virtually every system of the body. The following is a brief synopsis.

Digestive System   Alcohol is highly irritating to the stomach lining, and high levels of consumption are responsible for a specific type of gastritis. It is also very rapidly absorbed through the gastric mucosa into the portal system. The portal vein dumps the alcohol directly into the liver, from whence it enters the rest of the bloodstream. The effects of alcohol are felt until the liver has finished neutralizing the poison.

People who have pre-existing gastrointestinal problems are especially vulnerable to the worst effects of alcohol. It is implicated in the development of *cancer* (Chapter 11) in the upper gastrointestinal tract, especially in the esophagus, pharynx, larynx, and mouth. Alcoholism can cause *ulcers*, internal hemorrhaging, and pancreatitis. About 20% of long-term drinkers go on to develop *cirrhosis* (see Chapter 7).

Cardiovascular System   Alcohol use decreases the force of cardiac contractions and can lead to irregular heartbeats, or arrhythmia. Alcohol is also toxic to myocardial tissue and can lead to *alcoholic cardiomyopathy*. Alcohol tends to agglutinate red blood cells, making them stick together. This leads to the possibility of *thrombi* (Chapter 4) not only in the brain (*stroke*, this chapter), but in the coronary arteries as well (*atherosclerosis*, Chapter 4). Alcohol use can also have the opposite effect: liver damage can lead to poor vitamin K synthesis, which may result in uncontrollable bleeding.

Moderate alcohol consumption may actually help prevent cardiovascular disease by increasing high-density lipoprotein (HDL) levels (the "good" cholesterol) in the blood.

Nervous System   Memory loss frequently occurs for biochemical reasons and from agglutinated red blood cells getting stuck in the cerebral capillaries, causing brain cells to starve to death. Even some "social drinkers" sustain measurable brain damage from repeated agglutination. In the short term alcohol slows reflexes, slurs speech, impairs judgment, and compromises motor control. In the long term, the same effects can happen on a permanent basis in a condition known as *organic brain syndrome*. In advanced stages of cirrhosis, the blood has toxic levels of metabolic wastes that can cause brain damage.

Immune System   Prolonged alcohol use severely impedes resistance, especially to respiratory infections. Alcoholics are especially vulnerable to *pneumonia* (Chapter 6).

Reproductive System   Alcoholism can cause reduced sex drive, erectile dysfunction, menstrual irregularities, and infertility. Babies of alcoholic women are susceptible to fetal alcohol syndrome (FAS), the most common type of environmentally caused mental retardation in the United States. FAS affects 4000 to 12,000 babies every year.

Alcoholic Families   Children raised in homes with one or more alcoholic adults show a threefold increase in the risk of becoming substance abusers themselves. Their chances of developing depression, general anxiety disorders, and phobias are higher than the general population. Their health costs average 32% higher than other children.

Other Complications   Alcohol is a factor in almost half of all automobile fatalities. It is involved in 40% of all industrial accidents and up to 65% of adult drownings. It costs about $96.4 billion a year in lost productivity, health care costs, and death costs. It contributes to about 100,000 deaths every year.

Treatment

The first and most important step in treating any kind of chemical dependency is recognizing that a problem exists. Once a person has reached that point, most treatment programs have good success rates. It often seems to be a matter of finding which program best fits the personality of the patient. Treatment goals for chemical dependency are threefold: abstinence, rehabilitation, and prevention of relapses.

Most programs begin with a detoxification process, during which the drugs are expelled from the body. This may be ameliorated with sedatives, tranquilizers, or even less potent versions of the drug in question, until all chemical remnants have been processed out of the body. The length of time this requires varies according to the substance in question.

Detoxification is then followed by a process of rehabilitation, during which the patient is educated about the effects of chemical use and often trained in avoidance behaviors to give them some ammunition against the temptation to fall back into old habits.

Aftercare has been shown to be the most important part of treatment for chemical dependency. This sets up patients with a support system that can carry them through a lifetime choice of total drug abstinence.

Total abstinence is essentially the only successful conclusion to treatment for most chemical dependency, and it has traditionally been assumed to be the only successful outcome for alcoholism as well. Some medications have been developed that can help to suppress the craving for alcohol or that can cause violent physical illness when alcohol is consumed. Recently, some research has indicated that *some* alcoholism patients can learn to reset their levels of alcohol intake without completely abstaining from it, but the determination of who can handle alcohol successfully and who must completely avoid it is still difficult to make.

Massage?

Massage has a useful place in the treatment of chemical dependency. Some rehabilitation facilities employ massage therapists to help ameliorate withdrawal symptoms and reduce the need for tranquilizers and other drugs. A client with a history of alcohol or drug abuse is at high risk for secondary health problems. For this reason, it is important to work as part of a health care team and to beware of complications that are associated with "hard" drug use: staphylococcal or streptococcal infections, hepatitis B, AIDS, and heart problems.

Clients who are in long-term recovery with no lasting contraindications are good candidates for massage.

Clients who are under the influence of alcohol or other drugs at the time of their appointment should not receive massage.

Depression
Definition: What Is It?

Depression is a group of disorders that involve changes in emotional state. One of the best descriptions of this disease is, "A genetic-neurochemical disorder requiring a strong environmental trigger whose characteristic manifestation is an inability to appreciate sunsets."[f]

In other words, depression is a central nervous system disorder involving a genetic predisposition, chemical changes, and often a triggering event that results in a person losing the ability to enjoy life. Depression is more than a temporary spell of "the blues"; it can be a long-lasting, self-propagating, and ultimately debilitating disease.

[f]Salpolsky RM. Why zebras don't get ulcers: An updated guide to stress, stress-related diseases, and coping. New York, NY: W.H. Freeman and Company; 1998/1998:230.

DEPRESSION IN BRIEF

What is it?
Depression is an umbrella term covering a number of mood disorders that can result in persistent feelings of sadness, guilt, and/or hopelessness.

How is it recognized?
Symptoms vary according to the type of depression and the individual, but they usually include a loss of enjoyment derived from usual hobbies and activities, disappointment with oneself, hopelessness, irritability, and a change in sleeping habits.

Is massage indicated or contraindicated?
Most types of depression indicate massage, which can work in several ways to alleviate symptoms both temporarily and in the long run.

Demographics: Who Gets It?

Statistics on the incidence of depression in all its forms are hard to gather, because many affected people never seek help. Most estimates suggest that somewhere between 10 and 20% of the U.S. population experiences an episode of depression every year; this amounts to 11 to19 million people.

Women seem to be either more susceptible to depression or more likely to seek help, or both. The incidence of depression among women is about twice that among men.

Depression can affect people of any age. It has been observed in young children, up through senior adults, in whom its symptoms can mimic other specifically geriatric diseases. Depression in seniors can be misdiagnosed as early *Alzheimer's disease, Parkinson's disease* (this chapter), or other problems.

Etiology: What Happens?

What a great question. No one really knows how depression comes about. Several distinctive features have been noted in the brains and endocrine systems of depressive individuals, but whether these features *cause* the problem or are *caused by* the problem is still a mystery. Nonetheless, as more is learned about the chemical changes associated with depression, new methods of treatment can be attempted.

- *Neurotransmitter imbalance.* Three main neurotransmitters have been associated with depression: serotonin, norepinephrine, and dopamine. The assumption is that these neurotransmitters are in short supply, and if medical interventions make them more readily available, the patient will improve. Some research, however, points in a slightly different direction: that these neurotransmitters are actually present in *too much* concentration, and the brain builds up resistance to receiving them. Regardless, the drugs most often prescribed for depression change brain chemistry by increasing the accessibility of these important neurotransmitters.

- *Hormonal imbalance.* Neurotransmitter disruption leads to disruption in hormonal secretions, especially progesterone, estrogen, endorphins (which increase the sensation of pleasure), and cortisol (the hormone most closely related to long-term stress). It is also possible that this is a two-way street; in other words, that the hormonal shifts associated with long-term stress can disrupt neurotransmitter secretion.

- *Pituitary-adrenal axis.* This is the tight connection between the central nervous system and the endocrine system. The hypothalamus secretes corticotrophin releasing factor (CRF), which tells the pituitary gland to secrete adrenocorticotropic hormone (ACTH), which then stimulates the adrenal glands to secrete cortisol or epinephrine. Depressive people tend to secrete excessive amounts of CRF, meaning that they create more stress responses to minimal stimuli, and those responses tend to have a longer-lasting effect on the body.

Causes

Many contributing factors collide to initiate a depressive episode. Some of them are controllable, but many are not. Whether someone ends up in a depression depends on personal chemistry, genetics, and something much harder to quantify—personality.

- *Genetics.* The rates of various kinds of depression show higher-than-normal incidence among family members, pointing to a distinct genetic predisposition to this disorder. Because this is such a common and widely distributed disease, many different sites of genetic abnormality may be responsible.

- *Environmental triggers.* Most episodes of depression can be related to specific life events that initiate a slide into a depressed state. Sometimes the triggers are less clear, or they could be not recent. Triggers can range in severity from losing a loved one to losing a phone number. The more depressive episodes a person has had, the smaller the trigger may be to send the person into another.

- *Personality traits.* Some people, through their childhood experiences and family history, are simply more prone to depression than others. Psychological testing can identify people with a basically passive, "Things in my life happen to me; I don't make things in my life happen," kind of attitude. These people carry an increased risk for developing depression.

- *Chronic illness.* People who live with chronic illness show a much higher rate of depression than the general population. This is easy to understand, as chronic pain or the prospect of sliding into inevitable disability would naturally deprive a person of a sense of hopefulness or investment in life. Often the symptoms of depression can outweigh the symptoms of the chronic illness. If the depression can be resolved, then coping skills for the illness may also improve.

- *Other issues.* Several other issues can contribute to depression, but these are often much more easily controlled than the ones so far discussed. *Hypothyroidism* (Chapter 8), smoking, alcohol use, drug use, or side effects of medication can all create depressive symptoms. Also, certain nutritional deficiencies, notably vitamin B_{12} and folate, can contribute to depressive symptoms.

Signs and Symptoms

The signs and symptoms of depression depend partly on what type is present. Six leading symptoms are shared by the large majority of depression patients. They include a persistent sad or "empty" feeling; experiencing less enjoyment from usual activities (including sex) and hobbies; a deep sense of guilt or disappointment with oneself; a feeling of hopelessness—that things will never get better; irritability; and a change in sleeping habits (either the person sleeps very little or sleeps much more than usual).

Other signs and symptoms can include a decreasing ability to concentrate, weight changes (the person either eats much more than usual or loses all interest in food), a loss of energy, a feeling of helplessness, persistent physical pain that is unresponsive to treatment (headaches, digestive discomfort), and of course, suicidal thoughts or even suicidal attempts.

Other symptoms and their duration vary according to the type of depression.

Types of Depression

The *Diagnostic and Statistical Manual of Mental Disorders* (DSM) has officially recognized at least eight etiologically distinct types of depression. Five of them are relatively common and are discussed here:

- *Major depressive disorder.* This is the classic, debilitating "clinical depression." It involves the major symptoms listed above, in very severe form, for periods over 2 weeks. Left untreated, episodes of major depression may last anywhere from 6 to 18 months, and on average recur anywhere from 4 to 6 times over a lifetime. That means that someone who does not treat major depressive disorder can expect to spend up to 10 years of his or her life feeling hopeless, helpless, and worthless.

- *Dysthymia.* This is a less extreme version of depression, but it can last for years. Persons with dysthymia can function but will never feel normal or at their best.

- *Bipolar disease.* This is also called manic depression. It is marked by mood swings from major depression to mania: a state defined by heightened energy, elation, irritability, racing thoughts, increased sex drive, decreased inhibitions, and unrealistic or grandiose notions that lead to decisions made with extremely poor judgment. Someone in a manic state might spontaneously quit his job, buy a car, or make some other major life change without realizing the long-term implications—which will of course be waiting when the manic episode subsides.

- *Seasonal affective disorder (SAD).* This is a depression that seems to be related to absence of sunlight. Incidence of it in the general population goes up according to distance from the equator. SAD is thought to be related to low levels of melatonin, a neurotransmitter stimulated by exposure to sunlight. The key months for SAD to be prevalent are December, January, and February.

- *Postpartum depression.* The depression experienced by new mothers is different from other types. It is related to several factors, including sleep deprivation, vast hormonal shifts, and the challenge of matching expectations of parenthood with reality. A woman with postpartum depression has all the symptoms of major depression, along with the deep-rooted fear of having harm come, or of actually doing harm, to her baby.

Diagnosis

Depression is diagnosed with a combination of physical tests to rule out factors like hypothyroidism, vitamin deficiencies, or underlying disease, and psychological tests designed to identify exactly which type of depression might be present.

Treatment

Most types of depression are treatable; up to 90% of all depression patients eventually find some treatment option that significantly improves their quality of life. A combination of medical intervention and various types of psychotherapy seems to be the most effective way to treat most types of depression.

Antidepressant Drugs   Medications used for depression usually fall into one of three categories: SSRIs, MAOIs, or tricyclics. All of these classes of medication aim to make neurotransmitters more easily accessible in the mood-determining areas of the brain.

SSRIs, which include fluoxetine (Prozac) and sertraline (Zoloft), work by preventing the recycling of secreted serotonin into axon terminals. In other words, serotonin lingers in synapses for longer than it normally would, which reinforces its power to work. Tricyclic antidepressants, including amitriptyline (Elavil), do essentially the same thing, although they do not focus specifically on serotonin. MAOIs limit the action of an enzyme that would normally break down and clear away secretions of neurotransmitters. Phenelzine (Nardil) and tranylcypromine (Parnate) are examples of MAOIs.

Antidepressants are effective drugs for most people, but they have two major disadvantages: they take several weeks to establish any noticeable mood changes, and they tend to produce unpleasant side effects during that initial adjustment period. Side effects usually include dry mouth, dizziness, constipation, skin rashes, sleepiness or sleeplessness, and restlessness. Side effects generally subside within 4 to 6 weeks, which is about when the benefits of the medication begin to be felt.

Lithium is another drug used specifically with bipolar depression. Rather than altering levels of neurotransmitter reuptake or recycling, lithium works simply to "smooth out" mood swings.

Psychotherapy   Psychologists and psychiatrists may also use various types of "talk therapy" to help patients improve coping skills and reduce both the effects and the recurrence of depressive episodes. Three major approaches have been found to be most useful, depending on the personality and needs of the affected individual. *Cognitive-behavioral therapy* focuses on the patient's skills at managing their life and making choices that are beneficial. *Interpersonal therapy* focuses on how relationships color a person's life for better or worse. *Psychodynamic therapy* looks at how unresolved inner conflicts can affect the way a person makes choices and lives with those choices.

Psychotherapy in addition to medication often works better than medication alone, because it can help the patient take some control of the situation, a feeling many depressive people do not often have.

Other Therapies

Light Therapy.   Persons living with SAD may not need medication or talk therapy; they need sunlight. Exposure to broad-spectrum lights can help to reduce symptoms.

Electroconvulsive Therapy (ECT).   Some patients with depression have symptoms that do not respond to medication but persist and make their lives miserable. Electroconvulsive or "shock" therapy may be the best choice for these patients. Although this may bring up disturbing memories of *One Flew Over A Cuckoo's Nest*, modern ECT is conducted under light anesthesia and with muscle relaxants to limit uncontrolled contractions. It is not entirely clear why it works, but it can be a highly effective intervention for people who do not get relief from other options.

St. John's Wort. This herbal extract has received a great deal of attention as a mood enhancer without the side effects that other antidepressants carry. Early experiments indicate that it might work like SSRIs or tricyclic antidepressants by preventing the reabsorption of neurotransmitters at the synapses. The National Institute of Health recently began a 3-year study of St. John's Wort in comparison to amitriptyline for the treatment of mild dysthymia.

Complications

The most obvious and most serious complication of depression is suicide. Up to 15% of all major depression patients successfully commit suicide. Numbers on how many depression patients attempt suicide are unavailable.

In addition to suicide risk, a history of depression is now being found to have a statistical correlation to several other conditions, notably *heart attack* and other forms of cardiovascular disease (Chapter 4). Although the cause-and-effect relationship between depression and cardiovascular disease has not yet been established, an obvious connection can be made between depression and heart disease in terms of physical manifestations of long-term stress.

Massage?

The ways massage can help a depressed person are varied and many. Although some cautions must be borne in mind, most people with depression reap several benefits from bodywork.

Touch improves the efficiency of the pituitary-adrenal axis (see sidebar). Receiving non-sexual, nurturing, non-threatening touch is one of the most important ways humans and other mammals have of keeping a healthy stress response.

Massage moves people from a sympathetic into a parasympathetic state. This brings about several physiologic and chemical changes in the body, including an increase in serotonin secretion and a decrease in cortisol.

Research about how massage affects mood indicates a shift in electroencephalogram (EEG) activation from the right frontal lobe (usually associated with sad affect) to the left frontal lobe (usually associated with happy affect), or at least to a symmetrical reading.[g]

Receiving massage is one of the few distinctively pleasurable things people can do that is also really good for them. The act of scheduling and receiving this gift is a step toward self-determination that depressive people can take with little risk of having it backfire on them.

Some cautions about working with depression patients remain, however. Some clients who receive massage and enjoy its benefits may wish to stop taking their medication. Well-meaning massage therapists may view this as a successful outcome and encourage their clients to try it, but balancing medication for depressive people is a difficult business. The only ones who should get involved in changing doses are the depressed person and that person's physician.

Depression often accompanies complex emotional issues that a client may have trouble sorting out alone. Client-therapist relationships run the risk, in some cases, of becoming distorted when boundaries are not carefully respected. If a massage therapist has a client who is depressive in connection with other problems (e.g., recovering from emotional, physical, or sexual abuse), that relationship can be precarious, especially if the client is not getting adequate support outside the massage clinic. Therapists in cases like these have the obligation to refer clients for other kinds of help and to prevent the client-therapist relationship from becoming more central to the client's life than it should be.

DEPRESSION
Dave, Age 50
"Everybody wants to see the evidence!"

I don't know for sure when I first started to notice any symptoms of depression. Maybe when I was around 45. I remember I spent about a year trying to figure out what was wrong. I thought I had an infection or something, maybe a sinus infection that was making me feel tired all the time.

One day I went to get a physical, and my doctor asked me a couple of questions about things, about my life. I didn't think anything of it; I thought he was just making conversation. Then he said, "You know, Dave, you have depression." I laughed at him because there wasn't anything to be depressed about. My life was wonderful, I had no real problems, everything was good.

When I was first diagnosed, my problem was nowhere near its peak. After that, though, it got really bad. I couldn't concentrate on anything, and I spent weeks in bed. I couldn't respond to any questions, I didn't even know what was going on. When I did tune in, I had this indescribable horrible feeling. The only way I made it through that time was by asking Jesus to hold me. I just pulled the covers up over my head and asked God to just hold me. That gets me through the bad times.

I took short-term disability, for 6 months, from my job as a safety engineer. When it was over I tried to go back to work, but it wasn't any good. I used up all my sick leave, and one day the personnel officer came and told me I was through. I haven't worked since then. I got 18 months of disability, and they shut the door. If I'd broken my back, they would have paid disability for the rest of my life. But this kind of illness gets no respect. With mental illness, people think you're either slothful or you're insane. Slothful people are expected to get up and pull their own weight. Insane people are just ignored.

[g]Field T. *Touch Therapy*. London: Churchill Livingstone Press; 2000:65.

DEPRESSION—continued
Dave, Age 50
"Everybody wants to see the evidence!"

My illness is not the result of any outside situation; it is a chemical thing, an imbalance. I tried anti-depressant drugs. They're hard, though, because when you try one you have to give it a good 2 months before you know if it'll do any good. For about 90% of all people with depression, those drugs help them out. I'm in the 10% they don't help.

I've taken lots of tests in the past 2 years. My latest diagnosis is that I have schizoid-affective disorder along with depression. It's hard to categorize. Now I'm taking anti-psychotic drugs. I had a really bad episode about a month ago. I was in tears, tearing out my hair, just crawling out of my skin. I ended up in the hospital. I thought it was a reaction to the medication, but apparently the medication wasn't working yet. It was just my disease, hitting a big crest.

That's how it goes, in cycles. From day to day, hour to hour, week to week. It's impossible to predict, but it's always wave-like, never steady. Medications are a crap shoot. You take your meds and hope something happens. By now I've taken so many, and the combinations are so complicated, it's really hard to make any changes. I think I developed tolerance to all the anti-depressants. The anti-psychotics are new, and there are times when I feel pretty good.

The worst part of all this for me is that on my bad days I have no energy to do anything. I just lie there and sleep. I'm completely unreliable. I can't be sure I'll show up for church or for choir practice. It's a real bummer.

I get lots of support at home. My wife has an incredible burden, but she's been behind me 100% all the way. She knows that when I'm in bad shape there's nothing to do but wait until I'm feeling better. Then we just go on with life without dwelling on what we've missed— that's a good approach for me.

I know I'm in lots of people's prayers. I feel that's a powerful tool. I know the prayers being lifted up for me are helping, without a doubt. But when I'm feeling bad you can't come over and cheer me up, because that's not what I need. When people come visit me in the middle of the day and I've been in bed, I'm not showered or shaved, then I get so embarrassed, almost paranoid. It's not an atmosphere I like to see people in.

I don't think I'm at risk for suicide, although since I've had this disease I know more about why people do it. You get to a point where you say, " This. Is. Intolerable. This. Cannot. Go on." But it does. For now I don't see suicide being a danger for me.

At this point the only people who really understand depression are people in the medical profession, people who *have* it, or people who have someone in their family who has it. No one else really gets it. They all want to see the proof: where's the blood test, where's the x-ray, where's the *evidence*? I see a lot of the attitude that if you don't have the evidence, you must be faking it. I would like for everyone to understand that mental illness can be as debilitating as any other disease, and it deserves the same respect and concern that any other kind of disease gets.

Eating Disorders
Definition: What Are They?

Eating disorders include a variety of poor eating habits that may begin slowly but over time become difficult or even impossible to break. Eating disorders usually arise in response to specific kinds of emotional or physical stressors. They often begin as a coping mechanism but become a serious impairment to health.

- *Anorexia nervosa* is the use of fasting, severely restricted eating, and/or compensatory activities to drastically reduce the number of calories that enter the digestive system. It is essentially self-starvation.

- *Bulimia nervosa* involves normal or higher-than-normal calorie consumption, followed by compensatory activities to prevent the absorption of those calories.

- *Compulsive overeating* involves the consumption of food for reasons other than hunger. Those reasons may vary according to the individual. Eating is then *not* followed by compensatory activity, leading to rapid weight gain. Compulsive overeating has not been studied as a specific subset of eating disorders, but it happens so frequently and affects so many people, it is worth including in this discussion.

Stress Response System

The *stress response system* is the link between the central nervous system and the endocrine system that allows humans to respond to both short-term and long-term stressors. It is controlled by the hypothalamus-pituitary-adrenal axis (HPA): the communication between the hypothalamus, the pituitary gland, and the adrenals. A healthy stress response system allows immediate reactions that are appropriately gauged to the circumstances—big reactions to big threats, small reactions to small threats. When the stress response system works well, the chemical changes it brings about are transitory and quickly neutralized once the threat has passed.

Some people have a stress-response system that does not work well. The chemical messages issued first from the hypothalamus, then by the pituitary gland, are slow to leave the brain and reach the adrenals. This takes longer to have an effect on the body, decreasing the ability to respond quickly to threat. The stress reaction, once it takes hold, is tenacious. Its after-effects linger much longer than for someone who has a healthy stress response system. Furthermore, people who have a sluggish stress response system also tend to have *more* stress responses, *more* often, to *less threatening* stimuli, and those responses have longer-lasting effects on the body. This is a person who fumes in a long checkout line, who frets in heavy traffic, and who loses control when the kids leave their bikes in the driveway. This is someone who may have a sluggish but overreactive stress response, and this person has a high propensity to develop, among other things, depression.

What determines the health of the stress response system? Animal studies reveal one reliable predictor for a sluggish stress response: lack of tactile stimulation, or touch. Understimulated animals have consistently slower, longer-lasting, and more frequent stress responses than animals that had been regularly petted and fondled. Consider what this means for the average undertouched person in our society: the majority of us have low-functioning but long-lasting stress reactions, and they occur with unnecessary and unhealthy frequency. The good news is that the health of the stress response system can be improved with an abundance of healthy, nurturing touch.

Demographics: Who Gets Them?

The typical anorexia or bulimia patient is a young woman somewhere between adolescence and college age. Some estimates predict that up to 1% of all females in this age range may experience anorexia, and 3 to 10% of all girls may have bouts of bulimia. Although men may also have this problem, more than 90% of all eating disorder patients are female.

Eating disorders are found in all economic and social groups. The incidence among Hispanics and Whites is about even, but rates are slightly higher among Native Americans. Black women are more likely to be bulimic than anorexic.

Statistics on compulsive overeating are difficult to gather, but given the fact that over half of the U.S. population is overweight, it is reasonable to suggest that a high percentage of people have a less than functional relationship with food.

Etiology: What Happens?

Anorexia and Bulimia   The personality profiles of anorexia and bulimia patients point toward people with high expectations of themselves. They are often eager-to-please overachievers who do well in school and in athletics. Anorexia and bulimia are often control issues for a population that often feels powerless (adolescent girls in a culture that bombards them with impossible standards to meet). A young woman may not be able to control how people treat her, but she can at least control what goes into her mouth—for many, that feels like a major victory, at least in the short run.

Most people in this society are exposed to essentially the same cultural pressures, but not all young women develop eating disorders. This has led some researchers to look for organic causes in the chemistry of the brain. Not surprisingly, serotonin levels are found to be generally lower in eating disorder patients than in the general population. Whether this is a cause or a result of anorexia and bulimia is debatable, but it does open the door to some extra treatment options.

When a person begins to change the way she eats, ultimately it does not matter whether it is because of a neurotransmitter imbalance or because she is desperate to get on the track team. The impact her choices have on her body eventually change the way it functions. If her problems go on long enough, she may even reach the point at which it is impossible to go back; she can lose the ability to break down nutrients, absorb nutrition, and process waste. Anorexia and bulimia can be terminal illnesses.

Compulsive Overeating   The etiology of overeating is a complex mixture of physical and psychological issues. It has significance for massage therapists for several reasons.

- *Touch*. The experience of *touch* is a basic human need. Touch deprivation in infancy has been shown to lead to sluggish stress response systems and all manner of severe psychological dysfunction. When adults are deprived of touch they have weaker immune systems, higher incidence of chronic diseases, and shorter life spans. What does this mean for this undertouched society? It means that if a person does not get touch on the *outside*, she can at least get touch on the *inside*. Think of the digestive tract is a seamless continuation of the external skin. Eating to the point of satiation causes a specific snug, comforting feeling that may be in short supply for some people.

Eating for comfort can become a vicious circle, as our culture places a high premium on physical attractiveness (i.e., being slender), which means that overweight people may have a harder time making and keeping supportive touch-rich relationships. Massage therapists are in a position to provide nurturing, restorative, educated, and *nonjudgmental* touch to a population of people who may have little or no other access to this important sensory "food."

- *Protection*. Weight gain creates a physical barrier between a person and the world around her. This protective device may be a person's conscious or subconscious attempt to protect and distance herself from experiences she wants to avoid. For instance, it is common to see overeating and weight gain in people who are victims of sexual, physical, or verbal abuse.

- *Unattractiveness*. Again, abuse survivors may use overeating as a strategy to escape their abusers. If they can make themselves seem unattractive by gaining weight, they can hope to lose the sexual interest of the person who abuses them.

Many survivors of touch abuse are compulsive overeaters. Many survivors also eventually explore massage as a way to experience touch that is positive and nurturing. Massage therapists who work with this population must be very aware of how closely these clients' emotional state may be reflected in their physical state.

EATING DISORDERS IN BRIEF

What are they?
Eating disorders are a group of psychological problems involving compulsions around food and weight gain or loss. Anorexia, bulimia, and compulsive overeating are each distinct problems, although overlap between them frequently occurs.

How are they recognized?
Signs and symptoms of anorexia and bulimia may be hard to recognize in early stages, since these behaviors are usually done in private. Long-term consequences include esophageal and colon damage, tooth damage, arrhythmia and low cardiac stroke volume, electrolyte imbalance, hormonal disturbance, osteoporosis, and many other problems. Compulsive overeating is recognizable by eating habits in combination with significant weight gain, often in a short period.

Is massage indicated or contraindicated?
Massage may be very supportive and appropriate for all types of eating disorders, as long as the body's chemistry can keep up with the changes bodywork brings about. If a client is in an advanced stage of anorexia or bulimia, bodywork choices may need to change to respect the delicacy of the body's system.

Signs and Symptoms

Anorexia   As a person moves toward being anorexic, she may begin to avoid social eating situations in which people may notice her new habits. Anorexics often do not see themselves accurately. Seeing herself as fat, a pathologically thin woman may dress herself in large, shapeless, baggy clothes. These serve to hide her weight loss as well as they would to hide her perceived weight gain.

Anorexia has been divided into two varieties: *restrictive*, in which a person simply does not take in enough calories to sustain her, and *purge-type*, in which calorie intake may be adequate for sustenance but is negated by compensatory activities including vomiting, laxative use, diuretics, enemas, and excessive exercise.

In addition to being extraordinarily thin, advanced anorexics sometimes experience the growth of *lanugo* (fine, downy hair usually seen only in early infancy). This grows all over the body, possibly as an effort to compensate for the absence of any insulating fat in the superficial fascia.

Bulimia   Bulimia patients may appear to eat normally but then binge in private. Bingeing episodes are often triggered by emotionally stressful experiences: a fight with a loved one, a failed test, or some other disappointment.

The bingeing food is usually chosen to be self-indulgent. Bulimics do not binge on celery; they binge on candy bars. These episodes of drastic overeating are then followed by some kind of compensatory activity. *Purge-type* bulimics attempt to prevent calorie uptake by removing the food they have just eaten through vomiting, laxatives, diuretics, or enemas. In *non-purge type* bulimia, eating episodes are followed by excessive exercise or periods of fasting.

Bulimia patients do not experience the same weight loss that anorexics do; this can make it harder to recognize the disease in early stages. The complications they develop, however, can be more visible than those seen with anorexics.

Compulsive Overeating   Compulsive overeating may be done in public, in private, or both. The reasons behind it often have the same roots as the triggers for anorexia and bulimia: stress and a feeling that the person has little or no control over what happens to her. Because the overeating is not followed by excessive exercise, fasting, or purging, compulsive overeaters tend to gain a great deal of weight. If the behavior is related to a specific trauma or emotional problem, this can take place over a relatively short period. The good news is that the long-term physical damage and dangers to the body that arise from compulsive overeating are much easier to undo than those associated with anorexia and bulimia.

Complications

The complications associated with eating disorders can be divided into mental/emotional issues and physical issues. Many eating disorder patients struggle with *depression*, irritability, *sleep disorders*, and *anxiety disorders*, especially OCD (all in this chapter). Physical disorders vary according to eating behaviors.

Anorexia   Physical problems related to self-starvation include a slow heart rate (bradycardia), low blood pressure, and arrhythmia. Severely reduced caloric intake interferes with hormone secretion and leads to infertility and *osteoporosis* (see Chapter 2). Overuse of laxatives can cause colon dysfunction, and self-induced vomiting can lead to tooth damage, esophageal erosion, and dangerously upset electrolyte imbalances.

Bulimia   The physical complications seen with bulimia are all related to repeated self-induced vomiting or the use of laxative or enemas to empty the bowel. Advanced erosion of the enamel of molars is a hallmark of bulimia. The esophagus may develop ulcers, strictures (scar tissue that restricts movement), or it may rupture. The colon may progressively lose function when its work is done through laxative or enema use. Electrolyte imbalances brought about by vomiting and diarrhea may reach life-threatening levels. Eventually a bulimic person may find it difficult to keep food down even if she wants to.

Compulsive Overeating   Compulsive overeaters put themselves at risk for cardiovascular disease and other physical problems associated with being overweight if their eating habits are never modified. However, these patients do not create the same life-threatening chemical imbalances in their bodies that anorexic or bulimic patients do. If eating behaviors are changed, compulsive overeaters may sustain few if any long-term problems.

Diagnosis

The *Diagnostic and Statistical Manual of Mental Disorders* has identified four main criteria for the diagnosis of anorexia and five for the diagnosis of bulimia.[h] (Compulsive overeating has not been examined as an official eating disorder in this document.)

---

[h]Anorexia nervosa. MedicineNet, Inc.; 1996–2000. Available at: http://medicineNet.com. Accessed summer, 2001; and Bulimia. MedicineNet, Inc.; 1996–2000. Available at: http://medicineNet.com. Accessed summer 2001.

The four criteria for a diagnosis of anorexia are:

- Refusal to maintain weight at or above a normal level; weight is below 85% of normal for height.

- Intense fear of gaining weight.

- Distorted self-perception; the patient sees herself as heavier than she is.

- Menstrual periods stop (amenorrhea) for at least 3 months in a row.

The five criteria for bulimia are:

- Recurrent episodes of binge eating.

- A sense of lack of control; the patient could not stop eating even if she wanted to.

- Inappropriate compensatory behaviors including self-induced vomiting, laxative or enema use, or excessive exercise (persisting in exercise when exhaustion or injury are present).

- A binge/compensation pattern occurs at least twice a week for at least 3 months in a row.

- Behaviors are influenced by body image.

Treatment

Treatment for eating disorders is most successful when the emphasis is *not* on gaining or losing weight, but on resolving the issues that led to the behaviors in the first place. Although it is important to stabilize weight and educate patients about good eating habits, these interventions are generally unsuccessful until the patient's psychological and emotional issues have been addressed.

New research revealing neurotransmitter imbalances in the brains of many eating disorder patients has opened the door to medications that may help. Addressing some of the emotional and psychological complications of eating disorders can also help to stabilize a patient's emotional state so that she can begin to understand more clearly the consequences of her actions.

EATING DISORDERS
Jessica, Age 19
"Food was the one thing I thought
I could control completely."

I think my eating problems began when I was around 12 years old. I was an only child and a gymnast, and working hard in my program. All my coaches wanted muscle, muscle, muscle—no flab. At that time I got in the mindset that the more I worked out, the more muscle I'd have, so I started skipping meals to have more body building time. Having muscles and doing my routines perfectly were the only things on my mind.

I went on a pretty much just-rice diet. Rice doesn't have any fat, but lots of carbs to burn for energy. I'd have a bowl of rice and some water, which would make me feel really full. I think due to that my stomach shrank; just eating regular foods became really hard. Since I was always by myself, my parents didn't realize my problem. I always wore baggy clothes because I was constantly cold, and if I wore something tighter, my mother would say I looked fat; but in truth I was barely 5 feet tall and about 70–75 pounds. When I was in 7th grade I also got food poisoning from a school lunch. I ended up in the hospital. After that I couldn't eat lunch anymore until I was 18.

When I was 15 my grandfather, who had been the center of my life, died. I went into a deep depression. I had already lost gymnastics because of an injury. So I'd just go to school, home, go to sleep, get up for a little bit to eat, and go back to sleep to do it all over again. When I slept I had terrible dreams, and I heard voices when I was awake. I started to lose a lot of hair and have irregular menstrual cycles.

EATING DISORDERS—continued
Jessica, Age 19
"Food was the one thing I thought
I could control completely."

At this time, and up until I turned 18, I felt like my parents controlled everything: what I wore, who I spent time with, where I was, every minute of the day. Food was one thing I thought I could control completely. Sometimes I'd get up in the middle of the night and eat and eat like I was about to die. I would feel awful later, but I would never make myself throw up. I saw a movie on bulimia once, and saw how much damage it caused, so instead, I would not eat for a day or two after I binged. I still do that sometimes, but not as severely as I used to.

I had always been a straight-A student in school until my senior year in high school. That is when I learned of my eating problem. Several of my friends noticed how I never seemed to eat and started to help me break out of my cycle. The best thing I did was to go to Europe by myself. That gave me a chance to "break out of my box," which opened a whole new world of options to me. I'd say that was when I began to heal from both my depression and my eating problems.

Now I'm in massage school. I eat about 2-1/2 meals everyday. I was kind of surprised that getting massage was so easy for me. I did have some fears about laying supine on the table, but I'm over it. I have chronic back pain, and I enjoy deep massage. I still have some fears about long-term problems from anorexia. My periods were irregular then, and they're painful now. I lose a lot of blood every month; I'm definitely anemic.

Still, I know I was lucky. I was able to control my eating before it got so bad that I needed to be admitted to the hospital. My whole sense of who I am and what makes me feel good is different now. I still really like getting compliments. If I hear, "You look great," or "That shirt looks good on you," then I feel like I can eat a chicken sandwich or a bowl of ice cream without feeling guilty later. But for the most part, for stuff like the grades I get in school, or what courses I take, no one decides what I need now. I am my own person, and I am in control of my life once again. It feels really good.

Massage?

If a client with eating disorders is stable and her circulatory system is not overly taxed (as might be seen with an advanced anorexic client), massage can be a wonderful experience for a person who has a generally negative perception of her body. Overeaters, under-eaters, and people who interfere with the absorption of food can all benefit from time spent focused on how *good* they can feel. The main cautions for bodywork concern the possibility of cardiovascular weakness, and these can be circumvented by choosing modalities that do not focus on increasing circulation.

Nervous System Injuries

BELL'S PALSY

Sir Charles Bell (1774–1842) was a Scottish surgeon, anatomist, and physiologist. He pioneered neurologic research in several areas including damage to the facial nerve and the structure of the spinal cord (Bell's law states that the ventral horns of the spinal cord are for motor function while the dorsal horns are for sensory function).

Bell's Palsy
Definition: *What Is It?*

It is important for massage therapists to be familiar with this condition, because it is one of those things that a careless practitioner can actually induce, if the setting is right. This disorder is the result of damage to or impairment of cranial nerve VII, the facial nerve. This nerve is composed almost entirely of motor neurons and is responsible for providing facial expression, blinking the eyes, and providing some taste sensation (Fig. 3-6). It exits the cranium through a small foramen just behind the earlobe. This spot is palpable by *gently* putting the index finger just behind the earlobe and slightly opening the mouth.

Demographics: Who Gets It?

Bell's palsy is a fairly common condition that affects about 40,000 people per year in the United States. It is most common among young and middle-aged adults, although it has been seen in children. Men and women are affected equally.

Etiology: What Happens?

When a peripheral nerve is irritated or damaged, it ceases to function efficiently. Since the facial nerve provides most of the motor control for muscles of facial expression, damage to this nerve will result in weakness or total paralysis of the face on the affected side. The good news is that since the facial nerve is a peripheral nerve, it has a protective layer of neurilemma that allows it to regenerate. The facial nerve regenerates at a speed of about 2 mm per day.

Causes

Bell's palsy is a type of *peripheral neuritis*, that is, inflammation of a nerve, usually from some mechanical interference. Several contributing factors have been identified, but the majority of cases are evidently stimulated by a reactivation of the herpes simplex virus. The virus, which lays dormant in the nervous system until it becomes active again, stimulates the production of antibodies and elicits an inflammatory response. Usually the virus attacks nerves on the face (see *herpes*, Chapter 1). When an inflammatory response focuses specifically around where the facial nerve must pass through a narrow bony canal near the ear, the swelling damages the nerve and function is temporarily lost.

The stimulus for a resurgence of herpes activity varies from one person to another. Depressed immunity, lack of sleep, stress, and flares of autoimmune diseases are often

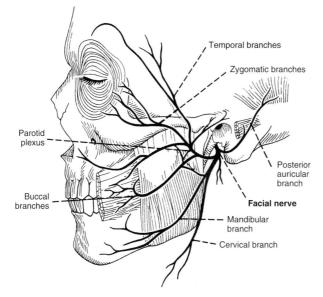

Temporal branches

Zygomatic branches

Parotid plexus

Posterior auricular branch

Buccal branches

Facial nerve

Mandibular branch

Cervical branch

Figure 3-6. The facial nerve

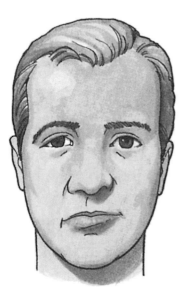

Figure 3-7. Bell's palsy: loss of motor function in one-half of the face

identified as triggers. Up to 75% of all recorded cases are preceded by an upper respiratory infection, which implies a weakened immune system and a golden opportunity for the herpes virus to attack.

Herpes is the leading factor in Bell's palsy episodes, but other problems can also put pressure on the facial nerve. Some possibilities include tumors, bone spurs at the foramen, severe middle ear infections, upper cervical subluxation, and *temporomandibular joint disorder* (Chapter 2), all of which can increase surrounding pressure on an already crowded area.

This condition is also associated with *diabetes* (Chapter 8), which can cause peripheral neuritis. *Lyme disease* (Chapter 2), *Guillain-Barré syndrome* (this chapter), exposure to certain toxins, and facial infections are also seen hand-in-hand with facial nerve damage.

Signs and Symptoms

Symptoms of Bell's palsy (flaccid paralysis and drooping and distortion of the affected side of the face) are brought about by the sudden loss of enervation to all the muscles on one side of the face (Fig. 3-7). It is difficult to eat, drink, and close the eye of the affected side. Sometimes the ear on that side becomes hypersensitive. The affected side may be painful, but it is not the sharp, electrical pain seen with *trigeminal neuralgia* (this chapter). This is a motor paralysis, not a sensory one (except for the facial nerve taste buds that may be affected), so sensation throughout the face stays intact.

Complications

Bell's palsy is usually a short-lived disorder with few serious complications. One serious problem to consider is corneal ulcers. These can occur if the lubrication and cleaning of the eyeball provided by blinking is impaired.

BELL'S PALSY
Jim S.
"No Dimple for a year!"

When I think about what may have precipitated my bout with Bell's palsy I remember one of the most stressful years of my life. I had recently moved to the Pacific Northwest and had to go back to school to receive Washington State licensure as a massage practitioner. I was working three jobs and going to school. I had also spent some days plunging into the cold water of a tributary of the Breitenbush river. I was overcooked!

When the paralysis started, I thought it was a temporary effect of some bodywork I had received. I was told to take Advil and ice my neck. I was given massage to help with the pain. But nobody recognized the seriousness of the symptoms. Within a day I had full-on Bell's palsy complete with hyperacusis (abnormal acuteness of hearing), full facial muscle paralysis, an eyelid that would not blink (with the inherent rolling of the eye up and out of danger when the lid would normally blink), and a distorted soapy beer taste on the affected side of my tongue.

It was clear in my subsequent research that these symptoms could not have been caused by a massage. With Bell's palsy, the location of impediment on the facial nerve is proscribed by the symptoms. In other words, if I had only had facial paralysis, I would know that the nerve was impaired at a point above the jaw line. As you add symptoms (hyperacoustic sensitivity, taste impairment), you trace further up proximal to the geniculate ganglion, located inside the area near the ear.

Because I neglected to see a neurologist for over a week, my facial nerve degenerated and it took almost a year for near full function to resume. I couldn't use my dimple for a year! I'm adamant about people seeing a neurologist immediately these days when I hear of a case of Bell's palsy.

The whole experience was generally frustrating because there's a lot of poor information out there, but it was a great emotional process; when you've used your face for a calling card all your life and suddenly it's not available to you anymore, you have to really deal with what's underneath.

Treatment

Treatment for Bell's palsy is usually conservative because most cases are self-limiting, that is, they resolve without interference. A combination of steroidal anti-inflammatories and acyclovir to slow down herpes activity are effective for up to 85% of Bell's palsy patients. A small number of patients do not experience full or close to full recovery, however. These patients, who can be identified early by nerve conduction studies to measure the extent of nerve damage, may benefit from a surgical intervention to release bony pressure on the nerve.

Prognosis

This condition almost always has a sudden onset (the textbook Bell's palsy patient will simply wake up with it one morning), and it also nearly always has a rapid recovery rate. Improvement is usually seen within 2 to 3 days, and complete restoration of function can be expected within weeks or months. Some cases take longer, however, and they often see a less complete recovery without some intervention to remove mechanical pressure on the facial nerve.

Massage?

Bell's Palsy is a flaccid paralysis with sensation left intact. If the underlying cause of the neuritis has been diagnosed to be safe for massage (i.e., not a tumor, Lyme disease, etc.), then massage is a very appropriate treatment choice. Massage keeps the facial muscles elastic and the local circulation strong. This sets the stage for a more complete recovery when nerve supply is eventually restored.

Cerebral Palsy

Definition: What Is It?

CP is a term that refers to many possible injuries to the brain during gestational development, birth, and early infancy. Several different types of CP have been identified, each involving damage to different parts of the brain.

Demographics: Who Gets It?

The incidence of CP in the United States is every 2 to 4 of 1000 live births. Around 500,000 CP patients live in the United States today, and about 1500 are born every year. Despite improved prenatal care, the rate of CP has remained unchanged for many years. The persons most likely to develop CP are infants who experience intracranial bleeding. Other high-risk populations are hard to identify, but statistics are highest among children of mothers who smoke, who live in poverty, who do not receive prenatal care, and who have previously had preterm babies.

Etiology: What Happens?

CP is the result of brain damage, usually to motor areas of the brain, specifically the basal ganglia and/or cerebellum. The damage can be brought about

---

CEREBRAL PALSY IN BRIEF

What is it?

Cerebral palsy (CP) is an umbrella term used to refer to a variety of central nervous system injuries that may occur prenatally, at birth, or in early infancy. These injuries usually result in motor impairment but may also lead to sensory and cognitive problems as well.

How is it recognized?

CP is usually diagnosed early in infancy when voluntary motor skills are expected to begin to develop. CP patients may have hyper- or hypotonic muscles, suppressed or extreme reflexes, poor coordination, and they may show random, involuntary movement.

Is massage indicated or contraindicated?

As long as sensation is intact and the patient is able to communicate with the therapist in some way, massage is appropriate and potentially very useful for persons with CP, as they work to maintain muscular elasticity and improve motor skills.

in a number of ways. For a long time it was believed that most cases of CP happened when a baby was deprived of oxygen for a dangerously long time during the process of childbirth. That myth has been dispelled by studies that show the majority of babies who experience *anoxia*, or oxygen depletion during childbirth, never develop brain damage, and the majority of CP patients had uncomplicated, uneventful births. The causes of most cases of CP are now being recognized to occur much earlier in pregnancy.

Causes

Causes of CP can fall into three groups, according to when they occur.

- *Prenatal causes.* Most cases of CP can be traced to problems during pregnancy, often due to maternal illness. Contributing factors include infections with herpes (Chapter 1) or toxoplasmosis, *hyperthyroidism*, *diabetes* (Chapter 8), or Rh sensitization (the mother's immune system attacks and destroys the red blood cells of her unborn child).

- *Birth trauma.* CP can result if the child experiences anoxia or asphyxia (lack of air from a mechanical blockage) during birth. Respiratory distress and head trauma (often from a difficult presentation or the use of forceps in delivery) may also increase the risk of brain damage.

- *Acquired CP.* This is CP that is acquired in early infancy. Causes include head trauma (often from car accidents or child abuse: "shaken baby syndrome"), infection with *meningitis* or *encephalitis* (this chapter), vascular problems (brain hemorrhages), or neoplasms in the brain that may lead to brain damage.

Regardless of the cause of brain damage, the child with CP will have some impairment of function. The problem could be so minor that only people who know what to look for may see it, or it may be completely debilitating both physically and mentally; it all depends on what part and how much of the brain has been affected.

Types of CP

CP is classified into four types: spastic, athetoid, ataxic, and mixed.

- *Spastic CP.* This is the most common form of the disorder, accounting for 50 to 80% of all CP patients. Spastic CP means that in some areas of the body muscle tone is so high that the tight muscle's antagonists have completely let go. This is called the "clasp knife" effect. (See more details on spasticity in the sidebar titled Nerve Damage Terminology, this chapter.)

- *Athetoid CP.* This variety is less common than spastic CP, accounting for up to 30% of all patients. It involves very weak muscles and frequent involuntary writhing movements.

- *Ataxic CP.* This rare variety of the disorder involves chronic shaking and tremors as well as very poor balance. Fewer than 10% of all CP patients live with ataxic CP.

- *Mixed CP.* Many CP patients live with combinations of the CP forms.

CP may also be classified by what part of the body is affected. These terms are consistent with those used for other central nervous system disorders: hemiplegic CP means the left or right side is affected; diplegic CP means either two arms or two legs are affected; and quadriplegic CP means all the extremities are affected to some extent.

Types of CP may come and go, or change entirely from one kind to another, as the child grows. CP is not a progressive disorder, however, and if symptoms seem to be getting significantly worse over time, a different kind of central nervous system dysfunction must be considered.

Complications

Damage to the motor systems of the body is only the beginning for many CP patients. Complications of this disorder include several other serious challenges. Many CP patients have partial or total hearing loss. Up to 75% of all CP patients have some amount of *strabismus* (eyes that do not focus on the same axis). This condition can be corrected to prevent further sight loss. Although CP does not necessarily imply cognitive problems, some 60% of CP patients experience some level of mental retardation. About 25% of all CP patients have *seizure disorders* (this chapter), which can require very powerful medication to control. Finally, the muscles of CP patients can become so chronically tight that they are replaced with tight, restrictive connective tissue; these are called contractures. Contractures can pull on the skeleton so constantly and so powerfully that the patient is at risk for developing pathologic levels of *scoliosis* (Chapter 2) that can make it painful to sit or stand and difficult to breathe.

Signs and Symptoms

Signs and symptoms of CP vary according to the location and extent of brain injury. Damage to the cerebellum produces different symptoms from damage to the frontal lobe, for instance. Some of the most common features of CP include hypertonicity, hypotonicity, poor coordination and voluntary muscle control, unusually weak muscles, random movements, and early hearing and/or vision problems.

Because infants do not develop voluntary motor skills until they are around 6 months old, CP may be difficult to diagnose before this point.

Treatment

CP is incurable and irreversible. Central nervous system damage is, at least at this point, permanent. CP is therefore managed, rather than treated, by providing skills and equipment to live as fully and functionally as possible. For some CP patients this means braces for one foot that is slightly weaker than the other; for others it could mean intensive occupational, physical, and speech therapy for many years.

Medication for CP is occasionally prescribed to help manage seizures and to reduce muscle spasm. Some surgical interventions have been developed to lengthen contracted muscles, to realign vertebrae that have become distorted by scoliosis, and to alter nerve pathways in the brain to reduce the severity of tremors.

Physical therapy is recommended for people with CP because the process of developing muscle contractures is slow and can be made even slower when muscles and joints are specifically stretched and manipulated to maintain flexibility. Patients may also be encouraged to use and strengthen their weaker limbs. It is important to note the many uses and benefits physical therapy has to offer CP patients, because massage therapy may also be a valuable adjunct in these cases.

Massage?

Massage therapy can have a valuable role in improving the quality of life of a person with CP. As stated above, if physical therapy is used to stretch and strengthen skeletal muscles, massage will also be a safe choice. The only caution is that people with very severe CP may not be able to communicate their wants or concerns clearly. If a massage therapist works with a client who cannot speak, other modes of communication, including nonverbal signals, become especially important. It is the responsibility of the massage therapist to make sure that his or her work is welcome and freely accepted at all times.

REFLEX SYMPATHETIC DYSTROPHY SYNDROME IN BRIEF

What is it?
Reflex sympathetic dystrophy syndrome (RSDS) is a chronic pain condition in which an initial trauma causes pain that is more severe and longer lasting than is reasonable to expect. The pain can become a self-sustaining phenomenon that becomes a lifelong affliction.

How is it recognized?
RSDS moves in stages, although symptoms may overlap. In early stages it involves redness, heat, sweating, and severe burning pain. In later stages the skin may turn bluish, and the nearby joints and muscles may atrophy. Bones in the area thin and become vulnerable to breakage. Late-stage RSDS can involve irreversible changes to the affected area and symptoms that spread to other parts of the body.

Is massage indicated or contraindicated?
Most RSDS patients have little or no tolerance for touch of any kind, at least in the area where the pain syndrome began. Physical therapy is often recommended to keep the affected joints moveable and functioning; massage may help to relieve some of the pain associated with this therapy. Massage within tolerance in other parts of the body may be welcome and supportive.

Reflex Sympathetic Dystrophy Syndrome

Definition: What Is It?

RSDS is a collection of signs and symptoms that involve changes to the skin, muscles, joints, nerves, and blood vessels of the affected areas. It usually (but not always) begins after some trauma or injury that initiates a reflex response (*reflex*). A problem in the sympathetic response leads to a chronic reinforcement of the initial pain (*sympathetic*). The chronic pain and resulting changes in blood flow lead to problems in tissue nutrition and growth (*dystrophy*). RSDS is classified as a variant of a broader phenomenon, *causalgia* (see sidebar).

Demographics: Who Gets It?

Statistics on RSDS have been difficult to gather, and different agencies quote contradictory numbers. Some estimates say that chronic pain follows after 2 to 5% of all peripheral nerve injuries and up to 21% of all hemiplegic injuries (see *stroke*, this chapter).

Although it has been observed in all age groups from babies to elderly adults, most RSDS patients are diagnosed when they are 40 to 60 years old. Estimates of the numbers of RSDS patients in the United States range from 5 to 7 million people. Some resources say that men are affected as often or more often than women; other resources suggest that women are diagnosed 3 or 4 times more often than men.

What these conflicting pieces of information reveal is that this condition is not well understood, that many people are not sure whether it is a real phenomenon, and that reliable standards for diagnosis have not yet been developed.

Etiology: What Happens?

When a person experiences a stimulus, a sensory neuron carries that information to the spinal cord where a reflex response begins. At the same time, that impulse travels up the spinal cord to the brain where the stimulus is interpreted at a conscious or subconscious level. The response might be regulated by the parasympathetic nervous system, for instance, if the stimulus was a soothing, confident effleurage stroke. The response is regulated by the sympathetic nervous system if the stimulus is interpreted as something threatening or painful.

In RSDS, the nervous system makes a mistake. An initial trauma (often to a hand or foot, but anywhere on the body can be affected) begins a pain sensation that is moderated by the sympathetic nervous system. RSDS is often associated with high-velocity traumas like bullet or shrapnel wounds, but it has also been seen with minor strains and sprains, as a postsurgical complication, along with cerebrovascular accidents, and sometimes with no identified causative trauma at all.

The pain, whatever its source, initiates a sympathetic response, which then reinforces the pain sensation. In other words, the pain becomes a self-fulfilling prophecy: a person hurts, which makes him or her feel stressed, which makes the hurt worse, and the normal healing processes that would interrupt this sequence are unable to overcome the power of the vicious circle.

Eventually the physiologic changes that occur when a specific part of the body is stuck in a sympathetic loop cause their own kinds of damage—damage that can be irreversible. This pain cycle also has the potential to spread proximally on the affected limb, to the eyes, internal organs, and even to the contralateral limb.

Signs and Symptoms

Four main symptoms have been observed in most RSDS patients: constant burning pain with little or no stimulus, local inflammation and sweating, spasm of both skeletal and smooth muscle in nearby blood vessels, and chronic insomnia (which gives rise to a number of other mental disorders including *depression* [this chapter]).

RSDS has been broken into three or four loosely defined stages. Overlap of these stages often occurs, so they are useful mainly as a time reference for how long a person has been affected by this condition, and what treatment options have the best chance of interfering with its progression.

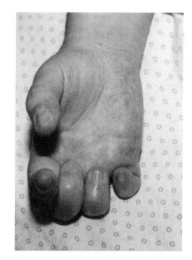

Figure 3-8. Reflex sympathetic dystrophy

- *Stage I.* Stage I signs and symptoms are prevalent during the first 1 to 3 months of pain. They include severe burning pain at the site of the injury, muscle spasm, reduced range of motion, excessive hair and nail growth if the injury is on a hand or foot, and hot, red, sweaty skin (Fig. 3-8), Color Plate 34).

- *Stage II.* In this stage changes in the growth pattern of the affected tissues can be observed. The swelling spreads proximally from the initial site, the hair stops growing, and the nails become brittle and easily cracked. Skin that was red in Stage I takes on a bluish tone in Stage II. In this intensely painful stage the muscles begin to atrophy from underuse, and the nearby joints may thicken and become stiffer. Stage II usually lasts from 3 to 6 months.

- *Stage III.* Stage III RSDS shows signs of irreversible changes to the affected structures. The bones become thin and brittle, the joints become immobile, and the muscles tighten into permanent contracture. The condition may spread proximally up the limb, to the contralateral limb, or anywhere else in the body.

- *Stage IV.* Some researchers maintain that Stage IV RSDS is different from the other stages because at this point the pain sensation is a self-sustaining phenomenon in the brain. In other words, the neurotransmitter balance and pain sensation centers in the brain are essentially incapable of letting go of this sensation.

Diagnosis

It is not difficult to identify RSDS, but this disease is not well recognized or understood, so it is probably underdiagnosed. This is a problem, because the long-term outlook for someone with this problem is significantly better if treatment can begin in Stage I, rather than if intervention is not tried until Stage IV.

Pain By Any Other Name . . .

In October 1864 a group of doctors compared their observations of Civil War soldiers recovering from gunshot wounds. Their comments were remarkably astute and constitute a vivid picture of the experience of the condition eventually termed "causalgia" from the Greek *kausis* (burning) and *algia* (pain).

> *In our early experience of nerve wounds, we met with a small number of men who were suffering from a pain which they described as "burning" or as "mustard red-hot" or as "red-hot file rasping the skin". . . Its intensity varies from the most trivial burning to a state of torture, which can hardly be credited, but which reacts on the whole economy, until the general health is seriously affected. . .* [i]

Over the years this condition has come to be known by many names. *Sympathetic maintained pain syndrome* is another name, as is *complex regional pain syndrome*. Causalgia itself is now considered the umbrella term for other chronic pain syndromes, and reflex sympathetic dystrophy, which is the name that has stuck, is a subtype under this heading.

[i]Reflex sympathetic dystrophy. RSDHope.org. Available at: http://rsd-hope.org. Accessed winter 2001.

Visible signs and patients' descriptions of symptoms are usually straightforward with this condition. Diagnosis can be confirmed with thermography, a test that measures blood flow and localized heat in the body. Radiographs or bone scans may be used to look for signs of osteoporosis at the site of injury.

Treatment

Treatment options for RSDS vary according to which stage the patient is in when the condition is diagnosed. The earlier in the process treatment begins, the better the chance for a full or nearly full recovery.

Stage I RSDS may be treated with simple analgesics: NSAIDs or short-term steroids if necessary. Patients get good benefit from heat, especially moist heat applications like paraffin baths or hot packs. Ice is absolutely out of the question for RSDS patients in any stage.

Stage II and III RSDS patients need to be more aggressive with their pain management. Morphine pumps that introduce morphine directly into the spinal canal are used with mixed results. TENS machines are successful for some people but not all. Calcium channel blockers may improve blood flow and relieve pain. Eventually a patient may consider a sympathectomy: the surgical severing of parts of the sympathetic nervous system to stop the endless cycle of repeating pain signals. This intervention can be successful, but many patients report that the benefits are short-lived and the pain comes back after surgery.

Massage?

RSDS locally contraindicates massage in affected areas, where any stimulus is painful and unwelcome. Some cases of RSDS are treated with physical therapy to limit bone and joint atrophy. Massage that is well tolerated may be appropriate in this context as well. If massage is perceived as pleasant anywhere else on the body, it could certainly add to the quality of life of a person who has some extreme physical challenges.

Spinal Cord Injury
Definition: What Is It?

The definition of SCI is self-evident. Damage to some percentage of nerve tissue in the spinal canal has occurred. How that damage is reflected in the body depends on where and how much of the tissue has been affected.

SCIs fall into one of three categories: *concussions*, in which tissue is jarred and irritated but not structurally damaged; *incomplete injuries*, in which only some of the neuron tracts in the spinal cord have been damaged; and *complete injuries*, in which all the ascending and descending tracts have been interrupted at a specific level or levels.

SPINAL CORD INJURY IN BRIEF

What is it?
Spinal cord injury (SCI) is a situation in which some or all of the fibers in the spinal cord have been damaged, usually by trauma but occasionally from other problems such as tumors or bony growths in the spinal canal.

How is it recognized?
The signs and symptoms of SCI vary with the nature of the injury. Loss of motor function follows destruction of motor neurons, but that paralysis may be flaccid or spastic depending on the injured area. Loss of sensation follows the destruction of sensory pathways. If the injury is not complete, some motor or sensory function may remain in the affected tissues.

Is massage indicated or contraindicated?
Mechanical types of massage are appropriate only where sensation is present and no underlying pathologies may be exacerbated by the work. Areas without sensation contraindicate massage that intends to manipulate and influence the elasticity of tissue.

An injury that affects the lower abdomen and extremities but leaves the chest and arms intact is called paraplegia. An injury that impacts the body from the neck down is called tetraplegia or quadriplegia. For more terminology in the context of central nervous system injuries, see the sidebar.

Demographics: Who Gets It?

Frequency of SCIs in the United States is estimated at about 10 to 11 thousand per year, excluding those persons who die at the scene of the accident. Between 183,000 and 230,000 people in the United States currently live with permanent spinal cord injuries. The average age at the time of injury is 32 years. Male patients outnumber females by more than 4 to 1.

Motor vehicle accidents cause 38.5% of all spinal cord injuries. Gunshot wounds and other acts of violence cause 24.5%. Falls are responsible for 21.8%, sports-related injuries contribute 7.2%, and other types of accidents cause 7.9%.

The neck is the most vulnerable part of the spine; about half of all injuries occur here. The levels most often injured, by order of frequency, are C5, C4, C6, T12, and L1. About 51.6% of SCI survivors are tetraplegic, and 46.3% are paraplegic.

Etiology: What Happens?

A primary injury to the spinal cord is usually a crushing blow (Fig. 3-9). The cord can also be injured through direct compression exerted by tumors, bone spurs, or cysts or by stretching the spinal column (this is most frequently seen in children). Gunshot wounds may lacerate the cord. Spinal cords are rarely completely transected, and when they are, the mortality rate is very high.

As researchers learn more about spinal cord injuries, some very exciting information has emerged: a large part of the damage to delicate central nervous system tissue is incurred not by the trauma itself, but by posttraumatic reactions in the body. These secondary reactions, which include excessive bleeding, localized edema, free radical activity, an overabundance of scar tissue formation, white blood cell attacks on healthy tissue, and gradual demyelination of healthy cells can be controlled and limited with appropriate early intervention.

A newly injured spinal cord goes through a period called "spinal cord shock." During this time many body functions are severely impaired: blood pressure is dangerously low, the heart beats slowly, peripheral blood vessels dilate, and the patient is susceptible to hypothermia. Any or all of the secondary reactions discussed above may set in at this time. These secondary responses can interrupt function up to two full levels above the primary injury, so it is vital that aggressive care is obtained during this window of opportunity.

During this acute phase of injury the affected muscles may be flaccid, or hypotonic. When the inflammatory process begins to subside (and this can mean days or weeks after the injury) the muscles supplied by damaged axons begin to tighten, and their reflexes become hyperreactive. Spasticity along with hyperreflexia is a hallmark of SCI. If muscles stay flaccid and reflexes are dull or nonexistent, the damage is probably to the nerve roots rather than to the spinal cord itself. Injuries to the low back often show this pattern, as the spinal canal is occupied by the cauda equina nerve extensions from T12 down to the sacrum. Depending on the nature of the accident, it is perfectly possible to sustain injury to both the spinal cord and the nerve roots simultaneously.

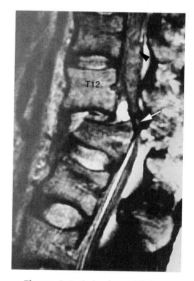

T12

Figure 3-9. Spinal cord injury

Signs and Symptoms

The motor and sensory impairment caused by SCI is determined by what parts of the cord are damaged and at what levels. Obviously, the higher the damage, the more of the body is affected. Injuries to the front part of the cord affect motor function, while damage to the posterior aspect affects the senses of touch, proprioception, and vibration. Damage to the lateral parts of the cord interrupts sensations of pain and temperature.

Complications

Spinal cord injuries can lead to many serious long-term complications. An SCI patient spends a great deal of time and energy in working to prevent, manage, or recover from these secondary problems.

- *Decubitus ulcers.* Also known as bedsores or pressure sores, *decubitus ulcers* (Chapter 1) can arise anywhere circulation is limited by mechanical compression of the skin. Because these wounds do not heal quickly or easily, they are highly susceptible to infection.

- *Heterotopic ossification.* This is the formation of calcium deposits in soft tissues. It is very similar to myositis ossificans (Chapter 2), but this particular process is seen only in SCI patients.

- *Deep vein thrombosis, pulmonary embolism.* The formation of blood clots in the venous system is a high risk for new SCI patients, but the risk decreases only slightly with the passage of time. Blood that goes into the legs, but that lacks the muscular support to get back up the leg veins, can pool and thicken, causing deep vein thrombosis. If a fragment of a clot breaks loose, it will inevitably go to the lungs, causing a life-threatening *pulmonary embolism* (Chapter 4).

- *Respiratory infection.* SCI patients are at high risk for respiratory infection, especially if the damage is higher than T12. When the chest cannot fully expand and contract and the cough reflex is limited, it is difficult to expel pathogens from the body. The leading cause of death for SCI patients is *pneumonia* (Chapter 6).

- *Urinary tract infection.* SCI patients who must use a catheter to urinate are at high risk for contamination and infection of the urinary tract. Left untended, the risk of these infections invading the kidneys is significant (see *urinary tract infection, pyelonephritis,* Chapter 9).

- *Autonomic hyperreflexia.* Damage to the spinal cord above T6 raises the risk of developing autonomic hyperreflexia, a condition in which a minor stimulus (e.g., a full bladder or bowel, a ridge of cloth caught under the skin, menstrual cramps) creates an uncontrollable sympathetic reaction. It causes a pounding headache, increased heart rate, sweating, and other flight or fight symptoms including dangerously high blood pressure. Autonomic hyperreflexia can be a medical emergency.

- *Cardiovascular disease.* Suddenly changing from being ambulatory to being confined to a wheelchair means a significant reduction in physical activity for most SCI patients. The risk of developing *hypertension, atherosclerosis,* and other cardiovascular problems (Chapter 4) is high for this sedentary population.

- *Numbness.* Most SCI patients experience some numbness or reduction in sensation, depending on which part of the spinal cord has been damaged. The absence of pain is a dangerous feature, because it allows for damage to occur without warning. Small cuts or abrasions can become infected and an SCI patient may never know.

- *Pain.* Some SCI patients experience various kinds of pain along with numbness and lack of sensation. Some chronic pain problems are generated in the spine itself but refer sensation to the damaged limbs; nerve root pressure may refer pain along the associated dermatome; pain may be generated by the development of calcium deposits (see *heterotopic ossification,* above); or pain may be related to musculoskeletal injury as a person must learn to use the arms and shoulders in new ways to propel a wheelchair and lift themselves into and out of it.

- *Spasticity, contractures.* As the muscles supplied by damaged motor axons begin to tighten, an SCI patient loses range of motion. Some spasticity may become a permanent feature of the injury. Chronically tight muscle fibers eventually atrophy, to be replaced by thick, tough layers of connective tissue; this is called a contracture. If any sensory or motor function is left in the limb, temporary episodes of spasticity may also be a problem. These may be caused by any kind of stimulus; the reflexes of active muscle fibers in SCI patients are very extreme and sensitive.

Treatment

If something is pressing directly on the spinal cord or cauda equina, emergency surgery to remove it is indicated. The other very important early intervention with these traumas is to limit inflammation and other secondary reactions that may damage uninjured tissue, so anti-inflammatory drugs and other medications that limit this kind of activity are usually administered as quickly as possible.

Some later treatments for SCI include the implantation of electrodes in muscles that are controlled from an external computer. These implants can provide pinching and gripping capabilities for people who otherwise would not have the use of their hands. Surgical transfer of healthy tendons can also be helpful. For some people the triceps muscle may be paralyzed while the deltoid is not. Surgically extending the posterior deltoid tendon and attaching it to the olecranon can provide these people with the power it takes to use a wheelchair.

Treatment for SCI survivors is targeted at providing them with the skills to live as fully as possible. Physical and occupational therapists specialize in helping these patients gain the skills they need to function; mental/emotional therapists are also critical, especially for those who are adapting to their paralysis as a new way of life. Ultimately, about 90% of all SCI patients are able to live independently with these new skills.

The focus of current research in SCI treatment is on influencing the growth of central nervous system neurons. It has been found that some proteins in cerebrospinal fluid

Nerve Damage Terminology

Nerve damage can manifest in several different ways. Familiarity with some of the vocabulary of nervous system damage can make it much easier to "talk shop" with clients and physicians dealing with these problems.

- *Paresthesia.* This is a technical term for any abnormal sensation, particularly the tingling, burning, and prickling feelings associated with "pins and needles."

- *Hyperkinesia.* This is excessive muscular activity.

- *Hypokinesia.* This is a condition involving diminished or slowed movement.

- *Hypertonia.* This is a general term for extreme tension, or tone in the muscles.

- *Hypotonia.* This is the opposite of hypertonia; it means an abnormally low level of muscle tone, as seen with flaccid paralysis.

- *Spasticity.* This is a type of hypertonia. It is a condition in which the stretch reflex is overactive. The flexors want to flex, but the extensors do not want to give way. Finally, the extensors are stretched too far and then they release altogether. This phenomenon is called the "clasp-knife effect."

- *Paralysis.* This comes from the Greek for "loosening." It means the loss of any function controlled by the nervous system.

- *Paresis.* This is partial or incomplete para-lysis.

- *Flaccid paralysis.* This is typically a sign of peripheral nerve damage. It accompanies conditions like *Bell's palsy* (this chapter). Flaccid paralysis involves muscles in a state of *hypotonicity.*

- *Spastic paralysis.* This indicates *central nervous system damage.* Spastic paralysis combines aspects of hypertonia, hypokinesia, and hyperreflexia. This situation is never resolved, which distinguishes it from mere *spasm* (Chapter 2).

Types of spastic paralysis:

- *Hemi*plegia means one vertical half (or hemisphere) of the body has been affected. This is the variation that most often accompanies stroke (this chapter).

- *Para*plegia means the bottom half of the body, or some part of it, has been affected. These patients still have at least partial use of their arms and hands.

- *Diplegia* is a symmetrical paralysis of both of the upper or both of the lower extremities resulting from injuries to the cerebrum.

- *Tetra*plegia, or *quad*riplegia, means that the body has been affected from the neck down. Tetraplegics can eat, breathe, talk, and move their heads because these functions are controlled by the cranial nerves, which are usually protected from injury.

inhibit neuronal growth, while others stimulate it. Further, it may be that different types of neurons require different chemical environments for repair. Eventually, through a combination of stem cell implantation, genetic manipulation, and the creation of highly conducive chemical environments, it may be possible for someone with extensive spinal cord damage to regenerate damaged tissue and emerge with full or nearly full function.

Massage?

Massage can be an important part of the life of people with spinal cord injuries, as long as the complications listed above are considered and respected.

These people have very different physical and emotional stressors than the rest of the population, but they are prone to the same kinds of injuries as anyone else. Imagine being in a wheelchair and having shoulder tendinitis: wouldn't it be a relief to get rolling pain-free again? It takes a lot of courage to work with SCI survivors; massage therapists may have fears of accidentally hurting them, physically or emotionally, by saying or doing the wrong thing. But within this group is a population of people waiting eagerly for the chance to receive bodywork.

STROKE IN BRIEF

What is it?
A stroke is damage to brain tissue caused either by a blockage in blood flow or by an internal hemorrhage.

How is it recognized?
The symptoms of stroke include paralysis, weakness, and/or numbness on one side; blurry or diminished vision on one side with asymmetrically dilated pupils; dizziness and confusion; difficulty in speaking or understanding simple sentences; sudden extreme headache; and possibly loss of consciousness.

Is massage indicated or contraindicated?
Most people who survive strokes are at high risk for other cardiovascular problems. Rigorous circulatory massage should be avoided with this group, although they may certainly benefit from other types of bodywork to augment their rehabilitative physical therapy.

Stroke

Definition: What Is It?

Stroke, also called brain attack or cerebrovascular accident (CVA), is damage to the brain due to oxygen deprivation.

Demographics: Who Gets It?

Stroke is the single most common type of central nervous system disorder. It is the third leading cause of death in the United States, coming in behind heart disease and cancer. It is the leading cause of adult disability.

About 600,000 people will have a stroke this year (1 every 53 seconds). Of them, 500,000 will experience their first attack, while 100,000 will have a repeat stroke. Close to 160,000 Americans will die of stroke this year. Of the survivors, 15 to 30% will be permanently disabled, and 20% will require institutionalized care. About 4.5 million stroke survivors are alive in the United States today.

More men have strokes than women, but more women tend to die of strokes than do men. The chance of having a stroke before age 70 is about 1 in 20. After age 70, however, the risk rises significantly each year, especially if risk factors are present.

Etiology: What Happens?

Oxygen deprivation in the brain can be caused by one of four things:

- *Cerebral thrombosis.* A clot becomes lodged in a cerebral artery and starves off nerve cells. These strokes account for up to 88% of all CVAs. They are closely related to *atherosclerosis* (Chapter 4). Cerebral thrombosis strokes usually occur during sleep or early in the morning.

- *Embolism.* This is much the same thing except that the origins of the obstruction are usually different. Emboli generally come from inefficient pumping of a heart with atrial fibrillations; incomplete and arrhythmic contractions allow blood in the left atrium to thicken and form clots before being forced out into the bloodstream. Emboli account for 8 to 14% of all CVAs.

These two problems are called ischemic strokes, as they have to do with oxygen in affected tissues and the subsequent death of those tissues (Fig. 3-10). Another type of stroke has to do with too much blood, although not within the proper blood vessels.

- *Cerebral hemorrhage.* This is the rupture of a blood vessel that can cause tissue death in the brain. Cerebral hemorrhages are often associated with aneurysms (Chapter 4), which may be a result of chronic hypertension, bleeding disorders, head trauma, or malformation of blood vessels.

- *Subarachnoid hemorrhage.* This is the rupture of a blood vessel on the surface of the brain rather than within the tissue itself. The leaking blood fills the space between the brain tissue and the arachnoid, eventually putting pressure against the cranium.

Ischemic strokes are distinct from but closely related to another phenomenon: *transient ischemic attacks* (TIAs). In a TIA a very tiny blood clot creates a temporary blockage in the brain, but it quickly disperses before any lasting damage can occur. Consequently, TIAs are associated with ischemic CVAs rather than hemorrhagic ones. Symptoms of TIA are very similar to those of stroke, except that they last only a few minutes or hours. They are, however, like the muffled rumblings of an incipient eruption; about one-third of all people who have a stroke had a TIA beforehand.

The amount of damage a stroke causes is determined primarily by the location and numbers of neurons that are damaged by oxygen deprivation. Secondary responses to tissue damage have also been seen to contribute heavily to stroke damage. Inflammatory reactions, free radical activity, and other factors can cause tissue damage that far exceeds the oxygen deprivation brought about by the stroke itself. The good news in this discovery is that these secondary responses can be interrupted and moderated if treatment begins quickly enough.

Risk Factors

Although a person can have a genetic predisposition toward a CVA, many factors contribute to the likelihood of stroke that are well within the reach of personal control.

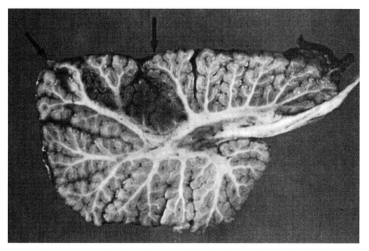

Figure 3-10. Stroke: damaged brain tissue is clearly visible

Risk Factors that Can Be Controlled

- *High blood pressure.* Untreated hypertension is the biggest single contributing factor to the risk of stroke (see *hypertension*, Chapter 4).

- *Atherosclerosis, high cholesterol.* This situation is another leading risk factor for cerebral thrombosis. It is closely tied to high blood pressure (Chapter 4).

- *Obesity.* Clinical obesity is often seen in conjunction with high blood pressure and atherosclerosis.

- *Smoking.* Nicotine constricts blood vessels and raises blood pressure.

- *Atrial fibrillation.* Left untreated, this condition can help to form the emboli responsible for some ischemic embolic strokes.

- *High alcohol consumption.* This is generally considered to be more than 2 drinks per day.

- *Sedentary lifestyle.* Lack of exercise leads to poor cardiovascular health and an increased risk of CVA.

- *Diabetes.* When this condition is untreated it can contribute to high blood pressure and atherosclerosis (see Chapter 8).

- *High-estrogen birth control pills.* Especially when taken by a smoker. No similar risk has been found with postmenopausal estrogen replacement therapy.

- *Overall stress.* Being stuck in a sympathetic state for prolonged periods drives up systemic blood pressure. Hypertension is often the starting point for many cardiovascular disorders as well as stroke.

Risk Factors that Cannot Be Controlled

- *Age.* Two-thirds of all stroke patients are older than 65 years of age. The incidence of stroke doubles each decade after 55.

- *Gender.* About 25% more men have strokes than women. However, women seem to have more severe strokes; 60% of all people who die of strokes are women.

- *Race.* African-Americans have a higher incidence of hypertension than Whites. They are about twice as likely to have a stroke as Whites and are almost twice as likely to die of it.

- *Family history.* Having a family history of stroke and cardiovascular disease can be a predisposing factor. Structurally weak blood vessels can be an inherited problem. However, in cases of ischemic strokes, the question needs to be asked, "What is inherited: the status of the blood vessels, or the diet and exercise habits?"

- *Previous stroke.* Having one stroke usually predisposes a person to having another. Predisposition is not predestination, however; by taking control of whatever factors are within reach, a person can take big steps toward reducing the chances that he or she will have another stroke.

Signs and Symptoms

It is important to be able to recognize the signs of stroke; the sooner treatment is administered, the less damage will occur. Surprisingly, a huge proportion of Americans do not recognize the major symptoms of stroke, which are as follows:

- Sudden onset of unilateral weakness, numbness, or paralysis on the face, arm, leg, or any combination of the three.

- Suddenly blurred or decreased vision in one or both eyes; asymmetrical dilation of pupils.
- Difficulty in speaking or understanding simple sentences; confusion.
- Sudden onset of dizziness, clumsiness, vertigo.
- Sudden very extreme headache.
- Possible loss of consciousness.

The symptoms of a TIA are very similar to those of a stroke. Although TIA symptoms may subside after a few minutes or hours, it is inappropriate to take a "wait and see" approach to any stroke symptoms. The effectiveness of stroke treatments depends on how soon treatment begins, so any symptoms should be immediately investigated.

After a debilitating stroke the extent of the damage depends on what part and how much of the brain has been affected. Occasionally progressive degeneration may continue over 1 or 2 days, but usually a stroke is complete within a few hours.

Motor damage from strokes can result in partial or full paralysis of one side of the body; this is called hemiplegia. Aphasia (loss of language), memory loss, and mild or severe personality changes may also occur. Sensory damage may result in permanent numbness and/or vision loss.

Diagnosis

When a person suspects that he or she may have had a stroke, the first priority is to determine whether it was an ischemic or hemorrhagic event, since these two phenomena require very different treatment approaches. A diagnosis may be reached through a combination of physical examination, CT scan, MRI scan, ultrasound, arteriography, and blood tests.

Treatment

The treatment of choice for ischemic stroke survivors is anticoagulant medication to minimize the risk of more clotting. Severe brain damage may be averted if the anticoagulants are administered within a few hours of the stroke. One anticoagulant called tissue plasminogen activator (tPA) has been found to be extremely effective for minimizing the blood clots involved in both stroke and *heart attack* (Chapter 4), if administered within the first few hours of onset.

If the CVA was from a hemorrhage, however, anticoagulant treatment could be dangerous or even deadly. A brain aneurysm caught before it ruptures may be treated with surgery to take the pressure off or strengthen the affected artery.

Once the dust has settled and it is clear how much function was lost during a stroke, therapy may begin to help a patient relearn how to do basic tasks like walking, speaking, eating, and performing self-care. Because the brain has a vast resource of back-up wiring, this is often a very successful part of the recovery process. It needs to be started very soon after the CVA to prevent the fibrosis and atrophy of muscle tissue that happen so quickly when nerve signals have been interrupted. Physical, occupational, and speech therapists may be enlisted in this process; massage, with respect for the risk of cardiovascular disease, may have a role also.

Carotid Artery Disease: Nowhere To Go but Up

The discussion of *atherosclerosis* (Chapter 4) points out that because of chronically high blood pressure, both the aorta and coronary arteries are particularly prone to the development of atherosclerotic plaque. The carotid arteries, which emerge from the aortic arch, are similarly vulnerable. Although they are further from the heart, blood pressure in the arteries that supply the head is ordinarily very high to ensure adequate blood flow to the brain. This puts the carotid arteries at risk for the same endothelial damage and plaque development seen with the aorta and the coronary arteries; this is called *carotid artery disease*.

The problem with carotid artery disease is that if any fragment of plaque or blood clot should break free, it has only one direction to go: straight up into the brain. When this happens in very tiny increments it is called transient ischemic attack (TIA). The presence of carotid artery disease significantly raises the risk of a major stroke—so much so that identifying this disorder often leads to aggressive treatment, in the shape of carotid endarterectomy (the artery is surgically opened, cleaned out, and closed up again).

Massage therapists working with clients who know they have carotid artery disease need to stay away from the neck, especially the anterior triangle, which is bordered by the sternocleidomastoid muscle, running superficially over the carotid arteries.

Limiting controllable risk factors is also important: stopping smoking, improving diet and exercise habits, and reducing stress are all important actions to take. If necessary, surgery may be performed either on the blood vessels leading to the brain or inside it to widen the lumenae and reduce the possibility of more clots being caught or formed inside.

Massage?

Massage can play a role in the recovery of a stroke survivor, but some cautions need to be considered. First, the client's general cardiovascular health must be considered. The vast majority of stroke patients have other circulatory problems. Therefore, it is very important to work as part of a client's health care team. Second, hemiplegia is a type of spastic paralysis, which carries specific cautions and guidelines for massage (see *nerve damage terminology* (sidebar) with *spinal cord injury*, this chapter).

Trigeminal Neuralgia

Definition: What Is It?

TN is neuro-algia ("nerve pain") along one or more of the three branches of cranial nerve V, the trigeminal nerve (Fig. 3-11). It is also called *tic douloureux*, which is French for "painful spasm" or "unhappy twitch."

Demographics: Who Gets It?

TN is a relatively rare disorder; its incidence is about 16 per 100,000. The average TN patient is a woman older than 50 years of age, although it has been documented among all ages.

Etiology: What Happens?

TN is usually classified as a primary or secondary problem. In either case, the trigeminal nerve is irritated, and the result is brief, repeating episodes of sharp, electrical, stabbing pain on one side of the face.

Primary TN is considered to be idiopathic. The cause or source of the nerve irritation may never be identified.

Secondary TN is due to mechanical pressure on the nerve or some other structural problem. Causative factors include tumors, bone spurs, a recent infection, complications of dental surgery, or *multiple sclerosis* (this chapter). Cervical misalignment or *temporomandibular joint disorder* (Chapter 2) may also contribute to symptoms. Perhaps the most common cause of TN is the growth of tiny blood vessels that may strangulate or otherwise irritate the nerve.

Episodes of trigeminal nerve pain can be triggered by speaking, chewing, swallowing, sitting in a draft, a light touch to the wrong spot, and sometimes by no stimulus at all. Episodes may happen several times a day for days, weeks, or months and then suddenly disappear—only to begin again months or years later. TN can be a debilitating lifelong condition if it is not treated.

Signs and Symptoms

Some people call the pain of TN among the worst in the world. It is often described as sharp, electrical stabbing or burning sensations. The words "hot poker" appear in much

---

TRIGEMINAL NEURALGIA IN BRIEF

What is it?
Trigeminal neuralgia (TN) is a condition involving sharp electrical or stabbing pain along one or more branches of the trigeminal nerve (cranial nerve V), usually in the lower face and jaw.

How is it recognized?
TN pain is very sharp and severe. Patients report stabbing, electrical, or burning sensations that occur in brief episodes but repeat with or without identifiable triggers. A muscular tic is often present as well.

Is massage indicated or contraindicated?
TN is intensely painful, and even very light touch may trigger an attack. It therefore contraindicates massage on the face, unless the client specifically guides the therapist into what feels safe and comfortable. Massage elsewhere on the body is appropriate, although TN clients may prefer not to be face down.

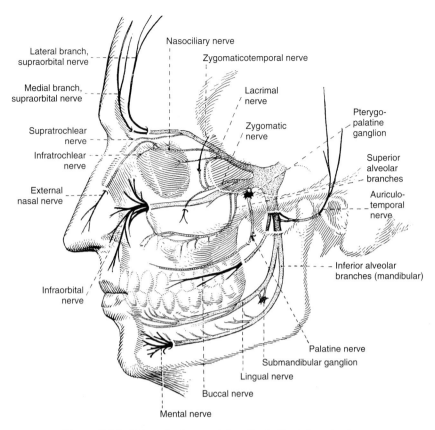

Figure 3-11. Trigeminal neuralgia affects the trigeminal nerve

of the literature associated with this condition. These episodes may last for 10 to 60 seconds, or several jabs may occur in rapid succession. A muscular tic sometimes develops along with the nerve pain.

Triggers of TN attacks may vary, or episodes may be completely spontaneous. The incidence of attacks may also vary. They can occur regularly, then disappear for a while, and then come back with renewed vigor.

Treatment

Treatment strategies for this problem depend on the source of the pain. Sinus and tooth infections can sometimes mimic TN, so an early step is to rule out those conditions. Cervical misalignment or temporomandibular joint problems can be sorted out by the appropriate professionals. Acupuncture often works well for TN, as it does for many problems with nerve conduction.

The mainstream medical approach to TN starts with painkillers and then proceeds to anti-seizure drugs that inhibit nerve conduction. Many patients do not tolerate these drugs very well, however, or they build up resistance and the drugs provide less and less relief.

Surgery for TN may focus on decompressing whatever vascular compression around the nerve may have occurred. If no vascular involvement can be found and the patient can no longer treat the problem with medication, a different type of

Other Cranial Nerve Disorders

Any damage or irritation to a cranial nerve can lead to symptoms in the face. TN and Bell's palsy are two of the most common disorders that may cause facial symptoms. Some other cranial nerve disorders are as follows:

- *Post herpetic neuralgia.* This is a complication of *herpes zoster* (this chapter). It may occur wherever the shingles blisters appeared but can outlast the visible lesions by several weeks or months.

- *Atypical face pain.* This is a condition similar to TN and in some cases may be a predecessor to it. It is characterized by pain that is less severe than TN but tends to be continuous rather than intermittent. The pain may also go up over the back of the head and into the scalp, and it may involve the occipital and the trigeminal nerve.

- *Hemifacial spasm.* This condition creates a painless tic that is related to blood vessel compression of the facial nerve rather than the trigeminal nerve.

surgery may be performed to carefully create a lesion on the part of the trigeminal nerve that transmits pain signals to the brain. The result is some permanent numbness but no other loss of function, and the debilitating TN symptoms can be completely interrupted.

Massage?

Clients who currently experience TN attacks will probably feel unsafe with any pressure or work on their face; massage therapists should respect this caution. Face cradles may also be uncomfortable; it may not be possible to work with TN clients in a prone position.

Massage anywhere else on the body is appropriate.

Other Nervous System Disorders

GUILLAIN-BARRÉ SYNDROME IN BRIEF

What is it?
Guillain-Barré syndrome (GBS) is a demyelinating disorder of peripheral nerves. It usually begins in the feet and moves proximally. It is probably autoimmune in nature, but the specific triggers have not been identified.

How is it recognized?
GBS is marked by sudden onset (symptoms usually begin quickly and peak within 2 weeks) followed by gradual remission (most patients have full or nearly full recovery within 18 months). Furthermore, GBS affects limbs symmetrically and moves proximally toward the trunk, which distinguishes it from other peripheral nerve problems.

Is massage indicated or contraindicated?
When a person has reached the peak of his or her GBS attack, physical and occupational therapy are often used to speed recovery and prevent muscle atrophy. Massage may be useful at this stage to improve circulation and to reduce fatigue and anxiety.

Guillain-Barré Syndrome

Definition: What Is It?

GBS is a condition involving acute inflammation and destruction of the myelin layer of peripheral nerves, specifically in the extremities. Its synonym is *acute idiopathic polyneuritis*, which is highly descriptive. It is a severe, extreme inflammation of multiple peripheral nerves, which comes about for reasons no one fully understands.

Demographics: Who Gets It?

GBS can affect anyone at anytime. Men with the syndrome slightly outnumber women, but it is seen in all ages and races. Although it is not a particularly common problem, affecting about 1 of every 100,000 people, it is the most frequently seen form of acute neuromuscular paralysis since the decline of polio in the Western hemisphere.

Etiology: What Happens?

GBS was first documented in 1916, but our understanding of how this disease comes about has not progressed a great deal since then. Many patients have an infection of the respiratory or gastrointestinal tract several days before developing GBS symptoms. It is believed that this preceding infection stimulates an immune system attack mistakenly directed against the myelin sheaths of peripheral nerves.

Some GBS patients do not experience a preceding infection. This disorder has also been seen in conjunction with immune system changes brought about by pregnancy, surgery, and as a reaction to certain vaccines, specifically the swine flu vaccine that was distributed in 1976.

Regardless of what initiates the disease process, the end result is that the myelin sheaths on peripheral nerves are attacked and destroyed. The damage progresses proximally and may also affect cranial nerves. This can be a life-threatening situation if the nerves that control breathing are damaged; many GBS patients require short-term use of a ventilator.

Signs and Symptoms

GBS is notorious for being unpredictable, but it has a few features that distinguish it from other peripheral nerve disorders. Onset is typically fast and severe; a patient may go from being fully functional to being in a hospital within a matter of hours or days. GBS is usually symmetrical, affecting both legs equally. Also, myelin damage progresses proximally, moving up toward the trunk rather than distally, which distinguishes it from other nerve problems.

When GBS first appears it often involves weakness or tingling in the affected limbs. Reflexes become dull or disappear altogether. Loss of sensation progresses proximally, although pain frequently develops in the hips and pelvis. If GBS affects cranial nerves of the face, facial weakness, pain, and difficulty with speech may develop.

GBS symptoms usually peak 2 or 3 weeks after onset and then they may linger for several weeks before they begin to subside. The amount of damage that accrues while the nerves are inflamed depends on what treatments are introduced at what times, and how soon the patient can begin to use the muscles after the paralysis resolves.

Diagnosis

The signs and symptoms of GBS are so distinctive that it is usually not difficult to diagnose. A lumbar puncture may be performed to look for elevated proteins in cerebrospinal fluid, and a nerve conduction test may be recommended to confirm that nerve transmission to the extremities is impaired.

Treatment

Because GBS is an idiopathic disease, no specific cure has been developed. Two treatment options have been successfully used to shorten recovery time: plasmapheresis ("blood cleansing") and injections of high concentrations of immunoglobulin or gamma globulin (donated antibodies).

Plasmapheresis is a process by which blood cells are removed from the patient's blood, placed in fresh donated plasma, and then replaced in the body. This removes autoimmune antibodies and reduces attacks against myelin. This procedure is most effective within 2 weeks of onset.

Intravenous doses of immunoglobulin or gamma globulin are believed to inhibit the patient's antibody and cytokine activity, thus limiting the autoimmune attack against myelin sheaths on peripheral nerves.

Clinical trials of both these treatment options show them to be about equally effective. They can shorten the duration of the recovery process by up to 50% compared with patients who do not receive these treatments.

Other interventions for GBS patients will be dictated by their individual needs. Many patients require the use of a ventilator for a time until the respiratory nerves regain full function. Anticoagulants may be used against the danger of blood clots in immobilized legs (see *deep vein thrombosis*, Chapter 4). Once the acute inflammation has passed, occupational and physical therapy are used to help the patient regain as much muscle function as possible.

Prognosis

The good news is that most people with GBS have a full or nearly full recovery, although the process may take 18 months or longer. A small number of patients (5 to 15%) have permanent disability because of the disease. Some people (about 5%) do not ever get better; their condition becomes a chronic inflammation that does not resolve. About 10% of all GBS patients experience a relapse later in life. About 3 to 4% of GBS patients die of instability of the autonomic nervous system that comes about with such rapid changes in functional levels.

Massage?

A person in the acute stage of GBS is unlikely to seek massage, and it would be wisest to avoid trying to mechanically stimulate the body while this immune system confusion is still raging.

Once the acute stage is over, physical and occupational therapy play a key role in the rehabilitation process of a person recovering from GBS. As long as sensation is present and accurate (i.e., the client can give feedback about pressure and comfort), massage could be a very useful adjunct in this long and frustrating process.

HEADACHES IN BRIEF

What are they?
Headaches are pain caused by any number of sources. Muscular tension, vascular spasm and dilation, and chemical imbalances can all contribute to headache. Headaches only rarely indicate a serious underlying disorder.

How are they recognized?
Tension-type headaches are usually bilateral and steadily painful. Vascular headaches are often unilateral and have a distinctive "throbbing" pain from blood flow into the head. Headaches brought about by central nervous system injury or disease are extreme, severe, and prolonged. They can have a sudden or gradual onset

Is massage indicated or contraindicated?
Headaches due to infection or central nervous system injury contraindicate massage. Persons experiencing vascular headaches generally avoid stimuli like massage, but tension-type headaches definitely indicate massage.

Headaches
Definition: What Are They?

Headaches are one of the most common physical problems in the range of human experience. Up to 90% of adults in the United States experience a headache each year; 10 million of them will see a doctor for relief. Although they can herald some serious underlying problems, most of the time headaches are self-contained, temporary problems that are only peripherally related to other conditions in the body.

Types of Headaches

New advances in headache research have uncovered similarities between headache types that had never been suspected. As more is learned about the physiologic processes of these disorders, the methods for classifying them may change. For the present, however, most headaches can be placed into one of four categories. Nevertheless, headaches do not fit into outlines well, because some headaches share qualities from more than one of these classifications.

- *Tension-type headaches.* By far the most common type of headache people experience (90 to 92%), these are triggered by muscular tension, bony misalignment, *temporomandibular joint disorder*, *myofascial pain syndrome* (Chapter 2), or other muscular problems.

- *Vascular headaches.* These include classic and common migraines, cluster headaches, and possibly sinus headaches. They account for about 6 to 8% of all headaches. Many vascular headaches are triggered by food sensitivities, alcohol use, or chemical shifts seen with the menstrual cycle.

- *Chemical headaches.* The triggers for these headaches can be any kind of chemical disturbance, including low blood sugar ("hunger headache"), hormone shifts, and dehydration, including the dehydration brought about by alcohol use ("hangover" headaches).

- *Traction- inflammatory headaches.* These are the rarest type of headache and the most dangerous, accounting for less than 2% of all headaches. They are indicative of severe underlying pathology such as tumors, aneurysm, or infection in the central nervous system.

Etiology: What Happens?

Although headaches are fairly easy to categorize by type, the actual pain-causing mechanisms of the various headache categories (which had always been assumed to be fundamentally different) are probably much closer than previously believed. Therefore, as more is learned about this phenomenon, the perceived differences between tension-type and vascular-type headaches may fade. This is good news, as a more thorough understanding of these mechanisms may lead to more effective ways to treat and even prevent the debilitating pain headaches can cause.

The common denominator that has been observed in tension and vascular headaches (by far the two most common types) has been the activity of serotonin, a neurotransmitter that has been implicated in a number of other nervous system disorders. Both migraine and tension headache episodes show significant drops in serotonin levels as blood vessels in the brain swell. This vasodilation puts pressure on the meninges, the main source of sensation for the brain, and also on the trigeminal nerve complex, the primary source of sensation for the head and face. The primary difference between migraine headaches and tension headaches, therefore, may simply be the triggers. Migraines are generally associated with chemical triggers like food sensitivities or hormonal shifts, whereas tension headaches are more often associated with mechanical triggers like tight muscles or misaligned vertebrae. Both types of triggers evidently may lead to serotonin shifts and intracranial vasodilation.

The specific changes brought about by headache triggers are discussed below.

Tension Headaches
Definition: What Are They?

Tension headaches are headaches triggered by mechanical stresses that initiate the central nervous system changes in serotonin levels and blood vessel dilation discussed above.

Etiology: What Happens?

The average head weighs about 18 to 20 pounds. The area of bone-to-bone contact where the occiput rests on the first cervical vertebra is about the same as two pairs of fingertips touching. The whole thing is kept in balance by tension exerted by muscles and ligaments around the neck and head. The muscles primarily responsible for the posture of the head form two inverted triangles just below the occiput (Fig. 3-12). It is not surprising, then, that when things can easily get a little out of balance, the resulting pain reverberates throughout the whole structure.

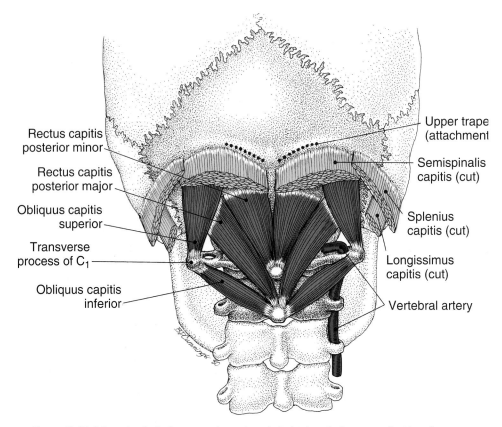

Figure 3-12. Muscular imbalance at the suboccipital triangle is a contributing factor in many headaches

Labels:
Rectus capitis posterior minor
Rectus capitis posterior major
Obliquus capitis superior
Transverse process of C₁
Obliquus capitis inferior
Upper trape (attachment
Semispinalis capitis (cut)
Splenius capitis (cut)
Longissimus capitis (cut)
Vertebral artery

Triggers

These are almost too numerous to list, precisely because staying pain-free involves such a delicate balance of muscle tension, bony alignment, and myriad other factors. Some of the major causes for tension headaches are listed below:

- *Muscular, tendinous, or ligamentous injury* to the head or neck structures can lead to headaches. The ligaments in the neck may be most easily injured; they are vulnerable to fraying and irritation with uncontrolled movement (see *whiplash*, Chapter 2).

- *Simple muscle tension* in the suboccipital triangle or the jaw flexors can cause headaches. These muscles are especially vulnerable to the effects of emotional stress. When people are worried or angry, they tend to clench their jaws and tighten their necks.

- *Subluxation or fixation* of cervical vertebrae can irritate ligaments and/or cause muscle spasms, both of which lead to headaches.

- *Structural problems* in the alignment of the cranial bones (which are not completely immobile) or in the temporomandibular joint can cause headaches.

- *Trigger points* in the muscles of the neck and head can refer pain all around the head. (see *myofascial pain syndrome*, Chapter 2).

- *Eyestrain*, the chronic contraction of muscles in the eye to focus on reading material or other visual input, can cause tension headaches. (These may be relieved when corrective eyewear successfully reduces eye muscle tension.)

- *Ongoing mental or physical* stress can change postural and movement patterns, which leads to muscle spasm, subluxation, fixation, and so on. Poor ergonomics, especially in repetitive work situations, are frequently the culprit behind chronic tension headaches.

Vascular Headaches
Definition: What Are They?

These are headaches that are often triggered by food sensitivities, hormonal shifts, alcohol use, or other factors that are difficult to identify. The pain they cause comes from excessively dilated blood vessels in the meninges. They are characterized by a pain that throbs with the patient's pulse.

Migraines
Demographics: Who Gets Migraines?

About 28 million people in the United States experience diagnosed migraines. This malady is responsible for an overwhelming $50 billion in lost wages and medical expenses every year.

Women get migraines more often than men. It is estimated that up to 18% of all women will have a migraine at some time in their lives, whereas about 6% of men will. Many migraines are genetically linked; 70 to 80% of migraine patients have family members with the same malady.

Etiology: What Happens with Migraines?

Migraine headaches begin with extreme vasoconstriction in the affected hemisphere, which one would expect to be painful, but it is not. Instead a sense of euphoria is felt, although it is mixed with dread that the worst is yet to come. The vasoconstriction is then followed by a huge vasodilation: a veritable flood of blood into the affected part of the brain. It is all still contained within the vessels, of course, but all the excess pressure presses against the vessel walls and meninges, which causes excruciating pain.

Triggers

No one has identified an exact reason for what sets up the process for migraines to take place. Some triggers have been identified, such as the consumption of certain kinds of foods, including cheese, chocolate, coffee, tea, and any kind of alcohol. Abnormal levels of stress can bring them on, as can hormonal shifts such as menstruation, pregnancy, and menopause. (These hormonal shifts can also make pre-existing migraines disappear.) The good news about migraines is that they usually subside by middle age. It is not unheard of, but quite uncommon, for mature people to experience migraines.

Signs and Symptoms

The word migraine comes from the French, hemi-craine, or "half-head." This is because migraine headaches have a characteristic unilateral presentation. In classic migraines the pain is preceded by blurred vision, the perception of flashing lights or auras, and even auditory hallucinations. Classic migraines comprise only about 15 to 20% of all migraines. Then, as with the aura-less common migraines (the other 80 to 85% of migraines), the patient experiences extreme throbbing pain on one side of the head, which may cause the affected eye and side of the nose to water. Hypersensitivity to light, nausea, and vomiting are all possible. Symptoms can persist for anywhere from several hours to several days.

Cluster Headaches
Definition: What Are They?

These are a fairly rare, not well-understood variety of vascular headaches. Cluster headaches affect men more often than women and affect less than 1% of the U.S. population. They come, one right after the other, for days or weeks at a time. Cluster headaches usually happen at night, with pain severe enough to wake a person out of a sound sleep. Like migraines, they cause the eye and nostril of the affected side to water. They may also cause facial swelling and unilateral sweating.

Reliable triggers for cluster headaches have not been identified. They may occur seasonally, once or twice in a year, or just once in a lifetime.

Sinus Headaches

Sinus headaches are mentioned among vascular headaches because they also have to do with too much fluid in the skull. The fluid is contained in the sinuses rather than the cranium itself. When a person has sinus-related allergies or sinusitis, their membranes can become irritated and inflamed. This will be discussed further in *sinusitis* (Chapter 6).

Chemical Headaches

Chemical headaches are triggered by a variety of chemical imbalances in the body. They are often warning signs that the person has too much or too little of some substance vital to maintaining homeostasis. Examples of chemical headaches can include:

- Headaches caused by very low blood sugar, indicating that the person needs to eat soon.
- Headaches caused by hormonal shifts like those seen with the menstrual cycle and childbirth (see *premenstrual syndrome* and *menopause*, Chapter 10).
- Headaches caused by extreme dehydration—both from physical exertion and from alcohol consumption.

Traction-Inflammatory Headaches

Headaches are occasionally a sign of a serious central nervous system injury or infection. Headaches in combination with extreme fever often have a bacterial or viral precipitator. They are usually short-lived, subsiding when the fever passes the crisis point. The time to become concerned is when headaches are severe, repeating, and have a sudden onset, or when they have a gradual onset but no remission. In other words, if a severe headache does not go away in 4 to 5 days on its own, it may be a symptom of some serious underlying condition. This is particularly true if the headache is accompanied by slurred speech, numbness anywhere in the body, and difficulties with motor control. The first things to investigate in cases like this are *encephalitis, meningitis, stroke* (this chapter), a tumor, or an *aneurysm* (Chapter 4).

Treatment

Avoiding or managing headache triggers is the most proactive and least invasive way to deal with this problem. People who experience chronic headaches of any type are usually encouraged to keep a "headache journal" to try to pin down their specific triggers for headaches.

As the understanding of the most common types of headaches changes, treatment options will likewise probably also shift. Currently, medical headache treatment falls into two categories: prophylactic treatment that works to prevent the headache from beginning, and abortive treatment that works to end the headache once it has begun. A class of medications developed for depression (SSRIs) are finding use in both categories to deal with migraine headaches. Other migraine treatments include beta blockers and calcium channel blockers, both of which work to interrupt the vasodilation phase of the headache reaction. Because migraines often involve vomiting, some medications are poorly tolerated when taken orally; nasal spray applications work well for some patients.

Tension-type headaches are still treated primarily with NSAIDs when medical intervention is required.

Massage?

The appropriateness of massage depends on what kind of headache the client has. If it is related to a serious underlying pathology, or to a bacterial or viral infection, any massage is obviously out of the question. If it is a vascular headache, the client may be most comfortable waiting until the acute stage has passed. Most common, tension-type headaches resoundingly indicate massage.

Seizure Disorders

Definition: What Are They?

A seizure disorder is any kind of problem that can cause seizures as one of its symptoms. Epilepsy, one type of seizure disorder, is one of the oldest conditions recorded in medical history. It was first described about 2000 years before Christ, but it was not studied as a specific problem other than "demonic possession" until the mid 19th century. Epilepsy is identified as a specific disorder when a person has two or more seizures that are *not* related to any identifiable cause such as head injury, stroke, infection, or fever. This rules out about 75% of all people who have a history of seizure.

Demographics: Who Gets Them?

Seizure disorders are the second most common type of central nervous system problem in the United States; *stroke* (this chapter) is the first. Approximately 1% of the population will experience a seizure at some point. About 25% of those people may eventually be diagnosed with epilepsy. In the United States, about 30,000 cases of epilepsy are diagnosed each year; approximately 4 million people currently live with epilepsy. Epilepsy occurs in males and females about equally.

Etiology: What Happens?

When interconnecting neurons in the brain are stimulated in a certain kind of way, a tremendous burst of excess electricity may stimulate the neighboring neurons. The reac-

---

SEIZURE DISORDERS IN BRIEF

What are they?
Seizure disorders are any condition that causes seizures. They are often related to some kind of neurologic damage (tumors, head injuries, or infection), although it may be impossible to delineate exactly what that damage is. Epilepsy is a subtype of seizure disorder.

How are they recognized?
Seizures may take very different forms for different people; they range from barely noticeable to life-threatening. Seizure disorders are diagnosed through physical examination, a description of symptoms, CT scans, MRI scans, and EEGs.

Is massage indicated or contraindicated?
Seizure activity itself contraindicates massage, but bodywork is certainly appropriate for patients with most kinds of seizure disorders at any other time.

tion is repeated and soon millions of neurons in the brain are giving off electrical discharge. This is the central nervous system "lightning storm" of the epileptic seizure, and it affects the rest of the body in a number of different ways.

For the most part, no one knows what starts the storm in the first place. Triggers vary for different people. For some, sudden changes in light level, from dark to light or vice versa, trigger a seizure. For others, flashing or strobe lights or the strobe effect created by ceiling fans, will be the trigger. For others, certain sounds or even particular notes of music may cause a seizure. High anxiety or other sicknesses like cold or flu can also lead to seizures.

Whatever the trigger, the result is uncoordinated neuronal activity that allows electrical signals to become progressively more extreme, sometimes to the point of collapse and loss of consciousness. Close studies of the synapses of seizure patients have revealed the possibility that these disorders may be linked to some important neurotransmitter imbalances; these patients have either underactive inhibitory neurotransmitters or overactive excitatory neurotransmitters, or both. This discovery has opened some new possibilities in seizure treatment.

Causes

In some cases the cause of seizures can be linked definitively to a mechanical or chemical problem in the brain. Birth trauma, skull fractures, shaken baby syndrome, brain tumors, and penetrating wounds can all cause seizures, as can some types of metabolic disturbances, infections, exposure to some toxins, and extreme hypotension or hemorrhage. Rarely, seizures can be traced to a hereditary problem. About 35% of all seizure disorder patients have idiopathic seizures that are untraceable to any identifiable problem.

Signs and Symptoms

Seizures take very different forms in each person they affect. From the original oversimplified categories of "petit mal" and "grand mal" seizures, more than 30 different classes of seizures have been identified. Seizures are classified by what parts of the brain they affect, when that information can be gathered. *Generalized* seizures affect the whole brain, whereas *partial* seizures involve abnormal activity in isolated areas. The most common types of seizures are as follows:

- *Partial seizures.* These are seizures that involve abnormal activity only in isolated areas. The motor cortex and the temporal lobes are the sites most often affected. Partial seizures come in two subtypes:

    - *Simple partial*   In this type of seizure the patient has no change in consciousness. He or she may become weak or numb, smell or taste things that are not there, have some changes in vision, or have temporary vertigo along with some muscular tics or twitching.

    - *Complex partial*   This type of seizure is specifically associated with temporal lobe dysfunction. The patient may exhibit repetitive behaviors like pacing in a circle, rocking, or smacking the lips. He or she may laugh uncontrollably or experience fear. Hallucinations and the perception of strange odors are other symptoms of complex partial seizures.

- *Generalized seizures.*   These seizures involve electrical signals that occur all over the brain. They may be very subtle or dramatic.

    - *Absence seizures*   These involve very short episodes of loss of consciousness. The patient does not fall to the floor but may simply "check out" for 5 to 10 seconds and have no memory of this lapse.

- *Tonic-clonic seizures*   These are what have traditionally been called "grand mal" seizures. They involve uncontrolled movement of the face, arms, and legs, followed by loss of consciousness and a fall to the floor. They may last for 5 to 20 minutes, and the patient is usually tired and disoriented after an episode.

- *Myoclonic seizures*   These involve bilateral muscular jerking, which may be very pronounced or almost unnoticeable. They are usually seen among very young patients.

- *Status epilepticus*   These are a life-threatening variation of tonic-clonic seizures. They last for a prolonged period, and can put such a strain on the body that they can cause death. Status epilepticus, or "static seizures," are a medical emergency.

Diagnosis

Epilepsy is usually diagnosed by an electroencephalogram (EEG), a test that measures electrical activity in the brain. Radiographs, CT scans, and/or MRI scans may be used to look for identifiable lesions. Tests are conducted in part to delineate seizures from other conditions that produce seizure-like symptoms including migraine headaches, stroke, fainting spells, heart arrhythmia, narcolepsy, hypoglycemia, some *anxiety disorders* (this chapter), and reactions to some medications.

Treatment

Seizures are generally treated with anticonvulsant medication, which acts to make neurons in the brain harder to stimulate. It can be difficult to find the right dosage of these powerful medications. Most patients can find an anticonvulsant that works for them, but some patients do not tolerate them well.

Some epilepsy patients find that their seizures are less frequent and less extreme when they follow a strict high-fat, low-fiber ketogenic diet.

Surgical intervention for seizure disorders is reserved for when an isolated and expendable mass (i.e., a tumor or clump of scar tissue) can be determined to be the cause of the seizures. Some patients who experience tonic-clonic seizures can successfully control them when their corpus callosum is severed.

One device that is successful for some patients for whom medications do not work is a vagus nerve stimulator. This mechanism is implanted in the vagus nerves in the neck and activated when the patient waves a magnet over the implant. It is believed that stimulating the vagus nerve in this way helps to activate some of the inhibitory neurotransmitters that these patients lack.

Massage?

It is inappropriate to try to massage someone who is in the midst of a seizure of any kind. In the event of a tonic-clonic seizure, the practitioner's job is to make sure the client is safe, call 911 or the local emergency number, and then wait until the seizure has subsided. If a client has a history of seizures, it is perfectly fine to work with him or her at any other time. Nevertheless, if the seizures tend to come on fast with no warning, the therapist should be alert to the possibility of this happening during an appointment.

Someone recovering from a severe seizure will probably find that they are sore and tender, as if they had been doing a great deal of unaccustomed exercise, which in fact is exactly what has happened. It is also very possible to sustain serious injury when these seizures happen in unprotected surroundings. Sprains, bruises, and even broken bones can happen during tonic-clonic seizures.

Sleep Disorders

Definition: What Are They?

Sleep disorders are any disorders that interfere with the ability to fall asleep, to stay asleep for an adequate period, or to wake up feeling refreshed. More than 70 different sleep disorders have been defined, but only the most common varieties are covered here: insomnia, sleep apnea, restless leg syndrome, narcolepsy, and circadian rhythm disruption.

Demographics: Who Gets Them?

Approximately 40 million Americans report chronic, ongoing problems with sleep every year, and another 20 million have short-term difficulties. Men tend to outnumber women with sleep problems by a small margin. The incidence of sleep disorders increases with age; elderly people are less likely to feel refreshed by sleep than younger people.

Etiology: What Happens?

To understand what happens when sleep is interrupted, it is useful to take a brief look at the phenomenon of sleep itself. Until recently sleep was considered to be a strictly passive, uneventful activity. As researchers have examined it more closely, they have found that sleep occurs in cycling stages, and each of those stages performs a specific function in keeping the body healthy. Although humans can adapt to live in colder or warmer temperatures or to live with more food or less, we simply *cannot* adapt to sleep deprivation. It is such a vital process that without the proper balance of the stages of sleep, people can end up with disorders that range from slowed reflexes and lower cognitive skills, to poor immune system efficiency, to *fibromyalgia syndrome* (Chapter 2), to chronic pain, and to *depression* (this chapter), hallucinations, and psychosis. The circular relationship between poor health and poor sleep is another complicating factor. If persons do not feel well and consequently do not sleep well, they will probably continue *not* to feel well *because* they do not sleep well.

The need for sleep is determined partly by the hormone melatonin, a secretion of the pineal gland, located deep within the brain. This hormone is secreted in the absence of full-spectrum sunlight. Melatonin contributes to a feeling of drowsiness. A standard rotation of wakefulness and sleepiness usually runs on a 24- to 25-hour cycle called the circadian rhythm.

Sleep occurs in five distinct phases or stages:

- *Stage I*. In this light sleep a person is easily wakened. Eye movement is slow. A phenomenon called *hypnic myoclonia* occurs in this stage—this is the feeling that a person is suddenly starting to fall.

- *Stage II*. In this stage the eyes stop moving. Brain waves slow down but still show occasional bursts of activity called "sleep spindles."

SLEEP DISORDERS IN BRIEF

What are they?
Sleep disorders are a collection of problems including insomnia, sleep apnea, restless leg syndrome, narcolepsy, and circadian rhythm disruption that make it difficult to get enough sleep or to wake up feeling rested and refreshed.

How are they recognized?
The primary symptom of sleep disorders is excessive daytime sleepiness. If this continues for a prolonged period, a weakened immune system, memory and concentration loss, and the risk of automotive or on-the-job accidents may increase.

Is massage indicated or contraindicated?
Sleep disorders indicate massage. Bodywork may not correct a mechanical or psychological dysfunction that leads to sleep deprivation, but it can improve the quality of sleep and can reduce the mental and physical stresses that may interfere with sleep.

- *Stage III.* Brain waves are much slower in Stage III. A particular "deep sleep" pattern called delta waves are intermixed with slightly faster brain waves during this stage.

- *Stage IV.* Only delta waves are emitted from the brain during this stage. Stage IV sleep is when the body secretes the hormones that enable new growth for children and adolescents and repair and regeneration for adults.

- *Rapid eye movement (REM) sleep.* In REM sleep breathing is rapid, shallow, and irregular. Eyes move quickly, but muscular activity in the limbs is usually absent. Heart rate and blood pressure approach waking levels. REM sleep is the stage in which dreams occur.

A person cycles through each of the five stages and then starts over again at Stage I. It takes about 90 to 100 minutes to complete a sleep cycle, although the amount of time spent in each stage varies according to the time of night. A person spends more time in Stages III and IV at the beginning of the night, and the majority of time in Stage I and REM sleep toward the morning. Overall, a healthy balance of sleep stages allows an adult to spend about 20% of sleep time in REM sleep, 50% in Stage II, and 30% in the other stages.

Types of Sleep Disorders

This section discusses 5 of the more than 70 different sleep disorders that have been documented.

Insomnia   Literally, this means "lack of sleep." Insomnia can involve difficulty falling asleep, difficulty in staying asleep, or difficulty in sleeping long enough for the body to get the rest it needs. Insomnia can be described as *transient*, in which case it occurs for less than 4 weeks, or *chronic*, in which case a person cannot sleep most nights for more than 1 month.

Transient insomnia is usually attributable to habits or environmental issues that are controllable. Caffeine taken too close to bedtime can ruin some peoples' sleep (for many people "too close to bedtime" means any time at all). Alcohol, while being a depressant, reduces the quality of sleep. Some medications, including diet pills, antihistamines, and antidepressants, can interfere with sleep or can reduce the time spent in REM stage. Cigarette smoking can cause a person to wake up too early due to nicotine withdrawal.

Environmental conditions can also contribute to insomnia. Having a room that is too cold, too hot, too loud, or too bright can make it hard to get to sleep or to stay asleep. Having a bed partner who snores or moves around a lot can interrupt sleep. Exercising too late in the day or not exercising at all can also make it hard to fall asleep.

Emotional stress is of course a major contributor to sleep loss. Ironically, the longer a person lays in bed feeling the need to sleep, the less likely he or she is to drop off—the stress of waiting for sleep ensures that it never comes.

Chronic insomnia is usually examined as a sign of some deeper medical or psychological problem. *Hyperthyroidism* (Chapter 8), fibromyalgia, depression, *kidney failure* (Chapter 9), *heart problems* (Chapter 4), or *chronic fatigue syndrome* (Chapter 5) are all possibilities when a person does not sleep well or long enough.

Sleep Apnea   "Apnea" means absence of breath. Sleep apnea is a disorder in which the air passage of a sleeping person temporarily shuts down, depriving the person of oxygen for up to 60 seconds. Repeated episodes may occur dozens or even hundreds of times each night, reducing the quality of sleep, but more importantly putting the person at risk for serious damage from oxygen deprivation.

Statistics on sleep apnea vary widely, with some estimates suggesting it affects up to 18 million Americans. Obstructive sleep apnea is a mechanical problem, in which the air passage collapses when muscles relax during sleep, so that oxygen cannot enter during inhalation. When oxygen levels fall sufficiently, muscles tighten slightly, and air reenters the passageway with a loud snort or gasp; loud snoring is one sign of possible sleep apnea. Other signs are excessive daytime sleepiness and morning headache from oxygen deprivation. Obstructive sleep apnea is a possible complication of obesity; excessive body weight can increase the tendency to block air passageways.

Central sleep apnea is a neurologic problem involving decreased respiratory drive.

Frequent waking leads to sleep deprivation and an increased risk of motor vehicle accident or on-the-job injury. Patients with sleep apnea also have an increased risk of *stroke* (this chapter) and *hypertension* (Chapter 4). In some extreme cases sleep apnea has caused sudden death from respiratory arrest during sleep.

Restless Leg Syndrome (RLS)   This is a disorder that often runs in families, although it can also be associated with *pregnancy* (Chapter 10), *diabetes* (Chapter 8), and *anemia* (Chapter 4). It involves a constant crawling, prickling, tingling sensation in the extremities, especially the legs, that is only relieved by rubbing and movement. It is closely related to another disorder called periodic limb movement disorder (PLMD), in which a person experiences repeated jerking movements of the legs every 20 to 40 seconds.

Although RLS is present at all times, its symptoms are most pronounced when a person lies still in an effort to sleep. It is relieved by movement, massaging the affected areas, or warm baths.

Some estimates suggest that RLS affects up to 12 million Americans, most of them elderly.

Narcolepsy   This chronic neurologic dysfunction gets its name from the Greek *narco* for stupor, and *lepsis,* for seizure. It involves unpredictable "sleep attacks" at inappropriate times, often in response to intense emotional reactions like laughing or anger.

Narcolepsy is generally diagnosed in adolescence; this is one sleep disorder that does not increase in incidence with age. It affects some 250,000 Americans.

During an episode, narcolepsy patients may experience a sudden loss in all muscle tone—they simply go limp and collapse. These events can last anywhere from several seconds to 30 minutes. Narcolepsy patients often experience poor nighttime sleep, which adds to a general problem with drowsiness during the day.

Circadian Rhythm Disruption   The circadian rhythm is the normal cycle of drowsiness and wakefulness that all humans experience. It is regulated by exposure to ambient light and the secretion of melatonin. Most people run through this cycle every 24 to 25 hours. They feel drowsy as the sun goes down and more awake as it rises. When people are forced to be physically or mentally active in a different cycle, their circadian rhythms are disrupted and the quality of their sleep, as well as the quality of their waking hours, is compromised.

Circadian rhythm disruption can occur in response to shift work, having to be awake all night for a graveyard shift, losing a night's sleep, or changing time zones through travel. Short-term difficulties associated with this problem are excessive sleepiness along with degenerating reflexes and mental functioning that accompanies exhaustion. Longer-term problems can include depression and other physical and psychological disorders brought about by sleep deprivation.

Some 25 million Americans do not work a "standard" daytime shift and are forced to adjust their sleep to accommodate a different schedule. Although numbers on how many of these people experience dysfunction are difficult to gather, it has been found that these workers carry a higher than normal risk for motor vehicle accidents and on-the-job injuries. They also have more colds, flu, hypertension, weight gain, irregular menstrual cycles, and digestive discomfort than the rest of the population.

Signs and Symptoms

The primary sign of someone with a sleep disorder is excessive daytime sleepiness. Chronic sleep deprivation can also cause irritability, decreased ability to focus or concentrate, mood changes, and poor short-term memory. Other symptoms are associated with specific disorders, as described above.

Complications

The National Highway Traffic Safety Administration estimates that about 1.5% of all motor vehicle accidents have excessive fatigue as a primary cause.[j] About 1500 fatalities and 71,000 injuries occur every year because of these accidents. In addition to car crashes, fatigue and sleep deprivation also contribute dangerously to on-the-job injuries that affect not only the sleep-deprived person but many others as well.

Deprivation of specific stages of sleep has also been associated with specific disorders. Lack of REM sleep over a prolonged period can lead to hallucinations and psychosis. Fibromyalgia syndrome patients do not get adequate Stage IV sleep, which means they do not secrete the hormones that stimulate healing and repair in adults.

Diagnosis

If a person experiences excessive drowsiness that makes it difficult to accomplish basic tasks, it is worth pursuing with a medical professional, on the chance that sleep apnea could be interfering with nighttime oxygen supply. Patients are often encouraged to keep a "sleep diary" in which they record activities in relation to how well they sleep. This is a useful tool to look for behavioral patterns that may interfere with a good night's rest. A physical examination is usually conducted to rule out other causes of insomnia, like hyperthyroidism. A *polysomnograph* is a sleep study conducted in a laboratory where a person's heart rate, respiratory rate, blood pressure, and other vital signs are measured while the person sleeps. How much time spent in each stage may also be measured.

These tests can yield useful information about the nature of an individual's sleeping problem along with possibilities for treatment.

Treatment

Cases of transient insomnia are treated with lifestyle changes that better support healthy sleep. This can mean changing diet and exercise habits, quitting smoking, adjusting temperature or sound levels in the bedroom, or other simple interventions. By the time insomnia has become a chronic problem it can be difficult to recondition the body to sleeping well, so the earlier intervention can be taken, the better.

Over-the-counter sleeping aids are generally discouraged, as they tend to create an imbalance in the time spent in each stage of sleep. Prescription sleeping aids can be helpful for short periods, but several can become habit-forming. Thus, long-term use is not a viable solution.

[j]Facts about drowsy driving. National Sleep Foundation. Available at: http://www.sleepfoundation.org/activities/daaafacts.html. Accessed summer 2001.

Sleep apnea can be treated in a variety of ways. Surgery to keep airways open may be performed, or a nose mask to provide continuous positive airway pressure may be used. Apnea patients should not sleep on their backs, and if they are obese they should work to lose weight and reduce their risk of apnea complications. It is especially important that sleep apnea patients not drink alcohol or use sleeping aids at night; these substances may interfere with their already challenged breathing mechanisms.

RLS is believed to be associated with dopamine deficiencies in certain brain areas. It is managed with dopamine agents, tranquilizers, and for very extreme cases, opioids and anticonvulsants. Less severe cases of RLS can be managed with mild exercise, warm baths, and massage.

Narcolepsy is treatable with some medications and by increasing exercise, which has been shown to reduce the number of sleep attacks.

Massage?

Most types of sleep disorders certainly indicate massage. Anyone who experiences restless nights and persistent daytime sleepiness appreciates the opportunity to "tune out" while receiving bodywork. Some studies indicate that massage increases the time spent in Stage III or IV restorative sleep,[k] which decreases pain sensation and speeds healing. Massage can improve the quality of sleep for insomniac clients. Although it does not reverse sleep apnea, a massage therapist may be the first person to bring the habit of not breathing and then gasping during sleep to a client's attention.

Chapter Review Questions: Nervous System Conditions

1. What is the difference between spastic and flaccid paralysis? Where in the nervous system does each indicate damage?

2. How can a person who has experienced spinal cord damage at C_6 still have control of his head and neck?

3. Why does Bell's palsy indicate massage, when most other types of paralysis contraindicate massage?

4. Is post-polio syndrome contagious? Why or why not?

5. Describe the safest course of action for a client who experiences an epileptic seizure during a massage.

6. A client who has multiple sclerosis comes for massage. The therapist performs a rigorous sports-massage type treatment and then recommends a soak in a hot tub. Is this a good idea? Why or why not?

7. Can a person who has had chicken pox catch herpes zoster from another person? Why or why not?

8. A person with reflex sympathetic dystrophy may have poor circulation and bluish skin in the affected area. Is it appropriate to massage her here? Why or why not?

9. List five types of depression.

10. A client is recovering from a major stroke. What are some of the key criteria on which to base a judgment about the appropriateness of Swedish massage?

---

[k]Field T. Touch Therapy. London: Churchill Livingstone Press; 2000:67.

Bibliography, Nervous System Conditions

General References, Nervous System

1. Dominico G, Wood E. *Beard's Massage.* Philadelphia, Pa: WB Saunders; 1997.
2. Damjanou I. *Pathology for the Health-Related Professions.* Philadelphia, Pa: WB Saunders; 1996.
3. Travell J, Simons DG. *Myofascial Pain and Dysfunction: The Trigger Point Manual.* Baltimore, Md: Williams & Wilkins; 1983.
4. Clemente CD. *Anatomy: A Regional Atlas of the Human Body.* 3rd ed. Baltimore, Md: Urban & Schwarzenburg; 1987.
5. Tortora GJ, Anagnostakos NP. *Principles of Anatomy and Physiology.* 6th ed. New York, NY: Harper & Row; 1990.
6. *Taber's Cyclopedic Dictionary.* 14th ed. Philadelphia, Pa: FA Davis; 1981.
7. *Stedman's Medical Dictionary.* 26th ed. Baltimore, Md: Williams & Wilkins; 1995.
8. Memmler RL, Wood DL. *The Human Body in Health and Disease.* 5th ed. Philadelphia, Pa: JB Lippincott; 1983.
9. Juhan D. *Job's Body: A Handbook for Bodywork.* Barrytown, NY: Station Hill Press; 1987.
10. Mulvihill ML. *Human Diseases: A Systemic Approach.* 2nd ed. Norwalk, Conn: Appleton & Lange; 1987.
11. Kunz JRM, Finkel AJ, eds. *The American Medical Association Family Medical Guide.* New York, NY: Random House; 1987.
12. Marieb EM. *Human Anatomy and Physiology.* Redwood City, Calif: Benjamin/Cummings; 1989.
13. Sapolsky RM. *Why Zebras Don't Get Ulcers: An Updated Guide to Stress, Stress-Related Disease, and Coping.* W.H. Freeman; 1998, NY/1998.
14. *Diagnostic and Statistical Manual of Mental Disorders-IV TR 2000.* Washington, DC.: American Psychiatric Press; 2000.

Alzheimer's Disease

1. Trafford A. Alzheimer's: No cure yet, but reasons for hope. *The Washington Post.* November 7, 2000:Z05. Available at http://www.washingtonpost.com/wp-dyn/articles/A28691-2000Nov7.html. Accessed winter 2001.
2. Alzheimer's disease. HealthAnswers.com, Inc.; 2000. Available at: http://www.healthanswers.com/centers/body/overview.asp?id=brain/+nervous+system&filename=522.htm. Accessed winter 2001.
3. What is Alzheimer's disease? Mayo Foundation for Medical Education and Research; 1998–2000. Available at: http://www.mayohealth.org/home?id=5.1.1.1.8#WhatIs. Accessed winter 2001.
4. Alzheimer's research: Protein links. Mayo Foundation for Medical Education and Research; 1998–2000. Available at: http://www.mayohealth.org/home?id=HQ00221. Accessed winter 2001.
5. Diagnosis of Alzheimer's disease. Mayo Foundation for Medical Education and Research; 2000. Available at: http://www.mayohealth.org/home?id=AZ00001. Accessed winter 2001.
6. Alzheimer disease power points. MedicineNet, Inc.; 1996–2000. Available at http://medicineNet.com. Accessed winter 2001.
7. Memory loss not always permanent. Mayo Foundation for Medical Education and Research; 2000. Available at: www.mayohealth.org/mayo/0005/htm/memoryloss.htm. Accessed winter 2001.
8. Alzheimer's: Unlocking the secret. Mayo Foundation for Medical Education and Research; 2000. Available at: www.mayohealth.org/mayo/9803/htm/article1.htm. Accessed winter 2001.
9. What is Alzheimer's disease? Meditopia!; 1996. Available at: http://www.meditopia.com/alzwhat.html. Accessed winter 2001.
10. Alzheimer's research. Mayo Foundation for Medical Education and Research; 1998–2000. Available at: http://www.mayohealth.org/home?id=HQ00221. Accessed winter 2001.
11. NINDS Alzheimer's disease information page. The National Institute of Neurological Disorders and Stroke, National Institutes of Health. Available at: http://www.ninds.nih.gov/health_and_medical/disorders/alzheimersdisease_doc.htm. Accessed winter 2001.
12. NINDS dementia with Lewy bodies information page. The National Institute of Neurological Disorders and Stroke, National Institutes of Health. Available at: http://www.ninds.nih.gov/health_and_medical/disorders/dementiawithlewybodies_doc.htm. Accessed winter 2001.
13. Cholinesterase inhibitors: Helping nerves communicate. PlanetRx, Inc.; 2000. Available at: http://www.alzheimers.com/health_library/treatment/treatment_01_cholin.html. Accessed winter 2001.
14. Aromatherapy massage. PlanetRx, Inc.; 2000. Available at: http://www.alzheimers.com/health_library/treatment/treatment_07_aromatherapy.html. Accessed winter 2001.
15. How Alzheimer's disease affects the brain. PlanetRx, Inc.; 2000. Available at: http://www.alzheimers.com/health_library/basics/basics_03_affect.html. Accessed winter 2001.
16. How common Is Alzheimer's disease? PlanetRx, Inc.; 2000. Available at: http://www.alzheimers.com/health_library/basics/basics_02_common.html. Accessed winter 2001.
17. Other conventional treatments. PlanetRx, Inc.; 2000. Available at: http://www.alzheimers.com/health_library/treatment/treatment_04_other.html. Accessed winter 2001.
18. The stages of Alzheimer's disease. PlanetRx, Inc.; 2000. Available at: http://www.alzheimers.com/health_library/basics/basics_04_stages.html. Accessed winter 2001.
19. Park A. The new science of Alzheimer's. *Time Magazine.* July 17, 2000:52–57.
20. Estrogen: Alzheimer's prevention and treatment for women. PlanetRx, Inc.; 2000. Available at: http://www.alzheimers.com/health_library/treatment/treatment_02_estro.html. Accessed winter 2001.
21. Antioxidants: Nutrients that can slow Alzheimer's. PlanetRx, Inc.; 2000. Available at: http://www.alzheimers.com/health_library/treatment/treatment_05_anti.html. Accessed winter 2001.

Amyotrophic Lateral Sclerosis

1. Fact sheet: Amyotrophic lateral sclerosis. Family Caregiver Alliance. Available at: http://www.caregiver.org/factsheets/diagnoses/als.html. Accessed winter 2001.
2. Vital statistics. ALS survival guide. Douglas E. Eshleman; 1998–2000. Available at: www.lougehrigsdisease.net. Accessed winter 2001.
3. Amyotrophic lateral sclerosis (ALS or "Lou Gehrig's disease"). MedicineNet, Inc. Available at: http://medicinenet.com. Accessed winter 2001.
4. Causes of ALS. ALS survival guide. Douglas E. Eshleman; 1998–2000. Available at: http://www.lougehrigsdisease.net/als_causes_of_als.htm. Accessed winter 2001.
5. Discovery suggests new strategies for ALS treatment. World Federation of Neurology; 1997–2000. Available at: http://www.wfnals.org/News/2000/caspasesscience.htm. Accessed winter 2001.
6. Mayfield E. Glimmer of hope for people with ALS. *FDA Consumer Magazine.* September 1996. Available at: http://www.fda.gov/fdac/features/796_als.html. Accessed winter 2001.
7. Myotrophin slows progression of Lou Gehrig's disease. P\S\L Consulting Group Inc.; 2000. Available at: http://www.docguide.com/news/content.nsf/News/25FA2D580143802D85256575005B7BEE?OpenDocument&id=48dde4a73e09a96985 2568880078c249. Accessed winter 2001.
8. NINDS amyotrophic lateral sclerosis information page. The National Institute of Neurological Disorders and Stroke, National Institutes of Health. Available at: http://www.ninds.nih.gov/health_and_medical/disorders/amyotrophiclateralsclerosis_doc.htm. Accessed winter 2001.
9. Potential test for Lou Gehrig's disease at hand. 2000 P\S\L Consulting Group Inc.; 2000. Available at: http://www.docguide.com.news/content.nsf/News/23D434113B67BC708525653F006D222F?OpenDocument&id=48dde4a73e09a96985256888007 8c249. Accessed winter 2001.
10. Revised criteria for the diagnosis of amyotrophic lateral sclerosis. World Federation

of Neurology; 1997–2001. Available at: http://www.wfnals.org/Articles/elescorial 1998criteria.htm. Accessed winter 2001.

11. Understanding ALS. ALSA. Available at: http://www.alsa.org/als/symptoms.cfm. Accessed winter 2001.

Multiple Sclerosis

1. Rao SM. Cognitive impairment in multiple sclerosis. Healthology, Inc.; 2000. Available at: http://www.understandingms.com/focus_article.asp?f=m_sclerosis&c=article_cogimpairms. Accessed winter 2001.

2. FDA approves Novantrone to treat progression in MS. The National Multiple Sclerosis Society; 2000. Available at: http://www.nmss.org/ publications/p-893282996/2000/oct/a-971450040.html. Accessed winter 2001.

3. Riskind P. Multiple sclerosis: The immune system's terrible mistake. *The Harvard Mahoney Neuroscience Institute Letter On the Brain*. 1996;5(4). Available at: http://www.med.harvard.edu/publications/On_The_Brain/Volume5/Number4/MSf.html. Accessed winter 2001.

4. Multiple sclerosis overview. Rose JW, Houtchens M, Lynch SG. Available at: http://www-medlib.med.utah.edu/kw/ms/prognosis.html. Accessed winter 2001.

5. Jacobs DA, Galetta SL. Multiple sclerosis: An overview. Healthology, Inc.; 2000. Available at: http://www.understandingms.com/focus_article.asp?b=understandingms&f=m_sclerosis&c=article_msoverview. Accessed winter 2001.

6. Multiple sclerosis. MedicineNet, Inc.; 1996–2000. Available at: \http://medicineNet.com. Accessed winter 2001.

7. Jacobs LD, Beck RW, Simon JH, et al. Intramuscular interferon beta-1a therapy initiated during a first demyelinating event in multiple sclerosis. *N Engl J Med*. 2000;343(13). Available at: http://www.nejm.com/content/2000/0343/ 0013/0898.asp. Accessed winter 2001.

8. NINDS multiple sclerosis information page. The National Institute of Neurological Disorders and Stroke, National Institutes of Health. Available at: http://www.ninds.nih.gov/health_and_medical/disorders/multiple_sclerosis.htm. Accessed winter 2001.

9. Multiple sclerosis and related disorders. Merck & Co., Inc.; 1995–2000. Available at: http://www.merck.com/pubs/mmanual_home/sec6/68.htm. Accessed winter 2001.

Parkinson's Disease

1. Ask the doc: New medications for Parkinson's disease. InteliHealth Inc.; 1996–2001. Available at: http://www.intelihealth.com/IH/ihtIH?t=24172&p=~br,IHW1~st,24479|~r,WSIHW000|~b,*|. Accessed winter 2001.

2. NIH researchers find first Parkinson's disease gene. American Association for the Advancement of Science; 1997. Available at: http://www. nhgri.nih.gov/DIR/LGDR/PARK2/media_release.html. Accessed winter 2001.

3. NINDS Parkinson's disease information page. The National Institute of Neurological Disorders and Stroke, National Institutes of Health. Available at: http://www.ninds.nih.gov/health_and_medical_disorders/parkinsons_disease.htm. Accessed winter 2001.

4. Online tutorials in neurology: Parkinson's disease. Available at http://medweb.bham.ac.uk/http/depts/clin_neuro/teaching/tutorials/parkinsons/parkinsons1.html. Accessed winter 2001.

5. Young R. Update on Parkinson's disease. American Academy of Family Physicians; 1999. Available at: http://www.aafp.org/afp/990415ap/2155.html. Accessed winter 2001.

6. Functional and stereotactic neurosurgery: Staging of Parkinson's disease. MGH Neurosurgical Service; 1999. Available at: http://neurosurgery. mgh.harvard.edu/pdstages.htm. Accessed winter 2001.

7. Treatment methods. National Parkinson Foundation, Inc.; 1996–2001. Available at: http://www.parkinson.org/treament.htm. Accessed winter 2001.

8. What the patient should know. National Parkinson Foundation, Inc.; 1996–2001. Available at: http://www.parkinson.org/pdedu.htm. Accessed winter 2001.

9. Mueller JM. Elderly Parkinson's patient—Feeling good. *Massage Ther J*. 1996;35(1): 28–42.

Peripheral Neuropathy

1. Diabetic Neuropathy. InteliHealth Inc.; 1996–2001. Available at: http://www.intelihealth.com/IH/ihtIH?d=dmtContent&c=233221&p=~br,IHW1~st,24479|~r,WSIHW000|~b,*|. Accessed winter 2001.

2. NINDS peripheral neuropathy information page. National Institute of Neurological Disorders and Stroke, National Institutes of Health. Available at: http://www.ninds.nih.gov/health_and_medical/disorders/peripheralneuropathy_doc.htm. Accessed winter 2001.

3. Peripheral neuropathy explained. Neuropathy Trust; 1998–2000. Available at: http://www.neuropathytrust.org/peripheral_neuropathy_explained.htm. Accessed winter 2001.

4. Shlay J, Chaloner K, Max MB, et al.; for the Terry Beirn Community Programs for Clinical Research on AIDS. Acupuncture and amitriptyline for pain due to HIV-related peripheral neuropathy: A randomized controlled trial. *JAMA*. 1998;280:1590–1595. Available at: http://www.ama-assn.org/special/hiv/library/readroom/jama98/joc80706.htm. Accessed winter 2001.

5. Peripheral neuropathy. Mayo Foundation for Medical Education and Research; 1998–2000. Available at: http://www.mayohealth.org/home?id=5.1.1.16.3. Accessed winter 2001.

Tremor

1. Charles PD, Esper GJ, Davis TL, Maciunas, RJ, Robertson D. Classification of tremor and update on treatment. *Am Fam Phys*. 1999. Available at: http://www.aafp.org/afp/990315ap/1565.html. Accessed winter 2001.

2. Essential tremor. The Parkinson's Institute. Available at: http://www.parkinsonsinstitute.org/movement_diorders/essential_tremor.html. Accessed winter 2001.

3. Tremor information page. The National Institute of Neurological Disorders and Stroke, National Institutes of Health. Available at: http://www.ninds.nih.gov/health_and_medical/disorders/tremor_doc.htm. Accessed winter 2001.

4. Tremor. MedicineNet, Inc.; 1996–2000. Available at http://medicineNet.com. Accessed winter 2001.

5. What is essential tremor? International Tremor Foundation; 2000. Available at: http://www.essentialtremor.org/essential_tremor.html. Accessed winter 2001.

Encephalitis

1. CDC answers your questions about St. Louis encephalitis. Division of Vector-Borne Infectious Diseases, National Center for Infectious Diseases, Centers for Disease Control and Prevention. Available at: http://www.cdc.gov/ncidod/dvbid/arbor/SLE_QA.htm. Accessed winter 2001.

2. Fact sheet: Arboviral encephalitis. Division of Vector-Borne Infectious Diseases, National Center for Infectious Diseases, Centers for Disease Control and Prevention. Available at: http://www.cdc.gov/ncidod/dvbid/arbor/arbofact.htm. Accessed winter 2001.

3. NINDS encephalitis and meningitis information page. The National Institute of Neurological Disorders and Stroke, National Institutes of Health. Available at: http://www.ninds.nih.gov/health_and_medical/disorders/encmenin_doc.htm. Accessed winter 2001.

4. Outbreak of West Nile-like viral encephalitis—New York, 1999. Available at: http://www.cdc.gov/epo/mmwr/preview/mmwrhtml/mm4838a1.htm. Accessed winter 2001.

5. West Nile virus. Division of Vector-Borne Infectious Diseases, National Center for Infectious Diseases, Centers for Disease Control and Prevention. Available at: http://www.cdc.gov/ncidod/dvbid/westnile/index.htm. Accessed winter 2001.

6. Platonov AE, Shipulina GA, Shipulina OY, et al. Outbreak of West Nile virus infection, Volgograd, Russia, 1999. *Emerg Infect Dis*. 2001;(7)1. Available at: http://www.cdc.gov/ncidod/EID/vol7no1/platanov.htm. Accessed winter 2001.

7. Rappole JH, Derrickson SR, and Hubálek Z. Perspectives. *Emerg Infect Dis J.* 2000;6(4). Available at: http://www. cdc.gov/ ncidod/eid/vol6no4/pdf/ rappole.pdf. Accessed winter 2001.
8. West Nile virus maps-2001. United States Geological Survey, Center for Integration of Natural Disaster Information. Available at: http://cindi.usgs.gov/hazard/event/west_ nile/west_nile.html. Accessed spring 2002.

Herpes Zoster

1. Herpes zoster (shingles) eye infections. Steen-Hall Eye Institute; 1996–2001. Available at: http://www.steen-hall. com/zoster.html. Accessed winter 2001.
2. Herpes zoster. American Academy of Dermatology; 1999. Available at: http://www.aad.org/ pamphlets/herpes-Zoster.html. Accessed winter 2001.
3. NINDS Ramsay Hunt syndrome type I information page. National Institute of Neurological Disorders and Stroke, National Institutes of Health. Available at: http://www.ninds.nih. gov/health_and_medical/disorders/ram-say1_doc.htm. Accessed winter 2001.
4. NINDS shingles information page. The National Institute of Neurological Disorders and Stroke. National Institutes of Health. Available at: http://www.ninds.nih. gov/health_and_medical/disorders/ shingles_doc.htm. Accessed winter 2001.
5. Varicella-zoster virus. Scientific Resources Program (SRP), National Center for Infectious Diseases (NCID), Centers for Disease Control and Prevention. Available at: http://www.cdc.gov/ncidod/srp/varicella. htm. Accessed winter 2001.

Meningitis

1. Meningococcal disease. Centers for Disease Control and Prevention, National Center for Infectious Diseases, Division of Bacterial and Mycotic Diseases. Available at: http://www.cdc. gov/ncidod/dbmd/disease-info/meningococcal_g.htm. Accessed winter 2001.
2. Viral (aseptic) meningitis. Centers for Disease Control and Prevention, National Center for Infectious Diseases, Division of Viral and Rickettsial Diseases, Respiratory and Enteric Viruses Branch. Available at: http://www.cdc. gov/ncidod/dvrd/virlmen. htm. Accessed winter 2001.
3. Viral meningitis (nonbacterial meningitis). New York State Department of Health communicable disease fact sheet. Available at: http://www. health.state.ny.us/nysdoh/ consumer/viral.htm. Accessed winter 2001.
4. Epidemic meningococcal disease. Fact sheet no. 105. WHO/OMS; 2000. Available at: http://www.who.int/inf-fs/en/ fact105.html. Accessed winter 2001.

Polio, Post Polio Syndrome

1. Public health dispatch: Certification of poliomyelitis eradication—Western Pacific Region October 2000. *MMWR.* 2001;50(01);1–3. Available at: http://www. cdc.gov/mmwr/preview/mmwrhtml/ mm5001a1.htm. Accessed winter 2001.
2. NINDS post-polio syndrome information page. The National Institute of Neurological Disorders and Stroke, National Institutes of Health. Available at: http://www. ninds.nih.gov/ health_and_medical/disorders/post_polio_short.htm. Accessed winter 2001.
3. Poliomyelitis, paralytic. Centers for Disease Control. Case definitions for infectious conditions under public health surveillance. *MMWR.* 1997;46(RR-10):26–27. Available at: http://www.cdc.gov/epo/mmwr/other/case _def/polio97.html. Accessed winter 2001.
4. Eulberg MK, Halstead LS, Perry J. Poliomyelitis. Patient Care; 1982. Available at: http://www.eastersealsco.org/postpolio/ poliomyelitis.html. Accessed winter 2001.
5. Ask the Mayo Physician, 08.20.99. Mayo Foundation for Medical Education and Research; 2000. Available at: http://www.mayohealth. org/mayo/askphys/qa990820.htm. Accessed winter 2001.
6. Eulberg M. Polio patient and MD. Available at: http://www.eastersealsco.org/post-polio/eulberg.html. Accessed winter 2001.
7. Update on the Outbreak of Poliomyelitis—Dominican Republic and Haiti, 2000—2001. MMWR. 10/5/01 50(39);855-6. Available at: http://www.cdc.gov/od/oc/ media/mmwrnews/n011005.htm#mmwr3. Accessed spring 2002.

Anxiety Disorders

1. Anxiety disorders. National Institute of Mental Health (NIMH). Available at: http://www. nimh.nih.gov/anxiety/anxiety. cfm#anx4. Accessed summer 2001.
2. Hsu K. Anxiety from emergency medicine/psychosocial. eMedicine.com, Inc.; 2001. Available at: http://www.emedicine. com/emerg/ topic35.htm. Accessed summer 2001.
3. The dangers of tranquilizer misuse. InteliHealth Inc.; 1996–2001. Available at: http://www.intelihealth.com/IH/ihtIH/ WSIHW000/8271/8558/191823.html?d= dmtContent. Accessed summer 2001.
4. Facts about anxiety disorders. National Institute of Mental Health (NIMH). Available at: http://www.nimh.nih.gov/anxiety/ adfacts.cfm. Accessed summer 2001.
5. Obsessive compulsive disorder. tAPir.; 1993–2000. Available at: http://www.algy. com/ anxiety/ocd.html. Accessed summer 2001.
6. Obsessive-compulsive disorder. InteliHealth Inc.; 1996–2001. Available at: http://www.intelihealth.com/IH/ihtIH/ WSIHW000/8271/8576/187891.html?d=d mtContent. Also at http://www.intelihealth. com/IH/ihtIH/WSIHW000/8271/8576/ 191824.html?d=dmtJHE#ocd1. Accessed summer 2001.
7. Anxiety disorders: Obsessive-compulsive disorder. National Institute of Mental Health (NIMH). Available at: http://www. nimh.nih. gov/anxiety/anxiety/ocd/ocdfac. htm. Accessed summer 2001.
8. Facts about post-traumatic stress disorder. National Institute of Mental Health (NIMH). Publication no. OM-99 4157. Available at: http://www.docguide.com/ news/content.nsf/news/. Accessed summer. 2001.
9. Post-traumatic stress disorder (PTSD). InteliHealth Inc.; 1996–2001. Available at: http://www.intelihealth.com/IH/ihtPrint/ WSIHW000/24479/9476.html?k= basePrint. Accessed summer 2001.
10. Social anxiety disorder: A common, under-recognized mental disorder. American Academy of Family Physicians; 1999. Available at: http://www.aafp.org/afp/991115ap/ 2311.html. Accessed summer 2001.
11. Social anxiety fact sheet. tAPir; 1993–2000. Available at: http://www.algy.com/anxiety/ social/fact.html. Accessed summer 2001.
12. Agoraphobia. tAPir; 1993–2000. Available at: http://www.algy.com/anxiety/agora. html. Accessed summer 2001.
13. Specific phobia. tAPir; 1993–2000. Available at: http://www.algy.com/anxiety/ phobia.html. Accessed summer 2001.
14. Facts about generalized anxiety disorder. National Institute of Mental Health (NIMH). Available at: http://www.nimh. nih.gov/anxiety/gadfacts.cfm. Accessed summer 2001.
15. Generalized anxiety disorder. tAPir; 1993–2000. Available at: http://www.algy. com/anxiety/gad.html. Accessed summer 2001.
16. Generalized anxiety disorder. InteliHealth Inc.; 1996–2001. Available at: http://www. intelihealth.com/IH/ihtIH/WSIHW000/ 8271/8558/187873.html?d=dmtContent. Accessed summer 2001.
17. Panic disorder. tAPir; 1993–2000. Available at: http://www.algy.com/ anxiety/panic. html. Accessed summer 2001.
18. Plewa MC. Panic disorders from emergency medicine/psychosocial. eMedicine.com, Inc.; 2001. Available at: http://www.emedicine.com/emerg/ topic766.htm. Accessed summer 2001.

Chemical Dependency

1. Substance abuse. American Psychiatric Association; 1988–1989. Revised 1994. Available at: http://www.psych.org/public_info/ sub_ab_1.cfm. Accessed winter 2001.
2. Diagnosis and treatment of drug abuse in family practice. National Institute on Drug Abuse (NIDA) and National Institutes of Health (NIH). Available at: http://www. nida.nih.gov Diagnosis-Treatment/ Diagnosis4.html. Accessed spring 2002.
3. Alcohol abuse and alcoholism. MedicineNet, Inc.; 1996–2000. Available at http://medicineNet.com. Accessed winter 2001.
4. Alcohol dependence: American description. Phillip W. Long; 1995–2000. Available at: http://www.mentalhealth.com/fr20.html. Accessed winter 2001.

5. Alcohol, substance abuse and addictions. Mayo Foundation for Medical Education and Research; 1998–2000. Available at: http://www.mayohealth.org/home?id=HQ 00201. Accessed winter 2001.

6. IV. Alcohol-related disorders: Treatment principles and alternatives. American Psychiatric Association, Clinical Resources. Available at: http://www.psych.org/clin_res/pg_substance_4.cfm. Accessed winter 2001.

7. Dopamine- A sample neurotransmitter. Addiction Science Research and Education Center, College of Pharmacy, The University of Texas. Available at: http://www.utexas.edu/research/asrec/dopamine.html. Accessed winter 2001.

8. Children of alcoholics: Important facts. National Association for Children of Alcoholics. Available at: http://www.health.org/nongovpubs/coafacts/. Accessed winter 2001.

9. National Institute on Alcohol Abuse and Alcoholism no. 48 July 2000. Alcohol alert. Available at: http://silk.nih.gov/silk/niaaa1/publication/aa48.htm. Accessed winter 2001.

10. Nationwide trends 13567. National Institute on Drug Abuse (NIDA), US Department of Health and Human Services, National Institutes of Health. Available at: http://165.112.78.61/Infofax/nationtrends.html. Accessed winter 2001.

11. When enough is enough: How to recognize a drinking problem. InteliHealth Inc.; 1996–2001. Available at: http://www.intelihealth.com/IH/ihtIH/WSIHW000/331/24290/261314.html?d=dmtContent. Accessed winter 2001.

12. Preidt R. Your brain can sober itself. Rx Remedy, Inc.; 2001. Available at: http://www.healthscout.com/cgi-bin/WebObjects/Af.woa/13/wo/Xj2000J5200 Md200M5/15.0.11.1.38.1.0.7.0.1 Accessed winter 2001.

Depression

1. Anxiety, depression, and manic depression. Phillip W. Long; 1995–2000. Available at: http://www.mentalhealth.com/book/p43-anx.html. Accessed winter 2001.

2. Cassem EH, Coyle JT. Depression. *The Harvard Mahoney Neuroscience Institute Letter on the Brain*. On The Brain. Vol. 2. Special Issue. Available at http://www.med.harvard.edu/publications/On_The_Brain/Volume2/Special/SPDepr.html. Accessed winter 2001.

3. Depression: New understanding, drugs help. Mayo Health Oasis, 1.04.99. Mayo Foundation for Medical Education and Research; 1995–2000. Available at: http://www.mayohealth.org/mayo/9901/depressi.htm. Accessed winter 2001.

4. Five top warning signals of depression identified. Available at: http://www.pslgroup.com/dg/c56fa.htm. Accessed spring 2002.

5. Castleman M. An Introduction to antidepressants. PlanetRx.com, Inc.; 2000. Available at: http://www.depression.com/tools/health_library/treatments/antidepressants.html. Accessed winter 2001.

6. Major depression and anxiety problems share many symptoms. PlanetRx, Inc.; 2000. Available at: http://www.depression.com.Accessed winter 2001.

7. Overview: Types of depression. PlanetRx, Inc.; 2000. Available at: http://www.depression.com. Accessed winter 2001.

8. Depression is a treatable illness: A patient's guide. Agency for Health Care Policy and Research (AHCPR) supported guidelines - online versions. Available at: http://www.mentalhealth.com/bookah/p44-dp.html. Accessed winter 2001.

9. Wysong P. Major depressive disorder: Little sleep loss goes a long way in depressed. *Medical Post*, June 4, 1996. Available at: http://www.mentalhealth.com/mag1/p5m-dp05.html. Accessed winter 2001.

10. The invisible disease—Depression. National Institute of Mental Health. Available at: http://www.nimh.nih.gov/publicat/invisible.cfm. Accessed winter 2001.

11. Depression. MedicineNet, Inc.; 1996–2000. Available at http://medicineNet.com. Accessed winter 2001.

12. Depression. NIH Publication no. NIH-99-3561. National Institutes of Health. Available at http://www.nimh.nih.gov/publicat/depression.cfm#ptdep1. Accessed winter 2001.

13. Understanding Depression. Mayo Foundation for Medical Education and Research; 2000. Available at: http://www.mayohealth.org/home?id=DP00001. Accessed winter 2001.

Eating Disorders

1. Anorexia nervosa. MedicineNet, Inc.; 1996–2000. Available at: http://medicineNet.com. Accessed summer 2001.

2. Bulimia. MedicineNet, Inc.; 1996–2000. Available at: http://medicineNet.com. Accessed summer 2001.

3. Eating disorders. Brain briefings. Society for Neuroscience; 2000. Available at: http://www.sfn.org/briefings/eating_disorders.html. Accessed summer 2001.

4. Eating disorders—Widespread and difficult to treat. Mayo Foundation for Medical Education and Research; 1998–2000. Available at: http://www.mayohealth.org/home?id=HM00016. Accessed summer 2001.

5. Leutwyler K. Treating eating disorders. Available at: http://www.sciam.com/explorations/1998/030298eating/index.html. Accessed summer 2001.

6. Understanding eating disturbances and disorders: A guide for helping family and friends. The Board of Trustees of the University of Illinois; 1998. Available at: http://www.mckinley.uiuc.edu/health-info/nutrit/eatdisor/und-ed-d.html. Accessed summer 2001.

Bell's Palsy

1. Bell's palsy information site. BPIS; 2000. Available at: http://www.bellspalsy.ws/. Accessed winter 2001.

2. NINDS Bell's palsy information page. The National Institute of Neurological Disorders and Stroke. National Institutes of Health. Available at: http://www.ninds.nih.gov/health_and_medical/disorders/bells_doc.htm. Accessed winter 2001.

3. Bell's palsy. Mayo Foundation for Medical Education and Research; 1998–2000. Available at: http://www.mayohealth.org/home?id=DS00168 . Accessed winter 2001.

4. Billue JS. Bell's palsy: An update on idiopathic facial paralysis. Springhouse Corp.; 2000. Available at: http://www.springnet.com/ce/j708a.htm. Accessed winter 2001.

5. LaRouere MJ. The current treatment of Bell's palsy. Michigan Ear Institute; 2000. Available at: http://www.michiganear.com/library/B/bellspalsy.html. Accessed winter 2001.

Cerebral Palsy

1. Cerebral palsy. WellnessWeb; 1995–2001. Available at: http://www.wellweb.com/INDEX/qcerebra.htm. Accessed winter 2001.

2. Cerebral palsy. HealthAnswers.com, Inc.; 2000. Available at: http://healthanswers.com/centers/body/overview.asp?id=brain/+nervous+system&filename=2662.htm. Accessed winter 2001.

3. Cerebral palsy. MedicineNet, Inc.; 1996–2000. Available at: http://medicineNet.com. Accessed winter 2001.

4. Causes of C.P. Anee Stanford; 1995–2000. Available at: http://www.geocities.com/HotSprings/Sauna/4441/index2.htm. Accessed winter 2001.

5. Cerebral palsy. ©Kathleen C. Boravitz, Children's Medical Center, University of Virginia. Available at: http://www.med.virginia.edu/cmc/tutorials/cp/index.html. Accessed winter 2001.

6. NINDS cerebral palsy information page. The National Institute of Neurological Disorders and Stroke, National Institutes of Health. Available at: http://www.ninds.nih.gov/health_and_medical/disorders/cerebral_palsy.htm. Accessed winter 2001.

7. Spasticity, rigidity, tone: What's it all mean? Anee Stanford; 1995–2000. Available at: http://www.geocities.com/HotSprings/Sauna/4441/index2.htm. Accessed winter 2001.

8. General information about cerebral palsy and types of cerebral palsy. Anee Stanford; 1995–2000. Available at: http://www.geocities.com/HotSprings/Sauna/4441/index2.htm. Accessed winter 2001.

Reflex Sympathetic Dystrophy Syndrome

1. Reflex sympathetic dystrophy syndrome. National Institute of Neurological Disorders and Stroke (NINDS). Available at:

http://www. ninds.nih.gov/health_and_
medical/pubs/rsds_fact_sheet.htm.
Accessed winter 2001.

2. NINDS reflex sympathetic dystrophy syndrome information page. National Institute of Neurological Disorders and Stroke (NINDS). Available at: http://www.ninds. nih.gov/ health_and_medical/disorders/ reflex_sympathetic_dystrophy.htm?format =printable. Accessed winter 2001.

3. Ask the Mayo physician. Mayo Foundation for Medical Education and Research; 2000. Available at: http://www. mayohealth. org/mayo/ askphys/qa970605. htm. Accessed winter 2001.

4. Reflex sympathetic dystrophy syndrome. Available at: http://rsdhope.org/Medical/ medical.asp. Accessed spring 2002.

5. Facts and fiction about RSD/CRPS. RSDSA; 1999. Available at: http://www. rsds.org/fact. html. Accessed winter 2001.

6. Reflex sympathetic dystrophy syndrome (RSDS). University of Washington; 2000. Available at: http://www.orthop. washington.edu/bonejoint/dzzzzzzz1_2. html. Accessed winter 2001.

Spinal Cord Injury

1. Carrano I. Acute management of spinal cord injury. Available at: http://www. spinalcord-injury.com/ spinalcordinjury.html. Accessed summer 2001.

2. Spinal cord injury facts and figures at a glance May, 2001. Board of Trustees University of Alabama; 2000. Available at: http://www.spinalcord.uab.edu/show. asp?durki=21446. Accessed summer 2001.

3. Hereotopic ossification- SCI infosheet #13. Board of Trustees University of Alabama; 2000. Available at: http://www.spinalcord. uab. edu/show.asp?durki=21485. Accessed summer 2001.

4. NINDS spasticity information page. The National Institute of Neurological Disorders and Stroke, National Institutes of Health. Available at: http://www.ninds. nih.gov/health_and_medical/disorders/spas ticity_doc.htm. Accessed summer 2001.

5. NINDS spinal cord injury information page. The National Institute of Neurological Disorders and Stroke, National Institutes of Health. Available at: http://www. ninds.nih.gov/ health_and_medical/ disorders/sci.htm. Accessed summer 2001.

6. Pain after spinal cord injury. Board of Trustees University of Alabama; 2000. Available at: http://www.spinalcord.uab. edu/show.asp?durki=41119. Accessed summer 2001.

7. Garcia R. Deep venous thrombosis and pulmonary embolism in spinal cord injury. Available at: http://www.geocities.com/ garciaronald/scidvtpe.htm. Accessed summer 2001.

8. Recent reports offer SCI statistics. Department of Rehabilitation Medicine, University of Washington; 1999–2000. Available at:

http://depts. washington.edu/rehab/sci/ update-statistics7-2.shtml. Accessed summer 2001.

9. Spinal cord injury complications. Blue Cross and Blue Shield of Massachusetts, Inc.; 2001. Available at: http://www. ahealthyme.com/topic/spinalinjury. Accessed summer 2001.

10. Spasticity following spinal cord injury- SCI infosheet #16. Board of Trustees of the University of Alabama; 1998. Available at: http://www.spinalcord.uab.edu/show.asp? durki=22455. Accessed summer 2001.

11. Schreiber D. Spinal cord injuries from emergency medicine/neurology. eMedicine.com, Inc.; 2001. Available at: http://www.emedicine.com/emerg/ topic553.htm. Accessed summer 2001.

12. Spinal cord injury: Emerging concepts. National Institute of Neurological Disorders and Stroke, National Institutes of Health. Available at: http://www.ninds. nih.gov/health_and_medical/pubs/ sci_report.htm?format=printable. Accessed summer 2001.

13. The facts about spinal cord injury and central nervous system disorders. Christopher Reeve Paralysis Foundation; 1999. Available at: http://paralysis.apacure.org/ progress/facts.html. Accessed summer 2001.

14. What happens in human spinal cord injuries? National Institutes of Health. Available at: http://science-education.nih.gov/ nihHTML/ose/snapshots/multimedia/ritn/ spinal/happens.html. Accessed summer 2001.

Stroke

1. Aneurysm. American Heart Association, Inc.; 2000. Available at:: http://www.americanheart. org/Heart_and_Stroke_A_Z_ Guide/aneurysm.html. Accessed summer 2001.

2. Carotid artery disease. Texas Heart Institute; 2001. Available at: http://www.tmc. edu/thi/ carotida.html. Accessed summer 2001.

3. NINDS cerebral aneurysm information page. The National Institute of Neurological Disorders and Stroke, National Institutes of Health. Available at: http://www. ninds.nih.gov/ health_and_medical/ disorders/ceraneur_doc.htm?format= printable. Accessed summer 2001.

4. NINDS stroke information page. The National Institute of Neurological Disorders and Stroke, National Institutes of Health. Available at: http://www.ninds.nih.gov/ health_and_medical/disorders/stroke.htm? format=printable. Accessed summer 2001.

5. NINDS transient ischemic attack (TIA) information page. The National Institute of Neurological Disorders and Stroke, National Institutes of Health. Available at:: http://www.ninds. nih.gov/health_and_ medical/disorders/tia_doc.htm?format= printable. Accessed summer 2001.

6. Stroke effects. American Heart Association, Inc.; 2000. Available at: http://www. americanheart.org/Heart_and_Stroke_A_Z _Guide/strokeef.html. Accessed summer 2001.

7. Stroke risk factors. American Heart Association, Inc.; 2000. Available at: http://www. americanheart.org/Heart_and_Stroke_A_Z _Guide/strokeri.html. Accessed summer 2001.

8. Stroke signs. American Heart Association, Inc.; 2000. Available at: http://www. americanheart.org/Heart_and_Stroke_A_Z _Guide/strokeef.html. Accessed summer 2001.

9. Stroke statistics. American Heart Association, Inc.; 2000. Available at: http://www. americanheart.org/Heart_and_Stroke_A_Z _Guide/strokes.html. Accessed summer 2001.

10. Stroke symptoms/warning signs. American Heart Association, Inc.; 2000. Available at: http://www.americanheart.org/Heart_and_ Stroke_A_Z_Guide/strokews.html. Accessed summer 2001.

11. Stroke. American Heart Association, Inc.; 2000. Available at: http://www.american-heart.org/ Heart_and_Stroke_A_Z_ Guide/stroke.html. Accessed summer 2001.

12. Strokes and CVA. tzartist http://www.sup-portpilot.com/stroke.html. Accessed summer 2001.

13. Stroke. Texas Heart Institute; 2001. Available at: http://www.tmc.edu/thi/stroke. html. Accessed summer 2001.

14. Tissue plasminogen activator (tPA). American Heart Association, Inc.; 2000. Available at: http://www.americanheart.org/ Heart_and_Stroke_A_Z_Guide/tpa.html. Accessed summer 2001.

Trigeminal Neuralgia

1. NINDS trigeminal neuralgia information page. The National Institute of Neurological Disorders and Stroke, National Institutes of Health. Available at: http://www. ninds.nih.gov/ health_and_medical/ disorders/trigemin_doc.htm?format= printable. Accessed summer 2001.

2. Microvascular compression syndromes: Treatment of trigeminal neuralgia, glossopharyngeal neuralgia, and hemifacial spasm. MGH Neurosurgical Service; 2000. Available at: http://neurosurgery. mgh. harvard.edu/mvd.htm. Accessed summer 2001.

3. Percutaneous stereotactic radiofrequency thermal rhizotomy for the treatment of trigeminal neuralgia. MGH Neurosurgical Service; 2000. Available at: http:// neurosurgery.mgh. harvard.edu/mvd.htm. Accessed summer 2001.

4. Trigeminal neuralgia. Trigeminal Neuralgia Resources /Facial Neuralgia Resources; 1995–2001. Available at: http://facial-neuralgia.org/conditions/tn.html. Accessed summer 2001.

5. What is trigeminal neuralgia? Trigeminal Neuralgia Association; 1996–2000. Available at: http://www.tna-support.org/Definition.htm. Accessed summer 2001.

Guillain-Barré Syndrome

1. What is Guillain-Barré syndrome (GBS)? Guillain-Barré Syndrome Foundation International. Available at: http://www.webmast.com/gbs/. Accessed winter 2001.
2. Sater RA. Acute inflammatory demyelinating polyradiculoneuropathy from neuro/neuromuscular diseases. eMedicine.com, Inc.; 2001. Available at: http://www.emedicine.com/ neuro/topic7.htm. Accessed winter 2001.
3. Guillain-Barré syndrome. MedicineNet, Inc.; 1996–2000. Available at: MedicineNet.com. Accessed winter 2001.
4. Guillain-Barré Syndrome. Mayo Foundation for Medical Education and Research; 1998–2000. Available at: http://www.mayoclinic.com/home?id=HO00076. Accessed winter 2001.
5. Guillain-Barré syndrome fact sheet. National Institute of Neurological Disorders and Stroke. Available at: http://www.ninds.nih.gov/ health_and_medical/pubs/guillain_barre.htm. Accessed winter 2001.
6. McGovern TV. Hard time. The Washington Post. September 5, 2000:Z10.
7. NINDS Guillain-Barré syndrome information page. National Institute of Neurological Disorders and Stroke (NINDS), National Institutes of Health. Available at: http://www.ninds.nih.gov/health_and_medical/disorders/gbs.htm. Accessed winter 2001.

Headaches

1. Q. How common are headaches? American Council for Headache Education; 2000. Available at: http://www.achenet.org/understanding/causes.php. Accessed winter 2001.
2. Headache types: Cluster. National Headache Foundation. Available at: http://www.headaches.org/educationalmodules/completeguide/clusindex.html. Accessed winter 2001.
3. Headache—Understanding the pain. Mayo Foundation for Medical Education and Research; 1998–2000. Available at: http://www.mayohealth.org/home?id=HQ00794. Accessed winter 2001.
4. Headache: Guide to types. Mayo Foundation for Medical Education and Research; 1998–2000. Available at: http://www.mayohealth.org/home?id=HQ00791. Accessed winter 2001.
5. Headache: Guide to treatments. Mayo Foundation for Medical Education and Research; 1998–2000. Available at: http://www.mayohealth.org/home?id=HQ00790. Accessed winter 2001.
6. Headache: Hope through research. InteliHealth Inc.; 1996–2001. Available at: http://www.intelihealth.com/IH/ihtIH/WSIHW000/20933/24815.html. Accessed winter 2001.

7. Headache types: Hormone. National Headache Foundation. Available at: http://www.headaches.org/educationalmodules/completeguide/hormindex.html. Accessed winter 2001.
8. Headache types: Migraine. National Headache Foundation. Available at: http://www.headaches.org/educationalmodules/completeguide/migrindex.html. Accessed winter 2001.
9. Migraine headache. MedicineNet, Inc.; 1996–2000. Available at http://medicineNet. com. Accessed winter 2001.
10. Troost BT. Migraine and other headaches. MEDMAN; 1996–1998. Available at: http://www.wfubmc.edu/neurology/migraine/migd.html#OTHER. Accessed winter 2001.
11. Packer-Tursman J. Treatment of choice. The Washington Post. June 13, 2000:Z23. Available at: http://www.washingtonpost.com/wp-dyn/articles/A46997-2000Jun13.html. Accessed winter 2001.
12. NINDS headache information page. The National Institute of Neurological Disorders and Stroke. Available at:: http://www.ninds.nih.gov/health_and_medical/disorders/headache.htm. Accessed winter 2001.
13. Other types: Rebound headache. National Headache Foundation. Available at: http://www.headaches.org/educationalmodules/completeguide/othindex.html. Accessed winter 2001.
14. Principles of headache diagnosis. SUNY Upstate Medical University; 2000. Available at: http://www.upstate.edu/neurology/haas/hpdxpr.htm. Accessed winter 2001.
15. What you should know about headache. American Council for Headache Education; 2000. Available at: http://www.achenet.org/understanding/definitions.php. Accessed winter 2001.

Seizure Disorders

1. Epilepsy in children. Mayo Foundation for Medical Education and Research; 2000. Available at: http://www.mayohealth.org/mayo/ 9612/htm/epilepsy.htm. Accessed summer 2001.
2. "Benchmarks" for epilepsy research. National Institute of Neurological Disorders and Stroke (NINDS). Available at: http://www.ninds.nih. gov/about_ninds/epilepsybenchmarks.htm. Accessed summer 2001.
3. NINDS epilepsy information page. The National Institute of Neurological Disorders and Stroke, National Institutes of Health. Available at: http://www.ninds.nih.gov/health_and_medical/disorders/epilepsy.htm?format=printable. Accessed summer 2001.
4. New device offers hope for epileptics. Available at: http://www.usc.edu/hsc/info/pr/1vol1/ 120/epileptics.html. Accessed summer 2001.
5. Generalized epilepsy. Institute for Neurology and Neurosurgery at the Beth Israel

Medical Center, New York. Available at: http://www. nyneurosurgery.org/cfr/epilepsy/types/generalized.htm. Accessed summer 2001.
6. Epilepsy/seizures. NeurologyChannel; 1998–2001. Available at: http://www.neurologychannel.com/seizures/. Accessed summer 2001.

Sleep Disorders

1. Brain basics: Understanding sleep. National Institute of Neurological Disorders and Stroke (NINDS). Available at: http://www.ninds.nih. gov/health_and_medical/pubs/understanding_sleep_brain_basic_.htm?format=printable. Accessed summer 2001.
2. Excessive daytime sleepiness. National Sleep Foundation; 1999. Available at: http://www. sleepfoundation.org/epworth/quizfaq.htm. Accessed summer 2001.
3. WellConnected: Dealing with stress. Wellsource, Inc.; 1998. Available at: http://www.mcmc.net/wellsource/stress/sleep.htm. Accessed summer 2001.
4. Insomnia. InteliHealth Inc.; 1996–2001. Available at: http://www.intelihealth.com/IH/ihtIH/WSIHW000/24597/24598/213075.html?d=dmtContent. Accessed summer 2001.
5. Phalen KF. Treatment of choice. The Washington Post. July 4, 2000;Z19. Available at: http://www.washingtonpost.com/wp-dyn/articles/A43739-2000Jul4.html. Accessed summer 2001.
6. Melatonin. American Academy of Family Physicians; 199. Available at: http://familydoctor.org/handouts/258.html. Accessed summer 2001.
7. Restless legs syndrome. InteliHealth Inc.; 1996–2001. Available at: http://www.intelihealth. com/IH/ihtIH/WSIHW000/24597/24598/195958.html?d=dmtContent. Accessed summer 2001.
8. Sleep apnea. InteliHealth Inc.; 1996–2001. Available at: http://www.intelihealth.com/IH/ihtIH/WSIHW000/24597/24598/201604.html?d=dmtContent. Accessed summer 2001.
9. Scientists pinpoint possible cause for debilitating sleep disorder narcolepsy. National Institute of Neurological Disorders and Stroke (NINDS). Available at: http://www.ninds.nih.gov/news_and_events/pressrelease_narcolepsy_082900.htm?format=printable. Accessed summer 2001.
10. The nature of sleep. National Sleep Foundation. Available at: http://www.sleepfoundation. org/publications/nos.html. Accessed summer 2001.
11. What are periodic limb movements in sleep (PLMS)? National Sleep Foundation. Available at: http://www.sleepfoundation. org/publicationhttp://www.sleepfoundation.org/publications/fact_plms.htmls/fact_plms.html. Accessed summer 2001.

12. What is restless legs syndrome? National Sleep Foundation. Available at: http://www.sleepfoundation.org/publications/fact_rls.html. Accessed summer 2001.

13. When you can't sleep. American Academy of Family Physicians; 1999. Available at: http://www.aafp.org/afp/991001ap/991001c.html. Accessed summer 2001.

14. Fatigue: When to rest, when to worry. Mayo Foundation for Medical Education and Research; 2000. Available at: http://www.mayohealth.org/mayo/9906/htm/fatigue.htm. Accessed summer 2001.

15. Facts about drowsy driving. National Sleep Foundation. Available at: http://www.sleepfoundation.org/activities/daaafacts.html. Accessed summer 2001.

Circulatory System Conditions

CHAPTER OBJECTIVES

After reading this chapter, you should be able to . . .

- Name two deficiencies that may cause nutritional anemia.
- Name the only destination for loose blood clots in the venous system.
- Name three possible destinations for loose blood clots or other debris in the arterial system.
- Name two signs or symptoms of deep vein thrombosis.
- Name what tissue is damaged first with chronic hypertension.

- Name three risk factors for the development of atherosclerosis.
- Name the difference between primary and secondary Raynaud's Syndrome.
- Name two factors that determine the severity of a heart attack.
- Name the most common causative factor for right-sided heart failure.
- Name the incidence of death from cardiovascular disease in the United States.

INTRODUCTION

Most of the diseases that contraindicate massage do so because of the way the circulatory system works. This introduction provides a brief overview of how this system feeds, cleans, and protects the body, with emphasis on the aspects of the system that are relevant to the conditions listed in this chapter.

The body's cells are highly specialized and complex in their functioning and metabolism. The large majority of them are fixed, that is, they are immobile (unable to move *toward* nutrition or *away* from toxic wastes). They depend on the circulatory system for the constant delivery of food and fuel and the constant carrying away of garbage. Suppose a person needed someone to run to the grocery store for him, *and* to flush his toilets, *and* take out his trash. How long would the person last if these services were interrupted? Massage can sometimes interrupt or interfere with circulatory service. If a massage therapist is going to make wise choices about to whom and when to give massage, he or she *must* have a strong understanding of how massage affects the cardiovascular system.

General Function: The Circulatory System

The body depends on the process of *diffusion*, the random distribution of particles throughout an environment, for the exchange of nutrients and wastes. For diffusion to happen, there must be a medium, an environment, that allows substances to move freely. What could be better than the combination of blood and lymph? Humans contain about 6 gallons of *liquid*. In every milliliter of it, particles are flowing this way and that, chemicals are reacting, and *life* is happening.

The circulatory system, through the medium of the blood, works to *maintain homeostasis*, the *tendency to maintain a stable internal environment*. It does this in a number of different ways.

- *Delivery of nutrients and oxygen.* The blood carries nutrients and oxygen to every cell in the body. If for some reason the blood cannot reach a specific area, cells in that area will starve and die. This is the situation in many disorders, including *stroke* (Chapter 3), *heart attack* (this chapter), and *decubitus ulcers* (Chapter 1).

- *Removal of waste products.* While simultaneously dropping off nutrients, the blood, along with lymph, picks up the waste products generated by metabolism. These include carbon dioxide and other more noxious compounds that, left to stew in the tissues, can cause problems. Again, if blood and lymph supply to an area is limited, the affected cells can "drown" in their own waste products and be damaged or even die.

- *Maintenance of temperature.* Superficial blood vessels dilate when it is hot, and they constrict when it is cold. Furthermore, blood prevents the hot places (the heart, the liver, working muscles) from getting too hot by flushing through and distributing the heated blood throughout the rest of the body. By keeping a steady temperature, the circulatory system maintains a *stable internal environment.*

- *Maintenance of clotting.* This is an often overlooked but truly miraculous function of the circulatory system without which people would quickly die. Every time a rough place develops in the endothelium of a blood vessel, a whole chain of chemical reactions happens that results in the spinning of tiny fibers that catch cells to plug any possible gaps. Unfortunately, under certain circumstances, this reaction is sometimes more of a curse than a blessing.

- *Protection from pathogens.* Without white blood cells there would be no defense against the hordes of microorganisms that are longing to gain access to the body's precious (and precarious) internal environment. For a closer look at what actually happens to those would-be invaders, see the introduction to *Lymph/Immune Conditions* (Chapter 5).

- *Maintenance of chemical balance.* The body has a very narrow margin of tolerance for variances in internal chemistry. A person can actually die if his or her blood gets even fifteen one-hundredths too alkaline or too acidic. Happily, blood components, including RBCs are supplied with enzymes and other mechanisms specifically designed to keep pH balance within the safety zone.

Structure and Function: The Blood
Red Blood Cells (Erythrocytes)

Almost all the blood cells, red and white alike, are born in the red bone marrow. Red blood cells (RBCs), or erythrocytes, are created at the command of a hormone secreted by the kidneys called *erythropoietin.* RBCs constantly are being produced and dying, at a rate of about 2 million per second. They comprise 98% of all blood cells. Their life span is about 4 months, and during that time they do a single job: deliver oxygen to the cells and carbon dioxide to the lungs. They are so devoted to this task they have given up their nuclei to make more room to carry their cargo. (One indicator of disease is the presence of nuclei in RBCs; it means they are being released from the bone marrow prematurely).

RBCs are tiny; one cubic milliliter of blood holds about 5 million of them. They are built around an iron-based molecule called *hemoglobin.* This molecule (there are 250 million of them in each RBC) is extremely efficient at carrying oxygen, slightly less so at carrying carbon dioxide. Much of the carbon dioxide in blood is suspended in plasma, like a carbonated drink (this once prompted a student to ask why, when we jump up and down, don't we fizz up and explode?). Another key quality to healthy RBCs is their shape: they are discs that are thinner in the middle than around the edges. They are very smooth and should be flexible enough to bend and distort themselves to get through the tiniest capillaries. If for some reason they are not round, smooth, and flexible, big problems ensue.

White Blood Cells (Leukocytes)

White blood cells (WBCs), or leukocytes, are not really white. They are more or less translucent. Unlike RBCs, which are all identical, different classes of WBCs fight off different types of invaders in different stages of infection. Types of WBCs include neutrophils, basophils, eosinophils, monocytes, and lymphocytes (Fig. 4-1). These are discussed in more detail in *Lymph/Immune System Conditions* (Chapter 5).

Platelets (Thrombocytes)

Platelets (thrombocytes) are not whole cells at all, but fragments of huge cells that are born in the red bone marrow. *Thrombo* means clot, and *cyte* means cell, so it is clear what thrombocytes do. As stated above, thrombocytes have the job of going through the system looking for leaks or rough places in the blood vessels. If they should find one, a series of chemical reactions occurs, which causes tiny threads of fibrin, a special protein, to be woven in the injured area. These act as a net to catch not only passing thrombocytes, but passing RBCs as well, forming a *crust* if it is on the skin or a *clot (thrombus)* if it is internal. This is a good thing. Clotting is very important and usually not a problem because other chemicals that *melt* clots also circulate in the blood; these are called *anticoagulants*. However, under certain circumstances this clotting mechanism has cause to overwork, which ultimately can become life threatening.

Structure and Function: The Heart

The heart is divided into left and right halves. The right half pumps blood to the lungs (the pulmonary circuit), while the left half pumps to the rest of the body (the systemic cir-

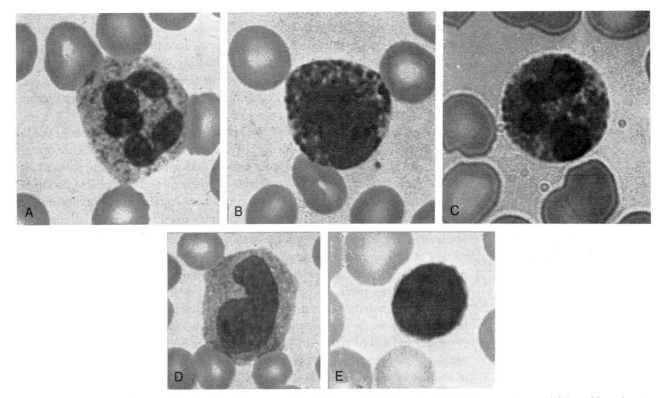

Figure 4-1. Varieties of white blood cells: (**A**) neutrophils, (**B**) basophil, (**C**) eosinophil, (**D**) monocyte, and (**E**) and lymphocyte

cuit). Each half of the heart is further divided into top and bottom. The small top chambers, where blood returning from the lungs and body enters, are called the atria (the singular form is *atrium* from the Latin for *entrance hall*), and the larger bottom chambers are the ventricles (from the Latin for *belly*). One-way valves separate the atria from the ventricles (the atrioventricular valves) and the ventricles from the blood vessels they pump into (the semilunar valves). The two part "lub-dup" of the heartbeat is produced by the closure of the atrioventricular valves first and the semilunar valves second.

The cardiac muscle of the atria is much thinner and weaker than that of the ventricles. This is because the atrial contraction needs to push blood only a few centimeters downhill into the ventricles. The cardiac muscle of the ventricles, however, is much thicker and stronger than that found in the atria, because the ventricular contraction pushes blood out into the circulatory system—through the pulmonary circuit to the lungs from the right ventricle, and through the systemic circuit to the rest of the body from the left ventricle. The differences in how hard various parts of the heart have to work have great implications for the seriousness of myocardial infarctions (heart attacks)—the location of the dead tissue determines how well the heart will function without it.

Structure and Function: Blood Vessels

The vessels *leaving* the heart are called *arteries* and *arterioles;* the vessels *going toward* the heart are called *venules* and *veins;* the vessels that connect them are called *capillaries.* Ideally this should be a closed system, that is, although WBCs are free to come and go through capillary walls, the RBCs should never be able to leave the 60,000 miles of continuous tubing that comprises the circulatory system. If they *do* leak out, it is because the system has an injury, and a blood clot should be forming.

Arteries and veins share the same basic properties of most of the tubes in the body. They have an internal layer of epithelium (called *endo*thelium here, because it is on the inside), a middle layer of smooth muscle, and an external layer of tough, protective connective tissue. This combination of tissues makes these tubes strong, pliable, and stretchy.

Capillaries are delicate variations of basic tube construction. As the arteries divide into smaller arterioles their outer layers get thinner and thinner. Finally, all that is left is one layer of simple, squamous epithelium: the capillaries. This construction is ideal for the passage of substances back and forth, because most diffusion happens readily through single-cell layers. Because capillaries lack the tougher muscle and connective tissue layers of the larger tubes, they are much more vulnerable to injury.

Blood cells leave the heart through the thick-walled arteries, crowd into arterioles, and line up one-by-one to squeeze through the capillaries. Once they have dumped their cargo of oxygen and picked up their carbon dioxide, they have more breathing room; now they are in the venules. Again the three-ply construction design is present, but with a difference. Much of the venous system operates against gravity. Blood flows upward in the legs, the arms, and the trunk partly by indirect pressure exerted by the heart on the arterial system, but also with the help of hydrostatic pressure and muscular contraction. To help the blood move along without backing up in the system, small epithelial flaps or *valves* line the veins. The smooth muscle layer here is present, but thinner and weaker than in the arteries, which have to cope with much higher pressure coming directly from the heart. Veins get wider, bigger, and stronger as they approach the heart, but they are never as strong as arteries. Fortunately, the force with which blood moves through them is never as strong either.

When blood returns from the body to the heart (the systemic circuit) it then goes to the lungs to be re-oxygenated (the pulmonary circuit) (Fig. 4-2). This chapter is the most self-referential portion of this book. Most of the conditions discussed here are caused by or are complications of (or both) other conditions in this chapter.

Circulatory System Conditions

Blood Disorders
Anemia
Embolism, Thrombus
Hematoma
Hemophilia
Leukemia
Thrombophlebitis, Deep Vein Thrombosis

Vascular Disorders
Aneurysm
Atherosclerosis
Hypertension
Raynaud's Syndrome
Varicose Veins

Heart Conditions
Heart Attack
Heart Failure

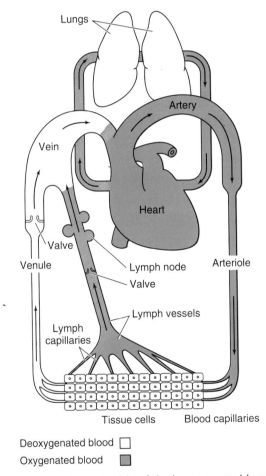

Deoxygenated blood ☐
Oxygenated blood ▨

Figure 4-2. The right side of the heart pumps blood to the lungs in the pulmonary circuit; the left side of the heart pumps blood through the rest of the body in the systemic circuit

Blood Disorders

Anemia

Definition: What Is It?

Anemia is the condition of having either an insufficient supply of RBCs, or an insufficient or somehow functionally impaired supply of hemoglobin within those cells, or both. In any case, "anemia" all by itself is not a diagnosis; it is a description. The diagnosis comes when one determines *why* a shortage of RBCs or hemoglobin has developed.

Etiology: What Happens?

Several different kinds of anemia are possible, each with different guidelines for treatment and the appropriateness of massage. Some of the most common varieties are examined here, with discussions of what is really happening in the body and how massage might positively or negatively affect it.

Idiopathic Anemias   These conditions, which have no well-understood cause, may be due to poor nutritional uptake because of how stress affects gastric juices, or to other more mysterious factors. Once other pathologies are ruled out, these anemias (which are usually comparatively mild) may respond well to massage.

Nutritional Anemias   These anemias occur because the body is missing something vital in its diet and no amount of massage, no matter how brilliantly administered, will replace it. However, most of these conditions will not be negatively affected by massage. The only exception to this rule is advanced cases of pernicious anemia.

- *Iron deficiency anemia.* Iron is the primary component of hemoglobin. An insufficiency of iron in the diet will lead to insufficiencies of hemoglobin and then to pathologically small RBCs and "iron poor blood." Iron deficiency anemia is the most common variety of anemia. It can come about from diets that are poor in iron, an inability to absorb iron from digestion, chronic bleeding, or lead poisoning. Iron deficiency anemia is estimated to affect about 2 in every 1000 Americans and up to half of all pregnant women.

- *Folic acid deficiency anemia.* Folic acid is a nutrient found in green leafy vegetables that is absolutely critical to the formation of RBCs. If a person does not get enough, it is impossible to produce the 2 million cells per second that it takes to keep up with the cells that are dying. Folic acid is also water-soluble. That means it cannot be stored for later use; a steady fresh supply is necessary. Folic acid anemia is usually related to dietary insufficiencies or malabsorption (often due to alcoholism or celiac sprue). It affects about 4 in every 100,000 Americans.

- B_{12} *deficiency anemia.* Vitamin B_{12}, or cobalamin, is another critical ingredient for the making of new RBCs. It comes *only* in animal food sources: meat and eggs. Vegans must supplement their B_{12} supply or they could end up with the much more serious *pernicious anemia.*

- *Pernicious anemia.* Of all the nutritional anemias, this is the most serious because it can lead to irreversible damage to the central nervous system. Vitamin B_{12} is necessary for the formation of RBCs. Very few people in the United States have a B_{12} deficiency, yet pernicious anemia does occur. This is because in order to *absorb* B_{12}, a special chemical in gastric secretions called *intrinsic factor* is needed. Without it a person may take in all the B_{12} he or she requires, but the body has no access to it, and the person will not produce enough erythrocytes to keep up with the body's needs.

  The causes behind reductions in intrinsic factor are not always understood. Genetic tendencies, alcoholism, tapeworms, and *Crohn's disease* (Chapter 7) may all interfere with intrinsic factor activity. Most often, though, it happens when some section of the stomach is surgically removed because of another condition. Whatever the reason, once it is gone, it is gone for good, and the affected person faces a lifetime commitment to supplementing B_{12} by injection.

  This pales in comparison to the alternative, however. B_{12} is also critical to the maintenance of the central nervous system. Without it, a person will experience the slow onset of paralysis and brain damage. This is often irreversible, and it contraindicates massage, especially if there is any impairment in sensation.

- *Other nutritional deficiencies.* Anemia can be the result of shortages of several other substances, notably copper and protein. Massage will not improve this condition, and if it is very advanced (with extreme shortness of breath, fatigue, and low stamina) massage could possibly tax the already overworking heart in a dangerous way. Anemia this advanced is relatively rare, however.

Hemorrhagic Anemias   Hemorrhagic anemias are those brought about by blood loss. It is usually from a slow leak, but occasionally it is from some trauma; this would be acute hemorrhagic anemia. The most common causes for hemorrhagic anemia are *ulcers* (Chapter 7), heavy menstruation, and large wounds. Obviously, bleeding ulcers and large wounds contraindicate rigorous circulatory massage. Heavy menstruation would not be badly affected unless the therapist worked deeply in the abdomen during flow, but it is a sign that something may be wrong, and the client should consult with her health care team to rule out other disorder like *endometriosis* or *fibroid tumors* (Chapter 10).

Hemolytic Anemias   These are a group of anemias that involve the premature destruction of healthy RBCs. In addition to the basic symptoms of anemia, splenomegaly will be present. This is the abnormal growth of the spleen as it works overtime to process all those dying RBCs. Another sign of hemolytic anemia is the presence of *reticulocytes* in the blood. These are simply immature RBCs that have not yet lost their nucleus and therefore are not equipped to carry the load of a normal mature cell. Reticulocytes are released from the bone marrow when it is sensed that the supply of erythrocytes is getting dangerously low.

In hemolytic anemias the RBCs may die for a variety of reasons, but they all leave their membrane or "ghost" behind while their hemoglobin leaks into the blood instead of being processed in the liver as it is supposed to. One consequence of this is the additional risk of blood clotting because of extra debris in the stream (see *thrombi*, this chapter). Furthermore, all that extra hemoglobin in the blood will break down into bilirubin, which may result in *jaundice*, which is a condition that can have a profound effect on the liver (see Chapter 7).

Causes of hemolytic anemia range from genetics (sickle cell anemia is an example of this), to allergic reactions to certain drugs, to malaria.

Sickle cell anemia is a special type of hemolytic anemia in which the hemoglobin molecules (250 million in each red blood cell) are not normal. They deteriorate after delivering their load of oxygen, which eventually leads to the collapse of the cell into the characteristic "sickle" shape (Fig. 4-3). Symptoms and complications of sickle cell anemia include blood that is viscous and prone to clotting; joint pain; *meningitis, seizures,* and *stroke* (all in Chapter 3); and several varieties of organ damage from blockages caused by blood clots. Trauma or infection can bring on extremely painful sickle cell "crises" when the body may experience yet more damage from the sticky, lumpy blood flow. Sickle cell anemia has no cure; treatment is limited to addressing the symptoms. The average age of death for men with sickle cell anemia is 42; for women it is 46.

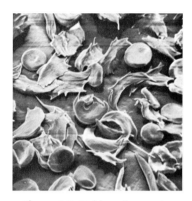

Figure 4-3. Sickle cell anemia

Any kind of hemolytic anemia contraindicates circulatory massage.

Aplastic Anemia   In aplastic anemia, bone marrow activity is sluggish or even nonexistent. The production of every kind of blood cell is slowed or suspended. When this moment's 2 million cells report to the spleen for destruction, no new RBC replacements are available. Likewise, no new WBCs are manufactured, so resistance to infection is impaired. Finally, the stream of thrombocytes has dried up too, making persons with aplastic anemia prone to uncontrolled bleeding.

Aplastic anemia can be caused by bone marrow tumors, autoimmune disease, renal failure, folate deficiency, certain viral infections, exposure to some types of radiation, and some poisons. Bone marrow transplants have proven fairly successful at solving the problem if it is caught early. See more under *leukemia* in this chapter.

Secondary Anemias   Anemia is a frequent complication of other disorders. Sometimes a direct cause-and-effect relationship is obvious, and sometimes the association is less clear but still present. The following is a partial list of some of the conditions that anemia frequently accompanies.

- *Ulcers.* Gastric, duodenal, and colonic ulcers can all bleed internally. This might not be very obvious but results in a steady draining of RBCs, which can impair general oxygen uptake and energy levels. This is a type of *hemorrhagic anemia,* discussed above.

- *Kidney disease.* The capillaries inside the kidneys have a tremendous workload. Not only are they filtering toxins and maintaining water balance, they are doing it under tremendous mechanical pressure from the renal arteries. Sometimes the kidney capillaries get damaged and leak RBCs into the urine. Again, it is a leak not a gush, but just as that dripping faucet will drive up a person's water bill, a leaking kidney will slowly but surely drain away viable RBCs.

    Furthermore, the kidneys secrete the hormone (erythropoietin, or EPO) that stimulates bone marrow to produce RBCs. When the kidneys are not functioning well, EPO levels drop, and RBC production goes down. See more on kidney dysfunction in Chapter 9.

- *Hepatitis.* The liver contributes vital proteins to the blood and is responsible, with the spleen, for breaking down and recycling the hemoglobin from dead erythrocytes. If liver function is disrupted for any reason, the quality and amount of hemoglobin available to new RBCs may suffer (see *hepatitis,* Chapter 7).

- *Acute infectious disease.* Anemia is sometimes a sign or indicator that the body is under attack. It is a frequent follower of pneumonia, tuberculosis, and rheumatoid arthritis. Infectious disorders often cause iron to be used elsewhere in the body, reducing the amount of hemoglobin available to new RBCs. Anemia in these cases usually clears up spontaneously once the primary condition has been resolved.

Signs and Symptoms

No matter what the cause, some signs and symptoms of anemia are consistent. These include:

- *Pallor.* Pallor is present because there is either a reduced amount of RBCs or a reduced amount of hemoglobin to carry the oxygen that gives the RBCs their color. Pallor is visible in the skin and also in mucous membranes, gums, and nail beds. In dark-skinned people, pallor shows as an ashy-gray appearance to the skin.

- *Dyspnea.* This is a fancy way of saying shortness of breath. This a symptom of anemia because with less oxygen carrying capacity, a person has to breathe harder and more often just to keep up. Another sign of anemia is a higher than normal respiratory rate.

- *Palpitations.* This does not mean the heart is beating irregularly; it means it is probably beating faster and harder, and a person is more *aware* of it. Another term for this is *tachycardia.*

- *Fatigue.* This is often the first noticeable symptom of anemia. Less oxygen is available to go around, so muscles wear out sooner, and stamina is nonexistent. Unfortunately, a host of other conditions may make a person feel worn out, so this is rarely enough to go on for a whole diagnosis.

- *Intolerance to cold.* Oxygen is needed for muscle contraction and for heat production (shivering). Someone who is in short supply of oxygen will run out of steam in a hurry.

Sickle Cell Anemia and Malaria: A Close Connection

A person will have sickle cell anemia if he or she inherits a gene for it from *both* parents. If a person inherits only one gene, that person is said to have the sickle cell *trait*, but not the disease. This is a crucial distinction because the sickle cell trait will usually *not* create any negative impact on the body, although some people experience mild anemia. However, the presence of this one gene *will* limit the rupturing of erythrocytes during an attack of malaria. Sickle cell genes are mostly found in populations (and descendants of populations) from the Mediterranean, subtropical Africa, and Asia—otherwise called the *malarial belt.* Isn't it an amazing world?

Massage?

The appropriateness of massage for clients with anemia varies according to the cause. Massage has been seen to increase RBC count, at least temporarily, but this is probably due to the action of pushing RBCs that were moving sluggishly back into circulation; these effects do not tend to last very long. Massage certainly will not provide needed nutrients, but the resulting parasympathetic response may improve uptake in the digestive system.

Anemia contraindicates massage when it accompanies other disorders that may be negatively affected. Specifically, if pernicious anemia has resulted in a decrease in sensation, or if the anemia were present because of acute infection, circulatory massage would be inappropriate.

Very advanced anemia of any kind is fairly rare. However, if the blood is especially low in hemoglobin or oxygen, the heart has to work extremely hard to pump the diminished supply through the body. For this reason, very advanced anemia of any kind contraindicates rigorous circulatory massage.

Embolism, Thrombus
Definition: What Are They?

An embolism is a traveling clot or collection of debris, and thrombus is a lodged clot (Fig. 4-4). Emboli and thrombi that form on the arterial side of the systemic circuit are part and parcel of the whole interrelated cardiovascular disease picture. Having them can cause heart trouble, and heart trouble can cause them.

Etiology: What Happens?

Blood leaves the left ventricle of the heart via the aorta and goes to its destination through smaller and smaller vessels: arteries, arterioles, and finally capillaries. Nutrient–waste exchange happens at the capillary level, and then the vessels get bigger and bigger as they zoom back toward the right atrium: venules, veins, and the vena cava. The same telescoping action happens in the pulmonary circuit: blood leaves the right ventricle through the huge pulmonary artery, and vessels going into the lungs get smaller and smaller. Oxygen and carbon dioxide are exchanged through capillaries in the lungs, and the freshly oxygenated blood goes back toward the heart through venules, veins, and finally the large pulmonary vein (Fig. 4-2).

Jagged-edged platelets constantly flow through the circulatory system looking for rough spots, which indicate injury. If they find anything to stick to (i.e., a disruption in the walls of the blood vessels), they will. Then they start releasing the chemicals that cause blood proteins to weave fibers, making a net to catch other blood cells, and a clot is formed. Clots can also form in places where blood does not flow quickly; the clotting factors will accumulate enough to thicken the fluid even without having platelets to initiate the action.

The construction of the circulatory system is such that clots cannot pass through capillaries; they either form on the arterial side of the systemic circuit or on the venous side. The kind of damage that ensues depends on the origin of the clot, its size, and where it finally gets stuck.

Pulmonary Embolism   The lungs are the one and only destination for clots formed anywhere on the venous side of the systemic circuit. When something, usually a sudden movement after prolonged immobility, knocks any clot in any vein loose, it will jet toward the heart in increasingly bigger tubes. It will make the rounds of the right atrium and ventricle, get into the pulmonary artery, and end up in the lungs. The extent of damage can vary from a temporary loss of a tiny bit of lung function to total circulatory collapse when suddenly little or no blood returns to the heart from the lungs.

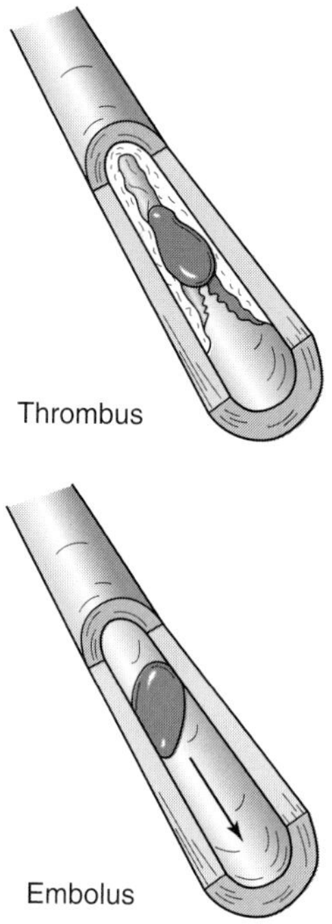

Every year about 600,000 people in the United States have a pulmonary embolism. Many of them resolve spontaneously, but anywhere from 50,000 to 200,000 people die of pulmonary embolism every year. This condition is usually related to *thrombophlebitis* or *deep vein thrombosis* (this chapter) that develops as a complication of surgery or trauma.

Risk Factors.   Risk factors for pulmonary embolism include other types of cardiovascular disease, recent trauma, extended bed rest, taking oral contraceptives, and any kind of surgery, although surgeries for femur and hip fractures have a particularly high embolism rate.

Women in advanced stages of *pregnancy* (Chapter 10) or who have recently given birth are also at high risk for pulmonary embolism, as the weight of the uterus on the femoral vessels can cause blood to pool and thicken in the legs, and hormonal changes associated with pregnancy and childbirth can also cause the blood to thicken.

Signs and Symptoms.   Some studies estimate that up to 80% of all pulmonary embolism cases show no discernible signs or symptoms until after lung damage has

---

EMBOLISM, THROMBUS IN BRIEF

What are they?
Thrombi are stationary clots; emboli are clots that travel through the circulatory system. Emboli are usually composed of blood, but may also be fragments of plaque, fat globules, air bubbles, tumors, or bone chips.

How are they recognized?
If venous thrombi break loose or *embolize*, they can only land in the lungs, causing pulmonary embolism. Symptoms of pulmonary embolism include shortness of breath, chest pain, and coughing up sputum that is streaked with blood. Many venous thrombi and pulmonary emboli are silent, that is, they cause no symptoms until the damage has been done.

Clots that form on the arterial side of the system can lodge anywhere their artery carries them. Some of the most common (and dangerous) locations for arterial clots to land are in the coronary arteries (heart attack), the brain (transient ischemic attack or stroke), and the kidneys (renal infarction).

Is massage indicated or contraindicated?
Any disorder than involves the potential for lodged or traveling clots contraindicates circulatory massage.

Thrombus

Embolus

Figure 4-4. A thrombus is a lodged clot; an embolus is a moving clot

occurred. Classic symptoms of pulmonary embolism include difficulty breathing, chest pains, and coughing with bloody sputum. Other symptoms that may be present are shortness of breath, lightheadedness, fainting, dizziness, rapid heartbeat, and sweating.

Treatment.   Treatment of non-life threatening pulmonary embolism situations is usually an aggressive course of anticoagulants and attention to the cause of the deep vein thrombosis. If it is a major embolism, surgery may be required to vacuum it out of the lung.

Prevention.   Pulmonary embolism is the leading cause of death due to surgical complication. Because this condition is very difficult to diagnose early, emphasis has shifted from treatment to prophylaxis, or prevention. Preventive measures include identifying patients who are at particularly high risk for developing clots, administering low-dose anti-coagulants starting shortly before surgery, having the patient wear tight stockings on the legs, elevating the legs, providing external compression on the legs, and providing early ambulation following surgery.

Arterial Embolism   This is one of the many complications of *atherosclerosis* (this chapter). Emboli in the arteries can also be a complication of bacterial infection, atrial fibrillation, or rheumatic heart disease, which can create clots inside the heart. Emboli can be made of some foreign object in the bloodstream like a bit of plaque, a bone chip, an air bubble or a knot of cancer cells.

The main difference between arterial emboli and venous ones is the final resting place. If the clot is somewhere in the systemic arterial system it could wind up virtually anywhere *except* the lungs. Therefore, the damage it will cause will be very different. The brain, the heart, the kidneys, and the legs are statistically the most common sites for arterial emboli to lodge.

Signs and Symptoms.   Symptoms of emboli in organs may be nonexistent until the affected tissue has significant loss of function. This is particularly dangerous in the kidneys, where many tiny clots can come to rest somewhere in the renal arteries, leading to progressive *renal failure* (Chapter 9). If clots lodge in the legs, however, symptoms will involve sharp, tingling pain, followed by numbness, weakness, coldness, and blueness. Left untreated, this tissue may become necrotic (i.e., it will start to die) in a matter of hours; immediate medical attention is necessary.

If the embolus lodges in the brain, it is called a *transient ischemic attack* if the symptoms are short-lived and a *stroke* (Chapter 3) if they are more serious. Finally, if it lodges in a coronary artery it is called a *heart attack* (this chapter).

Treatment.   If a person has a tendency to form clots easily, anticoagulant medications may be prescribed to circumvent the complications of heart attack or stroke.

Massage?

The tendency to form thrombi or emboli is a situation that systemically contraindicates rigorous circulatory massage. Lodged thrombi are a medical emergency. *If* a person knows an embolism is present in either the venous or arterial sides of the system, he or she should be under strict treatment. Clients who take anticoagulant medications require extra care from massage therapists, who must chose techniques that will not run the risk of overchallenging the circulatory system.

Hematoma
Definition: What Is It?

Technically, hematoma refers to extensive bleeding and pooling of blood between muscle sheaths. The simple leakage of blood from damaged capillaries that causes the familiar discoloration of the skin known as a bruise is called *ecchymosis*. Although the size and seriousness of these two conditions vary widely, their treatment guidelines are very much the same, so they will be considered together here.

Signs and Symptoms

Bruises are reddish or purplish (or black and blue) in the acute stage. They fade to yellowish green in the subacute stage, when the local macrophages have migrated in to clean up the debris. The processes for cleaning up capillary leaks deeper than the skin, for instance in a gastrocnemius that has been kicked, are invisible but otherwise identical.

Larger bleeds can involve quite a bit of inflammation along with discoloration. They can occur when an arteriole between deep muscle layers is injured. It will pour blood into an area until local pressure closes it off. A large acute hematoma feels like hot, half-congealed gelatin under the muscle layers, and it will be quite painful to the touch. They happen most often in large fleshy areas like the calf or buttocks.

A special variety of hematomas, subdural hematomas, happen in the brain; this is covered in *strokes* (Chapter 3).

Treatment

Small bruises require no medical intervention, although they respond well to alternating hot and cold applications, which stimulate macrophages to come into the area and flush wastes from the tissue damage away. Larger bleeds, however, can be more complicated. If they are caught relatively early they can be aspirated or drained, but if they're left too long they will have a tendency to congeal from the concentration of clotting factors in the blood. At that point only time, hydrotherapy, and gentle movement will help to break up the pooled blood into a form the body can reabsorb. An occasional complication of hematoma is *myositis ossificans* (Chapter 2).

Massage?

Hematomas and bruises contraindicate local massage in the acute stage because of pain and the possibility of disturbing blood clots. In the subacute stages (at least 2 days after the injury occurs) the local blood vessels will be sealed off. Gentle massage may be appropriate around the edges of the lesions, always within the tolerance of the client.

Hemophilia
Definition: What Is It?

This is a genetic disorder involving the absence of some plasma proteins that are crucial in the clot-forming process. Anyone who has studied Russian history has at least a vague idea about this disease. The last ruling family in Russia, the Romanovs, had it in their genes, and because it weakened the Royal Family, hemophilia changed the course oworld history.

Hemophilia is actually a collection of different types of genetic disorders, each one of them affecting a different clotting factor in the blood. Their presentations are all much the same, however, so the only people who need to know *which* type of hemophilia is

---

HEMATOMA IN BRIEF

What is it?
A hematoma is a deep bruise (leakage of blood) between muscle sheaths.

How is it recognized?
Superficial hematomas are simple bruises. Deep bleeds may not be visible but will be painful. If extensive bleeding has occurred, a characteristic "gel-like" feel will develop in the affected tissue.

Is massage Indicated or contraindicated?
Massage is at least locally contraindicated for acute hematomas because of the possibility of blood clots and pain. In the subacute stage (at least 2 days after the injury has occurred) when the surrounding blood vessels have been sealed shut and the body is in the process of breaking down and reabsorbing the debris, gentle massage around the perimeter of the area and hydrotherapy can be helpful.

HEMOPHILIA IN BRIEF

What is it?
Hemophilia is a genetic disorder in which certain clotting factors in the blood are either inactive or missing.

How is it recognized?
Hemophilia can cause superficial bleeding that persists for longer than normal or internal bleeding into joint cavities or between muscle sheaths with little or no provocation.

Is massage indicated or contraindicated?
Severe cases of hemophilia contraindicate bodywork that can mechanically stretch, manipulate, or accidentally injure delicate tissues. Milder cases of hemophilia may be safer for circulatory massage.

present are the patients themselves and the people who administer clotting factors after a bleeding episode.

Demographics: Who Gets It?

In the United States hemophilia affects about 15,000 men. The incidence is about 1 in every 10,000 males, and the disease appears equally among races and socioeconomic statuses. The disease is carried on the X chromosome of female genes, so female carriers pass the mutation on to their sons. It is possible that a girl could have hemophilia, if she got a positive X chromosome from both her father and mother, but this is a rare circumstance.

Etiology: What Happens?

Thrombocytes constantly cruise around the circulatory system looking for signs of damage. When they encounter any kind of rough spot inside a blood vessel, they stick to that spot and secrete a series of chemicals that cause plasma proteins to weave nets of fibers called *fibrinogen*. These nets then catch passing platelets and RBCs, forming a plug to limit loss of blood through the damaged vessel. The plasma proteins that weave the fi-brinogen have been identified as 12 distinct factors. Hemophilia occurs when a genetic mutation causes a deficiency in one or more of these clotting factors.

The most common variety of hemophilia is hemophilia A, which accounts for approximately 80% of all cases. It involves a deficiency in clotting factor VIII. Hemophilia B, also called Christmas disease, involves insufficient levels of factor IX. Hemophilia B affects about 15% of all hemophilia cases. Other clotting factor deficiencies are possible, but they are much more rare than hemophilia A or B.

If a person is deficient in clotting factor VIII, IX, or both, he will have difficulty in forming a solid, long-lasting clot. Hemophiliacs do not bleed *faster* than normal but they do bleed *longer*. Hemophilia is rated as mild, moderate, or severe depending on what percentage of normal levels of clotting factors the patient has. Severe hemophiliacs, who account for 60% of all hemophilia patients, have lower than 1% of normal levels of clotting factors.

Signs and Symptoms

Hemophilia first appears in early childhood, as babies begin to engage in physical activities that can involve mild bruising. These babies experience extensive bruising and bleeding with very mild irritation, and small scrapes and lesions tend to bleed for a long time.

As the person matures he will find that he is prone to subcutaneous bleeding (bruising), intramuscular hemorrhaging (see *hematoma*, this chapter), nosebleeds, blood in the urine (hematuria), and severe joint pain brought about by bleeding in joint cavities. Bleeding episodes may follow minor trauma or may occur spontaneously.

Complications

Bleeding into joint cavities is the main problem for people with hemophilia. Unless clotting factors are administered very soon after an episode, the blood inside the joint may collect and become very difficult for the body to reabsorb. This can lead to debilitating *arthritis* (Chapter 2).

Infected blood products have been another major worry for people with hemophilia. Before proper screening methods were used consistently, contracting human immuno-deficiency virus (HIV) was a significant risk for hemophiliacs. *Hepatitis* (Chapter 7) is another potential problem for people who receive blood products. Blood and plasma screening techniques are successful at filtering out most kinds of hepatitis viruses, but hepatitis A and hepatitis G can still get through. Hemophiliacs and other people who rely on blood products are recommended to be vaccinated against hepatitis A and B.

von Willebrand's Disease: An Equal Opportunity Mutation

The kinds of hemophilia that most people are familiar with involve X-linked genes that affect clotting factors VII or XI. However, these types of hemophilia affect a relatively small proportion of the population. It turns out that another type of genetic mutation causes another type of clotting factor deficiency, and it is *not* on the X chromosome, which means men and women can be affected equally.

The condition is called von Willebrand's disease, and it involves a deficiency or poor quality of von Willebrand factor: one of the last clotting factors to participate in the cascade of chemical reactions that cause the spinning of fibrinogen to make blood clots. Von Willebrand's disease is the most common type of genetically linked bleeding disorder in the world.

Von Willebrand's disease is usually very mild. Signs and symptoms include frequent bloody noses, bleeding from the gums, and, in women, heavy menstrual flow. A person may never be diagnosed until he or she has a tooth pulled, goes through childbirth, or undergoes some other experience that can lead to prolonged bleeding.

If a client knows he or she has von Willebrand's disease, no special precautions need to be taken for massage, other than to avoid bruises and other lesions—but these are precautions for all clients.

Treatment

Treatment protocols for people with hemophilia have taken gigantic leaps forward in the past 30 years. Before 1965, the only treatment available was transfusions of whole blood: a time-consuming and inefficient means of replacing clotting factors for someone experiencing internal hemorrhage. Consequently, most hemophiliacs were in wheelchairs by their teens, and their life expectancy was much shorter than the norm. In 1965 techniques were developed to isolate the specific missing clotting factors, allowing a much more efficient treatment. More recently, these clotting factors have been manufactured in a form that can be self-administered, which radically increases a hemophiliac's independence and ability to work and travel.

While the plasma products that are processed into concentrated clotting factor are as free from contaminants as it is possible to make them, another option is being explored with recombinant clotting factors. These are clotting factor proteins that have been genetically engineered from human and non-human DNA. Because they do not involve the use of blood or blood products, the risk of contamination with infectious diseases is eliminated.

Another step forward in hemophilia management has been the possibility of taking clotting factors prophylactically, just in case a spontaneous or trauma-related bleeding episode takes place. This is still a new option, and it remains to be seen whether taking clotting factors regularly will reduce the incidence of spontaneous bleeds and joint damage.

Massage?

Severe hemophilia contraindicates rigorous, mechanical, circulatory massage. People who have been diagnosed with mild or moderate cases should consult with their medical team about receiving bodywork. Although the mechanisms that cause spontaneous bleeds in hemophiliacs are largely unknown, massage therapists should not put themselves in the position of being even indirectly responsible for tissue damage to a client. Energetic and noncirculatory techniques may be appropriate and welcome.

Leukemia

Definition: What Is It?

Leukemia, or "white blood," is a cancer of WBCs that are produced in bone marrow. This distinguishes it from *lymphoma*, which is a cancer involving WBCs produced in lymph nodes. Lymphoma is discussed in Chapter 5.

Dozens of types of leukemia have been identified, but the four most common varieties are the focus of this section. These types of leukemia have much in common, but each has some unique features.

Etiology: What Happens in All Types of Leukemia?

White Blood Cells   All healthy RBCs and thrombocytes are virtually indistinguishable from each other. They look alike, they act alike, and they all perform the same function. The same cannot be said for WBCs. Leukocytes come in several shapes and sizes, each with a specific role to play in the effort to keep the body free from potential invaders.

Most WBCs are born in bone marrow. They develop from nonspecific stem cells into whatever type of cell is needed at the moment. WBCs from bone marrow fall into three categories: granulocytes, monocytes, and lymphocytes.

- *Granulocytes* are WBCs with *granules*—small spots that can be seen under microscopic examination. The WBCs known as neutrophils, basophils, and eosinophils are all types of granulocytes. They circulate through the bloodstream, looking for signs of invasion. They are often the first on the scene of new infections.

- *Monocytes* are closely related to granulocytes but behave differently. As monocytes mature, they migrate to tissues all around the body. They leave the circulatory system and enter their target tissues to become *macrophages*, or "big eaters."

- *Lymphocytes* are B-cells, T-cells, or natural killer cells, all of which are involved in specific immune system responses. Some lymphocytes are produced in lymphoid tissue, but some are produced in bone marrow. When bone marrow lymphocytes become cancerous, it is considered leukemia rather than lymphoma.

Types of Leukemia

Leukocytes are classified as *myeloid cells* (granulocytes and monocytes) or *lymphoid cells* (lymphocytes). Leukemia occurs when a mutation in the DNA of one or more stem cells in the bone marrow causes the production of multitudes of non-functioning leukocytes. These leukemia cells can crowd out the functioning cells in the bone marrow and in the blood. Leukemia can be aggressive and quickly progressive, involving the release of immature cells into the circulatory system ("acute"), or it can be slowly progressive, leading to the release of mature but non-functioning cells ("chronic"). The four most common varieties of leukemia are:

- *Acute myelogenous leukemia* (AML). Aggressive cancer of the myeloid class of cells (granulocytes or monocytes).

- *Chronic myelogenous leukemia* (CML). Slowly progressive cancer of the myeloid class of cells.

- *Acute lymphocytic leukemia* (ALL). Aggressive cancer of the lymphocytes (B-cells, T-cells, or natural killer cells).

- *Chronic lymphocytic leukemia* (CLL). Slowly progressive cancer of the lymphocytes.

Each of these is discussed in detail below.

a diferencia de

Unlike many types of cancer, leukemia spreads through the blood rather than the lymph. It can cause tumors in the lymph nodes (although not as readily as lymphoma) and also affects the liver, spleen, and central nervous system.

Left untreated, leukemia will result in death, usually from excessive bleeding or infection.

Signs and Symptoms of All Types of Leukemia

Signs and symptoms of all types of leukemia point back to bone marrow dysfunction. When the marrow is sabotaged by a genetic mutation that causes the overproduction of non-functioning cells, then functioning cells are produced in smaller numbers, if at all. A leading sign of leukemia is fatigue and low stamina due to *anemia* (this chapter): low numbers of RBCs are available to deliver oxygen to working tissues. A person with leukemia will often bruise easily, or he or she may experience bruises with no particular trauma. Small cuts and abrasions may bleed for long periods. Unusual bleeding or bruising comes about because platelet production is suppressed, and the person has limited ability to make blood clots. Finally, a person with leukemia will be susceptible to chronic infections—these can be skin infections like hangnails or pimples, or they can be respiratory infections like colds and flu. They can even be chronic urinary tract infections. Whatever the infectious agent, the person with leukemia has very limited resources to fight it because functioning WBCs are in short supply.

Other signs and symptoms of leukemia are unique to each type, and so are discussed in their individual sections.

Diagnosis

All types of leukemia are diagnosed by a combination of blood tests and bone marrow examinations. It is important to find out exactly which kinds of cells have been affected, and whether the cancer is an acute or chronic variety. Furthermore, each type of leukemia has subtypes that will respond differently to various treatment options.

Treatment of All Types of Leukemia

Chemotherapy   Leukemia treatment depends to a certain extent on what types of cells have been affected, how aggressive the disease is, and what kinds of treatments the patient has already undergone. Treatment usually begins with chemotherapy: the introduction of chemicals that are highly toxic to any cells that reproduce rapidly. Exactly which chemotherapy drugs are used depends on the type of cancer that is present. A course of chemotherapy for leukemia usually takes place in four stages:

* *Induction.* Chemotherapeutic drugs are introduced into the system, usually intravenously.

* *Central nervous system prophylaxis.* Some types of leukemia attack the central nervous system, but normal chemotherapeutic agents are blocked from these areas by the blood–brain barrier. To overcome this, chemotherapeutic drugs may be introduced via spinal tap directly into the central nervous system.

* *Consolidation.* Once the process has begun, chemotherapy will continue in high doses for several weeks or months in an effort to be sure that all cancerous cells have been killed.

* *Maintenance therapy.* Lower doses of chemotherapy are used over several years to maintain remission.

If a patient survives for 5 years with no signs of recurrance, he or she is said to be "cured," or cancer-free.

Other Treatment Options   If a person does not respond well to chemotherapy, or if his or her cancer keeps recurring (this is called "refractory leukemia"), it is necessary to explore other treatment options. These can include adding radiation therapy or surgery, especially if cancerous cells have aggressively invaded any particular organ or location.

The treatment options for leukemia (and other types of cancer) are broadening every day. The use of bone marrow transplants with closely matched donors (autogenic transplants) is useful for some leukemia cases, but the incidence of tissue rejection is high. Another option is to harvest some of the patient's own healthy bone marrow and freeze it, administer a very intensive course of chemotherapy, and then to replace the healthy bone marrow; this is called an autologous bone marrow transplant. It is also possible to harvest stem cells from the bloodstream, bone marrow, and even umbilical cords of healthy people and to transplant these "cellular blanks" into leukemia patients, so that they can make healthy, functioning blood cells.

Other research is closing in on the exact DNA mutation that causes certain stem cells to change. When this process is more clearly understood, it may become possible to design treatment options that may interfere with or even prevent the production of cancerous cells. Other research is examining the possibility of "training" healthy immune system cells to attack leukemia cells with radioactive antibodies.

Side Effects of Treatment   The treatment for leukemia, especially the acute varieties, can seem to take as hard a toll on the body as the disease itself.

Chemotherapy means introducing substances into the body whose functions are to kill off any rapidly reproducing cell. Unfortunately, this does not just mean cancer cells; it also means epithelial cells in the skin and the digestive tract, and, ironically, healthy blood cells. The side effects of chemotherapy on epithelial tissues include the development of ulcers in the mouth, nausea and diarrhea from gastrointestinal irritation, and hair loss as the epithelial cells in follicles are killed. One of the difficulties with digestive system disturbances is that if the patient cannot eat well, the whole system becomes weaker and less able to cope with the stresses of both the disease and its treatment.

Chemotherapy exacerbates symptoms of leukemia, as red and white blood cells and platelets are suppressed. Consequently, chemotherapy patients often experience anemia, blood clotting problems, and low resistance to infection—all signs of leukemia itself.

Acute Myelogenous Leukemia

Definition: What Is It?   Acute myelogenous leukemia (AML) is a rapidly progressive cancer of the myeloid group of WBCs, which includes granulocytes and monocytes.

Demographics: Who Gets It?   Statistics vary, but most agree that somewhere between 7000 and 10,000 new cases of AML are diagnosed every year in the United States. This variety of leukemia is associated with age. Most cases occur in people older than 50 years; the average age of diagnosis is 65.

Etiology: What Happens?   Like other forms of leukemia, AML begins with genetic damage to the DNA of specific stem cells. These cells then begin producing leukemic cells in great numbers. The new non-functioning WBCs are released into the circulatory system before they fully mature. These immature cells are called *blast* cells, which is why one synonym for AML is *acute myeloblastic leukemia*. (Other synonyms are *acute myelocytic leukemia* and *acute granulocytic leukemia*.)

The genetic damage that causes AML has been associated with certain specific environmental factors. High doses of radiation, chemotherapy for other types of cancer, and exposure to benzene all increase the risk of contracting AML in later years.

Signs and Symptoms: Suppression of normal bone marrow activity leads to shortages of normal blood cells. The result is anemia with fatigue, shortness of breath, and low stamina; persistent bleeding and easy bruising, indicating a shortage of platelets; and low resistance to infections due to a lack of functioning WBCs.

Treatment: A diagnosis of AML is only the first step in designing a treatment protocol. Each granulocyte or monocyte type responds best to an individualized course of chemotherapy drugs. Therefore, it is necessary to identify which subtype of AML is present.

Because this variety of leukemia is aggressive and rapidly progressive, it is important to start treatment as soon as possible. The steps in administering chemotherapy are outlined in the general treatment section above.

Prognosis: The prognosis for AML has improved drastically over the past 40 years, but even with all the treatment options available today only 14% of all AML patients make it to the 5-year remission goal. Children with AML tend to fare better; they have a 43% remission rate.

Leukemia: General Statistics

Leukemia in various forms is diagnosed in about 32,000 Americans every year. Although this is a disease many people associate with children, adult cases are far more common; about 29,000 adults are diagnosed, and just under 3000 children are diagnosed every year. About 142,000 leukemia patients are living in the United States today.

Research into new and better treatment options has drastically improved the outlook for most leukemia patients. In 1960 the survival rate for childhood cases was about 14%. Now it is 80% for ALL and 43% for AML. Death rates from leukemia among patients older than 65 have also gone down. Overall, the 5-year survival rate has tripled in the past 3 decades.

Nonetheless, leukemia kills about 22,000 Americans every year: about 12,000 are males and 10,000 are female. AML is at the top of the list, with 6900 deaths. It is closely followed by CLL with 5100 deaths. CML is next with 2300 deaths, and ALL comes in last with 1500 deaths. The remaining 6200 patients die of the several other less common forms of leukemia.[a]

[a]Leukemia. The Leukemia and Lymphoma Society. © The Leukemia & Lymphoma Society. Available at: http://www.leukemia.org/CMS/q?action=static&v=PF&pageID=14. Accessed winter 2001.

Chronic Myelogenous Leukemia

Definition: What Is It? Chronic myelogenous leukemia (CML) is a slow-growing cancer of myelogenous cells in the bone marrow. It is also called *chronic granulocytic leukemia* and *chronic myeloid leukemia*. It involves the myeloid class of WBCs: granulocytes and monocytes.

Demographics: Who Gets It? Approximately 5000 new cases of CML are diagnosed in the United States every year. Most patients are adults, but a small number of children contract CML as well.

Etiology: What Happens? The genetic mutations involved in CML may be the best understood of any kind of leukemia. Specific sites on the affected chromosomes have been identified; one of these sites is now called the *Philadelphia chromosome*, for the city in which researchers nailed down the exact location of the genetic anomaly.

Chronic leukemia involves the production of non-functioning WBCs, but unlike acute leukemia, these WBCs are produced relatively slowly and are released into the bloodstream when they are fully mature. These leukemic cells can interfere with and slow down normal immune system activity, but they do not usually bring it to a grinding halt like acute leukemic cells can do.

Signs and Symptoms: All the predictable signs and symptoms of leukemia are present in CML patients, but they tend to have a slow onset. In addition, CML patients often experience spleen enlargement and pain as leukemic cells congregate in this organ. Night sweats, unexpected weight loss, and a decreasing tolerance of warm temperatures are other signs and symptoms commonly experienced by CML patients.

Treatment: CML can often be controlled with chemotherapy. When it occurs in young patients, stem cell transplants or autologous bone marrow transplants may be able to eradicate the disease totally.

CML occasionally changes its pattern and becomes more aggressive. This is called an *accelerated phase* of the disease and is treated as if it were AML.

Prognosis: CML patients have a 32% chance of reaching the 5-year remission goal. Children have higher survival rates than adults; this is probably because young leukemia patients have better success with tissue transplants than do adults.

Acute Lymphocytic Leukemia

Definition: What Is It?   Acute lymphocytic leukemia (ALL) is a rapidly progressive, aggressive form of leukemia that involves DNA mutations in stem cells that produce bone marrow lymphocytes. Synonyms for ALL include *acute lymphoid leukemia* and *acute lymphoblastic leukemia.*

Demographics: Who Gets It?   This variety of leukemia affects young children more often than adults—until adults become older. The incidence of this disease peaks among 4 year olds and then subsides among older children and young adults. It becomes more common among people older than 50.

ALL is most common in developed countries and among higher socioeconomic groups. About 3000 new cases of ALL are diagnosed each year; about half of them are in children.

Etiology: What Happens?   ALL is an acute cancer of bone marrow lymphocytes. The affected cells can be B-cells, T-cells, or natural killer cells. Like with myelogenous leukemia, it is important to identify exactly which cells are cancerous, because different treatment options are used for the different cells.

As an acute form of leukemia, the genetic injury to a stem cell results in the rapid proliferation of non-functioning WBCs. This happens at such a rate that all other bone marrow activity is suppressed and immune system function is crippled. Leukemic lymphocytes (*lymphoblasts*) are released into the blood before they are fully mature.

Causative agents and risk factors for ALL are not clear, but this disease has been associated with high doses of radiation and exposure to toxic substances during gestation or in early childhood.

Signs and Symptoms: ALL symptoms follow the basic leukemia pattern: anemia, loss of blood clotting, and low resistance to infection. In addition to these, leukemic lymphocytes may gather in lymph nodes or may gain access to the central nervous system, where they accumulate and can cause severe headaches and vomiting.

Treatment: Treatment for ALL depends on several variables, including the age of the patient, the severity of the disease, and which type of cell is involved. Aggressive treatment with chemotherapy is usually recommended. Because this disease can invade the central nervous system, chemotherapeutic drugs may be directly injected into the cerebrospinal fluid.

Prognosis: The overall remission rate for ALL is 58%. Among children it is even higher; a child with ALL has an 80% chance of permanent remission.

Chronic Lymphocytic Leukemia

Definition: What Is It?   Chronic lymphocytic leukemia (CLL) is a slow-growing version of lymphocytic leukemia. Although it can involve T-cells or natural killer cells, 95% of all cases involve B-cell malignancies.

Demographics: Who Gets It?   CLL is a disease found primarily in elderly people. Up to 95% of all cases are among patients older than 50, and the incidence rises sharply with age. About 8000 cases of CLL are diagnosed every year.

Etiology: What Happens?   This a slowly developing cancer of bone marrow lymphocytes, usually B-cells. As normal working B-cells are replaced with cancerous cells, circulating levels of antibodies go down, making the CLL patient especially susceptible to infections.

Signs and Symptoms: This disease has a slow onset and may not be discovered until blood is tested for other problems. Signs and symptoms include many features that are automatically associated with old age: fatigue, low stamina, low immunity, and weight loss.

Treatment: Sometimes CLL is so stable and so non-threatening that no treatment is recommended. If numbers of functioning blood cells drop to dangerous levels, chemotherapy may be recommended, along with radiation to shrink enlarged lymph nodes. Bone marrow and stem cell transplants are seldom successful for CLL.

Prognosis: CLL has the best prognosis of all the types of leukemia: 71% of all patients make it to 5 years of remission.

Massage?

The question of whether massage is appropriate for all clients with cancer may never be settled. It seems clear that the benefits massage can bring (reinforcing a parasympathetic state, improving immune system function, and reducing pain perception) can be enjoyed with a minimum of risk, if simple precautions are taken.

Leukemia is a type of cancer that can spread through the circulatory system. It involves seriously impaired immunity and a tendency to bleed easily. Some types of bodywork, especially those that enlist the healing energies of the client rather than trying to impose outside forces on blood flow or tissue manipulation, may be helpful and supportive for a person going through a difficult and often painful treatment procedure. It is important in this situation to work as part of a well-informed health care team, so that the possibility of secondary infection or other complications can be carefully avoided.

If a client has a history of leukemia but has been in remission for 5 years or more, he or she is probably considered "cured," that is, free from the threat of more cancerous cells. In this case massage of any kind is appropriate.

For more guidelines about massage in the context of cancer and cancer treatments, see *cancer* in Chapter 11.

Thrombophlebitis, Deep Vein Thrombosis

Definition: What Is It?

Thrombophlebitis and DVT refer to inflammation of a vein caused by clots. These clots can form anywhere in the venous system, but they develop most often in the calves, thighs, and occasionally in the pelvis. Thrombophlebitis is a term used for clots in superficial leg veins (lesser and greater saphenous), whereas DVT is much the same problem in deeper leg veins, specifically the popliteal, femoral, and iliac veins.

Demographics: Who Gets It?

The clots of thrombophlebitis and DVT happen more commonly in women than in men, and they are especially associated with the elderly and the overweight. About 300,000 people are hospitalized with DVT every year.

THROMBOPHLEBITIS, DEEP VEIN THROMBOSIS IN BRIEF

What is it?

Thrombophlebitis and deep vein thrombosis (DVT) are inflammations of veins due to blood clots.

How is it recognized?

Symptoms of thrombophlebitis may include pain, heat, redness, swelling, and local itchiness as well as a hard cord-like feeling at the affected vein. Symptoms for DVT may be nonexistent or can be more extreme: possibly pitting edema distal to the site, often with discoloration, and intermittent or continuous pain that is exacerbated by activity or standing still for a long period.

Is massage indicated or contraindicated?

Thrombophlebitis and DVT contraindicate any kind of bodywork that may disrupt clots, which could lead to *pulmonary embolism* (this chapter).

Etiology: What Happens?

These conditions should be major concerns for well-trained massage practitioners. They involve thrombi, stationary clots, somewhere in the venous system where, if they break loose, nothing stops them from traveling straight into the lungs and causing pulmonary embolism (see *embolism, thrombus,* this chapter).

Causes

The causes of thrombophlebitis and DVT can be many and varied. Any circumstance involving venous stasis (slowed movement of venous blood), increased coagulability, or blood vessel damage will increase the chances of developing this problem. The following are a few of the most common precipitators of thrombophlebitis or DVT:

- *Physical trauma* is a predisposing factor; being kicked or hit in the leg can damage the delicate venous tissue, which will then be prone to clot formation. Athletes are particularly vulnerable to this problem.

- *Varicose veins* (this chapter) are another risk factor, since they too involve damaged tissue and the risk of clot formation. Fortunately, the clots that form in superficial veins tend to embolize or break loose much less frequently than those in deeper veins.

- *Local infection* can cause an inflammatory reaction leading to clot formation.

- *Reduced circulation,* either from physical restriction like too-tight socks or immobility can cause the clotting factors in the blood to accumulate in amounts that will cause coagulation even without damage to a vessel wall. People who must sit still for many hours at a time run the risk of developing DVT; this phenomenon has given rise to a new layman's term for this condition: "coach class syndrome."

- *Pregnancy* (Chapter 10) and childbirth can increase the risk of blood clotting. The weight of the fetus on femoral vessels slows blood return, and hormonal changes can cause the blood to thicken and become more viscous.

- *Blood diseases* that are particularly disposed to complicate into thrombophlebitis or DVT include polycythemia and *sickle cell anemia* (this chapter). Both of these involve blood that is viscous, sticky, and not free-flowing.

- *Surgery* is another major risk for DVT. In fact, thrombosis and subsequent pulmonary embolism is the leading cause of death due to orthopedic surgery, especially for knee and hip replacements. Heart and any kind of pelvic surgery also hold high risks for thrombosis.

- *High-estrogen birth control pills* can increase the risk of developing blood clots.

The majority of blood clots causing DVT or thrombophlebitis form in the lower legs, but the majority of clots that break off and go to the lungs originate in the thigh or pelvis. Sudden movement or change in position is often the factor that will cause part of a clot to detach and become a pulmonary embolism. Another alarming fact is that a patient who is immobile because of a leg injury is almost as likely to throw a clot from the *uninjured* leg as he or she is from the injured side. This is because lack of ambulation can thicken the blood systemically, even where no damage to blood vessels has occurred.

Signs and Symptoms

Thrombophlebitis can show the major signs of inflammation: pain, heat, redness, and swelling. Sometimes itchiness, a hard cord where the vein is affected, and edema with discoloration distal to the area will be present (Fig. 4-5). Thrombophlebitis that has become a chronic problem may result in poor blood flow to the skin, leading to flaking, discoloration, and skin ulcers. If it is caused by a local infection, fever and general illness may also be present.

DVT is considered the more dangerous of these two conditions. This is because the clots in deeper veins can be big enough to do serious damage in the lungs, and because clots in superficial veins usually melt under the influence of the body's own anticoagulants before they have a chance to break off and do any damage.

If DVT shows any signs (and it often does not), it may show more swelling and edema than thrombophlebitis, because the clot will inhibit more blood flow back to the heart. The affected leg may be puffier and notably warmer or cooler than the unaffected leg. The backup of blood forces plasma out of the capillaries and into the interstitial spaces, thus adding general edema to any localized swelling of the vein. The capillary exchange may become so sluggish that the edema will "pit," or leave a little dimple wherever it is touched. Pitting edema is a huge red flag for massage therapists. It is an indication that a person's circulation is absolutely not capable of dealing with the internal changes brought about by massage.

Diagnosis

Thrombophlebitis and DVT can be diagnosed in a few ways, each with inherent benefits and disadvantages. Ultrasound is a fast and noninvasive technique but tends to yield many false-positive results, leading to unnecessary prescriptions of anticoagulants, which can lead to risks of uncontrolled bleeding. Venography—injecting the blood vessel with dye and watching how it moves through the system—can be more accurate but is slow and the injection itself can damage delicate tissue.

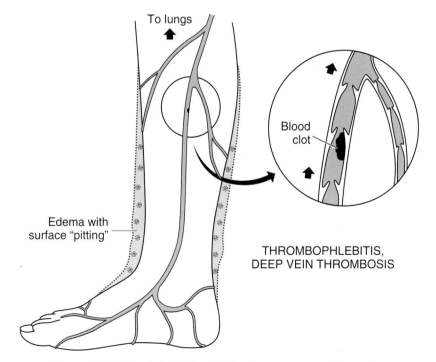

Figure 4-5. A blood clot lodged in the leg can cause pitting edema

One simple test is a fairly reliable indicator for blood clots in the legs: passive dorsiflexion of the foot will cause pain with DVT; this is called *Homans' sign.*

Treatment

The treatment of both thrombophlebitis and DVT is anticoagulants. The risk is that these chemicals will make a person very prone to heavy bleeding: another caution for massage. If the patient is bedridden, he or she may be given pneumatic compression (a machine will mimic the pumping action of exercise by inflating and deflating a tubular balloon around the affected leg). Support hose to prevent the accumulation of postoperative edema are also recommended.

People with thrombophlebitis in superficial veins are at much less risk for embolism than those with DVT. Self-care measures such as hot packs, analgesics, and gentle exercise may be recommended to resolve episodes of vein inflammation.

High-risk patients who have clotting disorders that make anticoagulants prohibitive may have a special filter implanted in the vena cava to prevent clots from reaching the lungs.

DEEP VEIN THROMBOSIS
Anne, 67 Years Old
"It was just a broken knee!"

Anne was a retired schoolteacher who spent her winters in Arizona and summers in the mountains of Colorado. In May, one week after she had moved to her summer home, she took a bad fall over a curb and sustained a lateral plateau fracture to the tibia of her left leg: a leg with which she had a history of varicose veins and phlebitis.

Because her health maintenance organization was out of state (in Arizona), it was reluctant to cover any treatment for conditions not considered "life threatening." For that reason Anne, a mildly overweight moderate smoker, spent 3 weeks sitting in a chair all day at 10,000 feet of altitude (which thickens the blood because there is less oxygen in the air). She was unable to move except with the use of a walker. Her broken knee was never set or seen by an orthopedist.

Eventually the swelling in the leg became so severely painful that she sought out a general practitioner in the Colorado town. He sent her to a local hospital for an ultrasound, which revealed a blood clot from her ankle to her groin. She was immediately admitted to the hospital and was given anticoagulant medication.

Four days later she was sent home. Still basically immobile, but taking anticoagulants, she returned to sitting in her chair with her leg elevated for 12 to 14 hours a day. On her second night at home, she woke in the night with severe chest pains and shortness of breath. The emergency medical team took her back to the hospital where it was revealed that she had thrown a large clot to the lung: a pulmonary embolism. At this point her condition was too severe to be treated at a small rural hospital. After 2 days in the intensive care unit, she was transferred to a larger facility about 100 miles away, where a filter was inserted into her vena cava to prevent any further clots from reaching her lungs.

When she checked out of the second hospital she was prescribed supplemental oxygen to compensate for the loss of lung function and the high altitude. She used an oxygen tank for several weeks and also had to quit smoking. Several months later, Anne had no severe pain in her knee but there was a constant achiness. She now limps when she gets tired, which happens easily; her energy level has never quite returned to what it used to be.

Massage?

A client who is at high risk for throwing a blood clot and developing pulmonary embolism is obviously not a candidate for Swedish, circulatory, rigorous massage. The trick is that although thrombophlebitis *may* show obvious signs, it may *not* as well, or the signs could be indistinct. A client may come in complaining of an ache deep in her calf that she really wants "worked out." This is a reasonable request—except that what the massage therapist may be "working out" is a blood clot that will land the client in the hospital with the other 600,000 pulmonary embolism cases this year.

Vascular Disorders

Aneurysm
Definition: What Is It?

An aneurysm is a permanent bulge in the wall of a blood vessel or the heart. The damage may be brought about by any combination of injury, genetically weak smooth muscle tissue, high blood pressure, atherosclerosis, and compromised connective tissue. If an aneurysm ruptures, the person can bleed to death in a very short time.

Demographics: Who Gets It?

About 200,000 aortic aneurysms are diagnosed in the United States each year, and about 15,000 of those patients die. Most aortic aneurysm patients are men older than 55 years. The risk of aneurysm rises with age; about 5% of all men older than 80 years have had an aortic aneurysm. Statistics show that the rate of aortic aneurysm in the United States has tripled in the past 40 years. This is probably due to an increase in the number of people who smoke and longer life spans.

> ### ANEURYSM IN BRIEF
>
> **What is it?**
> An aneurysm is a bulge or outpouching in a vein, artery, or the heart. They usually occur in the thoracic or abdominal aorta or in the arteries at the base of the brain.
>
> **How is it recognized?**
> Symptoms of aneurysms are determined by their location. Thoracic aneurysms may cause chronic hoarseness; abdominal aneurysms may cause local discomfort, reduced urine output, or severe backache. Cerebral aneurysms may be silent, or may cause extreme headache when they are at very high risk for rupture.
>
> **Is massage indicated or contraindicated?**
> If a client has been diagnosed with an aneurysm, circulatory massage will probably be contraindicated. Massage is also strongly cautioned for clients who fit the profile for aneurysms but have not been diagnosed.

Etiology: What Happens?

The three-ply construction of the arteries includes the endothelial inside layer, the smooth muscle middle layer, and the tough connective tissue outer layer. Blood pressure in the aorta, the largest artery, is very high. If the walls of the aorta have lost their elasticity, they can bulge wide with blood. This bulge is an aneurysm. As the aneurysm grows, the walls stretch and become weaker, increasing the risk of rupture and death.

Aneurysms happen most often in the abdominal aorta and at the base of the brain. Thoracic aneurysms are usually associated with specific diseases like Marfan's syndrome, which frequently exhibits a congenital weakness of the aorta. Aneurysms sometimes occur in more distal vessels, but those cases are generally much less serious because the blood pressure pushing on the vessels is much lower as it gets further away from the heart.

An occasional complication of a major heart attack is an aneurysm in the left ventricle of the heart itself. The damage to myocardium reduces elasticity to the point at which chronic pressure will cause the wall of the ventricle to bulge. The force of the contractions becomes weaker, and the risk of developing congestive heart failure is very high (see *heart attack* and *heart failure*, this chapter).

Causes

Several different factors can contribute to the chances of developing an aneurysm.

- *Compromised smooth muscle.* Atherosclerotic plaques invade and weaken aortal muscle (see *atherosclerosis*, this chapter). Aortic aneurysms are a serious complication of atherosclerosis and *high blood pressure* (this chapter).

- *Smoking.* The damage incurred to endothelium by carbon monoxide from cigarette smoke and a rise in blood pressure from nicotine make smoking a leading risk factor for aortic aneurysm.

- *Congenitally weak arterial wall muscle.* Sometimes the tissue simply is not strong enough to put up with normal blood pressure, and with no warning an aneurysm can rupture. This happens most often in the arteries at the base of the brain. When a high school basketball player drops dead on the court, this is usually the kind of situation that causes it (see *stroke*, Chapter 3).

- *Inflammation.* A few diseases, such as polyarteritis nodosa or bacterial endocarditis, can cause inflammation and weakening of the aortal tissue. Fortunately, these conditions are relatively rare; it is unlikely that someone with them will come looking for massage.

- *Trauma.* Mechanical trauma, like a car accident in which a person is injured by a steering wheel, may sometimes damage the outer layers of the aorta while leaving the inner one intact. This will result in the characteristic bulging and stretching of the most delicate arterial tissue.

Types of Aneurysms

Aneurysms come in a variety of shapes and sizes, some of which are particular to where the lesion occurs (Fig. 4-6).

- *Sacular.* These are usually the case with thoracic or abdominal aortic aneurysms. The aortal wall bulges like a small (or large) rounded sack, which throbs and pushes against neighboring organs and other structures.

- *Fusiform.* This is also common for aortic aneurysms; in this case the bulge is less round and more tubular, as if the aorta were widened like a sausage for a few inches.

- *Berry.* This is a term for several small aneurysms clustered together in the brain.

- *Dissecting.* This is the least common and most painful type of aneurysm. It happens again with the aorta, and in this situation the blood pressure actually *splits* the layers of the aorta. It can happen between the tunica intima (innermost layer) and the tunica media (muscular layer), or between the tunica media and the adventitia (outer layer). In some cases this type of aneurysm can seal itself off when the blood trapped inside the split coagulates and solidifies.

Common types of aneurysms

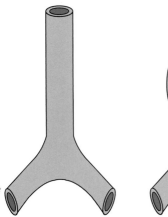

Normal artery

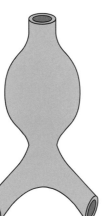

Artery with aneurysm

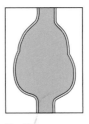

Saccular

Fusiform

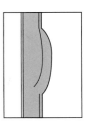

Dissecting

Figure 4-6. Several types of aneurysms

Signs and Symptoms

Aneurysms can be difficult to identify by symptoms because they often are not painful until they are actually a medical emergency. This is certainly true of cerebral aneurysms. With aortic aneurysms the swelling *might* create some warning signals; this usually happens when the bulge is pressing on something else or interfering with another organ's functioning. Thoracic aneurysms will sometimes create difficulty with swallowing (*dysphagia*), chest pain, hoarseness, and coughing that is not relieved with medication, because the protrusion is pressing on and irritating the larynx. Abdominal aneurysms will sometimes show as a throbbing lump, loss of appetite, weight loss, reduced urine output and, if it is pushing against the spine, severe backache.

This should be extremely alarming to massage therapists! How is a person supposed to tell if a client's backache is from a muscle spasm or an abdominal aneurysm? This is why it is vital to take a complete history before a first massage session. People with aneurysms will generally have a history of heart disease, atherosclerosis, and/or high blood pressure. If clients fit the profile for an aneurysm, it must be explained to them that medical clearance is not only in their best interest, but necessary before receiving rigorous circulatory massage.

Diagnosis

Physical examinations often show signs of aneurysm; the turbulent movement of blood through the wide area of the aorta makes a specific sound in stethoscopes. Large aneurysms in thin people can be palpated as a pulsating mass. Otherwise, aneurysms are diagnosed by ultrasound, computed tomography (CT) scans, and magnetic resonance imaging (MRI).

Complications

For those rare aneurysms that are *not* in the aorta or the brain, no serious complications may develop unless they get large enough to impede blood flow, which can lead to tissue death. The more typical aneurysm will at the very least press against its neighbors, which can be uncomfortable, or can even interfere with function. If blood pools in an aneurysm for any length of time, clots may form and then enter the bloodstream again (see *embolism or thrombus*, this chapter). Of course, a rupture would lead to hemorrhaging in the best case and shock followed by collapse of the circulatory system in the worst case. The vast majority (75 to 80%) of people whose aneurysms rupture die.

Treatment

Aneurysms *do not* spontaneously retreat, because the pressure that causes them never really lessens. They need to be repaired, either with open surgery or with endovascular surgery. Open surgery involves clamping off the artery above and below the lesion and attaching either a replacement graft or a Dacron substitute to the two ends. This is usually successful, but it has to be done *before* a rupture. Up to 10% of all aneurysm surgeries end in the death of the patient.

Endovascular surgery involves using a catheter through the femoral artery up to the aorta to insert a patch or stent at the aneurysm site. This is a much less invasive procedure with a lower risk of surgical complications, but it is new enough that long-term comparisons to open surgery cannot yet be made.

Some aneurysms do not require immediate intervention. Normal aortic size is about 2 cm; a dangerously distended aneurysm is about 5 to 6 cm. Many physicians recommend checking the growth of small aneurysms by ultrasound every 6 months until the benefits of intervention outweigh the risks.

Massage?

If a massage therapist works on a client who subsequently experiences a ruptured aneurysm and dies, it is conceivable that the therapist could be held responsible. Even if the aneurysm might have eventually ruptured regardless of massage, it is important to avoid raising even the *possibility* that massage might be responsible for a client's death.

Any condition involving damaged blood vessels requires extreme caution for circulatory massage. *Massage changes the internal environment.* It dilates some blood vessels and constricts others. It reroutes circulation, mechanically through compression and friction on the skin, via the parasympathetic nervous system, and by changing hormonal balance (reducing adrenalin), which will shift blood from the skeletal muscles (a sympathetic state) to the internal organs (a parasympathetic state). If a client cannot keep up with having the internal environment radically shifted in terms of blood vessel dilation, chemical distribution, and autonomic state, he or she is not a good candidate for circulatory massage.

If a client has been diagnosed with a stable aortic aneurysm and wants to receive massage, the therapist should choose modalities that aim to lower blood pressure and reinforce that parasympathetic state without putting undue mechanical force on the person's circulatory system.

ATHEROSCLEROSIS IN BRIEF

What is it?
Atherosclerosis is a condition in which the arteries become inelastic and brittle due to atherosclerotic plaques.

How is it recognized?
Atherosclerosis has no symptoms until it is very advanced. However, it is connected to several other types of circulatory problems, including hypertension, arrhythmia, coronary artery disease, cerebrovascular disease, and peripheral vascular disease.

Is massage indicated or contraindicated?
Advanced atherosclerosis systemically contraindicates rigorous circulatory massage, but other modalities may offer many benefits with a minimum of risks.

Atherosclerosis
Definition: What Is It?

Arteriosclerosis refers to a "hardening of the arteries" from any cause. Atherosclerosis is a subtype of arteriosclerosis. It is a condition in which deposits of cholesterol and other substances infiltrate and weaken layers of large blood vessels, particularly the aorta and coronary arteries. It is compounded by the fact that damage to these blood vessels can cause them to spasm, while blood clots will form at the site of these deposits. These features contribute to the occlusion of the diameter, or *lumen*, of the arteries as well as to the risk of creating and loosening blood clots on the arterial side of the systemic circuit.

Coronary artery disease (CAD) is atherosclerosis specifically located in the coronary arteries that supply the heart muscle (Fig. 4-7).

Demographics: Who Gets It?

Random samplings of arteries taken from autopsies of people who died of something other than heart disease reveal that the incidence of atherosclerosis is very high in the United States, although it does not always become symptomatic. Cultures exist in which this disease is completely unknown, but they are generally in countries where dietary diseases are related to famine rather than to excess.

Certain populations carry a higher possibility of developing atherosclerosis. This is discussed in detail in *Risk Factors* in this section.

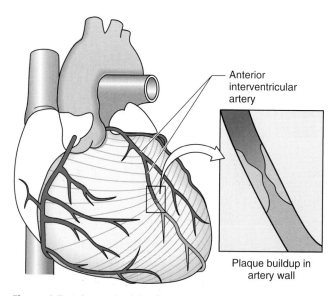

Anterior
interventricular
artery

Plaque buildup in
artery wall

Figure 4-7. Atherosclerotic plaque can deprive the heart
muscle of blood supply

Etiology: What Happens?

The process of developing atherosclerosis is a complex one that is not yet completely understood. Several theories have been formed, but as research reveals more and more about this condition the reality may turn out to be quite different from what people have always believed.

Theory 1   One theory for the development of atherosclerosis maps out various steps beginning with damage to the endothelial layer of the aorta. Deviations in the order of events in the disease process may occur for different people, but these are the basics:

- *Endothelial damage.* The inside layer of arteries is sometimes called the *tunica intima*. It is made of delicate epithelial tissue and subject to a great deal of abuse. A variety of things may cause the first insult at the tunica intima, including constant *hypertension* (this chapter) in the aorta and arteries surrounding the heart, carbon monoxide from cigarette smoke, and high levels of circulating low-density lipoproteins (LDLs) and triglycerides. Even a high level of iron in the blood may produce oxygen free radicals that begin the process of endothelial erosion.

- *Monocytes arrive.* These are small WBCs that are attracted to any site of damage in the body. The monocytes infiltrate the epithelial layer and turn into *macrophages* ("big eaters").

- *Macrophages take up LDL.* The reasons for this are unclear. As a quick overview, LDLs are the "bad guys" of the cholesterol world. Actually, they have an important job, which is to escort usable cholesterol to all the cells in the body. When those cells do not need any more cholesterol, they stop accepting it. This leaves those LDLs with nowhere to go. They are consumed by the WBCs in the tunica intima, which are then called "foam cells." This is the beginning of the development of fatty streaks that characterize atherosclerosis.

- *Foam cells infiltrate and damage smooth muscle tissue.* Foam cells secrete growth factors. This causes the smooth muscle cells in the arterial wall to proliferate all around them. The grayish-white lumps of plaque that are inside dissected arteries are made of these extra muscle cells and cholesterol-filled macrophages. Furthermore, these foam cells can release enzymes that damage arterial walls and cause bleeding and clot formation.

- *Platelets arrive.* Attracted by the changing texture of the arterial wall, platelets come and release their chemicals, which produce three unpleasant things:

  - *Growth factors* are secreted, which reinforces the proliferation of new smooth muscle cells.

  - *Clots form.*

  - *Vascular spasm* occurs because the chemical that inhibits it cannot get through all the plaque. This leads to a temporary lack of oxygen in the myocardium and the gripping chest pain called *angina pectoris*.

When vascular spasm and clots combine, partial or total occlusion of the artery can occur. Symptoms of this will depend on the location of the blockage and the amount of tissue that is affected.

Theory 2   Another explanation of the development of atherosclerosis begins with the deposition of LDL cholesterol in the subendothelial spaces of the arteries. There it undergoes some chemical changes (oxidation), which makes it impossible to leave the artery wall. Circulating monocytes are attracted to the LDL deposits. They infiltrate the arterial wall and literally gorge themselves on the embedded cholesterol, becoming foam cells.

The monocytes can eat so much they rupture, releasing their contents in the area. Among the chemicals released are growth factors that stimulate smooth muscle cell proliferation in the arterial wall. These sites become raised lesions or *plaques*. Calcium is eventually deposited there. The rough texture created by plaques attracts passing thrombocytes, which then contribute to clot formation and the subsequent dangers discussed above.

Risk Factors

Risk factors for atherosclerosis can be divided into situations that can be modified and others over which a person has little or no control.

Non-modifiable Risk Factors

- *Heredity, genetics.* This is one factor no one can control. Higher than average incidence of heart disease within families is clearly demonstrable. However, a family history is not a death sentence; controlling modifiable factors will significantly reduce the chance of developing problems.

- *Gender.* Simply being male increases the risk of atherosclerosis. Female hormones also seem to have some influence, as postmenopausal women have higher rates than premenopausal women.

- *Age.* The incidence of heart disease rises with age, but it is important to remember that nearly half of all those released from the hospital for cardiovascular problems every year are younger than 65 years of age.

- *Kidney disorders.* Atherosclerosis can sometimes lead to kidney problems. If the kidney problems predate the circulatory ones, high blood pressure brought about by kidney failure can be a precipitating cause of atherosclerosis (see *renal failure*, Chapter 9).

Modifiable Risk Factors

- *Smoking.* Carbon monoxide from cigarette smoke is extremely corrosive to endothelium. Furthermore, nicotine causes the release of epinephrine and norepinephrine, leading to vasoconstriction and high blood pressure. Studies show that cigarette smokers have a 2 to 4 times higher risk of dying of heart disease than the general public.

- *High cholesterol levels.* A predictable statistical link has been established between high cholesterol levels and the development of pathologic atherosclerosis. More than 52% of Americans have cholesterol readings above the recommended maximum of 200 mg/dL. More than 20% have readings over 240 mg/dL. For more details on cholesterol, see the sidebar "Cholesterol Facts."

- *High blood pressure.* Chronic uncontrolled high blood pressure will contribute to endothelial damage, which opens the door to the formation of plaques.

- *Sedentary lifestyle.* Perhaps more than any other factor, regular, moderate cardiovascular exercise can reduce the risk of atherosclerosis. It keeps arteries elastic and pliable, reduces weight, raises high-density lipoprotein (HDL) levels for the reduction of plaques, reduces the risk of diabetes, and lowers blood pressure.

- *Obesity.* The definition of obesity varies, but researchers agree that being significantly overweight is a risk factor for several diseases. Obesity often appears in combination with high cholesterol, high blood pressure, and a sedentary lifestyle and is a major contributor to developing CAD.

- *Diabetes.* People with uncontrolled diabetes are especially susceptible to atherosclerosis because of the way their bodies metabolize food. However, if diabetes is controlled, the risk of atherosclerosis is much lower.

Other risk factors are somewhat harder to quantify. The way a person responds to stress, for instance, has much to do with his or her health profile. If stress makes the person eat poorly and smoke more, and raises blood pressure, then this person's risk for developing atherosclerosis will be higher than for someone who deals with stress in different ways. Depression is another reliable predictor of heart disease. Surveys of men older than 65 years find that the risk of developing atherosclerosis is 40% higher when depression is also present.

Signs and Symptoms

What are the symptoms of atherosclerosis? Until the damage has progressed to dangerous levels, *there are none!* An artery has to be *75 to 80% occluded* before the person has any awareness of a problem. This is largely because the body does not depend on any single artery to do a job. Most parts of the body have two or three alternate vessels that can be pressed into service if one of them gets clogged.

Once signs begin to develop, they revolve around poor delivery of oxygen to the heart and consequently poor delivery of blood to the rest of the body. Low stamina, shortness of breath, and a host of predictable complications are all signs and symptoms of advanced atherosclerosis.

Complications

The complications of atherosclerosis are sometimes the first symptoms of the disease. They include but are not limited to the following:

- *High blood pressure.* Hypertension is both a cause and a result of this disease; it contributes to the original damage to the tunica intima, and it is made worse when the

Heart Disease in the United States: Sobering Statistics

The statistics for all varieties of cardiovascular disease are not generally separated from each other, since most of these conditions exist in a circular relationship. A person is unlikely to have atherosclerosis without high blood pressure, for instance, and a person is unlikely to have a heart attack without the predisposing factor of atherosclerosis.

Statistics for cardiovascular disease as a whole in the United States are sobering. About 2,600 people die of heart disease everyday. That amounts to 1 death every 33 seconds. This group of diseases is the leading cause of death in the United States today, accounting for 41.2% of all deaths.

The following is a breakdown of reported heart disease statistics[b]:.

Condition	Prevalence (number of cases within the population)
High blood pressure	50,000,000
Coronary artery disease	12,200,000
Myocardial infarct	7,700,000
Angina pectoris	6,300,000
Stroke	4,400,000
Rheumatic heart disease	1,800,000

When these numbers are adjusted for overlap, the prevalence of cardiovascular disease in the United States is about 59 million. This set of diseases accounts for 6 million hospitalizations per year. Although these conditions are often associated with advanced age, up to 6% of those who die of heart disease are younger than 65 years of age, and up to 43% of all heart disease patients released from the hospital are younger than 65.

[b]Cardiovascular Disease Statistics. © 2000 American Heart Association, Inc. Available at: http://www.americanheart.org/Heart_and_Stroke _A_Z_Guide/cvds.html. Accessed winter, 2001.

arterial walls are too brittle to adjust to the constant changes in blood volume flowing through them.

- *Aneurysm.* When the wall of an artery is rendered inelastic and defective, it can bulge, become thin and weak, and become susceptible to rupture (this chapter).

- *Arrhythmia.* Advanced atherosclerosis can contribute to the development of irregular or uncoordinated contraction of the cardiac muscle as blood supply through the coronary arteries is periodically interrupted. Arrhythmia can allow clots to form in the atria when the chamber does not empty completely. These clots can travel anywhere the aorta takes them.

- *Thrombus or embolism, peripheral circulatory damage.* A thrombus is a stationary clot; an embolism is a traveling clot. Thrombi are the link between atherosclerosis and *stroke* or transient ischemic attack (TIA) when they travel to the brain (see Chapter 3), and between atherosclerosis and *heart attack* when they lodge in the coronary arteries (this chapter). If a clot lodges in the renal artery, kidney damage and possible failure will ensue (see *renal failure,* Chapter 9). Clots on the arterial side of the system may also end up in peripheral blood vessels, where they can cause stasis dermatitis, skin ulcers, and necrosis.

- *Angina pectoris.* The process of developing atherosclerotic plaques also creates a higher risk of short-term vascular spasm, which can lead to intermittent heart and chest pain.

- *Heart attack.* When rough plaques form on smooth artery walls, they attract clotting factors. If a clot or fragment of a clot should break free from a plaque in the coronary artery, it will travel until its blood vessel becomes too small to let it pass. All the myocardium that should have been supplied by that artery will then die: a myocardial infarction, or heart attack.

Diagnosis

The traditional way to check for *stenosis,* or narrowing of arteries, is to inject them with dye and take a series of radiographs to watch the movement of fluid through the tubes in a procedure called an *angiogram.* Computer technology has produced a new, faster, less intrusive test called an ultrafast CT scanner, which takes very fast, clear pictures of the insides of arteries with about one chest radiograph's worth of radiation. It is not as complete a test as an angiogram, but it can be used to screen out high-risk patients who have no symptoms but want to find out at what stage their disease exists.

Treatment

Treatment for atherosclerosis starts simply. If the situation has been caught before it gets out of hand, it can often be dealt with by changing eating and exercise habits. Radically reducing the fat calories in the diet from 33% (the American average) to closer to 5% or 10%, along with mild exercise and stress reduction techniques, can yield success in reversing even advanced cases of atherosclerosis without surgery. The goal is to reduce serum LDL levels to less than 100 mg/dL to reverse the disease.

Some drugs and other substances, notably niacin and chromium, have been found to increase HDL levels and reduce LDL levels in the blood. Lipid-lowering agents can be successful, but they often have side effects. Unfortunately, plaques that have been long in place are only about 15% soluble fats; the rest are composed of cellular debris, connective tissue, foam cells, and smooth muscle cells.

More advanced cases, and more standardized medical approaches, will often involve drugs and/or surgery. The drugs are generally smooth muscle relaxants that will cause the blood vessels to dilate. Aspirin has been found to be useful, but many people experience stomach irritation with its use. Specially coated tablets that will not irritate the digestive system have been designed for the prevention of CAD.

Surgical intervention for atherosclerosis used to be automatic bypass surgery. That is, surgeons would remove the damaged piece of coronary artery and replace it with something else, often a graft from the internal mammary artery or a piece of femoral vein. A single, double, triple, or however-many bypass refers to how many sections of artery are being replaced.

Angioplasty is a less intrusive option that is useful for some patients. In this procedure the artery may first be treated with a laser, which vaporizes plaques (laser angioplasty), and then a small balloon is inflated to widen the artery (balloon angioplasty). Unfortunately, the scarring that occurs when the balloon is removed ("restenosis") can be a difficult, even dangerous complication of this procedure; new cells rapidly proliferate where the endothelium was scraped. Low doses of radiation inside the artery may be used to limit restenosis. A small rigid coil, called a *stent* is inserted to keep the artery widened, and in some procedures a laser heats up and "welds" the inside of the artery into a permanently smooth shape.

In yet another type of procedure, *catheter atherectomy*, a tiny rotating drill is inserted into clogged arteries to shave off plaque. The shavings are then trapped and removed. This is sometimes used for carotid arteries when the risk of stroke is high.

Cholesterol Facts

Cholesterol is a fatty substance that is produced in the liver and is also available in any animal product. Saturated fats are particularly rich in easily absorbable cholesterol.

Cholesterol by itself has no access to the body's cells. Just as glucose must be escorted into cells by insulin, cholesterol must be escorted by *lipoproteins*, other chemicals also produced by the liver. When a cholesterol measurement is taken, it is actually the lipoproteins that are being counted.

Three varieties of lipoproteins are involved with the movement of cholesterol: low-density lipoproteins (LDLs), high-density lipoproteins (HDLs), and triglycerides. The LDLs ("bad cholesterol") deliver cholesterol to the body's cells. They are only "bad" when the body's cells have no more need for their cargo. At that point the LDLs deposit the cholesterol in artery walls. The HDLs ("good cholesterol") are involved in a process called "reverse cholesterol transport." In this process cholesterol is moved out of the arteries and back to the liver for metabolic processing. The third variety, triglycerides, are chemicals that help to convert fats and carbohydrates into energy for muscles. Studies have shown that elevated triglyceride levels contribute to plaque formation, so it is desirable to keep their numbers down.

When a person has a cholesterol reading taken, it is useful to know not just what his or her overall levels are, but in what ratios the fat types occur. An ideal reading would find total levels below 200 mg/dL, with a relatively high proportion of HDLs (>35 mg/dL for men, and >45 mg/dL for women) and lower numbers of LDLs (<130 mg/dL) and triglycerides (<200 mg/dL).[c]

Unfortunately, in the United States less than half the adult population has ideal cholesterol levels. More than 98 million people have cholesterol readings greater than 200 mg/dL, and more than half of those people have levels greater than 240 mg/dL. The overall averages are 215 mg/dL for women and 211 mg/dL for men. Women have a slightly higher reading because menstruation tends to temporarily raise HDL levels.

Studies show that lowering cholesterol levels not only reduces the risk of developing atherosclerosis, but actually extends life expectancy. Men with cholesterol readings of 200 mg/dL or less live an average of 3.8 to 8.7 years longer than men with cholesterol readings greater than 240 mg/dL.

[c]Cholesterol. © Copyright 2001 Texas Heart Institute. Available at: http://www.tmc.edu/thi/choleste.html. Accessed winter, 2001.

With the exception of bypass surgery, all these procedures can be done by inserting special tubes into arteries in the arms or legs and guiding the equipment to where it needs to go. Obviously the amount of shock to the system is less and the recovery process is much easier than it used to be. In addition, new emphasis is being put on *maintaining* the structural changes brought about by intervention; if the patient reverts to former eating and exercise habits, his or her arteries can reach the same sorry state in just a few years.

Massage?

It is impossible to tell if a client has a subclinical build-up of plaque. The deciding factor is whether the client can adjust to the internal environment changes that massage will produce. In other words, if the client's ability to maintain homeostasis is going to be overly challenged by rigorous movement of fluid through the system, he or she is not a good candidate for circulatory massage.

If a client is taking *any* kind of medication for circulatory problems, it is important to clearly understand why and to adjust massage modalities to fit the circulatory limitations of the client.

HYPERTENSION IN BRIEF

What is it?
Hypertension is the technical term for high blood pressure.

How is it recognized?
High blood pressure has no dependable symptoms. The only way to identify it is by taking several blood pressure measurements over time.

Is massage indicated or contraindicated?
For borderline or mild high blood pressure massage may be useful as a tool to control stress and increase general health, but other pathologies having to do with kidney or cardiovascular disease must be ruled out. High blood pressure that requires medication may be inappropriate for circulatory massage, but may respond well to other modalities.

Hypertension
Definition: What Is It?

Hypertension is a technical term for *high blood pressure*. It is defined as blood pressure persistently elevated above 140 mm Hg systolic and/or 90 mm Hg diastolic.

Demographics: Who Gets It?

About 50 million people in the United States have high blood pressure (one in every four adults). It strikes men more often than women, until women reach the age of 65. Then it evens out and affects both genders equally. African-Americans have higher hypertension rates than other races. Age is a predisposing factor; about half of all people older than 60 years have high blood pressure.

Other predisposing factors include obesity, smoking, high cholesterol levels, atherosclerosis, and water retention. A genetic predisposition may raise the risk of high blood pressure, but sometimes it is hard to know what has been inherited—high blood pressure genes or high blood pressure habits.

Etiology: What Happens?

In hypertension, internal and/or external forces put pressure on the blood vessels. To understand how these forces can cause damage, it is necessary to take a brief look at the definition of blood pressure.

Anatomy Review A *sphygmomanometer* is an instrument that measures the pressure blood exerts against arterial walls at two different moments: ventricular contraction (systole) and ventricular relaxation (diastole). As a measure of the general health and resiliency of the cardiovascular system, it is clear that the *diastolic* pressure, taken at the moment of relaxation, gives more information than the *systolic* pressure, which is taken at the moment of contraction. The blood pressure cuff converts the pressure in the arteries to millimeters of mercury (mm Hg).

The variables involved in measuring blood pressure are four-fold: total blood volume, pressure from *inside* the vessel (which would be increased if there were any build-up of material inside), pressure from the *outside* the vessel (which would be increased by having excess fluid pressing all around), and blood vessel diameter. If any of these factors is out of balance, it will influence total body blood pressure, which will in turn influence the health and longevity of blood vessels.

Types of High Blood Pressure

Two types of high blood pressure have been identified: *essential*, which means that it is not due to some other pathology, and *secondary*, which is a temporary complication of some other condition such as pregnancy, kidney problems, adrenal tumors, or hormonal disorders. Secondary high blood pressure will clear up as soon as the precipitating cause is handled. Approximately 95% of all hypertension is essential. For both essential and secondary high blood pressure another variable is possible: *malignant hypertension*. In this condition the diastolic pressure rises very quickly, over a matter of weeks or months. It is extremely damaging to the circulatory system, is a high risk for ischemic or hemorrhagic *stroke* (Chapter 2), and is often fatal if left untreated. Malignant high blood pressure is a medical emergency.

Blood Pressure Readings   The following are some basic guidelines for rating the severity of hypertension in adults, based on the averages of more than two readings taken at each of more than two visits after an initial screening.[d]

Massage therapists are not generally required to take blood pressure measurements; these numbers are just an indicator of possible trouble. Be aware also that blood pressure can change significantly from hour to hour. It is not uncommon to see it shoot up from anxiety while a person is in a doctor's office; this is known as "white coat hypertension."

Category	Systolic BP (mm Hg)	Diastolic BP (mg Hg)
Optimal	<120	<80
Normal	<130	<85
High-normal	130–139	85–89
Hypertension		
Stage 1 (mild)	140–159	90–99
Stage 2 (moderate)	160–179	100–109
Stage 3 (severe)	>180	>110

Signs and Symptoms

This disease, which is often called "The Silent Killer," has few recognizable symptoms. A few subtle signs are occasionally observed, however, so they are included here: shortness of breath after mild exercise; headaches or dizziness; swelling of the ankles, especially during the daytime; and excessive sweating or anxiety. Any combination of these symptoms is an indicator that a visit to the doctor would be a good idea.

Complications

This is a very important list. Having high blood pressure can shorten a person's life span. Here's how:

- *Edema.* High blood pressure will force extra fluid out of the capillaries at the nutrient/waste exchange sites. This adds to overall levels of interstitial fluid, causing edema. In a typically vicious circle, edema will further raise the blood pressure by putting external force on blood vessels (see more in *edema*, Chapter 5).

- *Atherosclerosis.* Having blood pushing against arteries in an unceasing torrent will simply wear out the walls, especially when the arteries have naturally lost some of their resiliency from age. The moment there is the slightest damage for a

[d]The Sixth Report of the Joint National Committee on Prevention, Detection, Evaluation, and Treatment of High Blood Pressure. Nov, 1997. Available at: http://www.nhlbi.nih.gov/guidelines/hypertension/jnc6.pdf. Accessed winter, 2001.

platelet to cling to, the atherosclerotic process will begin. This will reinforce high blood pressure by narrowing arterial diameters (see more in *atherosclerosis*, this chapter).

- *Stroke.* Someone with hypertension is 4 times more likely to suffer a stroke than someone who does not have hypertension. The stroke may be from an embolism or from ruptured arteries in the brain (see more in *stroke*, Chapter 3).

- *Enlarged heart, heart failure.* Making the heart push against narrowed arteries will cause the left ventricle to grow considerably, but the coronary arteries will not grow with it to handle the extra load. The muscle fibers also lose elasticity. Therefore the contractions are actually weaker, because the muscle is not well supplied with blood and it cannot contract fully. This can also cause angina, or heart pain. When the ventricles of the heart are so overtaxed that they simply cannot keep up with the workload, the patient risks heart failure. This condition is 6 times more likely to happen to someone who is hypertensive than someone who is not (see more in *heart attack* and *heart failure*, this chapter).

- *Aneurysms.* This is the result of high blood pressure causing a bulge in the arteries (see more in *aneurysm*, this chapter).

- *Kidney disease.* In a way this is the most interesting complication of high blood pressure because of the circular relationship between hypertension and kidney dysfunction. Problems can start in either the kidneys or the circulatory system. If it starts with the circulatory system, here is the process: hypertension causes atherosclerotic plaques to form in the renal arteries, which are subject to *huge* blood pressure. This will cause reduced blood flow into the kidney, which will impair kidney function, leading to kidney damage, systemic edema, and yet more pressure exerted against vessel walls from that edema. If the problem starts in the kidneys, decreased kidney function will be an issue (see more under *renal failure*, Chapter 9). This will often be accompanied by extra release of *renin*, the kidney-based hormone that regulates some electrolyte balance. Excess renin results in vasoconstriction, water and salt retention, increased edema, increased blood volume, and high blood pressure.

- *Vision problems.* Chronic high blood pressure can damage the blood vessels that supply the eyes, causing them to become thickened and less elastic. Reduction of blood flow to the eyes results in permanent visual distortion.

Treatment

Hypertension is a highly treatable disease, but because it has virtually no symptoms until it has progressed to very dangerous levels, it is frequently untreated or incompletely treated (i.e., someone not taking medication because they feel fine).

Diet is the first way to manage this condition. The National Heart Lung and Blood Institute (NHLBI) recently conducted research about dietary factors and blood pressure. Their findings have led to the Dietary Approaches to Control Hypertension (DASH) diet: a combination of high-fiber, low-fat foods that provide higher than normal levels of calcium, magnesium, and potassium while cutting sodium by about 20%. Following the DASH diet (which is useful for anyone, not just hypertension patients) has been found to be just as effective as most varieties of blood pressure medication, without side effects or long-term health risks. The DASH diet reduces systolic readings by anywhere from 6 to 11 points, and diastolic readings from 3 to 6 points within 2 weeks of initiating the change in eating habits.

Some herbal remedies, especially garlic extracts, show promise in being able to help manage blood pressure levels.

Exercise is also crucial for the development of healthy new blood vessels and for weight control. Losing even a small percentage of body weight for obese or overweight patients can have a profound effect on blood pressure and cardiovascular health.

Medication, if called for, includes diuretics, vasodilators, and sometimes beta-blockers, which decrease the force of ventricular contraction. Medicating high blood pressure is a bit problematic. Because the disease itself has no strong symptoms and because the medicines often have unpleasant side effects (including dizziness, insomnia, impotence, and others), it has been difficult to get hypertension patients to be consistent with their medications. Recent statistics indicate that in the United States only one-third of the people who have hypertension are aware of it, and less than one-third of people diagnosed with hypertension treat it successfully.

Massage?

If a client knows that he or she has high blood pressure but is *not* required to take medication for it, circulatory massage is probably fine, especially if the client is physically active or encouraged to become physically active. Massage can help to lower general blood pressure and the stress that contributes to it. It is important, however, to rule out kidney and other advanced cardiovascular problems before beginning. Massage therapists should watch for signs that massage is overchallenging the body: clamminess, bogginess, and possible edema in the days after treatment.

If a client *is* taking medication for high blood pressure, circulatory modalities are strongly cautioned. Techniques that do not strongly influence fluid flow may be appropriate, but rigorous, fast-paced work may be too much of a challenge for an impaired ability to maintain homeostasis.

Regardless of whether the client is taking blood pressure medication, *deep abdominal work is contraindicated for high blood pressure.* This is because it is possible to accidentally trip the vaso-vagus reaction. Unintentionally overstimulating the vagus nerve can result in amplified parasympathetic reactions. This leads to systemic vasodilation and faintness from lack of blood to the brain. Another possibility is that the body could experience a sympathetic rebound effect. Ordinarily a vaso-vagus reaction is unpleasant but not dangerous—*unless* the blood vessels are not equipped to handle a rapid demand to dilate and constrict. Once again, a client's health is determined by the ability to maintain a stable internal environment during massage.

Raynaud's Syndrome
Definition: What Is It?

This is a condition involving the status of the arterioles in the hands and feet, although it can also affect the nose, ears, and lips. Primary Raynaud's disease is a simple vasoconstriction disorder, whereas secondary Raynaud's phenomenon is a complication of an underlying problem.

Demographics: Who Gets It?

Raynaud's that is unrelated to underlying conditions usually affects women between 14 and 40 years old; this population group makes up 75% of all primary Raynaud's patients. Secondary Raynaud's is often linked to autoimmune disorders, which women also expe-

RAYNAUD'S SYNDROME IN BRIEF

What is it?
Raynaud's syndrome is defined by episodes of vasospasm of the arterioles, usually in fingers and toes, and occasionally in the nose, ears, and lips.

How is it recognized?
Affected areas will often go through marked color changes of white or ashy gray for dark-skinned people, to blue to red. Attacks can last for less than 1 minute or several hours. Numbness and/or tingling may follow during recovery.

Is massage indicated or contraindicated?
Massage is indicated for Raynaud's syndrome that is *not* associated with underlying pathology. Otherwise, guidelines for the precipitating condition should be followed.

rience in greater numbers than men. Thus, women are more likely to be affected by either type of problem. Estimates vary, but it is projected that some variety of Raynaud's syndrome affects up to 5 to 10% of the general population.

Etiology: What Happens?

In both primary and secondary Raynaud's, the arterioles in the extremities experience *vasospasm* (contraction of smooth muscle tissue). It occurs in temporary episodes at first, but the vasoconstriction can become a permanent situation.

Causes (Primary)

Raynaud's disease is a primary problem, that is, unconnected to underlying pathology. It may be due to emotional stress (the autonomic nervous system will route blood away from the skin during emergencies), cold, or because of a mechanical irritation, such as operating machinery that influences blood vessel dilation. Pianists and typists are particularly vulnerable. Raynaud's disease generally has a very slow onset, and the attacks are less severe than when the symptoms occur as a secondary problem. If a person is prone to Raynaud's disease, both her feet and hands will tend to be affected.

Causes (Secondary)

Extreme vasoconstriction is occasionally a complication of some other disorder. In this case, the condition is called *Raynaud's phenomenon*. It will generally have a much faster onset than Raynaud's disease, and the risk of serious complications is much higher. Some conditions associated with Raynaud's phenomenon are:

- Arterial diseases that involve occlusions, such as *diabetes* (Chapter 8), *atherosclerosis* (this chapter), and Buerger's disease (another rare situation involving inflammation and blood clots in the arteries).

- Connective tissue diseases such as *scleroderma* (Chapter 1), *lupus* (Chapter 5), and *rheumatoid arthritis* (Chapter 2).

- Sensitivity to some drugs including beta-blockers and ergot compounds.

- Neurovascular compression, as seen with *carpal tunnel syndrome* (Chapter 2).

Signs and Symptoms

Raynaud's syndrome is usually bilateral. During an attack the skin will go through a characteristic cycle of colors: white, as the blood is shunted away from the area (on dark-skinned people the skin looks ashy gray); blue, as the cells are starved for oxygen; and red as the attack subsides, the arterioles re-open, and the blood returns to the affected area (Fig. 4-8, Color Plate 35).

Attacks of Raynaud's phenomenon can last anywhere from less than 1 minute to several hours. Secondary Raynaud's can be so extreme and long-lasting that a wasting of flesh and ulcerations on the starved skin may develop. The fingers may taper, and the skin can become thin, smooth, and shiny. Necrosis is a rare but possible complication for these extreme cases.

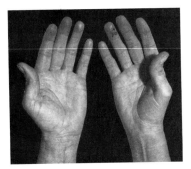

Figure 4-8. Raynaud's syndrome

Treatment

Treatment depends on whether the patient has a primary or secondary case of Raynaud's. Generally, a noninvasive approach is taken first, at least to primary Raynaud's disease. Quitting smoking, soaking the hands or feet in warm water, dressing appropriately for the weather, protecting the hands when working with cold or frozen foods, making sure that shoes are not too tight, and even moving to a warmer climate are all suggested before more intervention is attempted.

Because primary Raynaud's disease can be exacerbated by emotional upset, patients are often encouraged to find productive ways to manage stress. This can range from learning biofeedback techniques, to exercising regularly, to receiving massage.

If results are unsatisfactory, or if tissue damage from chronically impaired blood flow is a risk, the next step is medication to dilate the blood vessels. Other drugs work to counteract norepinephrine, the stress-related hormone that initiates vasoconstriction. Unfortunately, medical intervention is often unsuccessful for secondary Raynaud's phenomenon.

Massage?

The good news about Raynaud's is that although the primary version of the syndrome is fairly common, the secondary version is rather rare. If the Raynaud's is a part of lupus, scleroderma, or other vascular problem, the guidelines for massage must follow the cautions for the precipitating causes.

If any dangerous underlying causes for the vasoconstriction have been ruled out, primary Raynaud's syndrome indicates massage. Massage can work mechanically with local blood vessels and reflexively with the parasympathetic nervous system to stimulate vasodilation.

Varicose Veins

Definition: What Are They?

Varicose veins are distended, often twisted or "ropey" superficial veins. They are caused by damage to the internal valves whose job is to make sure that blood only goes one way—toward the heart. When blood backs up along the system, the affected vein is stretched, distorted, and generally weakened (Fig. 4-9). Varicose veins can happen at the anus (hemorrhoids), at the esophagus (esophageal varices), or at the scrotum (varicoles). Most often, however, they are in the legs, which is the focus of the rest of this discussion.

Demographics: Who Gets Them?

Women get varicose veins more often than men. This is largely due to estrogen, which can weaken venous walls, and to a history of pregnancy (a fetus can obstruct fluid return through the femoral vein, which can set the stage for later problems; see *pregnancy*, Chapter 10). It is estimated that about 1 in 10 people will have varicosities at some point, most after 50 years of age.

VARICOSE VEINS IN BRIEF

What are they?
Varicose veins are distended veins, usually in the legs, caused by vascular incompetence and a reflux of blood returning to the heart.

How are they recognized?
Varicose veins are ropey, slightly bluish, elevated veins that twist and turn out of their usual course. They happen most frequently in branches of the saphenous veins on the medial side of the calf, although they are also found on the posterior aspects of the calf and thigh.

Is massage indicated or contraindicated?
Massage is locally contraindicated for extreme varicose veins and anywhere distal to them. Mild varicose veins contraindicate deep, specific work but are otherwise safe for massage.

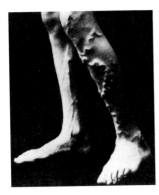

Figure 4-9. Varicose veins

Etiology: What Happens?

Anatomy Review   The veins in the legs have a fascinating construction that assists the heart in getting the blood from the toes all the way back to the chest. Small veins pick up the blood from the internal muscle capillaries. These veins tend to run on the superficial aspect of muscles. They feed into larger veins that perforate the muscle bellies and then into the really big deep veins that run under the muscles, close to the bones. When the leg muscles contract, the perforating veins are squeezed, sending their contents to the deep veins. When the leg muscles relax, the perforating veins draw in new blood from the smaller veins. The contraction and relaxation of the leg muscles (especially the soleus, the "sump pump of the leg") is crucial to blood return. The valves inside the perforating veins and the deep veins ensure that blood will not collect in the smaller, weaker superficial veins.

Causes

What can damage the valves in the veins? It could be simple wear and tear: being on one's feet for many hours a day, especially if the legs muscles are not allowed to fully contract and relax during that time, will weaken the veins. It could also be a mechanical obstruction to returning blood: knee socks that are too tight, a knee brace, or a fetus that presses on the femoral vein. Systemic congestion from kidney problems or liver backups has been seen to cause problems also. Finally, it could simply be congenitally weak veins. Once a valve sustains damage, blood will back up and put pressure on the next valve down. Vascular incompetence will ultimately cause the weakest superficial veins to become distorted, dilated, and twisted off their regular pathway. This weakening process seldom affects the biggest, deepest veins, because their walls are thicker and the leg muscles act as built-in support hose.

Signs and Symptoms

Varicose veins look like lumpy, bluish, wandering lines on the surface of the skin. They are often visible on the back of the calf, but more often they affect the great saphenous vein, where they show up anywhere from the ankle to the groin on the medial side. They may only be visible when the patient is standing.

   Varicose veins may itch or cause throbbing pain, especially at the end of the day when legs feel tired and heavy. They can contribute to edema around the ankles as fluid backs up in the lower leg.

Complications

Although varicosities are seldom anything more than annoying, they can occasionally create some unpleasant side affects. Chronically impaired circulation may result in varicose ulcers, which will not heal until circulation is restored. Skin irritation from poor circulation will occasionally lead to a type of *eczema* (Chapter 1) that will not be resolved until the varicosity is relieved. Interruptions in blood flow increase the likelihood of annoying night cramps (see *spasms, cramps,* Chapter 2). Stagnant blood in a distended vein may coagulate, raising the possibility of clotting. Most clots that form in varicose veins are superficial and melt easily, however, so they are less of a threat than clots that form in deeper leg veins (see *thrombophlebitis,* this chapter).

Treatment

Mild varicose veins are usually treated with good sense. Using support hose or elastic bandages can give extra help to damaged veins, and avoiding long periods of standing without full contraction and relaxation of the muscles is often recommended. Reclining with the feet slightly elevated will also reduce symptoms. Whether the veins can actually *heal* is somewhat controversial. If the damage has not progressed too far, relieving the mechanical stresses while strengthening the smooth muscle tissue (e.g., with hydrotherapy) can yield good results.

Surgery for mild varicose veins is not generally recommended as a purely cosmetic intervention. However, varicose veins are a progressive condition. They do not usually spontaneously reverse, and left untreated their complications can be serious. Therefore, a certain number of patients will eventually seek treatment for health, rather than cosmetic, concerns.

Several strategies for reducing varicose veins have been developed. The traditional approach is surgery to remove the affected vein ("stripping"). Ambulatory phlebectomy ("mini-stripping") is a similar treatment that removes only small sections of the affected veins. Sclerosing involves injections of chemicals (salt or sugar solutions) into the vein that cause it to close down completely. Laser treatments to heat up and collapse vein walls are also gaining popularity. In all these treatments, the body's remarkable ability to generate new blood vessels will quickly accommodate the closure or removal of the affected vein.

Massage?

Massage is a local contraindication for varicose veins, particularly for veins that are elevated from the skin and that have visibly been distorted from their original pathway. Not only is the tissue injured and delicate, it is inappropriate to push a lot of blood through vessels that may not be able to accommodate it. Heavy massage distal to these veins is cautioned also.

If the vein is only slightly darkened and not elevated or causing any pain, it is still wise to avoid local heavy pressure, but otherwise massage is safe. Tiny reddened spider veins (*telangiectasias*) are slightly dilated venules and are safe for massage.

Heart Conditions

Heart Attack

Definition: What Is It?

A heart attack is damage to some portion of the cardiac muscle as a result of ischemia, which starves and kills some of the muscle cells. The ischemia is usually caused by coronary artery disease (CAD) or *atherosclerosis* (this chapter) of the coronary arteries, which supply the cardiac muscle with oxygen and nutrition. If these arteries are completely occluded by plaque, thrombi, or any combination of the two, some piece of the muscle will die (Fig. 4-10). The muscle tissue will not grow back; it is replaced by inelastic, noncontractile scar tissue. The damaged area is referred to as an *infarct*. Another term for heart attack is *myocardial infarction*.

Demographics: Who Gets Them?

CAD and heart attack is the leading cause of death in the United States, claiming close to half a million lives every year, or 1 in every 5 deaths. Over a million heart attacks occur

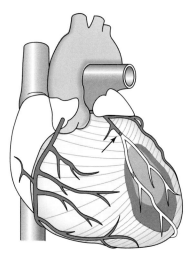

Figure 4-10. Heart attack

HEART ATTACK IN BRIEF

What is it?
A heart attack, or myocardial infarction (MI), is damage to the myocardium caused by a sudden obstruction in blood flow through the coronary arteries, which results in permanent myocardial damage.

How is it recognized?
Symptoms of most heart attacks include a sensation of great pressure on the chest, spreading pain, and lightheadedness, dizziness, and nausea. Sometimes symptoms vary, and occasionally a minor heart attack may occur with no symptoms at all.

Is massage indicated or contraindicated?
Patients recovering from recent heart attacks are not candidates for circulatory massage. After they have completely recovered they *may* be able to receive massage, depending on their cardiovascular health.

every year, and about 40% of them result in death. Not all heart attacks result in death, of course; about 12 million heart attack survivors are alive in the United States today.

Most people are familiar with the high-risk profile for heart attack victims: being sedentary, having *hypertension* (this chapter), having high cholesterol levels, being a smoker, and being overweight. Being male, having a family history of cardiovascular disease, or being a woman over 35 who takes birth control pills will increase the chances of a heart attack.

Etiology: What Happens?

A heart attack occurs when a portion of the cardiac muscle is killed off from lack of oxygen—an ischemic attack. The blockage in the coronary artery may be from a loosened blood clot or a broken or torn piece of atherosclerotic plaque.

Examinations of exactly which plaques pose the greatest risk of heart attack have yielded some surprising results. The size of the plaque seems to have little to do with its chances of breaking off or causing a heart attack. The more pertinent factor is the stability of the plaque. Older, harder plaques are relatively stable, but newer, softer plaques have a higher propensity to break open and let go of clots or atherosclerotic fragments that will then block the coronary artery.

When a portion of the cardiac muscle is killed by ischemic attack, the ability to contract with coordination and efficiency is badly damaged.

The seriousness of a heart attack is determined by the size and location of the blockage. If it is relatively small and blood flow is impaired to an area that does not have to work especially hard, the heart attack is not a serious one. If the infarct, or area of damaged tissue, is large enough to weaken the heart's ability to contract, or if the damaged tissue contains the electrical conduction system for the heart, major intervention will be necessary to aid in recovery. Because the right side of the heart pumps blood only to the lungs and back, while the left side pumps blood all over the body, left-sided infarctions are generally considered to be more serious than right-sided ones.

Signs and Symptoms

Heart attacks can have a variety of signs and symptoms, some of which are extremely subtle, and some of which feel "like an elephant sitting on your chest."[e] Three of the most common and dependable signs are:

- *Pressure, pain in the chest.*

- *Spreading pain.* This may spread to the shoulder, arm, neck, and jaw of the left side of the body: the referred pain pattern for the dermatome shared by the heart.

- *Lightheadedness, nausea, sweating.* These usually occur along with chest pain. When they occur *without* chest pain they may still indicate a heart attack, but it is a less common presentation.

[e]Taking Chest Pain Seriously. © 2000 Caresoft. Available at: https://www.thedailyapple.com/public/content/healthLibrary/printableArticles.jhtml?pArticleRepositoryID=%2Ftarget%2Fcs%2Farticle%2Ftda%2F100825.html&pArticleType=feature. Accessed winter, 2001.

Other symptoms can include shortness of breath with or without chest pain; unexplained nausea, anxiety, or weakness; fainting, palpitations, and a cold sweat. Even stomach and abdominal pain may sometimes be signs of a heart attack.

Angina pectoris (literally "chest pain") is one of the few early warning signs for the risk of heart attack. Angina is generally classified as "stable," in which episodes of pain follow a predictable pattern following activity; "unstable," in which a pattern suddenly changes in intensity or frequency; or "variant," which involves chest pain during rest rather than as a result of physical activity. Although an episode of angina does not necessarily signal a heart attack in progress, it is an indicator of an increased risk for myocardial infarct.

Complications

Several of these conditions are expounded upon elsewhere in this chapter; diseases of the cardiovascular system are highly interrelated. Furthermore, with heart disease it is hard to say what comes first—the infarct or the thrombus. In other words, the chronology of how these problems develop is often circular rather than linear.

- *Embolism.* A heart attack can cause blood clots to form in the heart. The clots then exit through the aorta and travel to wherever the bloodstream takes them. These are arterial emboli. They can land in the brain, causing a stroke, or the renal arteries, where they can contribute to *renal failure* (Chapter 9). Prolonged bed rest can also promote *deep vein thrombosis* (this chapter), which then carries a risk for pulmonary embolism (see *embolism or thrombus*, this chapter).

- *Atrial fibrillations.* These are rapid, incomplete, and weak attempts at contraction of the atria. They occur most often if any part of the sinoatrial node, the heart's electrical "pacemaker," has been damaged. These inefficient contractions allow blood to pool and thicken in the chambers of the heart and may contribute to the risk of *stroke* (Chapter 2). Ventricular fibrillations, because they interfere with blood flow to the entire body, may result in death if they are not treated quickly.

- *Aneurysm.* Weakened cardiac tissue can create a bulge in the heart muscle itself similar to *aortic aneurysms* (this chapter).

- *Heart failure.* Heart failure (this chapter) means that the muscle is no longer strong enough to do its work, and the body pays the price.

- *Shock.* In shock the circulatory system swings reactively from a sympathetic to a parasympathetic state, opening all the arteries to a maximum diameter in the process. The main danger with shock is loss of blood to the brain from radically decreased blood pressure.

Diagnosis

With all the new technologies that have been developed to deal with cardiovascular disease, the ability to identify and treat heart attacks *before* damage occurs is extraordinarily limited. Most of the time, the best that can be done is to wait until the heart attack is over and then evaluate the damage.

Screening for high-risk patients is usually conducted by angiogram. A flexible catheter is inserted into the femoral artery and snaked up to the coronary arteries. A contrast dye is injected into the aorta, and pictures are taken to see how blood flows through occluded arteries. This is an invasive procedure with somewhat limited accuracy. Although it can provide useful information about arterial diameter, it does not measure risk for heart attack.

Much emphasis is currently being put on imaging techniques that will help to identify who is at most risk for having a heart attack, and where that risk will come from *before* the heart is irrevocably damaged. Among the options that are becoming available are high-speed CT scans of the coronary arteries, contrast echocardiograms, and MRIs that can examine not only where plaques have developed, but how dense they are and how deeply they penetrate into arterial walls.

Treatment

The first priority with heart attack patients is to identify where the blockage is and to get rid of it as quickly as possible. This is done with thrombolytic agents: clot-dissolving drugs, which can take effect in 90 minutes or less, and with immediate balloon angioplasty, which can open up most clogged arteries in about 1 hour. The technical term for this procedure is *percutaneous transluminal coronary angioplasty* (PCTA). Other immediate care options include oxygen administration and pain management with nitroglycerin and/or morphine.

Later care usually includes more clot-dissolvers and nitroglycerin, which works to relax the smooth muscle tissue in the arteries. After the emergency has passed, the main treatment for heart attacks is observation. A barrage of tests is conducted to determine the location and extent of damage to the cardiac muscle. These tests will then indicate one of three future courses of action: that the infarct was minor and requires no further medical intervention; that prescriptive anticoagulants are indicated; or that a serious and permanent narrowing of a coronary artery requires surgery to open and repair it. This surgery may be a more complete version of the angioplasty, or it may be coronary by-pass surgery in which damaged sections of the coronary artery are replaced with grafts of healthy vessels from elsewhere in the body.

Treatment in heart attack and heart surgery recovery must also embrace the lifestyle changes that will support a healthier future: eating sensibly, exercising regularly, controlling high blood pressure, and quitting smoking are the most important factors.

Some studies have indicated that taking aspirin regularly can decrease the chance of a repeat heart attack for people with a history of heart disease. Specially coated tablets have been designed to minimize gastrointestinal problems, but this intervention carries a slight possibility of an increased chance of subdural hemorrhage, so patients must consider carefully all the implications of taking aspirin on a daily basis.

Massage?

The appropriateness of massage for heart attack survivors depends on the individual, the extent of the damage, and how long ago the damage occurred. Some survivors of mild heart attacks may make themselves healthier than they ever were before, whereas others will accumulate high levels of plaque on their arteries within just a few years of surgery. The safety of circulatory massage will depend on how easily the client can withstand those changes in internal environment that this work will produce.

Heart Failure
Definition: What Is It?

Heart failure is a term for the progressive loss of cardiac function that accompanies age and a history of cardiovascular disease. It does *not* mean that the heart has stopped working altogether (that would be "cardiac arrest"); it simply means that the heart cannot keep up with the needs of the body.

Demographics: Who Gets It?

The statistics on the incidence of heart failure in the United States are alarming but understandable, considering the changes in the health profile of the current population. Heart failure is on a dramatic rise in this country; it currently affects about 5 million people. About 400,000 new cases are diagnosed every year. The majority of those cases are among people who have survived other cardiovascular crises: heart attacks, CAD, aneurysm, and others. Where many years ago these problems would have killed these patients, they now survive and their hearts simply wear out from progressive damage to the cardiovascular system.

More men have heart failure than women, and it affects black men about twice as often as white men. The incidence for heart failure rises dramatically with age: it affects about 1% of the population at age 50 and up to 5% of the population at age 75 and older.

Etiology: What Happens?

When the heart is asked to pump hundreds of gallons of blood each day through vessels that are progressively narrowed and resistant, it will go through a series of changes that ultimately limit its ability to function. Unfortunately, the heart will enter early stages of heart failure with no signs or symptoms.

As resistance in the cardiovascular system increases, the heart actually grows; the muscle becomes bigger and the myocardial fibers thicken to overcome vascular narrowing. When this compensation is no longer adequate, the heart begins to beat faster, pushing less blood with each contraction. Finally, the muscle simply wears out and functions so inefficiently that blood flow to the rest of the body is insufficient for the most basic kinds of activities: climbing stairs, walking across a room, even getting out of bed.

Causes

Most cases of heart failure are related to underlying cardiovascular disease. A history of atherosclerosis or heart attack with resulting scar tissue in the heart muscle increases the risk of developing heart failure. High blood pressure, untreated *diabetes* (see Chapter 8), smoking, and alcohol and drug abuse can all be contributing factors as well. An especially potent set-up for heart failure is any combination of these risk factors (e.g., uncontrolled high blood pressure with smoking).

A smaller number of heart failure patients do not have a history of cardiovascular disease, but have sustained damage to the heart muscle for other reasons. Valve diseases, infections of the valves or heart muscle, or congenital problems may all be factors in these cases.

Types of Heart Failure

Heart failure is classified according to which side of the heart is affected. Signs, symptoms, and possible complications will vary according to which side of the heart is worn out the most.

HEART FAILURE IN BRIEF

What is it?
Heart failure is a condition in which the heart no longer can function well enough to keep up with the needs of the body. It is usually slowly progressive, developing over a number of years before any changes in function may be noticeable.

How is it recognized?
Different symptoms will be present depending on which side of the heart is working inefficiently. Left-sided heart failure results in fluid congestion in the lungs with general weakness and shortness of breath. Right-sided heart failure results in fluid back-ups throughout the system, which show as edema especially in the ankles and legs. Both varieties of heart failure will lead to chest pain; cold, sweaty skin; a fast, irregular pulse; coughing, especially when the person is lying down; and very low stamina.

Is massage indicated or contraindicated?
Circulatory massage is inappropriate for clients with heart failure, as it has the goal of pushing fluid through a system that is incapable of adjusting to those changes. Energy non-circulatory modalities are more appropriate to help clients lower stress and cope with the challenges of severely restricted circulation.

CORONARY ARTERY DISEASE
Bob, 49 Years Old
The Wake-Up Call

About 15 years ago my mom, who was 60 years old, had bypass surgery. I knew that having a female relative diagnosed with cardiovascular disease at 60 years old put me in a high-risk category for heart problems, especially since I've had type 2 diabetes for about 10 years. I know I didn't eat the healthiest diet in the world. At that time my regular lunch was a quarter-pounder and a bag of fries.

Last summer my mother went through a series of angina attacks followed by an angioplasty and having a stent inserted. After watching her, I began to seriously think of my own condition. I talked to my doctor, and he set me up with a low-cost onsite stress test that just used an exercise bike. He said if I could pass that I'd be okay. I took it, and in the words of the technician, "My heart was not happy with what I was doing to it." So my doctor scheduled me with a cardiologist for a full treadmill test.

After that first test I went out for what I knew would be my last double quarter-pounder with cheese.

I didn't last long on the treadmill. When it was over my blood pressure dropped and I had some really unpleasant symptoms, like dizziness, nausea, and a general feeling of crappiness. My doctor called my wife in from the waiting room and with both of us together he said, "My recommendation is to put you in the hospital now. We'll do an angiogram along with anything else that needs to be done."

"Well," I said, "I have a couple of things I need to finish up. Can I take care of them and then come right back?"

"I'd rather you didn't."

I checked right in.

I went in the hospital the Tuesday after Labor Day. On Wednesday I had the angiogram followed by an angioplasty. They found that the main section of the left coronary artery was 100% blocked. They had trouble pushing a wire through it, but when they got that done, they put in the balloon, and then a titanium stent. (They said it wouldn't set anything off, but I can't get into Target anymore without having all the alarms go off.)

They told me that they found evidence of a recent heart attack—one that was a fraction of an inch away from what they call a "widow-maker." This was amazing to me, because I have no memory of any chest pains. The only thing I can remember was when I went on a trip with my family at the beginning of the summer. I'd hiked around a little that day. That night in the motel I had a migraine headache, I felt sick, and threw up. I took some ibuprofen and went to bed. That's the only time I can think of that I might have had any symptoms at all.

Three days after the angioplasty I went home. They started my cardiac rehab right away. I go to the hospital to exercise under supervision. I am next door to an emergency room, and medical staff is in the room with me, so if anything happens, the response time will be really quick. When I first started I was hooked up to a heart monitor with four patches to measure my blood pressure before, during, and after my exercise. The first time I tried to exercise they made me quit, because I was about to go into ventricular fibrillation. Now I go exercise three times a week. I use the treadmill, the bike, weight machines, and free weights. I walk a lot at work, but I can't walk at home; it's too steep around my house. My doctors tell me I can't ever let my heart rate get over 120 beats per minute. If it gets any higher than that, I run the risk of forming clots around the stent.

I'm on several medications now. Some control my diabetes (I don't take insulin), and I'm also taking anticoagulants for 3 months, along with beta-blockers, and calcium channel blockers. And of course I've changed my diet. I eat so much chicken I feel like I'm growing feathers. It's all baked or grilled, and I take off the skin. We have little or no fried food, so no more french fries. Since I've made these changes my blood glucose has been much more under control—I average about 115 now, and normal is anywhere from 80 to 120.

This episode was a real wake-up call for me. I'm the youngest man at my job, and the last one they expected to have heart trouble. My identical twin went in for his own stress test, and came back fine, but he was a couple of years later than me in developing his diabetes, too, so he'll still have to keep an eye on it. I did some research about my situation and I found that what I had—silent ischemia—is especially common in diabetic men over 40. I hope any man with type 2 diabetes over 40 or 45 will be sure to get his heart checked. You never know what you might find.

- *Left-sided heart failure.* In this case a backup in the pulmonary circuit leads to the seepage of fluid back into the alveoli. This condition, if it becomes severe and is not corrected, leads to pulmonary edema. Symptoms of left-sided heart failure include severe shortness of breath and stubborn coughing, perhaps with bloody sputum. One serious complication of this condition is the risk of *pneumonia* (Chapter 6) in the functionally impaired lungs.

- *Right-sided heart failure.* In the absence of left heart failure, this is called *cor pulmonale*. It commonly results from pulmonary disease and high vascular resistance in the lungs. In other words, it becomes difficult to pump blood through the pulmonary circuit. Here the backup is felt through the rest of the body. Symptoms include severe *edema* (Chapter 5), especially in the legs. Someone with this type of heart failure will have ankles that look like they are spilling over the sides of the shoes. If the patient is bedridden, the edema may occur in the abdomen or low back, wherever gravity is pulling most. Right-sided heart failure is also closely linked to *renal failure* (see Chapter 9); as blood flow to the kidneys is reduced, the kidneys begin to retain water, which systemically increases blood pressure and makes the heart work even harder to push blood through narrow tubes.

- *Biventricular heart failure.* This is both left- and right-sided failure simultaneously. It is the end stage of the disease. If it does not respond to medications, the patient may be a candidate for a heart transplant or cardiomyoplasty.

Signs and Symptoms

Signs of heart failure depend on which side of the heart is dysfunctional, as described above. Along with shortness of breath (this is often exacerbated by lying down), low stamina, and distal edema, heart failure patients may also experience chronic chest pain, indigestion, arrhythmia, visibly distended veins in the neck, cold and sweaty skin, and restlessness.

⚠ WATCH FOR THIS

Chest Pain, Chest Pain, Chest Pain

Not all chest pain means heart attack, although in a culture where 42% of all deaths are related to cardiovascular disease, it seems logical to jump to that conclusion. What follows is a comparison of types of chest pain with some indications for what might be a heart attack and what probably is not. It is important to point out, however, that heart attack symptoms are notoriously variable and it is *always* a good idea to consult a health care professional when the source of chest pain is not clear.

	Angina	Heart Attack	Pulmonary Embolism	Other
Etiology	Chest pain triggered by activity It is caused by transient ischemia—the heart muscle does not get enough oxygen to function temporarily	Chest pain is caused by permanent ischemia—a blockage deprives cells of oxygen, and the heart is irrevocably damaged	Chest pain is caused by a blood clot in the lungs A small clot may have little impact; a large clot may lead to pulmonary and circulatory collapse	Chest pain is caused by any number of factors, including musculoskeletal injury or gastroesophageal reflux
Duration	Chest pain lasts several minutes and then subsides	Chest pain does not subside within several minutes; it gets progressively worse	Chest pain does not subside within several minutes; it gets progressively worse	Chest pain subsides in less than 1 minute
Alleviating factors	Chest pain stops when activity stops	Chest pain does not stop when activity stops; it continues to get worse	Chest pain does not stop when activity stops; it continues to get worse	Chest pain stops when the person drinks water, changes position, or takes a deep breath

Other Heart Conditions

Heart Murmurs

The heart can make several types of noises during its contractions. These are referred to as murmurs. They often, but not always, point to some type of valvular dysfunction within the heart. A client with a persistent heart murmur may have an inefficient pump and may not be able to keep up with rigorous circulatory massage.

Angina Pectoris

Literally "chest pain," this is a description of the symptoms that can occur when the heart muscle does not receive adequate oxygen. Angina pectoris is frequently a consequence of coronary arteries that are severely occluded, but other possible causes of chest pain include severe anemia or hyperthyroidism. This condition may involve severe pain or a feeling of heavy pressure around the chest, left shoulder and arm, and into the jaw and back.

Angina is typically brought on by periods of extreme stress or exertion. It is relieved by rest and drugs that dilate coronary vessels (nitroglycerin) and that reduce heart rate (beta-blockers) among others.

Angina itself does not imply that a heart attack is happening. However, it does suggest cardiovascular problems that may put a person at risk for MI.

Hypertrophy of the Heart

This condition, which is seen most dramatically in the left ventricle, is brought about by chronically high systemic pressure in the blood vessels. If the heart has to fight against constricted arteries to push blood through the body, it will hypertrophy, or grow larger. It may increase in strength as well, for a while, but as the need for oxygen outgrows the supply from the coronary arteries, the tissue will eventually experience ischemia, possible MI, and eventually congestive heart failure.

Another variety of hypertrophy occurs as a result of long-term volume overload. In this situation the left ventricle becomes enlarged but thinned and weak, like a big, baggy sack.

Congenital Heart Problems

Thirty-five different structural problems may affect the heart at birth, most of them focusing around valve function. Approximately 32,000 people a year are born with these problems, although new surgical techniques with infants (and even babies still in utero) are making it rarer and rarer to see adults with debilitating congenital heart defects.

Rheumatic Fever

Rheumatic fever is an autoimmune complication of exposure to streptococcus in which antibodies attack the heart valves, especially the mitral valve. It affects about 1.3 million Americans and is responsible for close to 6000 deaths per year. Mitral valve damage affects the way the heart can pump blood through the body. It can lead to arterial emboli or congestive heart failure.

Infectious Diseases of the Heart

Different varieties of streptococcus may prey on endocardium. If they find a way in (which can happen from something as innocuous as an abscessed tooth but is more often a complication of open heart surgery), they can cause valve damage and raise the risk of heart failure.

Massage?

Most of these conditions systemically contraindicate circulatory massage. Work that mechanically pushes fluid through the system will hinder rather than help these damaged structures.

Diagnosis

Heart failure is not difficult to diagnose. It is often done through observation of systemic edema and *auscultation* (listening to heart sounds and to the lungs for indications of fluid retention). A radiograph may be required to look for cardiac enlargement, and an electrocardiogram may be conducted to analyze the efficiency of the heartbeat. An echocardiogram can show valve function if damage to these structures is suspected.

Treatment

The treatment options for heart failure depend on its severity and which side of the heart has been affected. Early interventions include rest, changes in diet, and modifications in physical activity so that the heart can be exercised without becoming overly stressed. Drugs for heart failure may include beta-blockers, digitalis, diuretics, and vasodilators.

If the condition does not respond well to these noninvasive treatment options, surgery may be considered. Surgery can range anywhere from repair to damaged valves, to wrapping the latissimus dorsi around the heart and giving it a pacemaker (cardiomyoplasty), to a complete heart or heart-and-lung transplant.

Massage?

Heart failure means that the heart cannot function in a way that provides for essential needs. Most heart failure patients have other cardiovascular problems that contribute to their disease. Circulatory massage, which works with the intention of mechanically increasing blood flow through a basically healthy system, is inappropriate for clients whose blood vessels and heart cannot accommodate these changes in internal environment.

Energetic work that invites (rather than forces) the body to positive change may help to reduce blood pressure and perceived stress, and so may be useful for heart failure patients. However, it is not realistic to claim that massage can undo the extensive damage seen in these clients.

Chapter Review Questions: Circulatory System Conditions

1. Describe the process of the development of atherosclerosis.

2. Why is fatigue and low stamina a sign of anemia?

3. Where will all venous emboli go? Why?

4. Name three places arterial emboli can go to cause significant damage.

5. Do heart attacks involve blockages in the heart itself or in the coronary arteries?

6. Which chamber of the heart is the worst place to experience a myocardial infarct? Why?

7. Why is hypertension called "The Silent Killer"?

8. Describe the relationship between high blood pressure and kidney dysfunction.

9. Describe how a person may experience any three of the following conditions at the same time: high blood pressure, chronic renal failure, edema, atherosclerosis, diabetes, aortic aneurysm, and stroke.

10. A client has ropy, distended varicose veins on the medial aspect of the right knee. Distal to the knee the tissue is clammy and slightly edematous. Pressing at the ankle leaves a dimple, which takes several minutes to disappear. What cautions must be exercised with this client? Why?

Bibliography, Circulatory System Conditions

General References, Circulatory System

1. de Dominico G, Wood E. *Beard's Massage.* Philadelphia, Pa: WB Saunders; 1997

2. Damjanou I. *Pathology for the Health-Related Professions.* Philadelphia, Pa: WB Saunders; 1996.

3. Travell J, Simons DG. *Myofascial Pain and Dysfunction: The Trigger Point Manual.* Baltimore, Md: Williams & Wilkins; 1983.

4. Clemente CD. *Anatomy: A Regional Atlas of the Human Body.* 3rd ed. Baltimore, Md: Urban & Schwarzenburg; 1987.

5. Tortora GJ, Anagnostakos NP. *Principles of Anatomy and Physiology.* 6th ed. New York, NY: Harper & Row; 1990.

6. *Taber's Cyclopedic Dictionary.* 14th ed. Philadelphia, Pa: FA Davis; 1981.

7. *Stedman's Medical Dictionary.* 26th ed. Baltimore, Md: Williams & Wilkins; 1995.

8. Memmler RL, Wood DL. *The Human Body in Health and Disease.* 5th ed. Philadelphia, Pa: JB Lippincott; 1983.

9. Juhan D. *Job's Body: A Handbook for Bodywork.* Barrytown, NY: Station Hill Press; 1987.

10. Mulvihill ML. *Human Diseases: A Systemic Approach.* 2nd ed. Norwalk, CT: Appleton & Lange; 1987.

11. Kunz JRM, Finkel AJ, eds. *The American Medical Association Family Medical Guide.* New York, NY: Random House; 1987.

12. Marieb EM. *Human Anatomy and Physiology.* Redwood City, CA: Benjamin/Cummings; 1989.

13. Sapolsky RM. *Why Zebras Don't Get Ulcers: An Updated Guide to Stress, Stress-Related Disease, and Coping.* W.H. Freeman; NYC: 1998.

Anemia

1. Understanding the many types of anemia. *The Daily Apple.* Caresoft; 2000. Available at:. Accessed winter 2001.

2. B12 deficiency anemia. adam.com; 1999. Available at: http://www.adam.com/ency/article/000560.htm. Accessed winter 2001.

3. Phalen KF. Treatment of choice. *Special to the Washington Post.* November 21, 2000;Z19. Available at: http://www.washingtonpost.com/wp-dyn/articles/A47121-2000Nov21.html. Accessed winter 2001.

4. DeLoughery TG. Anemia: An approach to diagnosis. Oregon Health Sciences University; 2001. Available at: http://www.ohsu.edu/somhemonc/handouts/deloughery/printanemia.html. Accessed winter 2001.

5. Schwartz J. Drug prevents sickle cell anemia attacks. *Washington Post.* January 31, 1995;A1.

Embolism, Thrombus

1. Someren A. First renal CPC, June 1995. Available at: http://www.emory.edu/RENAL/ CPC/case1.95/cpc1.95.html. Accessed winter 2001.

2. Anderson FA, Jr., Audet AM. Best practices: Preventing deep vein thrombosis and pulmonary embolism. A practical guide to evaluation and improvement. Center for Outcomes Research, University of Massachusetts Medical Center; 1998. Available at: http://www.umassmed.edu/outcomes/dvt/ Chapt1-frameset.html. Accessed winter 2001.

Hemophilia

1. Hemophilia. InteliHealth Inc.; 1996–2001. Available at: http://www.intelihealth.com/IH/ihtIH?d=dmtContent&c=216738&p=~br,IHW1~st,244791~r,WSIHW0001~b,*1 Accessed winter 2001.

2. Hemophilia. Mayo Foundation for Medical Education and Research; 2000. Available at: http://www.mayohealth.org/home?id=5.1.1.8.22. Accessed winter 2001.

3. Introduction to hemophilia. The Web-Depot, Inc.; 1997. Available at: http://www.web-depot. com/hemophilia/

index.cgi/19970328.013255.21769. Accessed winter 2001.

4. What is hemophilia? National Hemophilia Foundation; 2000. Available at: http://www. hemophilia.org/. Accessed winter 2001.

5. What is hemophilia? World Federation of Hemophilia. Available at: http://www.wfh. org/. Accessed spring 2002.

6. What is von Willebrand disease? National Hemophilia Foundation; 2000. Available at: http://www.hemophilia.org/. Accessed winter 2001.

Hematoma

1. Bumps & bruises (contusions and ecchymoses). MedicineNet, Inc.; 1996–2001. Available at MedicineNet.com. Accessed winter 2001.

Leukemia

1. Leukemia. Mayo Foundation for Medical Education and Research; 2000. Available at: http:// www.mayohealth.org/ home?id=5.1.1.12.1. Accessed winter 2001.

2. Leukemia: What is it? American Cancer Society; 2000. Available at: http://www3.cancer.org/cancerinfo/ load_cont.asp?st=wi&ct=57& Language=ENGLISH#stats. Accessed winter 2001.

3. Acute lymphocytic leukemia: New treatments mean improved survival for many patients. Leukemia Society of America. Available at: http://www.leukemia.org/ CMS/q?action=static&v=PF&pageID= 29. Accessed winter 2001.

4. Acute myelogenous leukemia. Leukemia Society of America. Available at: http://www.leukemia.org/CMS/q?action= static&v=PF&pageID=29. Accessed winter 2001.

5. Childhood acute lymphoblastic leukemia. National Cancer Institute. Available at: http://cancernet.nci.nih.gov/cgi-bin/ srchcgi.exe?DBID=pdq&TYPE= search&SFMT=pdq_statement/1/0/0&Z2 08=208_00026P. Accessed spring 2002.

6. Chronic lymphocytic leukemia (CLL). Leukemia Society of America. Available at: http://www.leukemia.org/CMS/q?action=s tatic&v=PF&pageID=285. Accessed spring 2002.

7. Chronic myelogenous leukemia. The Leukemia & Lymphoma Society. Available at: http://www.leukemia.org/CMS/ q?action=static&v=PF&pageID=29. Accessed winter 2001.

8. Hairy cell leukemia. The Leukemia & Lymphoma Society. Available at: http://www.leukemia.org/CMS/q?action= static&v=PF&pageID=29. Accessed winter 2001.

9. Leukemia: What is leukemia? Mayo Foundation for Medical Education and Research; 1998–2000. Available at: http://www.mayohealth.org/home?id=5.1.1 .12.1. Accessed winter, 2001.

10. Leukemia: Reasons for hope. Originally published by Mayo Clinic Health Letter, November 1999. Available at: http://www.

mayohealth.org/mayo/9911/htm/ leukemia_hope.htm. Accessed winter 2001.

Thrombophlebitis, Deep Vein Thrombosis

1. Anderson FA, Jr., Audet, AM. Best practices: Preventing deep vein thrombosis and pulmonary embolism. A practical guide to evaluation and improvement. Center for Outcomes Research, University of Massachusetts Medical Center; 1998. Available at: http://www.umassmed.edu/outcomes/ dvt/Chapt1-frameset.html. Accessed winter 2001.

2. Peripheral venous disorders. Columbia University College of P & S Complete Home Medical Guide; 1997–2000. Available at: http://cpmcnet.columbia.edu/texts/guide/ hmg16_0007.html#16.27. Accessed winter 2001.

3. Deep vein thrombosis. K. Zwolski. Available at: http://www.pathoplus.com/dvt.htm. Accessed winter 2001.

4. Phlebitis & thrombosis. In Powell DR. *Chronic illnesses: Health at Home.* American Institute for Preventive Medicine; 1999. Available at: http://www.mcare.org/ healthtips/homecare/ PHLEBITI.HTM. Accessed winter 2001.

Aneurysm

1. Aneurysms. Texas Heart Institute; 2001. Available at: http://www.tmc.edu/ thi/aneurysm.html. Accessed winter 2001.

2. American Heart and Lung Institute's overview about aortic aneurysm: Surgery can stop this silent danger. American Heart and Lung Institute; 1996. Available at: http://www.best.com/~gek/Aneurys.htm. Accessed winter 2001.

3. Aortic aneurysm. Mayo Foundation for Medical Education and Research; 1998–2000. Available at: http://www. mayohealth.org/home?id=DS00017. Accessed winter 2001.

4. Aortic aneurysm. Surgical Care Associates. Available at: http://www.aorticaneurysm. com/sca-home.html. Accessed winter 2001.

5. FDA approves patch treatment for deadly abdominal condition. September 29, 1999. Cable News Network; 2001. Available at: http://207.25.71.29/HEALTH/9909/29/ aneurysm.alleviation/index.html. Accessed winter 2001.

Atherosclerosis

1. Angioplasty and cardiac revascularization treatments and statistics. American Heart Association; 2000. Available at: http://www.americanheart.org/Heart_and_ Stroke_A_Z_Guide/angioc.html. Accessed winter 2001.

2. Atherosclerosis. American Heart Association; 2000. Available at: http://www. americanheart. org/Heart_and_Strok e_A_Z_Guide/athero.html. Accessed winter 2001.

3. Beyond the headlines: Radiation shows promise for recurrent coronary arterial blockage. Mayo Foundation for Medical Education and Research; 1998–2000. Available at: http://www. mayohealth.org/ home?id=NE00221. Accessed winter 2001.

4. The basics: What is cholesterol? Caresoft; 2000. Available at: https://www. thedailyapple. com/public/cholesterol/ theBasics.jhtml. Accessed winter 2001.

5. Cholesterol in children. American Heart Association; 2000. Available at: http://www. americanheart.org/Heart_and_Stroke_A_Z _Guide/cholk.html. Accessed winter 2001.

6. Cholesterol statistics. American Heart Association; 2000. Available at: http://www .americanheart.org/Heart_and_Stroke_A_Z _Guide/chols.html. Accessed winter 2001.

7. Cholesterol. American Heart Association; 2000. Available at: http://www.american-heart.org/HeartandStrokeAZGuide/ chol.html . Accessed winter 2001.

8. Coronary artery spasm. American Heart Association; 2000. Available at http://www. americanheart.org/Heart_and_Stroke_A_Z _Guide/cas.html. Accessed winter 2001.

9. Headline watch: Younger men and cholesterol. July 19, 2000. Mayo Foundation for Medical Education and Research; 2000. Available at: http://www.mayohealth. org/home?id=NE00152. Accessed winter 2001.

10. Risk factors and coronary heart disease. American Heart Association; 2000. Available at http://www.americanheart.org/ Heart_and_Stroke_A_Z_Guide/riskfact. html. Accessed winter 2001.

11. About cardiovascular disease. Centers for Disease Control. Available at: http://www.cdc.gov/ nccdphp/cvd/ aboutcardio.htm. Accessed winter 2001.

12. Cardiovascular disease statistics. American Heart Association; 2000. Available at http://www.americanheart.org/Heart_and _Stroke_A_Z_Guide/cvds.html. Accessed winter 2001.

13. Cholesterol. Texas Heart Institute; 2001. Available at: http://www.tmc.edu/ thi/choleste.html. Accessed winter 2001.

14. The burden of chronic diseases as causes of death. Centers for Disease Control. Available at: http://www.cdc.gov/nccdphp/ statbook/pdf/section1.pdf. Accessed winter 2001..

15. Cigarette smoking and cardiovascular diseases. American Heart Association; 2000. Available at: http://www.americanheart. org/Heart_and_Stroke_A_Z_Guide/cigcvd. html. Accessed winter 2001.

16. Feeling down could raise the risk for heart disease. P\S\L Consulting Group Inc; 2000. Available at: http://www.pslgroup. com/dg/1e3bee.htm. Accessed winter 2001.

17. Preventing heart disease. August 4, 2000. Mayo Foundation for Medical Education and Research; 2000. http://www. mayohealth.org/ home?id=HO00119. Accessed winter 2001.

18. Iron and heart disease. American Heart Association; 2000. Available at: http://www.

americanheart.org/Heart_and_Stroke_A_Z_Guide/iron.html. Accessed winter 2001.

19. Preventing cardiovascular disease: Addressing the nation's leading killer. Centers for Disease Control. Available at: http://www.cdc.gov/nccdphp/cvd/cvdaag.htm. Accessed spring 2002.

20. Edelson E. Health scout reporter. Heart disease: Truly all in the family. Rx Remedy, Inc.; 2001. Available at: http://www.healthscout. com/cgi-bin/WebObjects/Af?ap=43&id= 107700. Accessed winter 2001.

21. Tests to diagnose heart disease. American Heart Association; 2000. Available at: http://www.americanheart.org/Heart_and_Stroke_A_Z_Guide/tests.html. Accessed winter 2001.

22. The link between physical activity and morbidity and mortality. Centers for Disease Control. Available at: http://www.cdc.gov/nccdphp/sgr/ mm.htm. Accessed winter 2001.

23. Women, heart disease and stroke statistics. American Heart Association; 2000. Available at:: http://www.americanheart.org/Heart_and_Stroke_A_Z_Guide/womens.html. Accessed winter, 2001.

Hypertension

1. Blood pressure. American Heart Association; 2000. Available at: http://www.americanheart. org/Heart_and_Stroke_A_Z_Guide/bp.html. Accessed winter 2001.

2. Phalen KF. Treatment of choice: Hypertension, silent and deadly, but treatable. *Special to the Washington Post.* July 18, 2000;Z27. Available at: http://www.washingtonpost.com/wp-dyn/articles/A61756-2000Jul18.html. Accessed winter 2001.

3. High blood pressure, why it is bad. American Heart Association; 2000. Available at: http://www.americanheart.org/Heart_and_Stroke_A_Z_Guide/hbpwhy.html. Accessed winter 2001.

4. Facts about the DASH diet. National Institutes of Health, National Heart, Lung, and Blood Institute. NIH publication no. 98-4082, September 1998. Available at: http://www.nhlbi. nih.gov/health/ · public/heart/hbp/dash/dashbody.htm. Accessed winter 2001.

5. High blood pressure statistics. American Heart Association; 2000. Available at: http://www. americanheart.org/Heart_and_Stroke_A_Z_Guide/hbps.html. Accessed winter 2001.

6. High blood pressure. American Heart Association; 2000. Available at: http://www.americanheart.org/Heart_and_Stroke_A_Z_Guide/hbp.html. Accessed winter 2001.

7. High blood pressure. Mayo Foundation for Medical Education and Research; 2000. Available at: http://www.mayoclinic.com/home? id=DS00100#WhatIs. Accessed winter 2001.

8. National Institute on Aging age page: High blood pressure a common but controllable disorder. National Institute on Aging. Available at: http://www.aoa.

dhhs.gov/aoa/pages/agepages/hibldpr.html. Accessed winter 2001.

Raynaud's Syndrome

1. Facts about Raynaud's phenomenon. National Institutes of Health. National Heart, Lung, and Blood Institute. NIH publication no. 93-2263. Available at: http://www.nhlbi.nih.gov/health/public/blood/other/raynaud.htm. Accessed winter 2001.

2. Questions and answers about Raynaud's. The National Arthritis and Musculoskeletal and Skin Diseases Information Clearinghouse. Available at: http://www.niams.nih.gov/hi/topics/raynaud/ar125fs.htm. Accessed winter 2001.

3. Raynaud's phenomenon. MedicineNet, Inc.; 1996–2001. Available at: http://www.medicinenet.com. Accessed winter 2001.

4. Barker EA. Raynaud's disease: Too much of a good thing. Cardiovascular Institute of the South; 1999. Available at: http://www.cardio.com/articles/raynaud.htm. Accessed winter 2001.

Varicose Veins

1. Feied CF. Sclerosing solutions. American College of Phlebology. Available at: http://www. phlebology.org/docmechanism.htm. Accessed winter 2001.

2. Varicose veins. InteliHealth Inc.; 1996–2001. Available at: http://www.intelihealth.com/ IH/ihtIH/WSIHW000/8059/23713/152194.html?d=dmtContent. Accessed winter 2001.

3. Varicose veins and spider veins FAQ's. Veinsonline.com. Available at: http://www.veinsonline.com/faq.html#What are varicose and spider. Accessed winter 2001.

4. Phalen K. Treatment of choice. *Special to the Washington Post.* June 20, 2000:Z27. Available at: http://www.washingtonpost.com/wp-dyn/articles/A25066-2000Jun20.html. Accessed winter 2001.

Heart Attack

1. Angina pectoris. American Heart Association; 2000. Available at: http://www.americanheart.org/Heart_and_Stroke_A_Z_Guide/angina.html. Accessed winter 2001.

2. Angina. Caresoft; 2000. Available at: https://www.thedailyapple.com/public/content/healthLibrary/featureArticle.jhtml?articleRepositoryID=%2Ftarget%2Fcs%2Farticle%2Fcs%2F100245.html. Accessed winter 2001.

3. Taking chest pain seriously. Caresoft; 2000. Available at: https://www.thedailyapple.com/public/content/healthLibrary/printableArticles. jhtml?pArticleRepositoryID=%2Ftarget%2Fcs%2Farticle%2Fda%2F100825.html&pArticleType=feature. Accessed winter 2001.

4. Atrial fibrillation. InteliHealth Inc.; 1996–2001. Available at: http://www.intelihealth.com/ IH/ihtIH?d=dmtContent&c=213152&p= ~br,IHW1~st,24479l~r,WSIHW000l

~b,*1. Accessed winter 2001.

5. Heart attack and angina statistics. American Heart Association; 2000. Available at http://www.americanheart.org/Heart_and_Stroke_A_Z_Guide/has.html. Accessed winter 2001.

6. Heart attack symptoms/warning signs. American Heart Association; 2000. Available at: http://www.americanheart. org/Heart_and_Stroke_A_Z_Guide/hasy.html. Accessed winter 2001.

7. Heart attack. American Heart Association; 2000. Available at: http://www.americanheart. org/Heart_and_Stroke_A_Z_Guide/ha.html. Accessed winter 2001.

8. Squires S. Secrets of the heart. *The Washington Post.* August 8, 2000:Z12. Available at: http://washingtonpost.com/wp-dyn/articles/ A53274-2000Aug8.html. Accessed winter 2001.

Heart Failure

1. Congestive heart failure. American Heart Association; 2000. Available at: http://www.americanheart.org/Heart_and_Stroke_A_Z_Guide/congest.html. Accessed winter 2001.

2. Congestive heart failure. Texas Heart Institute; 2001. Available at: http://www.tmc.edu/thi/ chf.html. Accessed winter, 2001.

3. Facts about heart failure. National Institutes of Health, National Heart, Lung, and Blood Institute. NIH publication no. 95-923. Available at: http://www.nhlbi.nih.gov/health/public/heart/other/hrtfail.htm. Accessed winter 2001.

4. Data fact sheet: Congestive heart failure in the United States: A new epidemic. National Heart, Lung, and Blood Institute. National Institutes of Health. Available at: http://www.nhlbi.nih.gov/health/public/heart/other/CHF.htm. Accessed winter 2001.

Lymph and Immune System Conditions

5

CHAPTER OBJECTIVES

After reading this chapter, you should be able to . . .

- Name one type of edema that indicates massage.
- Name three types of edema that contraindicate massage.
- Name two types of lymphoma.
- Name why lymphoma causes anemia.
- Name one risk for working with clients who have mononucleosis.

- Name two central nervous system components seen with most chronic fatigue syndrome patients.
- Name three benefits of not interfering with fever.
- Name the three stages of HIV infection.
- Name the most common symptom or complication associated with lupus.
- Name the four cardinal signs of inflammation.

INTRODUCTION

Lymph System

The lymphatic system is a critically important system for massage practitioners to understand. It is a bit peculiar; its components are not even vaguely symmetrical, and it functions as a sort of subsystem to both the circulatory and immune systems. The conditions listed under this heading may be influenced by either of the other two systems. The following is a brief reminder of how the lymphatic system works.

Lymph System Structure

As blood travels away from the heart it goes through progressively smaller tubes— the aorta branches into the arteries, which branch into arterioles, which finally divide into the very tiny and delicate capillaries. The pressure and speed with which blood travels decrease as it gets further away from the heart. Still, everything should keep moving at a good pace; a blood cell can complete its circuit through the body about every 60 seconds.

The walls of the capillaries are made of one-cell-thick squamous epithelium, designed for maximum efficiency of diffusion. The diameter, or lumina, of capillaries is so tiny that the red blood cells must line up one by one to pass through. This is the moment for the transfer of nutrients and wastes in the tissue cells. This is also where, having dropped off oxygen and picked up carbon dioxide, the vessels turn from arterial capillaries into venous capillaries. Finally, this is the moment when fluid from the arterial blood is squeezed out of the capillaries by external pressure. In other words, *this* is the origin of interstitial fluid.

Interstitial fluid is absolutely vital! It is the medium by which all the body's nutrients and wastes travel. It needs to keep moving. If it stagnates, toxins can accumulate there and cause problems. Interstitial fluid keeps moving through the system by flowing into a different type of capillary, a lymphatic capillary. Lymphatic capillaries are similar to circulatory capillaries in construction with one major difference—they are part of an *open* system. That is, interstitial fluid and even small particles can flow into lymphatic capillaries at almost any point along the length of that capillary. (Circulatory capillaries are *closed* to the extent that red blood cells are *not* able to come and go unless there has been damage to the vessel.)

When interstitial fluid is drawn into a lymphatic capillary it is officially called *lymph*. Lymph is composed mainly of plasma that has been pressed out of the bloodstream, loads of metabolic wastes that have been exuded by hardworking cells, and some chunks of particulate waste as well.

The new lymph is routed to a series of cleaning stations called *nodes* where the wastes are neutralized and any small particles are filtered out. The nodes are also home to most of the body's specific immune response cells, so if any pathogens have been picked up and marked by macrophages in the lymph, this is where the immune response really gets started. Eventually the cleaned-up fluid is deposited back into the circulatory system; this happens just above the right atrium of the heart where the right and left thoracic ducts empty into the right and left thoracic veins, respectively (Fig. 5-1).

Lymph System Function

Lymph flows through the lymphatic capillaries into bigger and bigger vessels, usually against the pull of gravity and without the aid of the heart's direct pumping action. What moves it along? Several things:

- *Gravity.* Gravity will help move lymph if the limb is elevated.
- *Muscle contraction.* When muscle fibers squeeze down around lymphatic vessels they push fluid through, just like a hand squeezes around a tube of toothpaste.

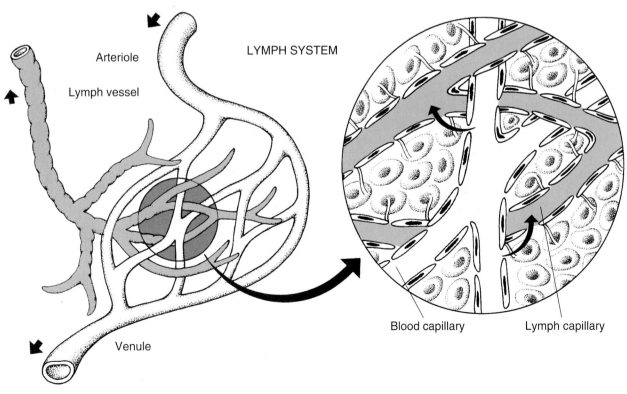

Figure 5-1. The origin of lymph

- *Alternating hot and cold.* Hydrotherapy applications can cause contractions in the smooth muscle tissue of lymphatic vessels to move fluid along.
- *Breathing.* Deep breathing draws lymph up the thoracic duct like an expanding bellows during inhalation and squeezes it muscularly during exhalation.
- *Massage.* Big mechanical manipulative strokes like petrissage and deep effleurage can increase lymph flow, but even small, extremely superficial reflexive strokes can cause stagnant fluid to be drawn into lymphatic capillaries.

If everything works well, fluid levels in the tissues should be constant but not stagnant. The amount of fluid squeezed *out* of circulatory capillaries should be almost equal to the amount being drawn *into* lymphatic capillaries; this is called Starling's equilibrium. A backup anywhere in the system could result in major changes in fluid balance. If lymph vessels or nodes are blocked, for instance, fluid will accumulate between tissue cells. The stagnant fluid quickly becomes a hindrance to diffusion and other chemical reactions, rather than the transfer medium it is designed to be. This is the problem with many of the diseases of the lymph system, and this is a serious situation for massage practitioners, who generally should *not* be trying to push fluid through a system that is already overtaxed.

Immune System Function

The immune system is unique in that it is not composed of a collection of organs each performing a task for a coordinated total effort, like the cardiovascular, muscular, nervous, or other systems in the body. Instead, it is a nebulous, incredibly complex collection of cells and chemicals stationed all over the body whose coordinated function is not to turn food into energy or to distribute oxygen, but to do something even more fundamental: to keep the whole organism safe. Because the immune system is composed of specialized cells rather than organs, this discussion focuses on the function rather than the structure of the system.

The primary function of the immune system is to distinguish what is "self" from what is "non-self" and to eradicate anything that is "non-self" as quickly as possible. Immune system devices range from being very general to highly specific in identifying exactly which pathogens they will attack. Some white cells will attack anything; others will simply ignore a pathogen if it is not their particular target. Most of the nonspecific immune devices like intact skin and the acidity of the gastric juices are not discussed here. Nevertheless, it is worthwhile to look at some of the *specific* immune machinery because when it is working well, it is positively miraculous; when it is *not* working well or when it makes mistakes, things can go terribly wrong.

T-Cells and B-Cells

The two interlocking branches of the specific immune responses are cellular immunity (T-cells) and humoral immunity (B-cells). Neither of these extremely complicated systems can work at all unless their target pathogen is displayed by a macrophage. So that is the first step in fighting off an infection: a macrophage must find, eat, and display a piece of the microorganism in question. Fortunately, macrophages are distributed generously all through the blood and interstitial fluid, and they are concentrated in places like the superficial fascia, lymph nodes, lungs, and liver, where the chance of meeting pathogens is especially high.

Consider what happens when someone touches a contaminated doorknob and then wipes his eye: rhinovirus 14 has just been introduced into the body. A passing macrophage eats the pathogen, and it is drawn through lymphatic capillaries into a nearby lymph node. A T-cell is waiting there. It just happens to be especially designed to recognize the flag of rhinovirus 14. The T-cell gets very busy, replicating itself into several different forms, which go out into the bloodstream in search of more viruses to attack. In the process, the original T-cell stimulates its B-cell partner. This B-cell clones, and the new cells start producing rhinovirus-14–specific antibodies at a mind-boggling pace of 2000 antibodies per second! Antibodies are *not* alive. They are Y-shaped chemicals that are forged especially to lock onto their target pathogen and "retire" it. This can happen in many different ways, depending on the pathogen and the antibodies involved.

Back when the T-cells and B-cells were first becoming active, they each made a few copies of themselves that would outlive the infection and circulate through the body on the lookout for future attempts by the same pathogen to invade. These are *memory cells*, and thanks to them people very seldom get sick with the same pathogen twice. If rhinovirus 14 gains access to the body again, an immune attack will mobilize against it so quickly that a person might never know that he or she was in danger.

The immune system is miraculous in how the T- and B-cells can somehow recognize their own special pathogen and launch just the right attack against it. It has even been shown that B-cells will produce antibodies that can disable *synthetic* pathogens that do not occur in nature. Now that's being prepared! However, the immune system occasionally makes mistakes. Sometimes it will launch a full-scale attack—with an inflammatory response, antibody production, and all the rest—against an antigen that is not really dangerous (e.g., cat dander or pollen). The other slip the immune system can make is to mistake a part of the body for a dangerous pathogen (i.e., it fails to distinguish self from non-self). Conditions involving this type of mistake are called autoimmune disorders.

Different White Blood Cells for Different Functions

White blood cells (leukocytes) come in different sizes, classes, and strengths. Each type of leukocyte has a specific role in the immune system and inflammatory response. As researchers learn more about how these cells work and communicate with each other, the ability to influence their activities is improved.

Neutrophils are the smallest, fastest, and most common of the white blood cells. They are produced in bone marrow, and chemicals that leak from damaged cells stimulate their production in even greater numbers. Neutrophils have a short life span; they can only disable potential pathogens once before they sacrifice themselves to the cause.

Monocytes begin as small white blood cells but they have the power to change. When they are released into the bloodstream from the bone marrow, they circulate until they reach a target tissue. Then they leave the circulatory system to infiltrate that tissue and grow into *macrophages* ("big eaters" that can devour pathogens and display bits of cell membrane that begin the specific immune response). Monocytes and macrophages move slowly; they are usually involved in the subacute or chronic phases of inflammatory response.

Eosinophils and *basophils* are not well understood inflammatory agents. They have been observed most often in the context of allergic reactions and responses against invading parasites.

Lymphocytes include B-cells, T-cells, and natural killer cells. These are manufactured in both bone marrow and lymphoid tissue and are most often engaged in specific immune system responses to pathogens. These are the agents that allow humans to develop immunity to infections.

Hypersensitivity Reactions

Autoimmune disorders and allergies are hypersensitivity reactions. They indicate immune system function that goes beyond the call of duty. Four types of hypersensitivity reactions have been classified. Because two of them can involve the skin and the other two can involve systemic disorders, it is useful for massage therapists to be familiar with them.

- *Type I.* A Type I hypersensitivity reaction is an immediate reaction to an antigen, or particle of "non-self." In this situation immunoglobulin E (IgE), a specific class of antibody, quickly sensitizes nearby mast cells to the presence of an "enemy"—which could be a fragment of pollen, the proteins from peanuts or shellfish, or a droplet of bee venom. The alerted mast cells then release histamine and other chemicals that create dramatic changes in vascular permeability and that attract other white blood cells to the area. This inflammatory response creates the symptoms that are associated with typical allergic reactions: redness, swelling, itching, weepy eyes, and runny nose with hay fever;

or nausea, vomiting, and diarrhea with certain food allergies. If the irritated mast cells are in the respiratory tract, the hypersensitivity reaction will occur as a bout of bronchial *asthma* (see Chapter 6).

One of the distinguishing features of a Type I reaction is that the IgE antibodies stay local in the affected tissues. The histamine and other chemicals that are released, however, may be carried through the bloodstream to other parts of the body. If enough of these chemicals are present and if the body's reaction is severe enough, the result may be *anaphylactic shock*. This happens when the vascular dilation stimulated by histamine and other inflammatory substances becomes so extreme and far-reaching that a person may be at risk of death from a combination of low blood pressure, pulmonary edema, and circulatory collapse.

Examples of Type I hypersensitivity reactions include hay fever, atopic dermatitis (also known as *eczema*, Chapter 1), *hives* (Chapter 1), and bronchial asthma.

- *Type II*. Type II hypersensitivity reactions are far less common than Type I. They involve inflammatory cytotoxic ("cell killing") reactions against a specific substance that may or may not belong to the body.

  Examples of Type II reactions include *myasthenia gravis* (Chapter 2), hemolytic *anemia* (Chapter 4), and reactions to the transfusion of mismatched blood.

- *Type III*. In Type III reactions antibodies bind with antigens, but the particles they form are too small to be phagocytized. These tiny conglomerates are eventually caught in the body's most delicate fluid filters: in the kidneys, the eyes, the brain, and the serous membranes surrounding the heart, lungs, and abdominal cavity. There they stimulate immune system activity that results in inflammation and damage to these very delicate structures.

  Examples of Type III reactions include *systemic lupus erythematosus* (this chapter), a specific type of *glomerulonephritis* (Chapter 9), and possibly *rheumatoid arthritis* (Chapter 2).

- *Type IV*. Type IV or "delayed" reactions are cell-mediated; they rely on T-cells to stimulate an immune response to an irritant. In some cases large clumps called *granulomas* are formed of immune system cells. In other cases an immune system overreaction occurs without the formation of granulomas.

  Contact *dermatitis* (Chapter 1) is an example of a Type IV hypersensitivity reaction. In this case, an inflammatory reaction appears on the skin after exposure to an irritating substance such as plant toxins (i.e., poison ivy), certain dyes, soaps, metals, or latex. This is usually a delayed reaction and may occur 24 to 48 hours after exposure.

The above summary of specific immunity is very brief. Much more is known now that was known just 20 years ago. One of the most exciting discoveries about immune system function is that immune system cells actually *talk* to each other, discussing in a language made of chemicals called cytokines what their strategies are in fighting off infection. These chemical messages are beginning to be deciphered, and some of them have been found to say things like "act like me," "come over here," and "eat this." This opens whole new treatment options, as researchers decipher these chemical codes and begin to manufacture medicines that can influence immune system behavior by mimicking specific cytokines.

Furthermore, it turns out that immune system cells do not just talk to each other. Some of the chemical messages they send out are picked up and acted on by other systems in the body, especially the nervous and endocrine systems. White blood cells have receptors for central nervous system chemicals, for instance. In other words, the nervous system can "talk" directly to the immune system. Some of the lymphokines secreted by white blood cells are similar, even identical to the neurotransmitters previously assumed to exist only in the central nervous system. Other lymphokines, specifically interleukin-1, are secreted by macrophages but relay information to the hypothalamus. This creates some major implications about how health and resistance to disease are related to mental and emotional state. Intuitively this makes a lot of sense, and now these theories are being supported with empirical evidence. A branch of science called psychoneuroimmunology has developed specifically to explore these relationships. Bit by bit, that imaginary division between mind and body is disappearing.

Hypersensitivity Reactions and Massage Oil

Type I hypersensitivity reactions typically occur within several seconds to a few minutes of exposure to an irritating substance. However, a late-phase Type I reaction can sustain allergic symptoms long after the irritation has been removed. *Arachidonic acid* is a substance associated with late-phase Type I reactions, especially in the form of bronchial asthma. The significance of this for massage therapists is that some types of massage oils can break down into arachinodonic acid on the skin. A client who is sensitive to this type of reaction may have no immediate skin symptoms, but may wonder several hours later why he or she is coughing, wheezing, and feeling short of breath.

Oils that are particularly prone to breaking down into arachidonic acid are composed mostly of omega-6–sized molecules. These include safflower, soy, almond, sunflower, and corn oils. Although they can be pleasant and convenient to use for massage, they are the most likely to cause skin irritation and allergic reactions. Therefore, when it is important to avoid potentially irritating oils for certain conditions, these are the ones to eliminate first.

Lymph and Immune System Conditions

Lymph System Conditions	Immune System Conditions
Edema	Chronic Fatigue Syndrome
Lymphangitis	Fever
Lymphoma	HIV/AIDS
Mononucleosis	Inflammation
Lupus	

Lymph System Conditions

Edema

Definition: What Is It?

Edema is the accumulation of fluid between cells. It may be associated with inflammation or poor circulation. In either case the stagnant fluid needs to be pulled into lymphatic capillaries and processed by the lymph system.

Etiology: What Happens?

The Starling equilibrium states that the forces that cause fluid to leave blood capillaries should *almost* equal the forces that cause fluid to be reabsorbed by blood capillaries, and that anything left over (which should be about 10%) should be taken in and processed by the lymph system. Lymph capillaries are perfectly designed to pick up excess interstitial fluid: each squamous cell is anchored to surrounding tissue by a collagen filament. When excess fluid accumulates in any area, these anchoring filaments pull back on the squamous cells, thus increasing the lymph capillary's ability to take in fluid. Sometimes, though,

EDEMA IN BRIEF

What is it?
Edema is the retention of interstitial fluid because of electrolyte or protein imbalances, or because of mechanical obstruction in the circulatory or lymphatic systems.

How is it recognized?
Edematous tissue is puffy or boggy. It may be hot, if associated with local infection, or quite cool, if it is cut off from local circulation.

Is massage indicated or contraindicated?
Most edemas contraindicate circulatory massage. This is especially true of pitting edema, in which the tissue does not immediately spring back from a touch. Edemas that indicate massage include those due to subacute soft tissue injury or temporary immobilization caused by some factor that does *not* contraindicate massage.

more fluid builds up in the tissues than the circulatory and lymph systems combined can take in, and this is called edema. This occurs in conditions in which blood return is somehow impaired, which pushes excess fluid out of the vessels around the capillaries. Edema is not generally noticeable until interstitial fluid volume is approximately 30% above normal.

Causes

Edema can have several causes; most of them are a combination of chemical and mechanical factors. Mechanical factors may involve a weakened heart or an obstruction of some kind. Chemical causes of edema usually have to do with the accumulation of proteins in the interstitial fluid, which causes the area to retain water.

Massage?

Most types of systemic edema, and *every* instance of pitting edema, contraindicate circulatory massage because of the impact this kind of bodywork has on fluid flow.

Contraindicated Edemas

- If the heart is overtaxed (i.e., *heart failure*, Chapter 4) and is not pumping the volumes it should be, fluid will accumulate in the tissues. Massage will not improve this situation and could quite possibly make it worse by putting an even greater load on the system.

- If the kidneys are not filtering blood fast enough or completely enough because of chemical imbalance or mechanical obstruction, edema will develop and massage could make the situation much worse (see *renal failure*, Chapter 9).

- If the liver is congested, the puffiness and bogginess of typical edema may be less visibly apparent, but the same rules apply: pushing blood through a system that is chemically or mechanically impaired will do only damage (see *cirrhosis*, Chapter 7).

- If edema accumulates because of local infection, it contraindicates massage because of the risk of pushing pathogens into the lymphatic and circulatory systems before the body has had a chance to marshal appropriate defenses (see *inflammation*, this chapter).

- Mechanical blockages anywhere in the circulatory system contraindicate massage because it can damage delicate structures, or worse, it could break loose a blood clot. Some examples of mechanical blockages include edema associated with *pregnancy* (Chapter 10), *thrombus*, *embolism*, or *deep vein thrombosis* (Chapter 4).

Indicated Edemas

All this is not to say that every kind of edema absolutely contraindicates every kind of massage under every circumstance. Edema is a red flag for massage therapists and calls for caution before proceeding. Nevertheless, if a client has fluid retention related to a subacute musculoskeletal injury, skilled massage is *very* appropriate and in fact could be vital to the healing process (see *sprains*, Chapter 2). Likewise, if a client is confined to bed or is even partially immobilized for some reason that does *not* contraindicate massage, bodywork can be valuable to the health of his or her injured tissues as long as the risk of blood clotting has been ruled out.

Bodywork modalities with minimal impact on fluid flow are more appropriate for edema than Swedish or other types of massage. However, even practitioners of energy work need to know *why* their clients are retaining water in order to make the best possible choices for their care.

Lymphangitis

Definition: What Is It?

Lymphangitis is an infection with inflammation in the *lymphangions* (lymphatic capillaries).

Demographics: Who Gets It?

People with depressed immunity and/or poor circulation are especially susceptible to lymphangitis and lymphadenitis (inflammation of the lymph nodes), because their white blood cell activity is likely to be sluggish while their colonies of bacteria are more than happy to take advantage of the opportunity to set up shop.

Massage practitioners have a much greater chance of developing lymphangitis than do most clients. This condition is an occupational hazard for bodywork professions because repeated immersions of the hands in soapy water may lead to hangnail formation and drying and cracking of nail beds.

> ### LYMPHANGITIS IN BRIEF
>
> #### What is it?
> Lymphangitis is an infection of lymph capillaries. If it gets into the nodes it is called *lymphadenitis*. If it gets past the lymphatic system it is called blood poisoning (*septicemia*) and can be life threatening.
>
> #### How is it recognized?
> Lymphangitis has all the signs of local infection: pain, heat, redness, and swelling. It may also show red streaks from the site of infection running toward the nearest lymph nodes.
>
> #### Is massage indicated or contraindicated?
> Lymphangitis contraindicates circulatory massage until the infection has been completely eradicated.

Etiology: What Happens?

In lymphangitis the lymph capillaries have become infected, usually with some of the colonies of streptococcus bacteria that congregate on the skin. This condition can be a complication of *erysipelas* or from a viral or fungal infection like *herpes simplex* or *ringworm* (Chapter 1). If the pathogens are successful, they can set up an infection in the lymph vessel before macrophages or other white blood cells can stop them. Infections that invade the lymph nodes themselves are called *lymphadenitis*.

Signs and Symptoms

Symptoms of lymphangitis start with signs of local infection: pain, heat, redness, and swelling. The infected lymph vessel often shows a visible scarlet track running proximally from the portal of entry, which is usually some lesion in the skin like a hangnail, a knife cut, or an insect bite (Fig. 5-2, Color Plate 36). If the infection is unchecked by white blood cells, it will quickly move further into the lymph system, leading to swollen nodes, fever, and a general feeling of misery. This can happen surprisingly quickly; lymphangitis can become a systemic infection in a matter of hours.

Complications

Lymphangitis is an infection of the *lymph* system, not the circulatory system. However, if even a few bacteria get past the filtering action of the lymph nodes, the infection *will* enter the bloodstream at the right or left subclavian veins. Then the situation changes to

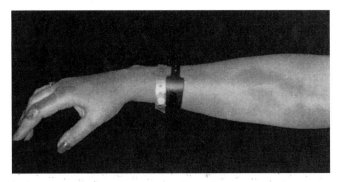

Figure 5-2. (CP 35) Lymphangitis: an infection of lymph capillaries

a much more serious one: septicemia, or blood poisoning, which is life threatening. This is why, if lymphangitis is a possibility, medical intervention is advisable at the earliest possible opportunity.

Treatment

Lymphangitis is usually treated successfully with antibiotic therapy. Treatment must begin soon after the infection has been identified, however, or the infection may complicate into blood poisoning.

Massage?

Lymphangitis patients feel so sick so fast that it is highly unlikely that an infected client would try to keep an appointment. Whereas a client who has lymphangitis is contraindicated to *receive* massage, a practitioner who has it is likewise contraindicated to *give* massage. Therefore, massage therapists must keep their hands clean and own a good pair of

---

LYMPHANGITIS
Rebecca, Age 24
"It was the most miserable night of my life."

There was a winter when I was working four jobs at once. I was tutoring for a massage school, I was setting up a small practice of my own, I was a nanny during the afternoons, and I was also working in a theatre company doing anything that needed doing, which was usually a lot.

I remember it was the week before Christmas, which was a really busy time for the theatre company—we went on tour doing shows for young children. I had also done several massage treatments that week, which was unusual for me. I was working in the light booth at the theatre one morning when I noticed that a hangnail on my right index finger suddenly seemed swollen, hot, and tender. There wasn't anything I could do about it. I remember sitting there for about an hour watching it get bigger, redder, and more painful.

That afternoon I had to leave town to be with my family over the holidays. The airport had been socked in with fog for 3 days, which delayed all the flights, so I missed my connection and had to spend the night on the floor of O'Hare Airport in Chicago. It was one of the most miserable times I can remember. I was feverish and shaking, and my hand hurt like hell.

By the time I finally reached D.C. all I wanted to do was go to bed. I spent practically the entire holiday flat on my back. The swelling at my finger finally subsided, but not before I broke out in intensely painful fever blisters all over my mouth. My doctor back home told me they were probably just an opportunistic outbreak while my defenses were low. All I know is they made it impossible to eat and I missed all my favorite Christmas foods.

I found out much later that I had probably had lymphangitis, and that I was very lucky it didn't develop into blood poisoning, especially since I didn't see a doctor until the whole thing was over. If I had it to do over again I'd make sure I never let myself get so run-down, and I'd be sure to cover any noticeable hangnails before doing massage. I wouldn't wish an experience like that on my worst enemy.

cuticle scissors. They must *not* allow hangnails and other lesions to go uncovered or untrimmed, and perhaps most importantly, they must *not* allow their health to degenerate to the point at which they are vulnerable to this kind of infection.

If a massage therapist has an open hangnail or other wound on a finger, the threat of lymphangitis is an excellent reason to cover it with a "finger cot" during appointments.

Lymphoma

Definition: What Is It?

Lymphoma is any type of cancer of the lymph nodes. Like *leukemia* (Chapter 4), lymphoma involves a mutation of the DNA in specific white blood cells. These cells are all based in lymph nodes rather than bone marrow, which makes the appearance and the progression of the disease very different from leukemia.

Lymphoma is usually categorized as Hodgkin's lymphoma (HL) and non-Hodgkin's lymphoma (NHL). Under the heading of NHL, many different subtypes of lymphoma have been identified.

Demographics: Who Gets It?

About 64,000 people in the United States are diagnosed with lymphoma every year (7200 with HL, and 56,800 with NHL). The incidence of lymphoma in general is rising at an alarming rate. It goes up by about 1.1% per year and has doubled since the 1970s.[a] The reasons for this are not clearly understood, although one subtype of NHL has a close association with infection with HIV and Epstein–Barr virus, both of which have become much more common in the past 3 decades.

Although lymphoma does occur in children, most patients are adults. HL most commonly affects adults in their 20s or those older than 50. NHL is most common among people 60 to 70 years old.

Lymphoma causes about 27,000 deaths per year (25,700 from NHL, and 1300 from HL).

Etiology

Lymphoma is cancer that originates in lymph nodes. Like leukemia, this disease begins with a mutation of the DNA of the affected cells, which in this case will be some type of T-cell, B-cell, or natural killer cell. The mutated cell begins to replicate, producing massive numbers of nonfunctioning lymphocytes. This causes the lymph nodes to enlarge, and it initiates the other symptoms associated with lymphoma (anemia, night sweats, itchy skin, and fatigue, among others).

The seriousness of lymphoma depends on what type of cell has mutated and how quickly it replicates. More than 30 different types of lymphoma have been identified and are categorized mainly by the appearance of the mutated cells.

LYMPHOMA IN BRIEF

What is it?
Lymphoma is any variety of cancer that grows in lymph nodes. Several types have been identified, some of which are aggressive and very threatening, others of which may progress more slowly.

How is it recognized?
Painless swelling of lymph nodes is the cardinal sign of lymphoma, along with the possibility of anemia, fatigue, low-grade fever, night sweats, itchiness, abdominal pain, and loss of appetite, all of which last for 2 weeks or more.

Is massage indicated or contraindicated?
Rigorous circulatory massage is generally not recommended for a person who is fighting lymphoma, although this may be a case-by-case decision. Persons who have been free from lymphoma for 5 years or more are considered "cured." Non-circulatory types of massage may be appropriate for lymphoma patients, although it is recommended that the therapist participate as part of an integrated health care team.

HODGKIN'S DISEASE
Thomas Hodgkin (1798–1866) was a British physician who documented this disorder.

[a]Hodgkin's disease. The Leukemia & Lymphoma Society (formerly Leukemia Society of America). Available at: http://www.leukemia.org/CMS/q?action=static&v=PF&pageID=17. Accessed winter 2001.

Types of Lymphoma

- *HL.* This disease involves the mutation of white blood cells into large, malignant, multinucleate cells called Reed–Sternberg cells. It is seen most often in the submandibular nodes but can also occur at the axillary and inguinal nodes. Eventually the growths metastasize to organ tissues, particularly the liver or bone marrow. HL accounts for about 10% of all lymphoma cases.

- *NHL.* These cancers, which account for 90% of all lymphomas, involve the mutation of lymphocytes into many different forms. They are classified as low-grade, intermediate, and high-grade lymphomas according to their aggressiveness. A short list of the 30 or so types of NHL includes the following:
    - *Low-grade lymphomas*
        A. Lymphocytic lymphoma
        B. Follicular cleaved-cell lymphoma
        C. Follicular mixed-cell lymphoma
    - *Intermediate lymphomas*
        A. Follicular large cell lymphoma
        B. Diffuse mixed cell lymphoma
        C. Diffuse large cell lymphoma
    - *High-grade lymphomas*
        A. Immunoblastic lymphoma
        B. Lymphoblastic lymphoma
        C. Burkitt's lymphoma
        D. Non-Burkitt's lymphoma

Risk Factors

The increasing incidence of lymphoma in the past 30 years has raised the distinct possibility that this cancer can be linked to environmental exposure. Some research finds statistical relationships between lymphoma and exposure to insecticides, herbicides, fertilizers, and even hair dye, but the direct cause-and-effect relationships have not yet been established.

Other environmental factors that increase the risk of developing certain types of lymphoma involve infection with specific pathogens. The incidence of lymphoma is 50 to 100 times higher among HIV-positive patients than it is among the general population. Epstein–Barr virus, which is associated with *mononucleosis* (this chapter), has been linked to Burkitt's lymphoma. Human T-cell lymphotropic virus (HTLV) is associated with T-cell lymphoma. Having the *Helicobacter pylori* bacterium (see *ulcers*, Chapter 7) raises the risk of developing lymphoma that originates in the stomach wall.

Signs and Symptoms

The primary symptom of any kind of lymphoma is painless, non-tender swelling of lymph nodes, especially in the neck, axilla, and inguinal area. (Fig. 5-3). Other symptoms include *anemia* (see Chapter 4), fatigue, weight loss, night sweats, itchy skin, and loss of appetite. If symptoms persist for 2 weeks or more, testing for lymphoma will probably be conducted.

Late stage lymphoma involves decreased immunity and susceptibility to secondary infection like shingles (see *herpes zoster*, Chapter 3), *flu*, or *pneumonia* (Chapter 6).

Diagnosis

The diagnosis of lymphoma begins with manual palpation of enlarged lymph nodes. If symptoms persist for 2 weeks or more, tests may be run to evaluate the node or nodes. Computed tomography (CT) scans or magnetic resonance imaging may be used to look for signs of growth in the chest or abdomen, so the cancer can be staged accurately.

Staging

Lymphoma is staged by its degree of progression. In addition to a numerical stage, lymphoma is also classified by whether symptoms other than enlarged glands accompany it. For example, Stage I-A means that the cancer is localized and not accompanied by fever, night sweats, or weight loss. Stage II-B means that the cancer has spread to nearby lymph nodes, and the patient also has fever, night sweats, and loss of appetite. The following is the staging scale for lymphoma:

I. The cancer is found in only one area, and that area is *not* the abdomen or the chest.

II. The cancer is found in only one area plus the nearest lymph nodes, *or* it is found in two sets of lymph nodes, but they are on the same side of the diaphragm, *or* the cancer is found in the digestive tract with or without lymph node involvement.

III. Tumors and affected lymph nodes are found on both sides of the diaphragm, *or* the cancer begins in the lymph nodes in the chest, *or* the cancer is in multiple places on both sides of the diaphragm, *or* the cancer is found in the central nervous system.

IV. The cancer is found in the bone marrow and/or in the central nervous system.

Recurrent lymphoma is cancer that reappears after a full course of treatment.

Treatment

Treatment choices for lymphoma depend on several factors, including exactly which type of cells are affected, the progression of the disease, and whether it is a Type A or Type B presentation.

Chemotherapy and radiation are the usual choices, but some other options are finding success in dealing with lymphoma, including allogenic and autologous bone marrow transplants as well as radioimmunotherapy (a process in which special antibodies that have been treated with radioactive iodine are injected into the body, where they attack and destroy cancer cells).

Prognosis

The prognosis for lymphoma depends on the type of cancer, the stage at which it is diagnosed, the age of the patient, and several other factors. Interestingly, the slower-growing types of lymphoma do not tend to respond as well to chemotherapy as the more aggressive varieties, which are considered more treatable.

Like leukemia, the "magic number" for lymphoma survival is 5 years. If a patient can make it that long with no signs of recurrent cancer, he or she is said to be cancer-free.

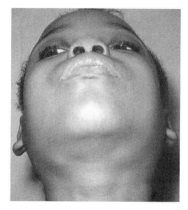

Figure 5-3. Hodgkin's lymphoma: cervical and submandibular lymph nodes are visibly enlarged

The overall 5-year survival rate for lymphoma is 51%, but the survival rate among children is as high as 78%. HL is considered the most survivable of all blood cancers; up to 80% of HL patients who are diagnosed early make it to the 5-year goal.

Currently, there are approximately 454,000 lymphoma survivors in the United States.

Massage?

Rigorous circulatory massage is inappropriate for clients whose lymph nodes may be malfunctioning, regardless of whether it is possible for massage to speed up metastasis. Non-circulatory work may be more appropriate, since the client may reap many supportive benefits without the risks of pushing a lot of fluid through a system that does not work smoothly. Nonetheless, it is always a good idea to work as part of a fully-informed health care team when a client is going through long-term, complicated, and even life-threatening challenges to health.

MONONUCLEOSIS IN BRIEF

What is it?
Mononucleosis is an infection, usually with the Epstein–Barr virus (EBV) but occasionally with cytomegalovirus (CMV) or other agents. The virus attacks epithelial tissue in the salivary glands and throat first and then invades B-cells and lymph nodes.

How is it recognized?
The three leading symptoms for mononucleosis are fever, swollen lymph nodes, and sore throat. Other symptoms may include fatigue, low stamina, enlarged spleen, and enlarged liver.

Is massage indicated or contraindicated?
Mononucleosis contraindicates circulatory massage in the acute stage when the body is fighting hard to beat back this viral attack. In later stages, as long as circulation is healthy and the spleen and liver are not congested, circulatory massage may improve recovery time, although abdominal work should be avoided. Non-circulatory types of bodywork may be appropriate, as long as the possibility of lymphatic congestion is considered.

Mononucleosis
Definition: What Is It?

Mononucleosis is a viral infection of the salivary glands and throat, which then moves into the lymphatic system by way of B-cells. The causative agent in about 90% of all cases is EBV, a member of the herpes family. Other pathogens that can cause mononucleosis are also members of Herpesviridae, specifically cytomeglovirus or CMV.

Demographics: Who Gets It?

EBV is everywhere. Random blood studies show that the rate of infection with EBV in the United States and elsewhere is about 90% by the time people reach 40 years old. Not everyone who has been exposed to EBV develops the symptoms associated with mononucleosis, or mono, however.

Mono is diagnosed in the United States at a rate of about 45 out of every 100,000 people. It is especially prevalent among adolescents and young adults; the vast majority of cases are found in people between 15 and 30 years of age. In college students the rate of infection is especially high; up to 3% of all college students are infected with mono every year.

Etiology: What Happens?

Mononucleosis from EBV spreads most efficiently through direct contact. This virus is fragile outside of a human host. Although it may remain viable for a short time on a dish or suspended in a droplet of mucus in the air, the most dependable way to catch it is through intimate saliva-to-saliva contact; it is not called the "kissing disease" for nothing.

Like many viral infections, mononucleosis moves through the body in two stages. In the first stage, the virus attacks epithelial tissue in the throat and salivary glands. It can take a long time for the infection to get established; incubation can last up to 60 days, during which time the patient is contagious but not strongly symptomatic. Once established well in the epithelial tissue of the throat, however, the virus moves on to infect B-lymphocytes and gain access to the lymph nodes.

The effect of the virus on its target B-cells is to make them immortal. That is, instead of dying at the end of a normal life span, the infected cells live on to replicate and produce a variety of antibodies, including antibodies to the virus itself, but also nonfunctioning antibodies called *heterophiles*. Changes to the infected B-cells cause them to resemble monocytes, an entirely different type of white blood cell. It is their resemblance to monocytes that led to the name *mononucleosis*.

As infected B-cells proliferate, the body responds by producing high numbers of cytotoxic T-cells. These T-cells eventually establish control over the rogue B-cells, and ultimately the virus becomes dormant in epithelial tissue of the throat. This process can take a long time, however; active virus has been found in the saliva of some patients many months after the acute stage of the infection had passed.

A resurgence of EBV after an initial infection is possible, but it is usually asymptomatic and easily quelled by T-cell activity.

Signs and Symptoms

Mononucleosis is notorious for presenting different symptoms in different patients. The younger the person is when exposed to EBV, the subtler the symptoms tend to be. Young children often go through exposure, infection, and recovery with no discernible symptoms at all.

In older patients, particularly adolescents and young adults, the symptoms are more dependable. The prodromic stage, as the infection is becoming established but creates no strong symptoms, may be marked by general fatigue and malaise; the patient often does not feel well but may not feel sick, either. This may last anywhere from a few days to several weeks. Then as the infection becomes more aggressive, the leading triad of symptoms appears: fever of 102 to 104°F, an extremely sore throat from the initial viral infection, and lymph nodes that are swollen from the production of massive numbers of B-cells and T-cells. The cervical lymph nodes are usually affected worst, but submandibular, axillary, and inguinal lymph nodes may also be palpably swollen and tender.

Puffy, swollen eyelids are a common complaint among mono patients. Splenomegaly (enlargement of the spleen) occurs in about half of all patients. About 20% also experience inflammation of the liver (see *hepatitis*, Chapter 7). Some mono patients develop a splotchy, measle-like rash, especially if they are concurrently taking amoxicillin or ampicillin (two penicillin-family antibiotics that could be prescribed for strep throat). A large majority of mono patients on these medications develop painful, alarming rashes.

Signs and symptoms of acute mononucleosis tend to last about 2 weeks before subsiding. Nevertheless, the whole infection is so wearing on the body that it can take several weeks or even months before a patient feels fully functional again.

Diagnosis

Diagnosing EBV is not difficult; the problem is in establishing the stage of the infection. Several features of this virus make it problematic to label. Mono presents differently in different patients, the incidence of EBV is nearly universal, and the virus can be present and active for many weeks or months after an infection. All these issues can make it difficult to definitively state that a person's symptoms are due only or even primarily to this particular virus.

The starting place for a diagnosis of mono is a Monospot test, which looks for signs of heterophile antibodies. Complete blood counts also reveal abnormally high lymphocytes: both atypical B-cells and extra T-cells to fight them.

Ultimately, since no medical intervention alters the course of mononucleosis, it is not important to know the exact phase of the infection. It is important, however, to rule out some conditions that mimic this infection but that are either more serious or more treatable. Some of these possibilities include rubella, *HIV/AIDS* (this chapter), diphtheria, measles, and strep throat (which is also a possible complication of the disease).

Complications

For most people, mono is an unpleasant but basically benign, self-limiting infection. It can cause a significant disruption in a person's life, just because it has such a powerful affect on stamina, resiliency, and general strength, but it is seldom a life-threatening situation. A very small number of patients, however, do develop serious complications. These can involve infections in the central nervous system (see *encephalitis* and *meningitis*, Chapter 3), infection of the heart, and breathing problems when lymph nodes get so inflamed that they block air passageways.

One fairly common complication of mono is a streptococcal infection of the throat. It is important to be clear about what infection is causing which symptoms in this case, because strep throat is easily treatable with medication, and mono is not.

Perhaps the greatest danger for most mononucleosis patients is the potential for damage to the spleen. This gland, which is sometimes described as "the body's largest lymph node," can become dangerously enlarged with lymphocytic activity. Since the spleen also breaks down and recycles dead red blood cells, it has a generous blood supply. If the enlarged organ should be injured by a fall or other trauma, it could rupture, which could lead to internal hemorrhage and rapid circulatory collapse. Persons recovering from mono are counseled to avoid contact sports for several months to reduce their risk of this kind of injury.

Treatment

Mononucleosis does not respond to antiviral medications. The typical approach is to treat the symptoms (acetaminophen to reduce fever and pain, good nutrition, and generous hydration) and wait for it to be over. At one time mono patients were confined to bed for several weeks. More recently it has been concluded that they simply need to curtail activities that exhaust them and to avoid situations that could put them at risk for damaging the spleen.

Massage?

A person in an acute stage of mononucleosis will have a fever, inflamed lymph nodes, and will feel generally sick and awful; all these features contraindicate circulatory massage. When a person is in recovery from this infection, lymphatic congestion may linger; this is also a caution for circulatory massage, any abdominal massage, and lymph drainage techniques. Energetic work that supports healing properties without taxing the lymph or immune systems may be a valuable addition to the lengthy healing process for mononucleosis.

Immune System Conditions

Chronic Fatigue Syndrome ✕

Definition: What Is It?

CFS is a recently recognized distinct collection of signs and symptoms that affect multiple systems in the body. It varies in severity from being mildly limiting to being completely debilitating.

This condition was officially named in 1988 by scientists at the Centers for Disease Control. They purposefully kept the name vague because this disease affects different people in very different ways, and by getting any more specific about causes or symptoms they feared they would exclude some people who are badly affected by this condition. Nonetheless, some people feel this title trivializes their condition, and CFS is therefore also called *chronic fatigue immune dysfunction syndrome* (CFIDS). In Europe this same condition is called *myalgic encephalomyelitis* (ME).

CFS has probably been around since at least the 19th century. Florence Nightingale suffered from debilitating fatigue for decades; it is suspected that she had CFS. This may also be the condition behind other vague diagnostic labels such as "neurasthenia," "iron poor blood," and more recently "yuppie flu."

> ### CHRONIC FATIGUE SYNDROME IN BRIEF
>
> **What is it?**
> Chronic fatigue syndrome (CFS) is a collection of signs and symptoms that affect many systems in the body and result in debilitating fatigue.
>
> **How is it recognized?**
> The central symptom to CFS is fatigue that is not restored by rest. It may be accompanied by swollen nodes, slight fever, muscular and joint aches, headaches, excessive pain after mild exercise, and nonrestorative sleep.
>
> **Is massage indicated or contraindicated?**
> CFS indicates massage; it can be a very helpful part of a treatment plan.

Demographics: Who Gets It?

Statistics on the incidence of CFS are notoriously difficult to gather for several reasons. First, it is probably drastically underreported, since not all people who are affected will attempt to be treated. Second, CFS looks like several other disorders, any of which may be happening simultaneously, so a definitive diagnosis is sometimes difficult to make. Third, statistics gathered from different cities show some vast differences in racial, gender, and age distribution of the disorder, which means that while diagnostic criteria have recently been redefined for clarity, some disparity still exists in when and where it is identified.

When all this disparate information is processed, estimates suggest that this disorder (or other CFS-like disorders) probably affects about 500,000 Americans. It is diagnosed most often in White women, but some areas report a higher incidence in other groups. CFS-like symptoms are sometimes observed in children, but it is assumed that these symptoms probably arise for other reasons in people younger than 12 years, and so it is not officially diagnosed among that population.

Etiology: What Happens?

CFS is not well understood. It seems clear that it arises from a combination of factors that may or may not involve infectious agents. In most cases it does *not* appear to be a contagious condition, but isolated incidents of whole communities coming down with CFS-like symptoms may point to exceptions to that rule.

Causes

Possible causes of CFS are a subject of intense scrutiny. Rather than focusing on any single causative factor, researchers have come to the conclusion that CFS is usually the result of a combination of triggers, which may vary significantly from one patient to another. The triggers may include viral exposure, stress, central nervous system problems, or any combination of mysterious factors.

For several years the leading theory was that a person was infected with a common virus (probably Epstein–Barr, the herpes family virus that causes most cases of *mononucleosis*, this chapter) and then the body simply continued to behave as though the infection were acute long after the danger had passed. Although blood studies of persons with CFS often show some immune system abnormalities (levels of an inflammatory cytokine called interleukin-1 are very high, while natural killer cell levels are unusually low), it now seems clear that not all CFS cases begin with a viral infection.

Other pathogenic exposures have been implicated in CFS, specifically *candidiasis* (see Chapter 7), mycoplasmas (a particular kind of bacteria-like pathogen), some enteroviruses, and other infectious agents. No single agent has been found to be present in a majority of CFS patients, however, and the majority of people who have been exposed to these agents do *not* develop CFS symptoms.

Two central nervous system components seem to be consistent problems for most CFS patients:

- *A hypothalamus-pituitary-adrenal axis (HPA) dysfunction.* This can lead to a sluggish but tenacious stress response (see sidebar under *depression*, Chapter 3) and eventually to adrenal depletion.

- *Neurally mediated hypotension.* This is a situation in which impulses from the brain to the circulatory system do not keep the blood vessels contracted enough to maintain normal blood pressure. This condition is connected to an inappropriate response to adrenaline.

A dysfunctional connection between the central nervous system and the endocrine system seems to be at the center of most CFS difficulties. People with CFS typically have lower than normal levels of cortisol in the blood, which indicates adrenal exhaustion as a part of the picture. Furthermore, many people with CFS report moderate to severe allergies, providing a further example of inappropriate immune response and adrenal depletion.

Signs and Symptoms

Fatigue is the central symptom of CFS—fatigue that is unending and not restored by sleep or rest. Other symptoms vary but may include general muscular or joint pain, low-grade fever, swollen lymph nodes, short-term memory loss, problems with concentration, sore throat, and nonrestorative sleep.

Other symptoms may include abdominal bloating, nausea, diarrhea, cramping, chest pain, irregular heartbeat, coughing, dizziness, dry eyes and mouth, weight loss, jaw pain, morning stiffness, night sweats, and psychological problems related to living with chronic illness (see *depression* and *anxiety disorders*, Chapter 3).

This list of symptoms points to an important feature of CFS: this condition closely resembles two other chronic stress-related conditions: *fibromyalgia syndrome* (Chapter 2) and *irritable bowel syndrome* (Chapter 7), and it frequently occurs along with them. In fact, so much crossover exists between these conditions that many people who experience aspects of all three disorders are simply diagnosed with whatever syndrome's primary features appear first (irritable bowel syndrome if it is gastrointestinal discomfort, fibromyalgia syndrome for leading muscle and joint pain, or CFS if the leading symptom is unrelenting fatigue).

Diagnosis

No particular marker in the blood identifies CFS. This condition is diagnosed first by ruling out other diseases with a similar profile. Once that has been accomplished, CFS is diagnosed based on the following criteria:

- The patient has unexplained persistent fatigue that is out of proportion to physical exertion. It is not alleviated by rest, it leads to a curtailment of normal activities, and the pattern of fatigue is different from previous experience.

- At least four of the following additional symptoms must be present. They must not predate the onset of fatigue, and they must be a consistent problem for 6 months or more:

    - Short-term memory loss
    - Confusion, difficulty with concentration
    - Sore throat
    - Tender lymph nodes
    - Muscle pain
    - Joint pain without inflammation
    - Pain that lasts for 24 hours or more after mild exercise
    - Nonrestorative sleep
    - Headaches of a new type or pattern since the onset of symptoms

Differential Diagnoses

One of the things that makes getting a clear diagnosis of CFS so difficult is that many other disorders can cause long-term unexplained fatigue. It is important to rule some of these out, since they may be more serious than CFS and sometimes can be successfully treated and resolved.

Some of the disorders that are ruled out when looking for a solid diagnosis include the following:

- Untreated *hypothyroidism* (Chapter 8)
- *Hepatitis B or C* (Chapter 7)
- *Lupus* (this chapter)
- *Post polio syndrome* (Chapter 3)
- *Lyme disease* (Chapter 2)
- *Sleep apnea or narcolepsy* (*sleep disorders*, Chapter 3)
- *Cancer* (Chapter 11)
- *Diabetes* (Chapter 8)
- *Eating disorders* (Chapter 3)
- *Bipolar disease* (Chapter 3)
- *Alcohol or substance abuse* (Chapter 3)
- Severe obesity

- Reactions to medications
- General autoimmune dysfunction
- Dementia (*Alzheimer's disease*, Chapter 3)

Treatment

The primary treatment for CFS is making lifestyle choices that support the body as fully as possible. This means avoiding stress as much as possible (here "stress" means any stimulus— emotional or physical— that requires that the body adapt to a change); moderating dietary choices to minimize stimulants (caffeine, sugar) and depressants (alcohol) as much as possible; and exercising *very* gently, within tolerance so as not to exacerbate symptoms.

Medical intervention can be helpful, but it is sometimes difficult to find exactly the right combination of drugs. Many CFS patients are extremely hypersensitive to chemicals, and they often find that one-quarter of regular dosage is adequate. A powerful combination for many people is immune-suppressant drugs combined with low-dose tricyclic anti-depressants.

Massage?

Massage stimulates a parasympathetic response, cleanses tissues, and stimulates circulation when exercise may be too much to handle. It can also relieve muscle and joint pain and improve sleep. Studies show that people diagnosed with CFS report lower levels of anxiety and better-quality sleep after receiving massage.[b]

FEVER IN BRIEF

What is it?
Fever is a controlled increase in core temperature, usually brought about by immune system reactions and often in response to pathogenic invasion.

How is it recognized?
Fever is identifiable by readings on a thermometer.

Is massage indicated or contraindicated?
Most fever contraindicates massage, as it is an indication that the body is fighting an infection. The body should be allowed to do its work undisturbed.

Fever

Definition: What Is It?

Fever is an abnormally high body temperature, usually brought about by bacterial or viral infection, but sometimes stimulated by other types of tissue damage. It is a controlled change in temperature, which distinguishes it from other types of hyperthermia (see sidebar). It is a condition that can be recognized at a glance (or touch). Massage therapists are not, by the way, usually required to keep thermometers in their offices.

Etiology: What Happens?

Several steps are involved in the development of a fever:

- A person is infected with some microorganism (e.g., bacteria).
- White blood cells find and eat those invaders.
- Some pieces of the bacterial cell membranes are displayed by the macrophages. They stimulate other white blood cells to secrete a lymphokine called interleukin-1. Other lymphokines and substances that are secreted include interleukin-6 and tumor necrosis factor (TNF).

---

[b]Field T. *Touch Therapy*. London: Churchill Livingstone; 2000:165.

- Interleukin-1 circulates through the system, ending up in the brain. It causes a series of chemical reactions involving prostaglandins that tell the hypothalamus to reset the body's thermostat to a higher level. In this situation interleukin-1 is acting as a pyrogen (a fever-starter).

- Orders from the hypothalamus ripple downward through the body, setting up the muscular and glandular reflexes that raise the core temperature. These reflexes include shivering, constriction of superficial capillaries, and increased metabolism.

The characteristic shivering and chills that go along with a rising fever are part of the mechanism to increase the core temperature. Once that goal has been met, the shivering stops, but the body processes keep working to maintain the increased temperature until the stress and stimulating chemicals have been removed. Reaching this peak is called the *crisis* of the fever. When the crisis has passed, the body's cooling mechanisms (sweating and capillary dilation) take over. That is the sign that the worst is over and the fever has broken.

This culture has a strange and troubling discomfort with discomfort. In general, people would rather *hide* a symptom than *feel* it and figure out what it is trying to tell them. This is particularly true with fever, which can be disagreeable and inconvenient. In rare cases it can get high enough to do some serious damage. For the vast majority of the time, however, fever is a sign that the body is working in the most efficient possible way to get rid of invading pathogens. Here's how:

- The presence of interleukin-1 and other cytokines will not only help to reset the body's thermostat, it will stimulate T-cell production. Increased T-cell production will then stimulate B-cells and antibodies.

- In the presence of fever, *interferon* (a powerful anti-viral agent) is much more active.

- Increased temperature limits iron secretion from the liver and spleen, starving off and slowing bacterial and viral activity.

- Increased temperature raises the heart rate (10 beats per minute per degree), which in turn increases the distribution of white blood cells throughout the body.

- Increased temperature increases cell wall permeability and speeds chemical reactions. This promotes faster recovery for damaged tissues.

Sometimes people will even use a sauna to induce an "artificial fever" in an attempt to stimulate immune system activity. Infection that is not accompanied by fever is considered to be much more serious than the fever itself. Aspirin, ibuprofen, and acetaminophen all work to inhibit fever by interrupting the action of prostaglandins on the hypothalamus to reset the thermostat.

Types of Hyperthermia

Fever is a systemic rise in body temperature that is carefully controlled by the hypothalamus. It has the advantages of speeding up immune system activity while slowing and starving infectious agents. Fever is an extraordinarily efficient system to fight infection.

Sometimes, however, a person's core temperature can rise without hypothalamic control. This generally occurs when a person generates more heat than he or she can release. In this case the body temperature continues to rise until external factors work to cool the person. If environmental factors do not allow this to happen, the person could be at risk for brain damage or even death.

The three signs of hyperthermia are heat cramps, heat exhaustion, and heat stroke. They are most commonly seen in people who are physically very active in warm, humid environments. Massage therapists who work at sporting events can expect to see any of these manifestations of hyperthermia.

- *Heat cramps.* Muscle cramping is a frequent result of the dehydration that accompanies excessive heat production. The body sweats in an attempt to lower its temperature, and the result is a deficit in interstitial fluid. This makes it more difficult for the calcium ions that stimulate muscle contractions to be reabsorbed into their storage containers. Consequently, muscle contractions are sustained and uncontrolled. Fortunately, massage along with hydration (drinking fluids) is an excellent way to mechanically move fluid back into the muscle bellies and stimulate the chemical and neurologic reactions that reduce the spasm.

- *Heat exhaustion.* This situation occurs when muscular activity generates more heat than a person can release. It is marked by excessive sweating, headache, vasodilation, and dehydration. Excessive sweating may lead to low blood pressure, light-headedness, and fainting.

- *Heat stroke.* Heat stroke is the final stage of hyperthermia. In this condition body temperature rises to dangerous levels (around 104°F for adults). Prolonged dehydration may lead to the lack of sweating and circulatory shock from loss of water and electrolytes. The person may become confused or delirious. Heat stroke can be fatal if the core temperature is not quickly but carefully reduced to safe levels.

- *Malignant hyperthermia.* This is not a sports-related problem, but rather a genetic anomaly that allows the body temperature to rise to dangerous, even fatal levels, with a minimum of muscular work. It is sometimes seen as part of an allergic reaction to anesthesia. Many people do not know they are at risk for this disorder until they have a dangerous episode.

Complications

Fever can occasionally complicate into a dangerous situation, particularly when the temperature rises over 104°F. The most common complications are *dehydration* (from prolonged sweating), *acidosis* (the blood gets too acidic), and once in a great while brain damage. Death from fever occurs somewhere around 112° to 114°F for adults. If a fever comes down too fast it can quickly dilate blood vessels. This situation can turn into *shock*, which can be dangerous, especially to older patients.

Massage?

Fever systemically contraindicates massage. Energetic techniques that do not affect blood flow may be helpful for someone having a hard time getting past the crisis point.

HIV/AIDS IN BRIEF

What is it?

Acquired immune deficiency syndrome (AIDS) is a disease caused by the human immunodeficiency virus (HIV), which attacks and disables the immune system. This leaves a person vulnerable to a host of diseases that are usually not a threat to uninfected people.

How is it recognized?

Most people with HIV experience a week or two of flu-like symptoms within a few weeks of being infected, followed by an interval with no symptoms. When the virus has successfully inactivated the immune system, infection by opportunistic pathogens like CMV or *Pneumocystis carinii* will occur.

Is massage indicated or contraindicated?

All stages of HIV infection indicate massage as long as the practitioner is healthy and does not pose any risk to the client, and the client is able to keep up with the changes that massage brings about in the body.

HIV/AIDS

Definition: What Is It?

AIDS was first recognized as a specific disease in the United States in 1981, but research indicates that it has been present here since 1979 and in Africa and the Caribbean long before that. This virus, which is called HIV, attacks various agents of the immune system with disastrous results.

Demographics: Who Gets It?

As of 2000, the World Health Organization estimates that worldwide 36.1 million people are HIV-positive; most are adults, but about 1.4 million HIV patients are children younger than 15 years of age. Women, formerly thought to be less at risk for the disease, now comprise 47% of the people infected.

About 5.3 million new HIV infections occur every year; that is 15,000 per day, or a little more than 10 new infections every minute. Sub-Saharan Africa has the fastest growing AIDS population in the world; 70% of new infections occur there. South and Southeast Asia is the site of 16% of new HIV infections. More than 80% of new HIV infections worldwide are the result of heterosexual intercourse.

As of 2000, cumulative worldwide deaths due to AIDS amounted to 21.8 million people. AIDS kills about 3 million people per year.

In the United States it is estimated that between 800,000 and 900,000 people are HIV-positive, although up to one-third do not know it. About 40,000 new infections begin every year in this country; 70% are among men, and 30% are among women. About half of all new infections are among people younger than 25 years of age.

Among men, 60% of new infections are the result of homosexual intercourse, 25% are the result of sharing contaminated drug needles, and 15% of new infections are from heterosexual intercourse. Among women, 75% of new infections are from heterosexual intercourse, and 25% are from drug use.

Rates of HIV infection decreased steeply in the late 1990s, but more recently they have leveled off to decrease at a rate of only 1% per year. AIDS is currently the fifth leading cause of death among people 25 to 44 years old. It follows accidents, cancer, heart disease, and suicide.

Etiology: What Happens?

HIV enters the body by way of body fluids: blood (including blood from contaminated transfusions and from shared needles), semen, vaginal secretions, and breast milk.

The first target of HIV is nonspecific macrophages and monocytes. From there it moves up the hierarchy of the immune system to infect helper T-cells. The virus' portal of entry to these cells has been a subject of intensive research. One entryway has been identified as a specific protein in cell membranes called CD4. The helper T-cells targeted by HIV are therefore sometimes referred to as CD4 cells.

These viral targets are significant for a few reasons. First, when the virus pools in macrophages before moving up in the immune system hierarchy, its presence does not immediately trigger the production of antibodies, which makes it difficult to identify in a blood test. Second, consider the consequences of a virus that targets, as its ultimate goal, the helper T-cells. Helper T-cells are the vital link between humoral and cell-mediated immunity. They tell the B-cells when to produce plasma cells and antibodies; they govern the activities of macrophages and monocytes through the secretion of lymphokines; they also stimulate killer T-cells and natural killer cells. Without helper T-cells, the entire immune system collapses and leaves the body vulnerable to a wide array of opportunistic diseases.

Most viruses invade active cells and enlist all that activity to produce new viruses. One of the more mysterious aspects of AIDS is that HIV works at a different pace. It invades *inactive* T-cells and lies in wait, its protein strands floating in the cytoplasm, until the day when the T-cell is activated by the presence of its target pathogen. Then the virus wakes up as well, invades the nucleus, and effectively disables the T-cell.

The core of HIV is RNA rather than DNA, which holds the blueprints for our cells. This retrovirus uses an enzyme called *reverse transcriptase* to convert its RNA to DNA. In the process, the virus is sometimes minutely altered—just enough to make it resistant to identification or treatment. Drug treatments for AIDS focus on interrupting the complex processes of viral transcription and replication inside the host cells.

Progression

Each stage of this disease is associated with decreasing numbers of active helper T-cells and increased viral titers (counts of virus). The typical pattern looks like this:

- *Phase 1.* A person is infected with HIV. The virus is present in the body but may be pooling in white blood cells rather than eliciting an immune response. Consequently, tests are negative, no symptoms are present, but the person can transmit the disease because the "viral load," that is, levels of virus in the blood, is very high. This incubation phase can last 1 year or more, although the average is 3 weeks to 6 months in sexually transmitted cases.

- *Phase 2.* In the acute primary HIV infection antibodies become detectable in blood tests. About 70% of people experience fatigue, swollen glands, fever, weight loss, headaches, drowsiness, and confusion within several weeks of exposure. These symptoms usually last about 2 weeks and are often mistaken for the *flu* (Chapter 6) or *mononucleosis* (this chapter).

- *Phase 3.* This is the inactive period of infection. No symptoms or opportunistic diseases are obvious. Although the virus is continuing to replicate while decimating immune system cells, the body is able to keep up with the process. It is during this phase that medical intervention limits viral growth and prolongs life expectancy. The length of the inactive phase varies widely, depending on the initial health of the person, what kind of treatment is given, and several other factors. It can last anywhere from 1 to 15 years, with a median average of 10 years.

- *Phases 4 and 5.* During this time symptoms of opportunistic diseases or AIDS-related cancers become apparent and eventually debilitating. A normal helper T-cell count is 800 to 1000 cells/µl of blood. AIDS is diagnosed when these levels drop to 200 cells/µl or below.

HIV Resistance

Recent research has focused on the variables that determine how long a person who is HIV-positive can keep the virus under control. Some people who are infected with HIV never develop symptoms or develop them much more slowly than most people. These "long-term nonprogressors" can provide important clues for how the virus may be fought once infection has been established. Three main factors have been identified.

- *Host resistance.* Some HIV patients have a genetic mutation in their immune systems that creates fewer receptor sites on their macrophages and T-cells for the virus to latch on to. It takes more exposure over a longer period to establish an infection in these people because the chance for a successful invasion is so much lower.

- *Immune system response.* When most cells are invaded by a virus, they display a fragment of that virus on their membrane. This serves as a signal to immune system agents that the cell is compromised and should be destroyed. HIV is capable of slowing down this "display" reaction or of hiding from it altogether by mimicking normal cell membranes. If the efficiency of the display mechanism is improved, immune system response is more aggressive.

- *Virulence of the virus.* HIV is sometimes partially weakened by medication or an immune system response but remains transmittable to another person. Infection with a weakened virus generally means the new host is better able to control it. Relative virulence of individual viruses is difficult to measure, however.

It seems clear that most long-term nonprogressors or very slow progressors have a combination of these factors working in their favor.

Signs and Symptoms

Signs and symptoms of HIV depend on the stage of infection. Specific guidelines are given in the discussion of phases of the disease above.

Complications

When HIV has virtually disabled normal immune function, the body is incapable of fending off attacks from pathogens that pose no problems for healthy people. A list of formerly obscure diseases are now so closely associated with AIDS that they are called "indicator diseases." Here are some of the most common and serious ones:

- *Pneumocystis carinii pneumonia* (PCP). This is a protozoal infection of the lungs.

- *Cytomegalovirus* (CMV). This member of the herpes family can cause retinitis and blindness, colitis, pneumonia, and infection of the adrenal glands.

- *Kaposi's sarcoma* (KS). This is a type of skin cancer (Fig. 5-4).
- *Non-Hodgkin's lymphomas* (NHL). HIV has been found to specifically initiate the cancer cell replication with a variety of lymphomas and KS.

Other opportunistic diseases associated with AIDS include *toxoplasmosis*, which can cause encephalitis or pneumonia; *candida*, a yeast infection that can cause thrush or esophagitis (Chapter 5); and *cryptococcus neoformans*, a fungal infection that can cause meningitis and pneumonia. In addition to these "indicator diseases," people with AIDS are highly susceptible to gastrointestinal disturbances, herpes simplex, shingles, tuberculosis, meningitis, cervical cancer, and many other conditions.

Diagnosis

Infection with HIV is determined by the presence of antibodies in the blood. This is a bit problematic since the peculiar nature of this pathogen prevents the body from tagging it and initiating antibody production until the virus is widespread. To get a truly dependable diagnosis, HIV tests must be conducted up to 6 months after the last incidence of high-risk behavior: sharing intravenous drug needles, unprotected sex with a potentially infected partner, or the use of blood or blood products.

Typically the first blood test given is an enzyme-linked immunosorbent assay (ELISA) test. Because this extremely sensitive test sometimes yields false-positive results, a positive reading is followed by a second ELISA test and/or a Western blot test. If both tests are negative and the person is clearly in a high-risk population and showing signs of being sick, tests may be conducted to look for signs of the virus itself in the blood, rather than antibodies to the virus.

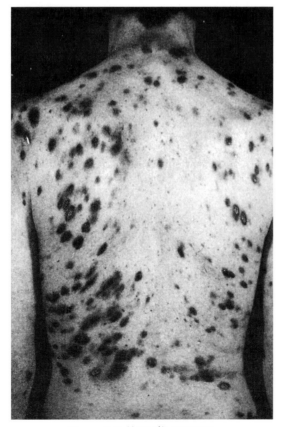

Figure 5-4. Kaposi's sarcoma

A Virus Primer

Viruses consist of a protein coat of variable complexity wrapped around a core of DNA or RNA. Outside a host cell, viruses have no metabolic functions and cannot replicate. Inside a host cell, the virus shoots its core into the nucleus and reprograms the functions of that cell to replicate more viruses. In other words, the host cell becomes a virus factory. When the factory is full of inventory it literally bursts at the seams, releasing hordes of new viruses in search of other hosts. Enormous amounts of damage occurs with any viral infection—not just to the cells attacked by the virus, but to the cells the body sacrifices to fight back.

Most viruses cause short-term acute infections that spread easily. The coughing and sneezing seen with respiratory tract infections like cold and flu are remarkably efficient distributors of virus. Likewise, the diarrhea that occurs with intestinal infections is an effective way to spread virus through fecal contamination. The immune system response to these viruses is severe and usually successful; most infections are curtailed and the viruses are expelled in short order.

A few viruses, however, cause long-term chronic infections instead of short-term acute illness. Hepatitis B and C, herpes, and HIV are notorious among these. For a virus to live in a body for a prolonged period, it must be able to hide from immune system cells to escape attack and destruction. It is precisely the ability of HIV to hide from typical immune system activity that makes it so difficult to fight. In addition to being good hiders, chronic infectious viruses have been seen to produce "decoy" particles that draw antibody attack away from themselves and to secrete "fake cytokines" (chemical messengers that confuse and slow immune system response).

As more is learned about how chronic infectious viruses pool in hidden reservoirs in the body, the ability to fight back will improve. These hidden invaders may someday be eradicated permanently.

Treatment

One of the things that makes finding a cure for AIDS so difficult is that in the process of converting its core from RNA to DNA, the virus can minutely change, just enough to make it resistant to drugs and to immune system activation. The answer to that problem has been to combine various drugs to anticipate the mutations of the virus. This has been highly successful in laboratory settings, but these drug combinations are often prohibitively toxic to patients.

The most successful AIDS treatments so far have involved interrupting viral replication. The use of *highly active antiretroviral therapy* (HAART) has slowed progression in many patients but cannot access the virus when it hides in long-lived cells like memory T-cells, which have a life expectancy of 60 years or more. Although the goal of fully eradicating the virus from an infected person is still a long way off, studies of patients who manage to control their infections efficiently will continue to point the way to better treatment options.

The picture for people with AIDS in the United States is rosier than it has been since the disease was identified in 1981. Although treatment can cost $15,000 to $20,000 per year, many people with AIDS in the United States at least have access to care. This is not the case in developing countries, where AIDS statistics are growing the fastest. Some 90% of the world's AIDS patients have little or no access to treatment.

Massage?

HIV is spread through the exchange of bodily fluids: semen, breast milk, blood, and vaginal secretions. No research has ever shown that it can be transmitted through sweat or casual contact. Obviously, the person most at risk for getting sick when an AIDS patient receives massage is not the therapist—it is the patient. Therefore, care must be taken that the practitioner does not carry active pathogens that may put a client with AIDS at risk.

HIV-positive clients who are asymptomatic are fine candidates for massage. Although in advanced stages of AIDS opportunistic diseases can make circulatory massage problematic, other types of work may reduce stress, which in turn strengthens the immune system. It can be a very appropriate treatment option and an important source of support and comfort for people who are often rejected, ignored, or actively persecuted by society.

Inflammation
Definition: What Is It?

Inflammation is a tissue response to the threat of bodily injury or invasion by antigens: bits of "non-self." The inflammatory response is controlled by chemical, cellular, and vascular functions that have the remarkable ability to adjust that response to the severity of the threat.

Etiology: What Happens?

When a person sustains tissue damage, cells are injured, ripped open, and destroyed. The damage may occur from mechanical or thermal stress (e.g., sprain, laceration, or burn), or it may be due to pathogenic invasion, or tissue may be injured by toxic chemicals. When cells are injured, a chain of events begins to minimize damage and threat of invasion. This chain of events is called inflammation: a reaction of injured tissue to defend and protect the body from invasion. The different aspects of this reaction are specifically designed to achieve three basic goals: to dispose of pathogens and cellular debris, to prevent the spread of pathogens in the body, and to prepare the injured area for healing.

Three components contribute to all stages of inflammation. The *chemical* components include inflammation mediators released from nearby cells like histamine and cytokines: chemicals that participate in cell-to-cell communication. The *vascular* components of inflammation involve vasodilation, vasoconstriction, and changes in the permeability of vessel walls to allow the migration of certain blood cells. The *cellular* component of inflammation includes platelet and white blood cell movement to the area of infection or injury, clotting, and phagocytosis as those white blood cells consume pathogens and debris.

> ## INFLAMMATION IN BRIEF
>
> ### What is it?
> Inflammation is a protective device in response to injury or infection. It involves localized vascular, cellular, and chemical reactions to isolate the area and to resolve the damage through immune system response.
>
> ### How is it recognized?
> The signs of inflammation are redness, pain, swelling, heat, and loss of function. These can be localized or systemic.
>
> ### Is massage indicated or contraindicated?
> Acute inflammation contraindicates circulatory massage, but bodywork may be appropriate for subacute situations, depending on the causative factors. Inflammation due to infection obviously carries a higher risk to the client and the practitioner than inflammation in response to musculoskeletal injury.

Progression:

Step 1: The Injury—Acute Vascular Response   For the sake of simplicity, consider a basic laceration or puncture wound as a model; the same principles hold true for any kind of local injury (Fig. 5-5). In the *very first moments*, especially if it was a very serious injury, vasoconstriction occurs. This is a protective mechanism against excessive bleeding. The vasoconstrictive stage is over within a few seconds for a minor injury and several minutes for a more serious one.

A period of capillary vasodilation follows vasoconstriction. This is the most important step in the inflammatory process. Stimulated cells, especially mast cells (which are stationed in superficial fascia and epithelial membranes), release a host of chemicals that cause increased permeability of blood vessel walls and capillary dilation.

Step 2: Immediate Cellular Response   When vasodilating chemicals have acted on local capillaries, substances can quickly get *out* of the bloodstream and *into* the damaged area. Specifically, neutrophils are usually the first white blood cells to arrive on the scene, but they are accompanied by antibodies, platelets, and clotting factors that are equally crucial in the inflammatory process. In addition to bringing new material in, this increased fluid flow also tends to flush wastes out, including dead cells and pathogenic toxins.

A complicated chain of events causes certain plasma proteins in the nearby capillaries to form fibrous nets. These nets serve a double purpose of making a clot to close off any broken blood vessels and to catch loose pathogens before they enter the bloodstream. Blood clots help to isolate infection from the rest of the body.

Step 3: Long-term Cellular Response   Slower moving white blood cells arrive later in the inflammatory process. They include monocytes, macrophages, and lymphocytes. These immune system agents are bigger than the neutrophils, have bigger ap-

THE LANGUAGE OF INFLAMMATION

Massage therapists are well trained in recognizing the basic signs of inflammation: pain, heat, redness, swelling, and sometimes loss of function. This litany has a long and venerable history beginning with the earliest practitioners of the healing arts. The traditional names for signs of inflammation come from Latin:

- *Dolor* (pain)
- *Calor* (heat)
- *Rubor* (redness)
- *Tumor* (swelling) and
- *Functio laesa* (loss of function)

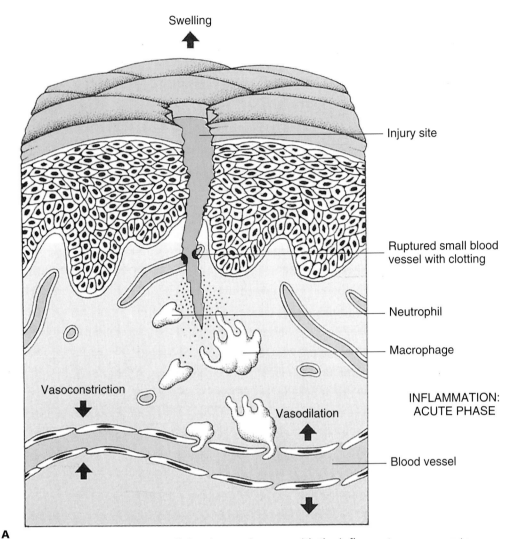

A

Figure 5-5. (**A** and **B**) Many cellular changes happen with the inflammatory response to keep the body safe from infection

petites, and can disable multiple pathogens (neutrophils can only serve once). Macrophages eat pathogens as well as clean up the body's own dead and damaged cells.

The result of all this cellular mopping up is the formation of tissue exudates. Exudates are any fluids that can be expressed from tissues that are in the process of healing. Pus is one example; it is composed of dead and living white blood cells along with whatever pathogens they have managed to kill. Pus is usually walled in by the thickened connective tissues surrounding the infection site. It can be expressed through the surface of the skin, aspirated, or, if left alone long enough, it is reabsorbed by the body (macrophages eventually clean it up).

Another type of cell that is drawn to areas of inflammation in this phase are fibroblasts, or collagen-producing cells. These lay down a weak, delicate version of collagen to begin knitting together damaged tissues. This collagen is reinforced and realigned later in the healing process.

Step 4: Resolution and Maturation   In this stage any residual blood clots are dissolved. New scar tissue becomes tougher and stronger and, depending on the type of tissue that was injured, it may align itself with the direction of forces put on it (see *sprains,*

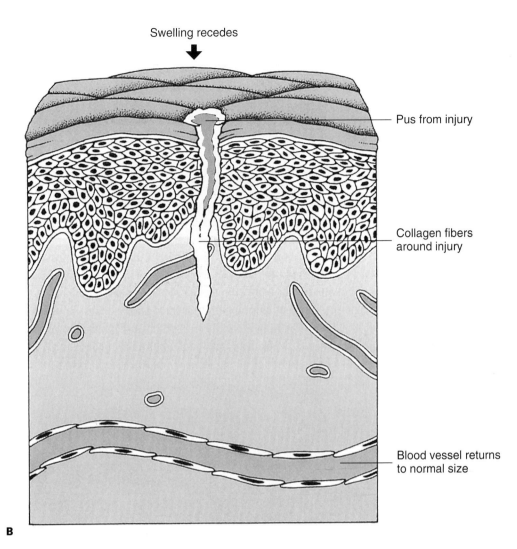

Figure 5-5.—continued

Chapter 2). The tissue is restored to as close to a normal state as possible.

Steps 1 and 2 happen in what would be considered the acute phase of infection: they begin within moments of the injury and remain the primary activity for up to 3 days, depending on the severity of the damage.

Steps 3 and 4 involve the rebuilding of damaged tissue. This usually begins 3 to 4 days after the injury and continues for 2 weeks or more. The maturation phase, when the scar tissue molds and changes according to the stresses put on it, can last up to 2 years, depending on the severity of the injury, the general health of the person, and other variables.

Signs and Symptoms

Every massage therapist should know this litany: the symptoms of inflammation are pain, heat, redness, swelling, and sometimes loss of function. Itching, clotting, and pus formation could be added to the list in some cases.

It is easy to see how each of these symptoms comes about. Vasodilation brings about the redness, heat, and swelling by drawing extra blood to a small area. Pain and itching can be the result of several factors including edematous pressure, damaged nerve endings, irritating pathogenic toxins, and irritating chemicals released by other cells. If the inflammation limits movement, the patient experiences loss of function. Clotting and pus formation have already been discussed. Not all these symptoms are present in all cases of inflammation.

With long-lasting infectious inflammations the types of white blood cells present vary, and it may take days or weeks to eradicate all traces of the pathogens completely. (Some pathogens are never completely eradicated but simply become dormant; see *herpes zoster*, Chapter 3.) Also, some types of pathogens cause a system-wide inflammatory reaction with *fever* (this chapter).

Treatment

The typical treatment of inflammation is no surprise—anti-inflammatories. These can be steroidal (e.g., cortisone) or nonsteroidal (e.g., aspirin). Regardless of their chemical impact on the body, anti-inflammatories may have significant impact on massage: they may hide the results of overtreatment, thus raising the risk that massage could cause injury. If a client is taking anti-inflammatories for a condition that does *not* contraindicate massage, the therapist should suggest that he or she make an appointment just as the dose is wearing off. That way, it will be possible to get much more accurate information about what massage is actually doing to the body.

Massage?

Acute localized infections at the very least locally contraindicate circulatory massage. Thickened fascial walls isolate the infection to a certain extent, but working anywhere around a badly infected knee may be asking for trouble. For a worst-case scenario, see *lymphangitis* in this chapter. If the infection is systemic, as in *influenza* (Chapter 6), it is also a systemic contraindication, at least in the acute stage.

Inflammation does not always imply the presence of infection. *Sprains* (Chapter 2) and *dermatitis* (Chapter 1) are two examples among many conditions in which an inflammatory process occurs without invading pathogens. When inflammation is present without infection, the general rule for circulatory massage is to wait for the subacute stage when bringing more fluid to the area is not likely to make matters worse. Lymph draining techniques may be safe and appropriate in earlier stages of non-infectious inflammation.

Bodywork may be helpful in flushing out debris and improving sluggish and congested circulation in the postacute stages of infection and inflammation.

Lupus

Definition: What Is It?

Lupus is an autoimmune disease in which the various types of tissues are attacked by the body's own antibodies. Although it only rarely becomes so, lupus has the potential to be life-threatening. In extreme cases this disorder can attack the heart, the lungs, the kidneys, and the brain, with devastating results.

Demographics: Who Gets It?

Statistics on this disease vary greatly. Population surveys estimate that the incidence of lupus in the United States is between 1.4 and 2 million people. African-Americans and Asians have higher rates than Whites, and Caribbean Blacks have the highest rates of all.

LUPUS

From the Latin word for "wolf," this name could have come about for a few reasons. It could refer to the characteristic "butterfly mask" on the face that looks like the facial markings of a wolf, or it could refer to the circular lesions that may appear on the face or elsewhere on the body that were thought to resemble wolf bites.

The incidence of this disease is between 40 and 50 of every 100,000 people. About 16,000 new cases of lupus are diagnosed in the United States every year.

Lupus affects people at any age, but it is most common in women of childbearing age. It affects women far more than men. Depending on the age group studied, women with lupus outnumber men by as much as 9 to 1.

Etiology: What Happens?

Three varieties of lupus have been identified: drug-induced lupus erythematosus, discoid lupus erythematosus, and systemic lupus erythematosus.

- *Drug-induced lupus* is a situation in which some rarely prescribed medications for high blood pressure, heart arrhythmia, and epilepsy can create lupus symptoms. These symptoms disappear when the medications are discontinued.

- *Discoid lupus erythematosus* (DLE) is a chronic skin disease. It can involve small scaly red patches with sharp margins that do not itch, or it can create the characteristic "butterfly rash" of redness over the nose and cheeks (Figs. 5-6 and 5-7, Color plates 36 and 37). The skin can become very thin and delicate, or lesions may become permanently discolored and thickened. If the lesions affect deep layers of the skin, scar tissue may lead to permanent hair loss. More commonly, acute flares lead to temporary hair loss. About 10% of people with DLE will eventually have SLE.

- *Systemic lupus erythematosus* (SLE) is a situation in which antibody attacks are launched against a variety of tissues throughout the body. This can result in *arthritis* (Chapter 2), *renal failure* (Chapter 9), *thrombosis* (Chapter 4), psychosis, *seizures* (Chapter 3), inflammation of the heart, and pleurisy. SLE can be a very serious disorder that can usually be controlled, but at this time it cannot be cured. SLE sometimes begins as DLE, but not always. The rest of this discussion will focus on SLE, which creates the most far-reaching and long-lasting symptoms of the three varieties of lupus.

Causes

The precise cause or causes of lupus are unknown. A genetic link is sometimes a factor, but a child of a parent with lupus has only a 5% chance of developing the disease. When one identical twin develops SLE, the other twin may not. This indicates that although a genetic susceptibility may be inherited, environmental factors also probably contribute to the development of the disease. Environmental factors may include exposure to certain viruses, ultraviolet light, certain medications, and high levels of estrogen. Women with lupus often report a change in symptoms with their menstrual cycle, and recent research shows that estrogen replacement therapy that is used to reduce the risk of *osteoporosis* (Chapter 2) can increase the risk of lupus for some women.

One new branch of research is examining the role of a specific enzyme whose job is to help clean up dead and dying cells. When this enzyme is weak or in low supply, the dead cells can trigger an autoimmune reaction against even healthy cells, which then becomes generalized throughout the body.

LUPUS IN BRIEF

What is it?
Lupus is an autoimmune disease in which antibodies attack various types of tissue throughout the body. Three distinct types of lupus exist, but systemic lupus erythematosus (SLE) is both the most common and the most serious.

How is it recognized?
Eleven specific criteria have been determined for a diagnosis of lupus. They include, among other things, arthritis in two or more joints, pleurisy, pericarditis, kidney dysfunction, and nervous system dysfunction.

Is massage indicated or contraindicated?
When lupus is in a state of acute flare, circulatory massage could exacerbate symptoms. When the condition is in remission, bodywork of any kind could be very helpful to reduce pain and anxiety and to help maintain flexibility.

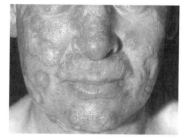

Figure 5-6. Discoid lupus

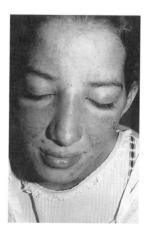

Figure 5-7. Systemic lupus erythematosus: malar rash

Signs and Symptoms

Lupus can affect virtually every system in the body. Sometimes the problems associated with lupus are not serious or even detectable. At other times they can be life-threatening. Because some of the features of this disease make profound changes in health, it is worth looking at how SLE affects several systems.

- *Integumentary system.* The characteristic butterfly or discoid rash that is seen with lupus has already been mentioned. These rashes, which can appear anywhere on the body, may be exacerbated by sunlight in a condition called *photosensitivity.* Lupus can also cause ulcers in the mucous membranes, particularly in the nose, throat, and mouth. Lupus-related rashes may be acute or subacute. Subacute rashes tend to be photosensitive but do not leave permanent scars. Photosensitive rashes can be prevented with the use of sunscreen.

  When SLE causes superficial blood vessels to become inflamed, symptoms may appear on the skin in the shape of welts, red lines, and painful bumps.

- *Musculoskeletal system.* Arthritis eventually develops in 80 to 90% of all people with lupus. Joint pain usually occurs at the hands and feet and seldom in the spine. Interestingly, even someone with longstanding lupus will not usually show signs of internal joint damage.

  Nonspecific muscle pain is another common symptom, and many lupus patients may also meet the criteria for *fibromyalgia* (Chapter 2).

- *Nervous system.* Twenty-five percent of people with lupus have some nervous system dysfunction. This can range from extreme headaches, to psychosis, to high fever, to seizures, depending on which part of the brain is being adversely affected by blood vessel inflammation. When the clotting disorders that may accompany this disorder occur in the brain, the result is cerebrovascular accident or *stroke* (Chapter 3).

- *Cardiovascular system.* Lupus can lead to inflammation and damage of major blood vessels, opening the door to *atherosclerosis* (Chapter 3). It is also associated with a specific clotting disorder that involves slow clot formation and slow clot dissolving. This problem can lead to *thrombophlebitis* or *pulmonary embolism* (Chapter 3).

  In addition to blood vessel damage, lupus may also affect the serous membranes of the heart. This results in inflammation, arrhythmia, and severe chest pain.

  Anemia (Chapter 3) is a frequent complication of long-term inflammation and bone marrow suppression. Thrombocytopenia, or a shortage of platelets, may occur when lupus antibodies have attacked thrombocytes. *Raynaud's phenomenon* (Chapter 3) is a sign of vasculitis (inflammation of the blood vessels).

- *Respiratory system.* A common complication of lupus is pleurisy: inflammation and fluid accumulation in the serous membranes that line the lungs. This causes pain on inhalation and restricted movement of the lungs.

- *Excretory system.* Tissue damage in the kidneys leads to *glomerulonephritis* (Chapter 9), a condition seen in 50% of people with lupus. Kidney damage can accumulate without symptoms until the kidneys are on the brink of renal failure.

- *Reproductive system.* The clotting disorder associated with lupus can make it difficult to carry a child to term. Repeated spontaneous miscarriages are sometimes the first sign of the disease which leads to a diagnosis. Pregnant women with lupus face special challenges as the medications that control symptoms are sometimes not safe for the baby.

Diagnosis

It is clear from this long and varied list of symptoms that lupus can look like many different diseases. Fortunately, it leaves some specific clues in the blood that can help to identify it. Unfortunately, those clues are sometimes present in people *without* lupus, so they cannot be used as a definitive diagnosis.

A collection of 11 signs and symptoms has been developed as a diagnostic criterion.[c] If any four of these criteria are present at any time, a positive diagnosis of lupus can be made. The four signs do *not* need to be present simultaneously.

- Malar (butterfly) rash
- Discoid skin rash (can cause permanent scarring)
- Photosensitivity
- Mucous membrane ulcers, particularly in the mouth, nose, or throat
- Arthritis in more than two joints, specifically in the hands or feet (not in the spine)
- Pleurisy and/or pericarditis
- Kidney problems (blood or protein in the urine)
- Brain irritation (seizures or psychosis)
- Blood count abnormalities (low red blood cell, white blood cell, or platelet counts)
- Immunologic disorders (special antibodies and/or lupus anticoagulants present in the blood)
- Antinuclear antibodies (ANA) present in the blood

This condition, like other autoimmune conditions, is exacerbated by certain kinds of stimuli. Exposure to certain drugs (including penicillin, sulfa, and tetracycline) may initiate an attack as will excess exposure to ultraviolet light, emotional stress, injury, infection, or trauma. Someone who has lupus must identify those stimuli that are particularly potent for her and avoid them carefully.

Treatment

The treatment strategy for lupus is to minimize the negative impact of inflammation during flares. Lupus patients have essentially four levels of medical recourse in the effort to manage this condition. Each intervention has inherent risks, however, which must be weighed against the benefits.

If the case is not very severe, it may be managed with nonsteroidal anti-inflammatory drugs. These drugs are inexpensive, easily accessible, and often effective against inflammation. Unfortunately, they are also associated with chronic stomach irritation (see *ulcers*, Chapter 7), and long-term use can also irritate and damage the kidneys. The latter is of greater concern for lupus patients, many of whom end up sustaining kidney damage from the disease process and do not want to speed that progression with medication.

Steroidal anti-inflammatories are sometimes prescribed for short-term use, especially during flares. These are very powerful anti-inflammatories, but they are also associated with many dangerous side-effects including mood changes, weight gain, liver damage,

[c]Systemic Lupus Erythematosus. American College of Rheumatology; 2000. Available at: http://www. rheumatology.org/patients/factsheet/ sle.html. Accessed winter 2001.

bone thinning, and osteonecrosis (death of bone and joint tissue), especially in the hips and shoulders.

Anti-malarial drugs have produced success in treating some of the symptoms of lupus, especially skin rashes and ulcers of mucous membranes. Some anti-malarial drugs cause changes in eye function, so an ophthalmologist must closely monitor their use.

In very severe cases of lupus, cytotoxic drugs that entirely disable the immune system may be recommended. This of course leaves the patient vulnerable to secondary infections because her immune system has been suppressed to keep it from attacking her own tissues.

Other treatment options for lupus depend on the presenting symptoms. Acute rashes may be treated with topical steroid creams or ointments. If a patient is experiencing blood clotting problems, anticoagulants may be administered. It is a high priority to treat lupus symptoms quickly as they arise; early intervention can reduce the amount of damage that accrues during flares and keeps the body functioning at normal levels during periods of remission.

The treatment options for lupus sound alarming, but in truth this disease is usually manageable. When this disease was first recognized, most patients died within 5 years of diagnosis. Now, thanks to these medical interventions, 80 to 90% of all lupus patients can expect a normal life span.

Massage?

Active flares of lupus mark periods of inflammation that can damage the heart, lungs, kidneys, and joints. Circulatory massage during these acute episodes may exacerbate symptoms and put unhealthy stress on an inflamed cardiovascular system. Energy work during these episodes, however, may be supportive and helpful.

Circulatory massage is more appropriate during remission, especially as a treatment strategy against the stress that can trigger attacks. However, care must be taken to ensure that the circulatory system is capable of handling the changes in internal environment that massage produces.

Chapter Review Questions: Lymph and Immune System Conditions

1. What is an allergy?

2. What is an autoimmune disease? Give two examples.

3. What are lymphokines? What do they do?

4. What type of cell is the primary target for HIV?

5. Who is most at risk for getting sick when a massage therapist works with an AIDS patient? Why?

6. What is the link between chronic fatigue syndrome and the central nervous system?

7. Describe how the inflammatory process causes pain, heat, redness, and swelling.

8. What are the dangers of working with a client who is taking anti-inflammatory drugs?

9. How is lupus generally treated medically? Why?

10. Why are massage therapists particularly at risk for lymphangitis?

Bibliography, Lymph and Immune System Conditions

General References, Lymph and Immune System

1. de Dominico G, Wood E. *Beard's Massage.* Philadelphia, Pa: WB Saunders; 1997
2. Damjanou I. *Pathology for the Health-Related Professions.* Philadelphia, Pa: WB Saunders; 1996.
3. Travell J, Simons DG. *Myofascial Pain and Dysfunction: The Trigger Point Manual.* Baltimore, Md: Williams & Wilkins; 1983.
4. Clemente CD. *Anatomy: A Regional Atlas of the Human Body.* 3rd ed. Baltimore, Md: Urban & Schwarzenburg; 1987.
5. Tortora GJ, Anagnostakos NP. *Principles of Anatomy and Physiology.* 6th ed. New York, NY: Harper & Row; 1990.
6. *Taber's Cyclopedic Dictionary.* 14th ed. Philadelphia, Pa: FA Davis; 1981.
7. *Stedman's Medical Dictionary.* 26th ed. Baltimore, Md: Williams & Wilkins; 1995.
8. Memmler RL, Wood DL. *The Human Body in Health and Disease.* 5th ed. Philadelphia, Pa: JB Lippincott; 1983.
9. Juhan D. *Job's Body: A Handbook for Bodywork.* Barrytown, NY: Station Hill Press; 1987.
10. Mulvihill ML. *Human Diseases: A Systemic Approach.* 2nd ed. Norwalk, Conn: Appleton & Lange; 1987.
11. Kunz JRM, Finkel AJ, eds. *The American Medical Association Family Medical Guide.* New York, NY: Random House; 1987.
12. Marieb EM. *Human Anatomy and Physiology.* Redwood City, Calif: Benjamin/Cummings; 1989.
13. Sapolsky RM. *Why Zebras Don't Get Ulcers: An Updated Guide to Stress, Stress-Related Disease, and Coping.* New York, NY: W.H. Freeman; 1998.

Lymph System Conditions

Edema

1. Hipps J. Edema and water retention. The Country Doctor; 1998. Available at: http://www.thecountrydoctor.com/edema.htm. Accessed winter 2001.
2. Hong J. Edema: The wonderful world of edema. Available at: http://www.science.mcmaster.ca/Biology/4S03/EDEMA.HTM. Accessed winter 2001.

Lymphangitis

1. Rowland BM. Acute lymphangitis. Gale Research, Inc.; 1999. Available at: http://www.buildingbetterhealth.com/article/gale/100084992. Accessed winter 2001.
2. Lymphadenitis and lymphangitis. adam.com; 1999. Available at: http://webmd. lycos.com/content/asset/adam_disease_lymph_gland_infection. Accessed winter 2001.

Lymphoma

1. Adult Hodgkin's disease. Lymphoma Information Network; 1996–2000. Available at: http://www.lymphomainfo.net/hodgkins/description.html. Accessed winter 2001.
2. Adult Hodgkin's disease: Diagnosis. Lymphoma Information Network; 1996–2000. Available at: http://www.lymphomainfo.net/hodgkins/diagnosis.html. Accessed winter 2001.
3. Adult Hodgkin's disease (PDQ). National Cancer Institute. Available at: http://cancernet.nci.nih.gov/cgi-bin/srchcgi.exe?DBID=pdq&TYPE=search&UID=208+00003&ZFILE=patient&SFMT=pdq_treatment/1/0/0. Accessed winter 2001.
4. Hodgkin's disease incidence. Lymphoma Information Network; 2000. Available at: http://www.lymphomainfo.net/hodgkins/incidence.html. Accessed winter 2001.
5. Hodgkin's disease. The Leukemia & Lymphoma Society. Available at: http://www.leukemia.org/all_page?item_id=8312. Accessed spring 2002.
6. NCI/PDQ patient statement: Adult Hodgkin's disease-updated 11/2000. University of Pennsylvania Health System; 2001. Available at: http://cancer.med.upenn.edu/pdq_html/2/engl/200003.html. Accessed winter 2001.
7. Childhood non-Hodgkin's lymphoma (PDQ). National Cancer Institute. Available at: http://cancernet.nci.nih.gov/cgi-bin/srchcgi.exe?DBID=pdq&TYPE=search&UID=208+00915&ZFILE=patient&SFMT=pdq_treatment/1/0/0. Accessed winter 2001.
8. Lymphoma. Available at: http://www.leukemia.org/CMS/q?action=static&v=PF&pageID=15. The Leukemia & Lymphoma Society. Accessed spring 2002.
9. Lymphomas (Hodgkin's disease and non-Hodgkin's lymphoma). InteliHealth Inc.; 1996–2001. Available at: http://www.intelihealth.com/IH/ihtPrint/WSIHW000/8096/24763.html?k=basePrint. Accessed winter 2001.

Mononucleosis

1. Infectious mononucleosis. MedicineNet, Inc.; 1996–2000. Available at: MedicineNet.com. Accessed winter 2001.
2. Mononucleosis. HealthAnswers.com, Inc; 2000. Available at: http://www.healthanswers.com/centers/disease/overview.asp?id=blood+disorders&filename=337.htm Accessed winter 2001.
3. Eichner ER. Infectious mononucleosis: recognizing the condition, 'reactivating' the patient. *Phys Sportsmed.* 1996;24(4). Available at: http://www.physsportsmed.com/issues/apr_96/eichner.htm. Accessed winter 2001.
4. Omori M. Mononucleosis from emergency medicine/infectious diseases. eMedicine.com, Inc.; 2001 Available at: http://www.emedicine. com/emerg/topic319.htm. Accessed winter 2001.
5. General health encyclopedia: Infectious mononucleosis (CMV). A.D.A.M. Software; 1998. Available at: http://www.healthcentral.com/home/home.cfm. Accessed winter 2001.
6. Infectious mononucleosis. InteliHealth Inc.; 1996–2001. Available at: http://www.intelihealth.com/IH/ihtPrint/WSIHW000/24479/10351.html?k=basePrint. Accessed winter 2001.
7. Infectious mononucleosis. National Institute of Allergy and Infectious Diseases, National Institutes of Health. Available at: http://www.niaid. nih.gov/factsheets/infmono.htm. Accessed winter 2001.
8. Novitt-Moreno A, KidsHealth at the AMA staff. Mononucleosis. The Nemours Foundation; 2000. Available at: http://kidshealth.org/ parent/general/infections/mononucleosis.html. Accessed winter 2001.
9. Epstein-Barr virus and infectious mononucleosis. National Center for Infectious Diseases, Centers for Disease Control. Available at: http://www.cdc.gov/ncidod/diseases/ebv.htm. Accessed winter 2001.

Immune System Conditions

Chronic Fatigue Syndrome

1. CFS definition: The revised case definition (abridged version). Centers for Disease Control and Prevention. National Center for Infectious Diseases. Available at: http://www.cdc.gov/ncidod/diseases/cfs/defined/defined2.htm. Accessed winter 2001.
2. CFS definition: Screening tests for detecting common exclusionary conditions. Centers for Disease Control and Prevention. National Center for Infectious Diseases. Available at: http://www.cdc.gov/ncidod/diseases/cfs/defined/defined5.htm. Accessed winter 2001.
3. Treatment. Centers for Disease Control and Prevention. National Center for Infectious Diseases. Available at: http://www.cdc. gov/ncidod/diseases/cfs/treat.htm. Accessed winter 2001.
4. CFS information. Centers for Disease Control and Prevention. National Center for Infectious Diseases. Available at: http://www.cdc.gov/ncidod/diseases/cfs/info.htm. Accessed winter 2001.
5. Chronic fatigue syndrome. Available at: http://www.intelihealth.com/IH/ihtPrint/WSIHW000/9339/9715.html?k=basePrint. Accessed winter 2001.
6. Bombardier B., Buchwald D. Chronic Fatigue, Chronic Fatigue Syndrome, and Fibromyalgia. Disability and healthcare use. Med Care 1996;34(9):924–930. University of Washington, Seattle. Available at: http://www.sonic.net/cnds/impact.html. Accessed spring 2002.

7. Do you suffer from persistent pain? Aching? Fatigue? The Chronic Syndrome Support Association; 2000. Available at: : http://www.cssa-inc.org. Accessed winter 2001.

8. Chronic fatigue syndrome. National Institute of Allergy and Infectious Diseases fact sheet. Available at: http://www.niaid.nih.gov/factsheets/cfs.htm. Accessed winter 2001.

9. Nightingale Research Foundation. Paper presented by Byron Marshall Hyde, MD. sage http://www.nightingale.ca/ICaustralia2.html. Accessed winter 2001.

10. Ask NOAH about: Chronic fatigue syndrome. Nidus Information Services, Inc; 2000. Available at: http://www.noah-health.org/english/wellconn/chronicftge.html. Accessed winter 2001.

11. Chronic fatigue syndrome fact sheet. The CFIDS Association of America; 2000. Available at: http://www.cfids.org/news/factsht.html. Accessed winter 2001.

Fever

1. Drakos N. 2.1 Regulation and control of body temperature. Computer Based Learning Unit, University of Leeds; 1993–1994. Available at: http://nic.savba.sk/logos/books/scientific/node49.html. Accessed winter 2001.

2. Severine JE. Advances in temperature monitoring: A far cry from shake and take. *Nursing99.* 1999. Available at: http://www.springnet.com/ ce/temp.htm. Accessed winter 2001.

3. Why fever? Princeton University. Available at: http://plpk04.plpk.uq.edu.au/webtuts/SDL_skin/fever.htm#Why do we maintain body temperature. Accessed winter 2001.

HIV/AIDS

1. Blakeslee D. HIV's silent reservoirs. *JAMA.* 2000. Available at: http://www.ama-assn.org/ special/hiv/newsline/briefing/reserv.htm. Accessed winter 2001.

2. Blakeslee D. HIV fitness and disease progression. *JAMA.* 2000. Available at: http://www.amaassn.org/special/hiv/newsline/conferen/iac00/fitness.htm. Accessed winter 2001.

3. HIV/AIDS statistics. Fact sheet. National Institute of Allergy and Infectious Diseases. Available at: http://www.niaid.nih.gov/factsheets/ aidsstat.htm. Accessed winter 2001.

4. Blakeslee D. Long-term nonprogressors. *JAMA.* 2000. Available at: http://www.ama-assn.org/special/hiv/newsline/briefing/ltnps.htm. Accessed winter 2001.

5. Questions and answers: HIV is the cause of AIDS. Centers for Disease Control & Prevention, National Center for HIV, STD, and TB Prevention. Available at: http://www.cdc.gov/ hiv/pubs/cause.htm. Accessed winter 2001.

6. Blakeslee D. HIV and cancer. *JAMA.* 2000. Available at: http://www.ama-assn.org/special/ hiv/newsline/briefing/hivcan.htm. Accessed winter 2001.

7. Landy AL, Levy JA, Basic science: Report from the 13th International AIDS Conference. *JAMA.* 2000. Available at: http://www.ama-assn.org/special/hiv/ newsline/ conferen/iac00/basicsci.htm. Accessed winter 2001.

Inflammation

1. Kannus P. Immobilization or early mobilization after an acute soft-tissue injury? *Phys Sportsmed.* 2000;28(3). Available at: http://www. physsportsmed.com/issues/2000/03_00/kannus.htm. Accessed winter 2001.

2. Slavkovsky P. 1.1 Principles of inflammation. Computing Center of the Slovak Academy of Sciences; 1995. Available at: http://nic.savba.sk/logos/books/scientific/node43.html. Accessed winter 2001.

3. Thornton JS. Pain relief for acute soft-tissue injuries. Phys Sportsmed. 1997;25(10). Available at: http://www.physsportsmed.com/issues/1997/10oct/thornton.htm. Accessed winter 2001.

Lupus

1. Systemic lupus erythematosus. American College of Rheumatology; 2000. Available at: http://www.rheumatology.org/patients/factsheet/sle.html. Accessed winter 2001.

2. Commonly asked questions about lupus. Lupus Foundation of America. Available at: http://www.lupus.org/lupusfaq.html#1. Accessed winter 2001.

3. Discoid lupus erythematosus. New Zealand Dermatological Society; 1997–1999. Available at: http://www.dermnet.org.nz/index.html. Accessed winter 2001.

4. Grisolia JS. Systemic lupus erythematosus from neurology/inflammatory and demyelinating diseases. eMedicine.com, Inc.; 2001. Available at: http://www.emedicine.com/neuro/topic360.htm. Accessed winter 2001.

5. Edelson E. Genetic clue to lupus found. Rx Remedy, Inc.; 2001. Available at: http://www. healthscout.com/cgibin/WebObjects/Af?ap=43&id=107754. Accessed winter 2001.

6. Stevens MB. Joint and muscle pain in lupus. Lupus Foundation of America; 1995. Available at: http://www.lupus.org/topics/arthritis.html. Accessed winter 2001.

7. Klippel JH. Kidney disease and lupus. Lupus Foundation of America; 1995. Available at: http://www.lupus.org/topics/kidney.html. Accessed winter 2001.

8. Belmont HM Lupus clinical overview. 1996–1998. Available at: http://cerebel.com/ lupus/overview.html. Accessed winter 2001.

9. Matsen F III, ed. Lupus erythematosus. University of Washington; 2000. Available at: http://www.orthop.washington.edu/bonejoint/lzzzzzzz1_2.html. Accessed winter 2001.

10. What is lupus? Mayo Foundation for Medical Education and Research; 1998–2000. Available at: http://www.mayohealth.org/home?id=5.1.1.12.3. Accessed winter 2001.

11. Patient information sheets. National Institute of Arthritis and Musculoskeletal and Skin Diseases (NIAMS), National Institutes of Health (NIH). Available at: http://www.nih.gov/niams/ healthinfo/lupusguide/chppis1.htm. Accessed winter 2001.

12. Tuffanelli DL. Photosensitivity and lupus erythematosus. Lupus Foundation of America; 1995. Available at: http://www.lupus.org/topics/photosens.html

13. Signs and symptoms which may signal that a lupus flare is beginning. A selection from the Lupus Foundation of America Newsletter Article Library. Lupus Foundation of America; 1995. Available at: http://www.lupus.org/topics/flaresigns.html. Accessed winter 2001.

14. Provost TT. Skin disease in lupus. Lupus Foundation of America; 1995. Available at: http://www.lupus.org/topics/skin.html. Accessed winter 2001.

15. Lupus definition. Lupus Foundation of America; 1995. Available at: http://www.lupus.org/ info/general.html. Accessed winter 2001.

16. Wallace DJ. Systemic lupus and the nervous system. Lupus Foundation of America; 1995. Available at: http://www.lupus.org/topics/nervous.html. Accessed winter 2001.

17. Schwartz RS. Blood disorders in SLE. Lupus Foundation of America; 1995. Available at: http://www.lupus.org/topics/blood.html#3. Accessed winter 2001.

Respiratory System Conditions

6

CHAPTER OBJECTIVES

After reading this chapter, the reader should be able to . . .

- Name what percentage of calories a healthy person invests in the act of respiration while at rest.
- Name three muscles involved in respiration.
- Name the difference in causative factors between acute and chronic bronchitis.
- Name two differences between influenza and common cold.
- Describe why the flu vaccine does not impart life-long immunity.

- Name three causative agents for pneumonia.
- Name what percentage of tuberculosis exposures turns from primary to secondary disease.
- Name three risk factors for developing emphysema.
- Describe why persons with asthma, chronic bronchitis, or emphysema are often encouraged to be vaccinated against the flu.
- Name the average 5-year survival rate for lung cancer.

INTRODUCTION

Structure

The easiest way to discuss the structure of the respiratory system is to follow a particle of air through it (Fig. 6-1). Take a deep breath. Air drawn in through the nose encounters mucous membranes. Mucous membranes line any cavity in the body that communicates with the outside world (the respiratory, digestive, and reproductive and urinary systems). In the respiratory system the mucous membranes start inside the nose and mouth; they line the sinuses and throat, all the way down into the smaller tubes in the lungs. The wet, sticky mucous membranes in the respiratory system are responsible for warming, moistening, and filtering all the air that passes by.

Once past the nose and mouth, air enters first the pharynx, then the larynx, the trachea, and then the bronchi. The bronchi are asymmetrical. The right bronchus is bigger, wider, and straighter, leading into the three right lobes of the lungs. The left bronchus is smaller in diameter and curves off to the side to reach the two lobes of the left lung. This is significant because if anything should ever get inhaled into the lungs, it almost always follows the path of least resistance to the right side. The next section of tubing is the bronchioles, which subdivide 23 times until finally ending in microscopic alveoli. These little grape-shaped clusters of epithelium are like tiny balloons surrounded by blood capillaries. Gaseous exchange occurs through the alveoli. If for any reason they are impaired or not functioning correctly, the body will not be able to make an efficient trade of carbon dioxide for oxygen.

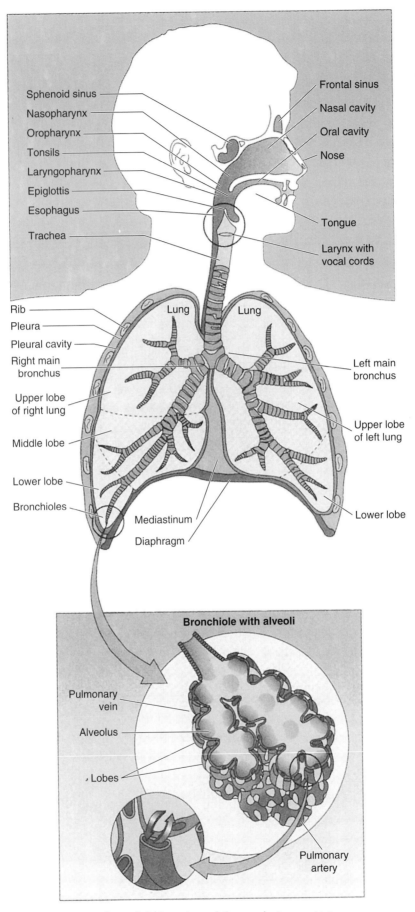

Figure 6-1. Overview of the respiratory system

The structure of the lungs themselves is well suited for fighting off infection. Each lung has two or three separate lobes, and each of those lobes has smaller separate segments. This isolation of different areas makes it difficult for pathogens to infect the whole structure. The whole tract is lined with mucous membrane, which traps pathogens and other particles. Then the "mucus blanket" slowly creeps toward the mouth and nose for expulsion. Smooth muscle tissue lines all of the tubes down to the smallest bronchi; once an irritant has gotten into these tubes a healthy cough reflex quickly moves it out of the body.

Function

Air cycles through the lungs anywhere from 12 to 20 times per minute. The lungs themselves do not have any muscle tissue to make them fill up or empty; they are simply two limp-walled sacs that inflate or deflate according to the air pressure inside and outside of them. Changes in air pressure are brought about by changing the shape of the thoracic cavity. If the cavity is made larger (i.e., when the diaphragm contracts), the air pressure inside will be low until air rushes in to equalize it. In other words, the act of inhaling is simply filling a vacuum. When the pressure inside and outside the lungs has been equalized, air eases out again (exhalation). Exhalation is usually a passive process when a person is at rest; it does not involve muscular activity unless a person specifically tries to remove air from the lungs.

The kinds of conditions examined in this chapter mostly have to do with how vulnerable the respiratory system can be to infection. Fortunately, thanks to the sticky mucous membranes and lungs that have carefully isolated segments, those infections seldom get a strong enough grip on to do lasting damage.

What Does "Lung Capacity" Mean?

In a normal, healthy person at rest, the act of breathing consumes approximately 5% of the energy he or she uses. This percentage rises when structural or functional problems develop in the respiratory system; the act of breathing, of providing the tissues with oxygen, can become an exhausting labor.

Massage does not change the structure of the lungs, but it *can* affect the efficiency of the muscles of inspiration. Work with the diaphragm, the scalenes, and the intercostal muscles can make the act of breathing easier, which in turn can make a person feel generally more energetic.

The size of a person's lungs depends largely on his or her height and general build. An average male can hold up to 6 L of air, but only a small portion of that total is exchanged with each breath.

- *Tidal volume* is the amount of air moved in and out of the lungs during normal resting breathing. It involves about 500 mL of air.

- *Inspiratory reserve volume* is the amount of air that can be consciously inhaled beyond tidal volume inhalation. It averages about 3100 mL.

- *Expiratory reserve volume* is the amount of air that can be consciously exhaled beyond tidal volume exhalation. It averages about 1200 mL.

- *Vital capacity* of the lungs is all the air that is possible to consciously inhale and exhale. That is, vital capacity is tidal volume, plus inspiratory reserve volume, plus expiratory reserve volume. Vital capacity accounts for a total of about 4800 mL.

- *Residual volume* is the amount of air left in the lungs after a maximum exhalation. This volume is necessary to prevent the alveoli from collapsing. Residual volume is about 1200 mL in a healthy adult.

Thus, total lung capacity is the vital capacity plus the residual volume, about 6000 mL, or 6 L, for an average adult male in good health.

Highly trained athletes work to increase the accessibility of oxygen to their tissues. They look for a balance between breathing deeper and faster to bring more air in, and expending a minimum of energy on the act of breathing. Massage therapists can influence this balance by working with the muscles of respiration to reduce resistance and increase efficiency.

Respiratory System Conditions

Infectious Respiratory Disorders

Acute Bronchitis
Common Cold
Influenza
Pneumonia
Sinusitis
Tuberculosis

Obstructive Pulmonary Diseases

Asthma
Chronic Bronchitis
Emphysema

Other Respiratory Disorders

Lung Cancer

Infectious Respiratory Disorders

ACUTE BRONCHITIS IN BRIEF

What is it?
Acute bronchitis is an infection and inflammation of the bronchiole tree anywhere between the trachea and the bronchioles. If inflammation extends into the bronchioles and alveoli, it is called bronchopneumonia.

How is it recognized?
The hallmark of acute bronchitis is a persistent productive cough along with sore throat, nasal congestion, fatigue, and fever. Whereas other symptoms generally subside within 10 days, the cough may last for several weeks while the bronchi heal.

Is massage indicated or contraindicated?
Acute bronchitis, like all acute infections, contraindicates circulatory massage. If the infection has passed and the cough is the only lingering symptom, massage may be appropriate as long as the client is comfortable on the table.

Acute Bronchitis
Definition: What Is It?

Acute bronchitis is a self-limiting infection and inflammation of the respiratory tract, specifically of the bronchial tree. It is usually a complication of the *common cold* or *flu* (this chapter), but the causative factors are often difficult to identify. Acute bronchitis is a self-limiting disorder; it is usually resolved within 10 days to several weeks of onset. This helps to distinguish it from *chronic bronchitis* (this chapter), which is an irreversible condition.

Demographics: Who Gets It?

It is estimated that somewhere between 7 and 12 million cases of acute bronchitis are diagnosed every year in the United States. Most cases are identified among young children, but adults are certainly susceptible. Adults who smoke or work in environments with dust, fumes, or other pollutants are at higher risk for developing acute bronchitis than others.

Etiology: What Happens?

When the bronchi are irritated or infected by any kind of pathogen, an inflammatory response ensues. The tubes swell, the cilia are damaged, excessive mucus is produced, and the result is coughing and wheezing as air moves through obstructed passageways. The big mystery with infectious acute bronchitis is the source of the infection. Most cases are complications of a cold or flu, in which the viruses simply move from the upper respiratory system to the bronchial tubes. Other causative agents may include a variety of bacteria, fungi, or noninfectious irritants such as fumes, air pollutants, and other contaminants.

A surprising and somewhat alarming development in recent studies of acute bronchitis among some adults is the presence of pertussis bacteria; this is the causative agent for whooping cough. In adults this infection is not serious, but in young children it can be life-threatening. Therefore, it is important that infected adults not be exposed to non-immunized children while this pathogen is active.

Signs and Symptoms

The primary sign of acute bronchitis is a persistent productive cough. Sputum may be clear or opaque. Wheezing, nasal congestion, headache, low fever, muscle aches, chest pain, and fatigue may also be present. Most of the symptoms of acute bronchitis subside within about 10 days of onset, but the cough may persist for several weeks while the delicate lining of the bronchial tubes heals.

Diagnosis

Acute bronchitis is usually diagnosed by the presence of its distinctive symptoms. However, several other respiratory disorders can create similar symptoms. Bacterial *sinusitis*, mild *pneumonia*, and *asthma* (this chapter) can all involve wheezing and productive coughs. These disorders should be ruled out to be sure that treatment options are as effective as possible.

Treatment

The best treatment options for most cases of acute bronchitis are the same as those for cold or flu: plenty of rest, lots of fluids, and warm, humid air to liquefy mucus and aid in its expulsion. Antibiotics are not effective in most cases of acute bronchitis, but they are appropriate when the causative agent has been identified as bacterial, especially in the case of pertussis.

Bronchodilators and cough suppressants can help to ameliorate some of the symptoms of acute bronchitis, but they will not eradicate the infection or speed recovery.

Massage?

Circulatory massage is inappropriate for someone in the acute stage of a bronchial infection. When the infection has passed, however, and the person is left with a persistent cough while the bronchial tubes heal, massage may be appropriate as long as the client is comfortable on the table.

Common Cold
Definition: What Is It?

This condition is brought about by any of about 200 different viruses. Over the course of a lifetime people are exposed to multitudes of pathogens. They get sick, they establish immunity to that particular pathogen, and they move on to the next infection. Much of this happens in childhood; by adulthood people have encountered the majority of what they are likely to see, and the frequency of infections generally subsides. Nevertheless, no single infectious agent causes the so-called common cold, and the viruses themselves keep mutating and changing. This is why an effective cure for this condition may never be found.

Demographics: Who Gets It?

It is difficult to project just how common the common cold really is. One estimate suggests that about 1 billion infections with common cold virus occur in the United States in an average year. Children are most at risk for these infections until their immune systems have built up a collection of resistant antibodies. Children have an average of 6 to 10 colds a year, and adults generally have 2 to 4 per year. People older than 60 years may have fewer than 2 colds per year.

Colds are a major cause of school and work absenteeism and cost untold millions of dollars in health care and lost productivity.

COMMON COLD IN BRIEF

What is it?
The common cold, or upper respiratory tract infection (URTI), is a viral infection from any of approximately 200 different types of viruses.

How is it recognized?
The symptoms of colds are nasal discharge, sore throat, mild fever, dry coughing, and headache. Symptoms last anywhere from 2 days to 2 weeks.

Is massage indicated or contraindicated?
Colds indicate circulatory massage only when the acute stage has passed. Even then, massage may exacerbate symptoms as the healing process may be accelerated.

Etiology: What Happens?

The viruses that cause the common cold have a specific target cell: mucous-producing cells that line the throat and respiratory tract. When a virus gains access to its target, it infiltrates that cell and takes over its processes until the cell literally bursts with new viruses.

Although the damage that cold viruses cause is substantial, it pales in comparison to the damage caused by the immune system when it is fighting off a cold virus. Special signals released by infected cells attract immune system agents, which cause the area to be flooded with inflammatory chemicals and aggressive immune systems cells. It is the immune system response to a viral threat that causes most of the discomfort that is associated with common cold symptoms.

Contrary to popular belief, being cold has nothing to do with catching a cold. Extensive research has shown that a person's susceptibility to a cold virus has little to do with temperature, diet, exercise, or even whether the tonsils are enlarged. Instead, the leading risk factors for catching a cold are being under psychological stress, having respiratory allergies that make mucous membranes vulnerable to infection, and the stage of the menstrual cycle.[a]

Signs and Symptoms

The symptoms of a cold are probably familiar to everyone—runny nose, sneezing, sore throat, dry coughing, headache, and perhaps a mild fever. Colds are typically limited to the respiratory tract, which is why they are sometimes called *upper respiratory tract infections* (URTIs). Symptoms generally last less than 2 weeks, although the virus may be present in the body for up to 3 days before symptoms begin. This incubation period is also a contagious period, which can make the spread of infection hard to control.

Complications

Colds are seldom dangerous except when they complicate into another disorder. The compromised integrity of the membranes and the accumulations of mucus, a perfect growth medium, leave the body vulnerable to a bacterial onslaught that can include middle ear infections (otitis media), laryngitis, *acute bronchitis*, *sinusitis*, and *pneumonia* (this chapter).

Prevention

Cold viruses can live for up to 3 hours outside the body. The viruses are airborne after an infected person coughs or sneezes. However, they are much more easily spread when someone gets a virus on their hand or face, and the virus finds access into the body through a portal of entry (mouth or nose). Picking up a virus on the hands or from a face pad, a doorknob, or a piece of money, and then rubbing the nose is a very efficient way to spread the disease.

The best way to prevent the spread of colds and other infectious diseases is by frequently washing the hands, focusing on the cuticles and nails, using soap or detergent, and scrubbing for 10 seconds or more before rinsing.

[a]The common cold fact sheet. National Institute of Allergy and Infectious Diseases, National Institutes of Health. Available at: http://www.niaid.nih.gov/factsheets/cold.htm. Accessed spring 2001.

Treatment

Because these are viral infections, antibiotics are useless for treating colds. Getting extra rest, drinking lots of fluids, and isolating oneself away from family, classmates, and co-workers who could get infected are all high priorities. Using a humidifier may relieve some of the irritation to mucous membranes, although it is important to be aware that some types of humidifiers can be breeding grounds for bacteria and it is important to keep them scrupulously clean. Over-the-counter drugs can relieve the symptoms of a cold but they do *not* reduce recovery time. In fact, by inhibiting the ways a body fights off infection (reducing fever, drying up the sinuses), over-the-counter drugs have been shown to actually increase the amount of time the infection is present in the body. Some research shows that aspirin can also increase the concentration of virus shed in nasal secretions, thus increasing the possibility of spreading the disease.[b]

Concerns have arisen over the prescription of "just in case" antibiotics. Only about 20% of colds develop into bacterial infections. Frequent administration of needless antibiotics does not improve recovery time, but can contribute to the creation of new and more drug resistant strains of bacteria.

Alternative health-care strategies for dealing with colds include plenty of vitamin C, echinacea, lysine (an amino acid with antiviral properties), zinc lozenges (also antiviral), and perhaps licorice root as an expectorant. Some of these interventions have been shown to reduce recovery time, but their efficacy as cold preventatives has yet to be proven. Hydrotherapy options include artificial fevers to boost immune function (see *fever*, Chapter 5) and cold double-compresses or packs.

Massage?

Circulatory bodywork is appropriate for colds only in the subacute phase. If someone receives massage in the acute stage of a cold, it can spread it through the body *much* more effectively than would happen naturally, and that is *not* a benefit. On the other hand, if someone is on the post-acute side of an infection, massage may help to speed recovery time. It is important to ask permission though, because this may sometimes make people feel like they are having a relapse. It is, after all, squeezing 3 days of recovery into one day of feeling crummy again.

Influenza

Definition: What Is It?

Influenza or "flu" is a viral infection of the respiratory tract. Most of the time it is a relatively benign, self-limiting infection, but it can become life-threatening if an aggressive virus infects a vulnerable patient.

Demographics: Who Gets It?

Everyone can get the flu and probably does at least a few times over a lifetime. It is estimated that anywhere from 10 to 20% of the population has at least one bout of flu each year. For most people it is a significant inconvenience but not a serious

INFLUENZA IN BRIEF

What is it?
Influenza ("flu") is a viral infection of the respiratory tract.

How is it recognized?
The symptoms of flu include high fever and muscle and joint achiness that may last for up to 3 days, followed by a runny nose, coughing, sneezing, and general malaise.

Is massage indicated or contraindicated?
Flu indicates circulatory massage during the subacute stage only.

[b]The common cold fact sheet. National Institute of Allergy and Infectious Diseases, National Institutes of Health. Available at: http://www.niaid.nih.gov/factsheets/cold.htm. Accessed spring 2001.

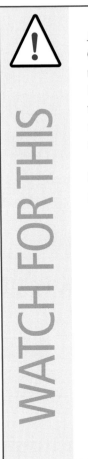

Is It a Cold? Is It the Flu? Does It Matter?

Colds and flu are both caused by viral attacks on mucous cells in the respiratory tract. They have similar symptoms and carry similar cautions for working with clients who have these infections. Still, flu infections can be much worse than colds. They are more contagious and can linger in the body much longer. Therefore, it is useful to have a clear idea of which pathogen a client is battling.

PRESENTATION	COMMON COLD	INFLUENZA
Duration	Usually less than 1 week	Could be 10 days or more
Fever	Usually low (less than 102°F) and short-term (resolves within 48 hours)	Usually high (more than 102°F) and long-term (may persist for 3 days or more)
Location	Symptoms are strictly in the upper respiratory tract	Symptoms may be felt systemically as muscle and joint pain, inflamed lymph nodes, and debilitating fatigue
Complications	If complications occur, they are usually sinus or ear infections	If complications occur, they usually affect the lower respiratory tract as bronchitis or pneumonia
Communicability	Cold virus is usually spread by hands contacting contaminated surfaces; colds are contagious but do not usually create widespread epidemics	Flu virus is usually spread by inhalation of airborne virus; flu viruses are often highly virulent and may infect high proportions of the population
Resolution of the infection	Cold viruses are quickly eliminated from the body; when symptoms are over, it is no longer contagious	Flu virus may linger in the body several days after symptoms have abated; it continues to be communicable at this time

problem. For the very young, the very old, people with chronic heart or lung disease, people who are immune suppressed, or people who spend a great deal of time in hospitals or long-term care facilities, an outbreak of flu can be deadly. Flu kills about 20 thousand Americans each year.

A synonym for flu is grippe, from the French gripper, to seize.

Etiology: What Happens?

Flu viruses work in the usual way of infectious agents: they gain access to the body (flu virus is usually inhaled as airborne particles) and then they invade and attack their target cells, in this case, mucous-producing cells that line the respiratory tract. Once the infection becomes established, the immune system response is what causes most of the extreme symptoms. White blood cells attack infected mucous cells, causing sore throat and coughing. They also release the chemicals that stimulate *fever* (Chapter 5). It can take 2 or 3 days for symptoms to appear, but the person is shedding virus in oral and mucous secretions all the time. The peak of communicability is usually around day 4 of the infection. The person continues to shed virus throughout the acute and subacute stages, up to 7 days after symptoms have subsided.

Three different classes of flu virus have been identified. The type A viruses are the most virulent and are responsible for the major epidemics that claimed millions of lives in the early part of the 20th century (see sidebar). Type A viruses mutate quickly and so can cause repeated infections in the same person. Type B flu viruses can also spread but are not as aggressive or widely spread as Type A viruses. Type C flu viruses are not associated with epidemics and are relatively stable. They create much less severe symptoms than the other types.

Type A flu viruses are remarkably adaptable. They can infect several species in addition to humans, including birds, pigs, seals, whales, and horses. It usually appears that the flu passes from one species to another and undergoes some minor changes to its enzymes that allow it to invade its new host. In some cases the transmission may occur directly from animals to humans without mutation. So far, only Type A viruses have been seen to be capable of this process.

Flu viruses also have the ability to mutate as they develop resistance to attack. This makes it impossible for the body to establish permanent immunity; each time it is exposed, the pathogen is different.

Signs and Symptoms

Flu symptoms can range from being subtle to causing death within hours or days. For most common infections the symptoms look like a really bad cold: respiratory irritation with runny nose and dry cough, and a long-lasting high fever (it is not unusual for flu-related fevers to go over 102°F in adults, and they may last for 3 days or more). Most flu infections cause symptoms that affect more than the upper respiratory tract, however. Many patients experience aching muscles and joints as well as debilitating fatigue. (One area that flu viruses generally *will not* attack, however, is the gastrointestinal tract. What is commonly referred to as "stomach flu" is far more likely to be infection with rotavirus or a case of food poisoning; see *gastroenteritis*, Chapter 7.) For more information on how the flu differs from the common cold, see the side bar "Is it a Cold? Is it the Flu?"

Flu symptoms usually appear about 3 days after exposure to the virus and may persist for up to 2 weeks. If they persist longer than that, or if the coughing begins to produce a large amount of phlegm, it is time to consider that the original viral infection has complicated to a secondary bacterial infection of the lungs.

Complications

The greatest danger with flu is the possibility of an opportunistic bacterial infection in the shape of *pneumonia* or *acute bronchitis* (this chapter). This is a particular danger for high-risk populations (i.e., the very young, the very old, heavy smokers, diabetics, people who are immune-suppressed, people who are living in long-term care facilities, or people with chronic lung or heart problems).

Treatment

As a viral infection, flu is unaffected by antibiotics. Good sense measures include rest, liquids, alternative regimens, and lots of chicken soup. Over-the-counter drugs may abate the symptoms but do not speed healing. They can be useful, however, if the symptoms are preventing a person from getting the sleep needed to heal.

A new class of antiviral medications is finding use among flu patients. Amantadine can reduce the duration of symptoms of flu if they are caused by a type A virus, but it is associated with central nervous system side effects including sleeplessness, restlessness, and confusion, especially among elderly patients. A closely related medication, rimantadine, usually has fewer side affects. Neither amantadine nor rimantadine is effective against type B or C viruses, and both medications have been seen to allow the mutation of flu virus into more dangerous drug-resistant strains.

We Are All Under the Influence: The History of Flu

Symptoms of the infectious disease now called flu have been documented since the 5th century BC. It was observed in those early days of medicine that this disorder could spread throughout a population, but symptoms sometimes would not appear for a few days after exposure. In addition, it continued to spread for several days after all symptoms were gone among the original patients. Because its course seemed so mysterious, it was assumed that this disease was controlled by the influence of the planets and stars. Then in the early 1500s, the Italian term for influence ("influenza") became the common name for this disorder.

The first recorded pandemic of flu virus is known from records from Europe from 1580. The 20th century saw four pandemics of flu infections and a near miss of a fifth.

- 1918: The "Spanish Lady" was a flu virus that swept across the globe. In the course of 3 years it killed half a million people in the United States and 20 million people worldwide.
- 1957: The Asian Flu.
- 1968: The Hong Kong Flu.
- 1977: The Russian Flu. These flu viruses killed a total of 1.5 million people worldwide.
- 1997: In Hong Kong another new flu virus was identified. This one had a previously unknown feature: it seemed to be directly communicable from birds to people. It infected 18 people and killed 6, but if it had escaped Hong Kong it could have killed millions more. It was controlled largely by an aggressive public health effort that ended in the slaughter of all of Hong Kong's domestic poultry to limit the potential spread of the virus.

Today flu is not considered much of a threat by the majority of the population, but for those people who live in confined situations like nursing homes or other long-term care facilities, those who live with chronic lung or heart disease, or those who are immune suppressed, flu can be a life-threatening infection.

Research is now being conducted into a medical intervention that would interfere with how the virus moves from one cell to the next. Weakening a specific viral enzyme can slow the proliferation of the virus, shortening the duration and reducing the severity of infection.

Every year the Food and Drug Administration distributes a vaccine to fight a combination of type A and type B viruses. These vaccines are created about a year ahead of when "flu season" (late fall to early spring) hits. Consequently, the vaccine may or may not be effective against the viruses that are circulating when it is administered. Furthermore, because viruses mutate so quickly, flu vaccines need to be updated every year. Nonetheless, flu vaccines are highly recommended for high-risk populations.

Massage?

Persons who have the flu and receive circulatory bodywork in the early stages of infection may find themselves with a much more serious infection than they would have otherwise. Persons who receive massage after the infection has peaked may find that they recover more quickly. Two cautions must be kept in mind, however. One is that squeezing several days of recovery into one or two days may make clients feel sick again; they should know that this is a possibility. The other is that persons who are recovering from the flu may still be shedding virus up to 7 days after symptoms have disappeared. This puts the massage therapist at risk for getting sick.

Pneumonia
Definition: What Is It?

Pneumonia is a general term for inflammation of the lungs, usually due to an infectious agent.

Demographics: Who Gets It?

Pneumonia can affect the entire age range of the population, from infants to senior adults. Because it is an opportunistic infection that takes advantage of weak immune systems, it is the sixth leading cause of death in the United States. Every year between 3 and 5 million people in the United States get pneumonia; half a million of them receive hospital care, and about 84,000 die. Severity of the infection ranges from being not much worse than a bad cold to being a cause of death within 24 hours.

Etiology: What Happens?

The alveoli are the most vulnerable structures in the lungs. They are the tiny air balloons with walls made of squamous epithelium. They are surrounded by the capillaries of the pulmonary circuit for the exchange of oxygen and carbon dioxide in the bloodstream. When an infection strikes in the lungs, these tiny air balloons fill up with dead white blood cells, mucus, and fluid backed up from the capillaries. Eventually, diffusion of gases

PNEUMONIA
The Greek root of this word is *pneumon*, which means lung. The suffix *-ia* indicates "condition."

is impossible. Abscesses may form, and capillary damage may occur, allowing red blood cells into the alveoli and eventually into the sputum.

In some forms of pneumonia, fibrin, a blood protein responsible for clotting, begins to thicken the fluid in the alveoli until it becomes a gelid mass. This is known as *consolidation*. In most cases the alveolar exudate remains liquid but is still a hindrance to diffusion. Edema is not always limited to the alveoli. In extreme cases fluid may be found between the visceral and parietal layers of the pleurae. This can lead to *pleurisy* (scarring and limitation of movement between the pleurae during breathing).

Causes of Pneumonia

Several infectious agents can cause pneumonia. Each one of them has a different symptomatic profile, including what kind of sputum they create and how they appear on chest radiographs. It is also possible for more than one type of pathogen to be present at a time, a fact that sometimes makes diagnosis and treatment of this condition a challenge.

- *Viruses.* Viral infections account for about half of all pneumonia cases. *Influenza A* and *B* (this chapter) and syncytial virus are the most common culprits. Other viruses include cytomegalovirus, *herpes simplex* (Chapter 1), and adenovirus. The incubation period of viral pneumonia is 1 to 3 days. Viral pneumonia tends to be short-lived and not serious. It appears most frequently in children.

- *Bacteria.* Bacterial pneumonia can be caused by staphylococcus or streptococcus. The bacteria often live harmlessly in the throat, but when resistance is low they may invade the lower respiratory tract to set up an infection in the lungs. The toxins released by the bacteria initiate an inflammatory response, leading to edema in the alveoli and a reduced ability to draw oxygen into the system. This kind of infection usually responds well to antibiotics.

- *Mycoplasma.* Mycoplasma are the smallest free-living agents ever found. They are sometimes classified as a type of bacteria, but they have no clearly defined cell wall. They also have several invasive properties that most bacteria do not. The incubation period for mycoplasma pneumonia is quite lengthy (1 to 4 weeks). Because it tends not to be as severe as bacterial or viral types of infection, it is sometimes called "walking pneumonia." Fortunately, like bacterial pneumonia, mycoplasma pneumonia responds well to antibiotics.

- *Pneumocystis carinii.* This is a protozoan infection almost exclusively associated with immunosuppressed patients such as those with *AIDS* (Chapter 5) and those receiving cancer chemotherapy or immunosuppressive drugs to prevent the rejection of organ transplants.

- *Others.* Other pathogens that can cause pneumonia include chlamydia, rickettsia, and tuberculosis bacilli.

Forms of Pneumonia

Pneumonia appears in several forms. Each one may have different presentations or cautions, so it is worthwhile to be familiar with the most common types.

PNEUMONIA IN BRIEF

What is it?
Pneumonia is an infection in the lungs brought about by bacteria, viruses, or other pathogens.

How is it recognized?
The symptoms of pneumonia include coughing that may be dry or productive, high fever, pain on breathing, and shortness of breath. Extreme cases may show *cyanosis* or a bluish caste to the skin and nails.

Is massage indicated or contraindicated?
Depending on the causative factor and the general resiliency of the person, massage may be indicated in the subacute stage.

- *Primary pneumonia* is relatively rare. In this case no predisposing factor has weakened the patient; it is simply an attack directly on the lungs.

- *Secondary pneumonia* is by the far the most common situation. In this a pathogenic assault on lung tissue is successful because the body's immune system is weakened by another disease. Even if the primary disease is viral, the accumulation of mucus is a perfect growth medium for bacteria, leaving the patient vulnerable to this kind of infection.

Under the headings of primary or secondary, pneumonia may also be classified by the location of the infection.

- *Bronchopneumonia.* This type starts as a bronchial inflammation and spreads into the lungs. It appears in a patchy pattern all over the lungs, not segregated to a specific area.

- *Lobar pneumonia.* This type is restricted to one lobe of the lungs. Consolidation occurs there, and gradually the whole lobe may be affected.

- *Double pneumonia.* This affects both lungs. It can be bacterial or viral.

A final classification for pneumonia determines the source of the infectious agent.

- *Community acquired pneumonia* is the most common form and is usually a bacterial infection of *Streptococcus pneumoniae* (also called *pneumococcus*), *Haemophilus influenzae*, or influenza Type A or B.

- *Nosocomial or hospital-acquired pneumonia* is an infection in a person who has been a hospital inpatient for at least 72 hours or within the previous 1 to 3 weeks.

Signs and Symptoms

Symptoms of pneumonia can vary widely, depending on the causative factor and how much of the lung is affected. Some of the possible symptoms of pneumonia include coughing, very high fever, chills, sweating, delirium, chest pains, cyanosis, thick and colored sputum, shortness of breath, muscle aches and pains, and pleurisy.

Pneumonia can have a sudden or gradual onset. Very often it follows the same course as flu, but instead of getting better, the respiratory symptoms get rapidly worse, along with fever up to 104°F.

Diagnosis

Pneumonia is usually diagnosed by clinical examination and a description of symptoms. Both viral and bacterial pneumonia have sudden onset with a rapid development of symptoms, whereas mycoplasma pneumonia may take weeks for symptoms to reach their peak. Different types of bacterial pneumonia produce different colors of sputum, from opaque green to rust-colored to "currant jelly" sputum, so these are often helpful diagnostic clues. Throat and sputum cultures are rarely taken unless a nosocomial infection is suspected, as they take a long time to grow and are often incorrect.

A diagnosis is sometimes confirmed with a radiograph, which shows where areas of the lungs have become pathologically dense. Again, different types of lung infections have particular patterns in radiographs, so this is another helpful diagnostic clue.

Treatment

Treatment depends on what type of pneumonia is present. Bacterial and mycoplasma pneumonias generally respond well to antibiotics, but viral infections do not respond to these medications.

Symptomatic relief and supportive therapy include breathing humidified air, drinking ample fluids, and supplementing oxygen if necessary. Physical therapy or massage therapy to percuss the rib cage and help loosen phlegm is sometimes recommended. Practicing good hygiene by preventing any contact with expectorated material is especially important in these situations.

Prevention

Two main methods exist to prevent some of the most common types of pneumonia infections. Flu vaccines, if they are effective against the circulating flu viruses of the year, can prevent flu infections from complicating into viral or bacterial pneumonia. A vaccine has been developed against the most common type of bacterial pneumonia, *Streptococcus pneumoniae*. This vaccine is recommended mainly for high-risk patients and for people who live or work in long-term care facilities or hospitals.

Prognosis

Considering the delicacy of the epithelium in the lungs, it is amazing that if a pneumonia infection is short-lived, it is completely reversible. The body can re-liquify and absorb the consolidated matter in affected alveoli, as it can reabsorb the fluid from any inflamed part of the lung. If a patient is basically healthy, he or she can expect to recover fully within 2 weeks.

In long-standing cases in which fibrosis and scar tissue accumulate, permanent damage to the elasticity of the epithelial tissue may occur, or the freedom with which the lungs move in the pleural cavity may be compromised. This can raise the risk for future infections.

When people develop this condition as a complication of a more serious underlying disorder, pneumonia can be life-threatening. Secondary pneumonia is an opportunistic disease. It kills more people every year than any other kind of infection because it takes advantage of low defenses. It is often the final complication of other serious diseases, even noninfectious ones. People who have had a stroke, heart failure, alcoholism, or cancer die of pneumonia more often than any other disease. People who are bedridden or paralyzed are susceptible too, because their cough reflex is often impaired; they cannot expel mucus easily. Having a pre-existing chest problem like flu, bronchitis, emphysema, or asthma is an open invitation. Finally, being immune-suppressed because of tissue transplants, AIDS, steroids, leukemia, or cytotoxic drugs makes a person particularly vulnerable to pneumonia.

Massage?

This is a serious and complicated condition that frequently accompanies other serious conditions. Under the right circumstances pneumonia can respond very well to the mechanical impact of percussive massage. Tapotement on the chest and back can help to move mucus from the alveoli into the bronchial tubes, where muscle action can take over to expel it from the body. Massage therapists working with pneumonia patients would do well to be part of a well-informed health care team, rather than working alone.

SINUS
From the Latin for channel, hollow place, or tunnel.

Sinusitis
Definition: What Is It?

Sinusitis, as the name implies, is a condition in which the mucous membranes that line the sinuses become inflamed and swollen.

Demographics: Who Gets It?

Sinusitis statistics are rising quickly. It is estimated that about 37 million sinus infections occur in the United States each year, and that up to 15% of the population experiences chronic sinusitis at one time or another.

Etiology: What Happens?

Sinuses are hollow areas located lateral to, above, and behind the nose (Fig. 6-2). Sinuses are meant to be hollow. They provide resonance for the voice and lighten the weight of the head considerably. The mucous membranes lining sinuses are provided with cilia, the tiny hairs that move the mucous along so that trapped pathogens and particulate matter can be expelled before reaching the lower respiratory system.

When the cilia break down, often as a result of viral infection or environmental irritants, pathogen-laden mucous lingers over delicate epithelial cells, stimulating an inflammatory response. Soon the hollow areas fill with sticky, pus-filled mucus that cannot drain. Inflamed, infected sinuses can be a source of tremendous pain and discomfort.

Alternatively, the cilia may remain intact and highly functional, but the mucous membranes are stimulated to respond to oak pollen or cat dander as if they were life-threatening organisms. Inflammation ensues, with itchiness, production of huge amounts of thin, runny mucous, puffy, itchy eyes, and all the symptoms associated with allergic rhinitis or "hay fever."

Causes

Sinusitis comes in two varieties: noninfectious and infectious. Noninfectious sinusitis may also be called allergic rhinitis. Infectious sinusitis involves a pathogenic invasion followed by an inflammatory response that creates a vicious circle: the body creates excessive mucus to help remove infectious agents, but the inflamed tissues make drainage of that mucus (which is an ideal growth medium for many types of bacteria) impossible.

- *Noninfectious sinusitis: allergic rhinitis.* Hay fever also causes inflammation of the sinus membranes, but it happens without underlying infection. Hay fever is often distinguished from infectious sinusitis by the lack of congestion and by the quality of the nasal discharge (it tends to be thin and runny rather than thick and sticky). Hay fever is the only variety of sinusitis that may be treated safely with antihistamines.

  It is always a possibility that the irritation to sinuses caused by hay fever can open the door to a secondary bacterial infection, which makes the sinusitis infectious and allergic.

- *Infectious sinusitis: causative agents.*
  - *Viruses and bacteria*
    The most common types of infectious sinusitis begin as viral infections (see *common cold*, this chapter). When defenses are low, the bacteria that normally

colonize the skin and mucous membranes take advantage of the situation and begin to multiply. The bacteria most commonly associated with these infections are *Streptococcus pneumoniae* and *Haemophilus influenzae*. Dental work may very occasionally cause sinusitis if the contents of an abscessed tooth are somehow released into the nasal cavity.

- *Structural problems*

  A deviated septum or the growth of nasal polyps can obstruct the flow of mucus out of the sinuses. This is not an infectious situation to begin with, but mucus held back from normal flow is a perfect growth medium for bacteria. Therefore, what begins as a simple structural anomaly can become a true infection.

- *Fungi and bacteria*

  Recent research has revealed that a high percentage of people with chronic sinusitis have significant amounts of fungal growth in their sinuses. One theory is that sensitivity to fungi stimulates an inflammatory response that then allows naturally occurring bacteria to grow and cause a chronic infection.

- *Other fungal infections*

  These are particular dangers for persons who are immune-suppressed. Fungi such as *Aspergillus* or *Curvularia* are not threats to most people, but can be sources of sinus infection to AIDS patients or others whose immune systems are compromised.

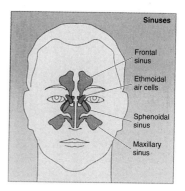

Figure 6-2. Sinusitis

Infectious sinusitis can be acute, in which cases symptoms develop just as a respiratory infection subsides and continue to get worse for 6 to 8 weeks. It can also be a chronic situation in which symptoms may be less severe but more prolonged. Episodes of chronic sinusitis can last 8 weeks or more and can happen several times a year.

Signs and Symptoms

Symptoms of sinusitis vary according to the cause of the inflammation and which sinuses are involved. Severe headache is a key feature, especially upon waking. Bending over makes it much worse, because that position increases pressure on already stressed membranes. The affected area may be extremely painful to the touch, and swelling or puffiness around the eyes or cheeks may be visible. Fever and chills may accompany an acute bacterial infection. Sore throat, coughing (caused by post-nasal drip), and congestion or runny nose may appear with any type of sinus irritation. Regardless of whether it is an infectious or allergic situation, people with sinusitis are likely to experience fatigue and general malaise because the body is fighting hard to cast off an invader.

The mucus expressed with a sinus infection is likely to be streaked or completely opaque in shades that range from pale green to yellow to brown. It tends to be thick and sticky. The mucus expressed with hay fever, on the other hand, tends to be thin, runny, and clear.

Complications

It is rare but not unheard of for sinus infections to spread and become very serious situations. The infection can infiltrate facial bones, causing osteomyelitis and permanent bone damage, or it can gain access to the central nervous system and cause *meningitis* (Chapter 3).

Treatment

Treatment of sinusitis begins with self-help measures. Staying in humid air or breathing steam to help moisturize and liquefy the clogged mucus is an important step. Increasing daily water intake and reducing the use of alcohol, caffeine, and other diuretics may also help to soften and loosen thick, sticky mucous. Using air filters to remove irritating particles from the air can also help.

Drugs prescribed for this disorder begin with antibiotics if the infection is bacterial. Sinuses are difficult to access, and the bacteria associated with most cases of sinusitis tend to be drug resistant, so this condition often requires long-term courses of specialized antibiotics.

Decongestants are sometimes recommended to shrink the mucous membranes, but these are only appropriate for short-term use because they can create a terrible "rebound effect" when use is stopped. Corticosteroids in nasal spray form can reduce swelling, but they are also best used in short-term doses. In very extreme cases surgery is recommended. This involves inserting a tube through the nose and enlarging sinus passages, removing polyps, repairing a deviated septum, and doing anything else that may assist the mucous to drain freely.

Antihistamines are specifically avoided with sinus infections. These substances simply dry up the mucus and allow it to cling to the membrane walls, thus improving bacterial access. Allergies *without* signs of infection may be treated with antihistamines to limit the inappropriate immune response that causes inflammation.

Massage?

Massage is fine for allergic sinusitis, because the client has no bacterial or viral infection to spread, catch, or complicate into a more serious condition. However, it can be uncomfortable for the client to be completely horizontal for extended periods.

When a client has an acute sinus infection, however, and especially if he or she is feverish and achy, circulatory bodywork is inappropriate.

Chronic sinus infections are probably safe for most types of bodywork, as long as the client is comfortable. Face holes or cradles may put pressure on sensitive parts of the face and exacerbate symptoms.

Tuberculosis

Definition: What Is It?

"Tubercle" means *bump*, as in the greater tubercle of the humerus. Tuberculosis (TB) is a disease involving pus and bacteria-filled *bumps* usually in the lungs, but sometimes in other places too.

Demographics: Who Gets It?

The World Health Organization reports that TB affects one-third of the world's population. Eight million people are infected with it every year and 3 million people die. That is more than the deaths from AIDS, malaria, and all tropical diseases combined.

In the United States TB was considered virtually conquered, because in the 1950s a series of antibiotics was developed that finally managed to kill it. It steadily declined until 1986 when suddenly it began to rise again. Between 1986 and 1993, U.S. TB statistics rose alarmingly. When public health efforts became more focused, rates of new TB infection began to decline. However, about 15 million Americans are infected with the dis-

TUBERCULOSIS

From the Latin *tuber*, a swelling or bump (or potato), plus *-osis*, condition. The word *tubercle*, an anatomical term denoting a bump or protrusion has the same root.

ease, and about 17 thousand have it in the active phase, during which it is highly infectious.

The distribution of TB in the United States is not demographically even. It occurs in highest numbers among the poor, people of color, people with limited access to health care, people in prisons or homeless shelters, and recent immigrants. For more information on TB statistics, see the sidebar.

Etiology: What Happens?

TB is an airborne disease. It is caused by *Mycobacterium tuberculosis*. This is a microorganism with a peculiar waxy coat that gives it many advantages over regular bacteria. This pathogen exists quite happily outside the body. When a person with an active infection coughs or sneezes, bacteria are expelled into the air. The tiny bacteria, protected from drying out by their waxy covering, simply drift around until another host comes along. Ordinary antiseptics and disinfectants will not affect it if it does not land on a surface. The only thing that will dependably kill *M. tuberculosis* is prolonged exposure to direct sunlight.

Progression

TB moves in the body in two phases.

- *Primary phase.* A person inhales some bacteria. (It usually takes prolonged exposure to begin a new infection, as these bacteria grow slowly.) The bacteria travel all the way to the alveoli, where they are engulfed by macrophages. The waxy coating on the pathogens makes them resistant to the macrophage's digestive enzymes. Instead, they take up residence inside the macrophages and slowly build up colonies of bacteria. Unable to expel these invaders, the body instead builds a protective fibrous wall around the site of infection—a tubercle. Tubercles are usually found in the lungs, but if some of the bacteria seep out into the bloodstream or lymph, they will set up the same process elsewhere in the body. Kidneys and bones are the most common other choices.

  A single capsule in the lung is where it all stops for most people. This is TB infection but *not* the active disease. Within a few weeks, T-cells will be activated and a specific immune response will ensue. Antibodies are produced that will react to another contact with the bacillus, as in the "scratch test" that looks for past exposure. The inhaled bacteria remain stuck inside their tidy fibrous package until something happens to set them free, usually a future depression in immune system function.

- *Secondary phase.* Approximately 10% of persons exposed to TB develop the active disease later in life. The bacteria eventually escape and spread into other areas in the lungs or wherever else in the body they may be stationed. The body attempts to surround the new sites with bigger and bigger fibrous capsules, which can cause permanent scarring. Pleurisy, the scarring and sticking of the pleurae, is nearly always a complication of TB. Inside the capsules, the bacteria are destroying cells; the tissue is necrotic, or dead (Fig. 6-3).

  New tubercles eventually take up enough room in the lungs to impede function. A cough begins and gradually produces bloody sputum; this phlegm actually

TUBERCULOSIS IN BRIEF

What is it?
Tuberculosis is a bacterial infection that usually begins in the lungs but may spread to bones, kidney, lymph nodes, or elsewhere in the body. It is a highly contagious airborne disease.

How is it recognized?
Infection with the tuberculosis bacterium may produce no initial symptoms. If the infection turns into the active disease, symptoms may include coughing, bloody sputum, fatigue, weight loss, and night sweats.

Is massage indicated or contraindicated?
Active tuberculosis disease systemically contraindicates massage, unless the client has been consistently taking medication for several weeks and has medical clearance. Massage for clients with tuberculosis infection but no disease is fine, but these people should be under medical supervision as well.

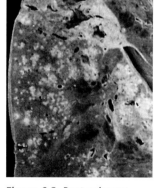

Figure 6-3. Post-primary tuberculosis

contains detached pieces of the bacteria-infested tubercles, which is why TB is so contagious. If several of the tubercles join together, their necrotic centers can cause a cavity in the lung. Surrounding blood vessels may hemorrhage into the cavity, leading to coughing up blood. Similar cavities can develop in the kidneys if the tubercles form there. Infections in the bones tend to destroy articular cartilage.

Risk Factors

The major risk factor for TB infection without active disease is any kind of long-term exposure to someone with active disease. Travelers to parts of the world where TB is most common are at risk, as are people who spend time with immigrants from those same areas. Also at risk are those living or spending a great deal of time in prisons, nursing homes, and homeless shelters.

Once a person has been exposed to TB, the next question is what will increase his or her risk of developing the active infection. Several risk factors for this process have been identified.

Human immunodeficiency virus (HIV) puts people very much at risk for active tuberculosis. In an otherwise healthy person, the bacterium would enter the body and be largely controlled by the immune system. People with TB who are not HIV-positive have a 1 in 10 *lifetime risk* of developing active TB. If a person who is HIV-positive is exposed to TB, his or her chance of developing the disease goes up 7 to 10% *per year* of being infected. TB infection turns into TB disease in 1 of every 2 or 3 people who are HIV-positive. These people can then, in turn, infect others. In fact, TB is the only airborne sickness that AIDS patients can transmit to healthy people *(See* HIV/AIDS, Chapter 5).

Other risk factors for progressing to active TB infection include other conditions in which the immune system is compromised such as poor nutrition, substance abuse, alcoholism, advanced age, and limited access to health care.

Factors that contribute to the prevalence of TB in the United States include the vulnerability of HIV-positive patients, high numbers of immigrants from countries with high rates of TB (42% of the U.S. population with TB are immigrants), increasing levels of poverty, intravenous drug use, homelessness, poor compliance with treatment plans, and growing numbers of elderly people living in long-term care facilities.

Signs and Symptoms

The primary phase of tuberculosis is so benign that persons may never know they have been exposed. The symptoms, if any occur, are the same as for a mild flu. Nevertheless, the active disease shows much more severe symptoms. They include fever, sweating, weight loss, and exhaustion. Chest pain and shortness of breath are common. A stubborn cough that starts dry and becomes productive of bloody or pus-filled phlegm is a cardinal sign. Other symptoms arise if other organs have been infected as well.

Diagnosis

It is not difficult to identify people who have been exposed to the TB bacterium. Within several weeks of infection, enough antibodies to the pathogen will have been produced that a scratch test will create a characteristic welt.

When the disease becomes active, it becomes surprisingly difficult to catch early, because its symptoms mimic pneumonia, lung abscesses, and fungal infections. Radiographs can reveal the tubercles in the lungs, but it is not until bacteria are expelled in bloody sputum that the disease can be reliably identified and the pathogens analyzed for which medications will be most effective.

Treatment

In the past, TB patients were sent to sanitaria where it was hoped that sunlight, rest, and good food would enable them to outlive their infection. That is still a good approach, but it is even better when combined with the right antibiotics. More than 90% of TB patients experience a full recovery if their treatment is completed.

Anyone who has been exposed to TB, regardless of whether the infection is dormant or active, can receive successful antibiotic treatment. The problem is that these antibiotics need to be taken with unfailing consistency. In addition, several different types of antibiotics may be prescribed to circumvent the bacteria's resistance to any single variety. This can mean up to 13 pills a day for many months. Not surprisingly, studies indicate that approximately one-third of all patients do not take their medication as directed.

Multi-drug—resistant TB

When patients do not take all their TB medication properly, the bacterium may mutate into a form that most drugs cannot affect. Whoever is infected with this new strain is likewise difficult to treat. This mutation is called multi-drug–resistant TB, or MDR-TB.

It costs about 10 times more to treat MDR-TB than to treat regular TB. It requires 18 to 24 months of intensive drug therapy that is highly toxic and has many unpleasant side effects. The death rate of MDR-TB that is treated in this way is about the same as the death rate for completely untreated regular TB: 40 to 60%.

MDR-TB has been reported in 43 states and the District of Columbia.

Directly Observed Therapy, Short-Course

In a study done of directly observed therapy, short-course (DOTS)—that is, when social workers directly observed their clients taking every dose of their medication—the rate of acquired drug resistance sank to 2.1%, down from 14%. DOTS is now considered the gold standard for TB treatment. Fortunately, although progress is slow, DOTS is being used more and more frequently. By 1998, 43% of the world had at least nominal access to a DOTS program, and 21% of all TB patients received treatment under this protocol.[c] Thanks to DOTS, some of the countries on the World Health Organization's list of at-risk locations were able to move off the list; several more are on the brink.

Tuberculosis: Worldwide and U.S. Statistics

TB has a long history in medical and cultural tradition. It was called "consumption" and "the white plague" for many years because it literally consumed its victims with fever and bacterial invasion, causing them to become ghostly pale in the process. In the 19th century it was the leading cause of death by infectious disease in the United States. It was such an integral part of the cultural scene that it appeared in opera, literature, theatre, and music, from *La Boheme* to *A Long Day's Journey Into Night*.

For years the only dependable treatment for TB was to retire to a sanatorium, often a luxurious retreat where patients who could afford it would be given excellent food, good rest, and lots of sunshine for several months. If they outlived their disease, they were able to return home. Many sanatoria that began as TB treatment centers are now health and spa resorts.

The causative agent for TB, *M. tuberculosis*, was first isolated and identified in 1882. In the 1950s the development of a series of antibiotics that could successfully eradicate the disease completely changed its place in the medical community. From being a life-threatening scourge, it became all but unknown in the United States.

The confluence of several events has led to a resurgence of TB both in the United States and especially in developing nations, where antibiotic therapy is harder to access. The national and worldwide statistics on TB are cause for concern, but also point out that with the right kinds of intervention, the "white plague" can indeed become a thing of the past.

Worldwide Statistics

- About 2 billion people have been infected with TB. That is a worldwide incidence of approximately 1 in 3.

- Approximately 4.4 million of those infections are among HIV-positive patients, in whom the risk of active infection and contagion is very high.

- More than 8 million new infections occur every year. TB has become the leading cause of death from AIDS around the world, but especially in sub-Saharan Africa and Southeast Asia.

The institution of DOTS treatment protocols limits the spread of both regular and multi-drug–resistant TB. Since this has been implemented in several key countries, some have moved off the World Health Organization's high-risk list; others are very close.

U.S. Statistics

- Approximately 15 million Americans are infected with TB. Recent immigrants comprise 42% of all U.S. TB infections.

- About 17,000 Americans have active TB infections.

- About 100,000 Americans have coexisting HIV and TB infections.

Multi-drug–resistant TB has been reported in 43 states and the District of Columbia.

Between 1984 and 1993, the rates of TB in the United States rose by 16%. They are now consistently going down.[d]

[c]World Health Organization fact sheet no. 104. Tuberculosis. WHO/OMS; 2000. Available at: http://www.who.int/inf-fs/en/fact104.html. Accessed spring 2001.

[d]Tuberculosis summary. WHO/OMS; 2001. Available at: http://www.who.int/gtb/publications/globrep01/summary.html. Accessed spring 2001.

A successful DOTS program depends on several factors, including governmental commitment, reliable detection of infection, a dependable and affordable source of medication, and a good reporting system. Populations that are mobile, like war refugees and homeless people, are difficult to track and treat successfully.

Massage?

TB is an infection that can travel in the blood and lymph. If a client has the active disease, massage can spread it through the body and help to set up tubercles where they would not otherwise have occurred. TB is also contagious. Therapists will not do their clients much good if their own careers are cut short by this condition. However, if a client has been exposed to the bacterium and is taking medication, or if a client has had the active disease but has been taking medication for several weeks, massage may be appropriate, with medical clearance to assure that the risk of contagion has been eliminated.

Obstructive Pulmonary Diseases

Asthma
Definition: What Is It?

Asthma is a chronic inflammatory disorder that may be triggered by external factors like allergens, but is also directly linked to internal factors like emotional stress. The result is bronchospasm, excess mucus production, and the narrowing of airways.

Asthma is considered by some to be part of a classic trio of lung problems called *obstructive pulmonary disease* because, like *chronic bronchitis* and *emphysema* (this chapter), one of its symptoms is resistance to exhalation: it becomes very difficult to move air *out* of the lungs. In some extreme cases it can cause structural changes in the lungs that may also open the door to these other problems. In most cases, however, asthma does not cause irreversible damage to the lungs.

Demographics: Who Gets It?

Asthma affects some 17 million people in the United States, from young infants to elderly people. It accounts for 3 million lost workdays per year, and about $12 billion in direct and indirect costs.

Close to half a million people are hospitalized with asthma attacks per year. Asthma is responsible for about 5000 deaths per year: a statistic that has almost doubled in the past two decades.

Children are more often affected by asthma than adults. Persons who have asthma as a child are very likely to continue to have symptoms well into adulthood.

Etiology: What Happens?

Rising asthma statistics over the past two decades have drawn much attention to the quality of indoor air. As buildings become "tighter" to conserve energy, the amount of air-

---

ASTHMA IN BRIEF

What is it?
Asthma is the result of spasmodic constriction of bronchial smooth muscle tubes in combination with chronic local inflammation and excess mucus production.

How is it recognized?
Asthma attacks are sporadic episodes involving coughing, wheezing, and difficulty with breathing, especially exhaling.

Is massage indicated or contraindicated?
Massage is a good idea for anyone with asthma, as long as he or she is not in the throes of an attack. Between episodes massage can be useful to reduce stress and deal with some of the muscular problems that accompany difficulty with breathing.

borne irritants in them can accumulate to levels that are dangerous to some people. Specific substances like pet-related allergens, cockroach wastes, cigarette smoke, and dust mites have been found to be especially potent asthma triggers.

Other factors evidently contribute to the development of this disorder as well. Protection from exposure to common pathogens in early childhood seems to raise the risk of developing asthma and other respiratory allergies later in life. Statistically, children who are in daycare settings or who have older siblings—in other words, children who are exposed to other children very early in life (before 6 months of age)—have much lower levels of asthma and allergic rhinitis.

All bronchioles are sensitive to foreign debris, but asthmatics' bronchioles are extremely irritable. Furthermore, the bronchiole tubes of a person with asthma appear to be in a state of constant inflammation, always ready to begin an attack when appropriately stimulated. When the right trigger comes along, an asthmatic person's bronchioles first dilate (a sympathetic reaction), and then the body overcompensates by sending the bronchioles into spasm. The irritated membranes lining these tubes swell up and secrete extra mucus (Fig. 6-4). People with asthma find it very difficult to breathe, especially to exhale, during an attack.

Three common types of asthma have been identified, along with a few others that occur more rarely.

- *Extrinsic asthma.* This is a typical example of a type 1 hypersensitivity reaction. In this situation the mast cells that are thickly distributed in the mucous membrane secrete excessive histamine. Histamine causes vasodilation, increases cell permeability, and, in the respiratory system, initiates excess mucus production. What counteracts histamine? Cortisol is the best chemical neutralizer available, but asthmatics, along with many allergy sufferers, seem to be short on this important adrenal hormone.

- *Intrinsic asthma.* This situation is more common in adults than in children. It involves attacks that may have no known origin, or which may be related to exercise, upper respiratory tract infection (see *common cold*, this chapter), or emotional stress.

- *Mixed asthma.* This combination or extrinsic and intrinsic factors is probably the most common situation.

- *Others.* A few other types of asthma exist but are less common They include *occupational asthma*, which is a reaction to work-related substances such as detergents,

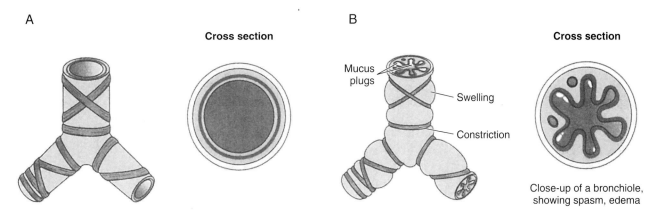

Figure 6-4. (A) Normal bronchiole and **(B)** bronchiole under asthma attack

plastics, resins, and fumes, and *cardiac asthma*, which is related to *congestive heart failure* (Chapter 4) and the resulting excess fluid in the lungs.

Signs and Symptoms

Symptoms of asthma include dyspnea (shortness of breath), wheezing (the sound of air moving through tightened and clogged bronchioles), and coughing that may or may not be productive. It feels especially difficult to *expel* air; the bronchioles are constricted, so the alveoli do not empty easily.

Asthma can show symptoms in several ways. *Bronchial asthma* is a typical episode with tight-bronchioles with excess mucus production and wheezing. *Exercise-induced* asthma occurs with physical exertion. *Silent asthma* shows no symptoms leading up to an episode, and then patients suddenly find themselves dangerously short of breath. *Cough variant asthma* shows coughing alone as its primary symptom.

If symptoms are extreme and prolonged, the asthmatic person may start to feel panicky, adding sweating, increased heart rate, and anxiety to the list of symptoms. In emergency situations the lips and face may take on a bluish cast (cyanosis) when access to oxygen is severely restricted.

Asthma attacks are sporadic, lasting anywhere from a few minutes to a few days. Between attacks the lungs are generally normal. Someone who has had asthma for a long time may develop structural changes in the lungs that raise the risk of other respiratory disorders, particularly *chronic bronchitis* and *emphysema* (this chapter).

ASTHMA
Richard, Age 52

I didn't contract asthma until I was 22, after I got back from Viet Nam. I was living in Los Angeles and I got real bad bronchitis. I was diagnosed then with just a common smog problem.

Then I moved to Corvallis, Oregon, and ran into the Willamette Valley Crud: they have pollination 10 months out of the year there. I saw an allergist who gave me skin tests, and I came up positive to 95% of the things he tested me for. Then I realized it wasn't just the smog; I had a lung problem.

At that time I started taking desensitization shots. I did that for about 5 years, but it didn't really help. I ended up quitting and just medicating myself with aspirin, Sudafed, and over-the-counter inhalants. I didn't have any really bad episodes that I couldn't handle, but I was working in construction, and I knew that I couldn't be sawing or working in a closed room because I would stop breathing; my lungs would just shut down.

Then I moved to Bellingham, Washington, and went into a roofing business. I was working with hot tar, and this stuff called "torch down" that's pretty fume-y. A couple of times I ended up in the emergency room with breathing problems. They gave me a prescription inhalant and prednisone.

When I moved to Seattle, I wound up with a asthma specialist who's been really good for me. I've had a few bouts down here; one time a cold put me in the hospital for about a week. I work in a shipyard now. I can stay away from the worst of the fumes, but about once a year I get a bad attack and go on prednisone until it clears up.

I've been doing massage since the 1960s but just recently went to school and got licensed. I'm really sensitive to perfumes, and massage schools are 90% female, so I'd always choose where to sit, to be away from anyone wearing perfume. But I never thought about massage oils until we got into it. I knew to stay away from oils and lotions that are scented at all. When I got a massage with almond oil I noticed my skin would turn really red, but it wasn't until someone worked on my chest and back that I noticed about an hour later my breathing was affected. Since then I only use unscented lotion, and no almond oil.

Asthma affects my life in all kinds of ways. My lung capacity is only about 65% of normal. I like to go listen to music, but the venues where the good bands play are always too smoky. I have to stay away from stale flower shops. It was almost impossible to go into a mall because you have to walk past the perfume counter to get through the big department stores, but that seems to be less of a problem now. Asthma really limits my social life too. When someone asks us over to dinner, our first question has to be, "Do you have any pets?"

As my massage clientele builds I'm able to cut back at the shipyard. Eventually I'll be able to do massage full time. My focus now is on controlling my environment—keeping out the things I know will trigger an attack and trying to stay as healthy as possible.

Treatment

Treatment for asthma begins with managing the stimuli that are known to trigger attacks. Other interventions include stress management techniques like biofeedback. Some studies have shown that asthma patients trained in biofeedback can learn to control their attacks to the point that they need less medication and have better pulmonary function than other asthmatics.

Medical intervention is available in two forms: anti-inflammatories that can quell the inflammatory nature of the bronchioles, and bronchodilators that relax the smooth muscles of the bronchiole tubes.

Both of these interventions must be used carefully, as frequent use can lead to side effects or can make the body resistant.

Massage?

A person who has asthma can derive great benefit from massage, as long as he or she is not having an attack. No one who is fighting for breath will be comfortable on a massage table. Someone who struggles with this problem will probably have a number of different muscular reflections of it that massage can help. Therapists should watch for hypertonic intercostals, scalenes, serratus posterior inferior, and diaphragm with asthmatic clients. These muscles of inspiration are chronically tight for someone who does not breathe easily, and that tightness further interferes with breathing.

Chronic Bronchitis

Definition: What Is It?

Chronic bronchitis is part of a lung problem called chronic obstructive pulmonary disease (COPD). Chronic bronchitis, as its name implies, involves long-term irritation of the bronchi and bronchioles, which may occur with or without infection. It is a progressive disorder that may be halted or slowed, but not reversed.

Demographics: Who Gets It?

About 8 million people in the United States have chronic bronchitis. Men have it more often than women, and it appears more frequently in Whites than any other racial group.

Smokers are more vulnerable to COPD than non-smokers. About 15% of all smokers develop chronic bronchitis.

COPD, in which chronic bronchitis coexists with emphysema, is the fourth leading cause of death in the United States, killing more than 100,000 people every year.

Etiology: What Happens?

This disorder is the result of long-term irritation to bronchial tubes. When the delicate lining of the respiratory tract is chronically insulted with cigarette smoke (first- or second-hand), air pollutants, industrial chemicals, or other contaminants, an inflammatory response ensues. Attacks against the bronchial lining can lead to the destruction of elastin fibers, overgrowth of mucus-producing cells, excessive pro-

CHRONIC BRONCHITIS IN BRIEF

What is it?
Chronic bronchitis is a long-term inflammation of the bronchi with or without infection, leading to permanent changes in the bronchial lining. Chronic bronchitis frequently occurs as a prelude to or simultaneously with *emphysema* (this chapter). The presence of both chronic bronchitis and emphysema constitutes a diagnosis of chronic obstructive pulmonary disease.

How is it recognized?
Chronic bronchitis is diagnosed when a person experiences a productive cough that occurs most days for 3 months or more, for at least 2 consecutive years. Other common signs are a susceptibility to respiratory tract infections, cyanosis, and pulmonary edema.

Is massage indicated or contraindicated?
Massage can be appropriate for chronic bronchitis patients, as long as they are not fighting acute respiratory infection at the time, and as long as heart function is not compromised.

duction of mucus, and increased resistance to the movement of air in and out of the system. Eventually the damage is permanent; chronic bronchitis is an irreversible progressive disorder.

As resistance to air flow in the bronchi increases, less oxygen enters the body with each breath. The heart has to work harder to push enough blood into the lungs to supply the body with fuel. At the same time, erythrocyte production may increase, in an effort to provide more access to any oxygen that can seep into the capillaries. The blood may become thicker with excess erythrocytes (this is called *polycythemia*), so the heart has to work even *harder* to push it through the pulmonary circuit. Eventually *right-sided heart failure* (Chapter 4) may develop, leading to *edema* (this chapter), especially in the legs and ankles.

Signs and Symptoms

Signs and symptoms of chronic bronchitis develop slowly, often taking months or years before they are severe enough to attract attention. The process usually begins with a mild cough, perhaps following a typical flu or cold. The cough lingers long after the infection has cleared. It is present most days for 3 months or more and produces thick, clear sputum. This pattern occurs for at least 2 consecutive years.

The person with chronic bronchitis may be aware that he or she must clear the throat very often, especially in the morning. This reflects the excessive production of mucus in the lungs. Shortness of breath gets progressively worse, and the patient becomes highly vulnerable to any respiratory infections. Later in the process, the chronic bronchitis patient may develop signs of oxygen deprivation such as cyanosis and eventually edema from right-sided heart failure.

Complications

Complications of this situation are obvious. Bronchi that are chronically inflamed and producing loads of mucus are highly vulnerable to viral or bacterial infection. A person with chronic bronchitis can develop *pneumonia* from *cold* or *flu* viruses (this chapter) much more easily than the general population.

The long-term risk of right-sided heart failure has already been discussed. This serious prognosis is the reason it is important to try to stop the progression of chronic bronchitis as soon as it can be recognized.

Diagnosis

Chronic bronchitis is diagnosed through a variety of methods including patient history, physical examination, and a test of pulmonary function called *spirometry*. In this test the patient exhales into a mouthpiece connected to a device that measures air volume. Additional tests may be conducted to measure levels of oxygen and carbon dioxide in the blood.

Treatment

People with chronic bronchitis are especially susceptible to viral and bacterial infections of the respiratory tract. If a bacterial infection arises, aggressive treatment with antibiotics may be recommended to prevent the situation from developing into life-threatening pneumonia. Chronic bronchitis patients are encouraged to be vaccinated against *pneumococcus* pneumonia and to get yearly flu shots for the same reason.

Other than preventing worse infections from happening, chronic bronchitis treatment focuses on halting the progression of the damage and keeping the patient as comfortable as possible. Quitting smoking, if that is an issue, is the single most important step a chronic bronchitis patient can take. Patients should avoid polluted air and known triggers of bronchial spasm. Bronchodilators in spray or pill form may be prescribed to keep the smooth muscle tissue of the respiratory tract relaxed and open. Oxygen may be supplemented in a medical emergency, but most chronic bronchitis patients do not need to supplement oxygen on a regular basis.

Massage?

If a chronic bronchitis patient has a healthy circulatory system and no current infections, massage, including circulatory massage, should probably be fine. Someone in an advanced stage of the disease may not be able to keep up with the internal changes to blood flow that circulatory modalities produce. These clients require bodywork that does not intend to move a lot of fluid, and they may have some special requirements for positioning to keep them comfortable.

WATCH FOR THIS

Acute Bronchitis, Chronic Bronchitis, or Bronchiectasis: Which is Which?

The lungs are particularly vulnerable to infection, stationed as they are at the receiving end of everything that enters the body through the nose. They have some structural features that make it easy to isolate sites of infection, and they are well stocked with stationery immune system cells to fight off incoming invaders. Nevertheless, they are susceptible to a variety of infectious disorders that can cause both short-term and long-term damage.

Acute bronchitis often accompanies upper respiratory infections or flu. This is a viral attack directly on the bronchi, although it can also complicate into a bacterial infection. Chronic bronchitis involves long-term irritation to the bronchial lining, all the way down to the terminal bronchioles. This irritation can cause the lining to become permanently thick with excessive mucous production that can make it difficult to breathe. Finally, bronchiectasis is a disorder brought about by repeated lung infections that cause structural changes to the bronchial tubes (they become permanently widened). When the bronchi become unable to move mucus out of the body, it pools in the lungs, creating a risk for further infection and more structural damage.

If a lung disorder is present, it is useful for the massage therapist to have a clear idea of the situation, so that the client may be made as comfortable as possible on the table, and so that the risk of spreading infection is minimized.

	ACUTE BRONCHITIS	CHRONIC BRONCHITIS	BRONCHIECTASIS
Cause	Viral attack on lungs; often accompanies cold or flu	Long-term lung irritation (e.g., cigarette smoke, pollution, particles in the air)	Usually a history of multiple lung infections, including acute bronchitis and pneumonia; could also be triggered by a history of pulmonary collapse, aspiration of a foreign body, congenital weakness of the bronchial walls, or other factors

	ACUTE BRONCHITIS	CHRONIC BRONCHITIS	BRONCHIECTASIS—continued
Symptoms	A productive cough with clear sputum (if the sputum is colored, suspect a secondary bacterial infection) along with fever, aches, and pains	A productive cough with clear sputum (if the sputum is colored, suspect a secondary bacterial infection). Excessive mucus production, requiring lots of throat clearing Susceptibility to lung infections Wheezing, shortness of breath, cyanosis	A frequent cough with a large amount of green or yellow sputum, especially when lying down; sputum may also be bloody (hemoptysis) Chronic hypoxia occasionally leads to "clubbed" fingers (fingers become thick and wide, with shiny, curved nails)
Prognosis	If the patient is basically healthy, full recovery with no long-term problems	If the irritation to the lungs is halted, the problem may not progress, but it is not reversible If it does progress, it may develop into right-sided heart failure, respiratory failure, or emphysema	Patient must avoid lung irritants and the possibility of further lung infections, which may cause further damage to the bronchi Damage caused by bronchiectasis is usually not reversible
Implications for massage	This client should not receive massage until the infection has been resolved	This client may receive massage, as long as he or she can be positioned on the table in a way that does not exacerbate symptoms Care must be taken to rule out the possibility of circulatory stress	This client may receive massage, as long as he or she can be positioned on the table in a way that does not exacerbate symptoms Circulatory problems are not generally associated with bronchiectasis

EMPHYSEMA IN BRIEF

What is it?
Emphysema is a condition in which the alveoli of the lungs become stretched and inelastic. They merge with each other, decreasing surface area, destroying surrounding capillaries, and limiting oxygen-carbon dioxide exchange.

How is it recognized?
Symptoms of emphysema include shortness of breath with mild or no exertion, a chronic dry cough, rales, and susceptibility to secondary respiratory infection. Late stage emphysema patients will show cyanosis and pronounced weight loss as well.

Is massage indicated or contraindicated?
Emphysema indicates massage with caution for circulatory complications, secondary infection, and positioning the client for maximum comfort.

Emphysema
Definition: What Is It?

Emphysema, along with chronic bronchitis, is a contributor to COPD. The name emphysema means "blown up" (as in inflated, not exploded), and this is a very apt description of the disease process.

Demographics: Who Gets It?

It is estimated that 32 million Americans have some form of COPD. About 2 million people have emphysema. Most emphysema patients are between 65 and 75 years of age. More than 80% of emphysema cases can be traced to cigarette smoking. Others may be due to occupational hazards: working with grain dust, in coal mines, or quarries can increase risk. A small percentage of emphysema patients have a genetic lack of the alpha-1 antitrypsin protein that protects alveolar walls. These people generally develop the disease before they are 50 years old.

Etiology: What Happens?

When the delicate epithelium that lines the respiratory tract is constantly irritated (cigarette smoke and air pollution are the two biggest culprits) the cilia, which are supposed to trap pathogens and particles, eventually disintegrate. Then the bronchioles produce excess mucus in an effort to fight off environmental irritations: this is chronic bronchitis, and it involves damage proximal to the terminal bronchioles. When the damage spreads further, or when it originates distally to the terminal bronchioles, the delicate alveoli are vulnerable.

The 300 million alveoli in the lungs provide sites for oxygen–carbon dioxide exchange. Each one has a circulatory capillary to allow the exchange of oxygen and carbon dioxide. All alveoli need a specific substance called alpha-1 antitrypsin (AAT). This is a protein that protects the delicate tissue from damage by environmental forces. Long-term exposure to cigarette smoke or other pollutants can overcome the protective abilities of AAT, resulting in the destruction of the alveolar elastin fibers. The alveoli become less elastic and they fill up with mucus, which interferes with their ability to exchange oxygen and carbon dioxide. Instead of emptying and filling with every breath, they only partially empty or stay altogether full. This usually begins in a small area, but if the irritation continues it will spread throughout the lung. The alveolar walls eventually break down and merge with each other, forming larger sacs, called *bullae*. These sacs have less volume and less surface area for gaseous exchange than the uninjured alveoli did (Fig. 6-5).

As the alveoli fuse and surface area for gaseous exchange is lost, the emphysema patient has to work much harder to move air in and out of the lungs. A person with healthy lungs expends about 5% of his or her energy in the effort of breathing. A person with advanced emphysema puts closer to 50% into this job, every minute, 24 hours a day.

Less gaseous exchange means reduced oxygen levels in the blood, or *hypoxia*. This situation is toxic to brain cells. It also causes the epithelial walls of the alveoli to thicken into tough fibrous connective tissue, which allows even less diffusion. As breathing becomes more difficult (the emphysema patient must *consciously* exhale—it no longer happens spontaneously), the respiration rate slows. This leads to even higher concentrations of carbon dioxide in the blood. The blood vessels supplying the damaged alveoli also sustain dam-

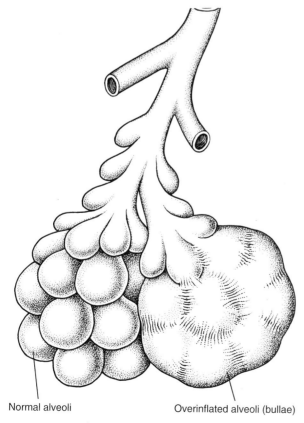

Normal alveoli   Overinflated alveoli (bullae)

Figure 6-5. COPD/emphysema

age; it becomes harder to pump blood through the pulmonary artery. Hypoxia also leads to spasm of pulmonary blood vessels. All these factors may contribute to pulmonary hypertension and *right-sided heart failure*, or cor pulmonale (Chapter 4). Eventually the untreated emphysema patient will experience respiratory and circulatory collapse.

Signs and Symptoms

It can take many years for emphysema to advance to a stage when a person seeks medical help. Because it usually affects people older than 65 years of age, early symptoms are often assumed to be normal signs of aging. Symptoms of emphysema include pain with breathing, shortness of breath, dry cough, and wheezing. Weight loss often occurs as a person who must exert so much energy in breathing has little interest in eating. Rales, a characteristic bubbling, rasping sound of air moving through a narrowed passage, may occur with some cases. Difficulty in exhaling is also shown in spirometry, a test that measures expiration volume. Exhalation takes longer, and the patient may develop a habit of pushing air out through pursed lips. This is an attempt to push against increasing back pressure in the lungs. Because the lungs no longer deflate normally with each breath, the diaphragm becomes permanently flattened. The emphysema patient often develops "barrel chest;" that is, the intercostals lock into a position that holds the rib cage out as wide as possible.

Complications

Emphysema patients are extremely vulnerable to *influenza* and *pneumonia* (this chapter) because they have lost much of the ability to resist secondary infection. Another complication occurs if the bullae should rupture. This allows air into the pleural space (which is supposed to be a vacuum) and ends in total lung collapse or *atelectasis*. If the lungs sustain this kind of damage, the stress on the circulatory system is very great. The right ventricle, trying to pump blood through the partially collapsed pulmonary circuit, enlarges and heart failure may eventually develop. The risk of blood clots forming somewhere in the circuit is also high, which may result in *pulmonary embolism* (Chapter 4).

Treatment

Emphysema is an irreversible disease. If it is found and treated early, further damage can be avoided. Once the alveoli have begun to break down, however, they cannot be rebuilt. The first course of action, of course, is to remove the irritating stimulus, which is usually cigarette smoke. Drugs may be administered to dilate the bronchi and take pressure off the alveoli, to remove mucus and edema from the lungs, and to ward off potential lung infections. Oxygen supplementation may be recommended during sleep or following exercise. Surgery called "lung volume reduction surgery or "lung shaving" removes only damaged portions of the lung. This increases thoracic capacity for the diaphragm to work and improves circulation. Statistics on how it affects longevity, however, are not yet available. In rare cases a heart and lung transplant may be necessary.

Patients with emphysema and/or other obstructive disorders are often strongly urged to be vaccinated against *pneumococcus* pneumonia and to get a yearly flu shot, since they are at higher risk for serious lung infections than the general population.

Massage?

If a client is in the early stages of this disease, if the tissues are healthy and responsive (i.e., the skin shows signs of normal blood flow by appropriate temperature and color

EMPHYSEMA
Roberta, Age 68

Roberta is 5'2" and weighs 100 lb. She started smoking in 1947 and quit in 1984. She first experienced pulmonary symptoms in the mid-1980s. She noticed that she was frequently short of breath, she had low energy, and she had consistent headaches on rising each morning. She was unable to walk far or fast. In an effort to catch her breath she hyperventilated easily, which only made matters worse. She experienced a lot of stress and frustration that breathing was so difficult, and that she could no longer accomplish the things she wanted to do.

Roberta's original doctor diagnosed her with COPD and chronic bronchitis. She then saw a pulmonary specialist who diagnosed her with emphysema. This finding was based on a number of tests, including a chest radiograph, spirometry (a measurement of respiratory gases), an analysis of arterial blood gases, and a measurement of the air volume she was able to expel.

Emphysema makes it hard for Roberta to do anything. The activities of daily living are difficult, and all daily routines have to be altered to accommodate the disease. Stairs and hills are especially difficult. Emphysema dulls the thinking by depriving the brain of oxygen. It reduces the appetite, and the lack of oxygen reduces the benefit from what food is eaten. It also strains the heart, because it has to work harder to push more blood, which contains less oxygen, through the body.

When Roberta was x-rayed for emphysema it was found that she also has some degree of osteoporosis. This condition, in combination with her breathing difficulties, has significantly altered her posture. Her shoulders rise to her ears in an attempt to get more air. Also the shoulders tend to roll forward. Because of the increased tension Roberta experienced while trying to breathe, some muscle stiffness and pain was occasionally a problem.

Another aspect of Roberta's experience with emphysema is how it has seriously affected her resistance to disease. Some medicines Roberta takes to help her breathe weaken her immune system, so it is harder for her to ward off respiratory ailments. In March 1997 she had a crisis that hospitalized her for 10 days. At that time she began supplementing oxygen by nose. She was in a rehabilitation facility for 2 weeks, working with physical and occupational therapists who taught her ways to accomplish more with less energy.

In June 1997 she had a bad cold, which put her in the hospital for 4 days.

In January 1998 Roberta contracted pneumonia, which was confirmed by chest radiography. She was in the hospital for 5 days. The pneumonia was cured by antibiotics, and she returned home.

Roberta is now feeling improved. She still supplements oxygen, and her daily activities have become a little easier. She tries to keep up with her exercises, eat properly, and reduce stress. She also attends Better Breathing Club meetings sponsored by the American Lung Association to keep up with new information about techniques to deal with her disease, and she sees her pulmonary specialist regularly.

changes with massage), and if the client has no heart problems or secondary infection, massage may be very beneficial. Back, neck, and chest massage may be especially helpful to help reduce any muscular resistance to the movement of air in and out of the body.

Advanced cases in which a client is experiencing difficulty with breathing and shortness of breath may not be appropriate for rapid, vigorous Swedish strokes, but calming reflexive work may be excellent for dealing with anxiety and the stress of quitting smoking, as well as the inevitable fatigue these people experience. Massage can also address the muscular contribution to barrel chest. Emphysema and other COPD patients often cannot tolerate lying completely prone or supine; they may be more comfortable receiving work in a reclining chair or on a massage chair.

Other Respiratory Disorders

Lung Cancer
Definition: What Is It?

Lung cancer is the growth of malignant cells in the lungs. These cells eventually form tumors. Because they have extremely easy access to both the circulatory and lymph systems, they are capable of spreading before tumors are detectable.

LUNG CANCER IN BRIEF

What is it?

Lung cancer is the development of malignant cells in the lungs. These cells have easy access to blood and lymph vessels, and quickly spread to other organs in the body.

How is it recognized?

The early symptoms of lung cancer are virtually indistinguishable from normal irritation from cigarette smoke: a chronic cough, blood-stained sputum, and recurrent bronchitis or pneumonia.

Is massage indicated or contraindicated?

Sadly, most people diagnosed with lung cancer do not survive. Massage has a place in cancer recovery care and in terminal care, but these situations call for specific precautions to achieve maximum benefit with minimal risk.

Lung cancer is an example of epithelial cancer that tends to grow where tissue is vulnerable to repeated irritation and damage.

Demographics: Who Gets It?

Statistics in the United States vary, but it is estimated that about 175,000 new cases of lung cancer are diagnosed, and about 160,000 people die of this disease each year. Whereas it was once considered a "men's disease," the social acceptability of women smoking has led to rising numbers of women being diagnosed with lung cancer; the statistics for men are beginning to decline. The average lung cancer patient is a man or a woman in the sixth to seventh decade of life, who has smoked for 20 years or more.

Cancer in general is the second leading cause of death in the United States, and lung cancer accounts for nearly 30% of all cancer deaths. Some statistics show that it is the cause of more deaths than breast, colon, and prostate cancers (the next three runners-up) combined.

Etiology: What Happens?

Lung cancer occurs in epithelial cells that are chronically irritated by environmental contaminants. Although cigarette, pipe, and cigar smoke are responsible for 85 to 90% of all cases of lung cancer, other causes have also been identified. Exposure to radon, a naturally occurring radioactive gas that is released when rocks and soil are moved for construction, is the second leading cause of lung cancer; it is especially dangerous in combination with smoking or in very high concentration. Exposure to asbestos, uranium, arsenic, and other carcinogens follow radon exposure as leading causes of lung cancer.

When the epithelial cells that line the respiratory tract have a long history of exposure to these highly toxic substances, their orderly pattern of replication and repair is finally disrupted. Abnormal cells begin to accumulate in uncontrolled and disorganized patches. A rich supply of blood and lymph vessels allows mutated cells to travel out of their immediate area before a detectable tumor appears; this is why lung cancer is seldom caught before metastasis.

The lymph nodes in the mediastinum are often the first site of metastasis for lung cancer. From there the cells have access to distant places in the body. The liver, bone tissue, skin, adrenal glands, and brain are frequently invaded.

Types of Lung Cancer

Different types of lung cancer tend to grow at different rates and in different parts of the lung. Several types of lung cancer have been identified and are broken down into two basic groups: small cell carcinoma and non-small cell carcinoma.

- *Small cell carcinoma.* This is also called oat cell carcinoma. It is responsible for about 25% of all lung cancers. Small cell lung cancer grows fast, spreads quickly, and is rarely operable. The 5-year survival rate for small cell carcinoma is less than 1%.

- *Non-small cell carcinoma.* This includes several different types of cancers, depending on which cells they affect first. Non-small cell carcinomas account for

75% of all lung cancers (Fig. 6-6). They include squamous cell carcinoma, adenocarcinoma, large cell carcinoma, and several others. Most of these grow more slowly than small cell carcinoma, but the symptoms they create are so subtle that diagnosis does not usually happen until long after the cancer has spread beyond its original area. The 5-year survival rate for non-small cell carcinoma is less than 30%.

Risk Factors

The most obvious risk factor for lung cancer is smoking. Cigarette smoke contains more than 40 known carcinogens, and the tar in cigarettes holds the damaging chemicals close to the delicate linings of the lungs. Light smokers are about 10 times more likely to get this disease than non-smokers; heavy smokers are 25 times more susceptible. Almost 90% of all lung cancer patients are smokers or people exposed to second-hand or side-stream smoke. (Side-stream smoke is the smoke coming directly from lit cigarettes; not from the smokers.) An estimated 3000 Americans die every year of lung cancer due to second-hand smoke; that is more deaths than from all other air pollutants combined.

Lung cancer is also an occupational risk for people working with asbestos insulation, coal miners, and people who work with other toxic chemicals. Exposure to radon, excessive radiation, or a history of TB or other lung infections can also increase risk.

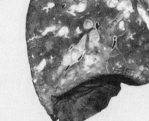

Figure 6-6. Lung cancer (bronchiolar carcinoma)

Signs and Symptoms

One of the biggest problems with lung cancer is that it is extremely difficult to identify early. The growth of abnormal cells in bronchial linings or mucous membranes stimulates virtually no changes in function or sensation. A persistent "smoker's cough" is one early sign, along with blood-stained phlegm, chest pain, and possibly shortness of breath. None of these symptoms is particular cause for alarm, since a smoker or someone who works with irritating chemicals probably has them regardless of the health of their respiratory cells.

Later signs of lung cancer may be more revealing. If a tumor is growing near the apex of the lung it may put mechanical pressure on the brachial plexus, leading to symptoms that look like *thoracic outlet syndrome* (Chapter 2). A tumor that presses on the superior vena cava may cause facial swelling and dilated blood vessels in the neck and face when the vena cava cannot drain easily; this is called *superior vena cava syndrome*. If a tumor protrudes on the esophagus or larynx, a person may experience chronic hoarseness.

Diagnosis

Once a tumor has formed in the lung it is not hard to find; any imaging technique, from radiography to computed tomography to magnetic resonance imaging, can locate growths. An analysis of sputum might reveal abnormal cells, but then again it might not. Radiographic studies of bronchiole tubes can show where obstructions are growing, and needle biopsies of suspicious areas can help to pinpoint a diagnosis. The problem is that this type of cancer often metastasizes *before* detectable tumors have grown. This makes it difficult to identify the condition in time to stop it. In fact, only 20% of all detected lung cancers are caught before they have spread elsewhere in the body. About 25% of all diagnoses occur then the cancer is still in the thorax but may be in both lungs. More than 55% of all patients have tumors growing in distant areas at the time of diagnosis.

Treatment

Lung cancer treatment depends on what kind of cancer is growing and how far it has progressed. For the lucky few that find their cancer while it is still localized, surgery followed by radiation may be adequate. The surgery could involve the removal of a small section of lung tissue (wedge resection), the removal of an entire lobe (lobectomy), or even the removal of an entire lung (pneumonectomy). These are options for non-small cell carcinoma.

Small cell carcinoma grows so fast and spreads so quickly that it is generally treated with radiation and chemotherapy alone. Surgery usually has no chance of containing the extent of the growth.

New therapies for lung cancer are still in the experimental stage, but some are showing promise. They include injecting specially sensitized antibodies that attack cancerous tissue, artificially stimulating interferon and interleukin-2 (naturally occurring cancer-fighting chemicals), and providing photodynamic therapy (a process in which a laser-sensitive chemical is injected into the cancerous area, absorbed into abnormal cells, and then activated by a laser, which causes the chemicals to destroy the cancerous cells).

Even when all the identified abnormal cells are caught and removed or destroyed, the chance of lung cancer recurrence is high. Many lung cancer patients are deficient in vitamin A. Supplementing this nutrient has been seen to reduce the chance for recurrent cancer. Nonetheless, despite many advances in cancer identification and treatment, the prognosis for most lung cancer patients remains very poor.

Massage?

Massage can be a useful stress reliever for a person undergoing cancer treatment because it stimulates immune system activity, reduces pain and fatigue, and generally adds to the quality of life. Fears about the possibility of spreading cancer cells through the circulatory or lymph systems can be allayed by using non-circulatory techniques. Of course, certain cautions must be observed when working with people who are receiving radiation or chemotherapy or who have had recent surgery. For more details, see *cancer* in Chapter 11.

If a client's condition is terminal, massage still has a useful place in comfort care protocols. Even when a person is too fragile to receive most types of bodywork, energy work, gentle stroking of hands and feet, or simple laying on of hands can all contribute to feelings of peace and well-being. In these situations the massage therapist may want to teach the patient's family members and loved ones some simple techniques that may enrich their time together.

Chapter Review Questions: Respiratory System Conditions

1. What is the purpose of mucous membranes? Where are they found?

2. How does the structure of the lungs work to limit the spread of infection?

3. Explain the sympathetic/parasympathetic swing that occurs with asthma.

4. What is the best defense against catching or spreading the cold virus?

5. What is the danger associated with taking antibiotics "just in case?"

6. What are the repercussions of having alveoli fuse together, as happens with emphysema?

7. Why is the prognosis for lung cancer generally so poor?

8. What feature of the tuberculosis bacterium distinguishes it from most other pathogens?

9. What happens when prescriptions of antibiotics for tuberculosis (or other bacterial infections) are not completed as directed? Why is this a particular danger in tuberculosis?

10. A client has sinusitis. Her mucus is thick, opaque, and sticky. She has had a headache and a mild fever for several days. Is she a good candidate for massage? Why or why not?

Bibliography, Respiratory System Conditions

General References, Respiratory System

1. de Dominico G, Wood E. *Beard's Massage.* Philadelphia, Pa: WB Saunders; 1997.
2. Damjanou I. *Pathology for the Health-Related Professions.* Philadelphia, Pa: WB Saunders; 1996.
3. Travell J, Simons DG. *Myofascial Pain and Dysfunction: The Trigger Point Manual.* Baltimore, Md: Williams & Wilkins; 1983.
4. Clemente CD. *Anatomy: A Regional Atlas of the Human Body.* 3rd ed. Baltimore, Md: Urban & Schwarzenburg; 1987.
5. Tortora GJ, Anagnostakos NP. *Principles of Anatomy and Physiology.* 6th ed. New York, NY: Harper & Row; 1990.
6. *Taber's Cyclopedic Dictionary.* 14th ed. Philadelphia, Pa: FA Davis; 1981.
7. *Stedman's Medical Dictionary.* 26th ed. Baltimore, Md: Williams & Wilkins; 1995.
8. Memmler RL, Wood DL. *The Human Body in Health and Disease.* 5th ed. Philadelphia, Pa: JB Lippincott; 1983.
9. Juhan D. *Job's Body: A Handbook for Bodywork.* Barrytown, NY: Station Hill Press; 1987.
10. Mulvihill ML. *Human Diseases: A Systemic Approach.* 2nd ed. Norwalk, CT: Appleton & Lange; 1987.
11. Kunz JRM, Finkel AJ, eds. *The American Medical Association Family Medical Guide.* New York, NY: Random House; 1987.
12. Marieb EM. *Human Anatomy and Physiology.* Redwood City, Calif: Benjamin/Cummings; 1989.
13. Sapolsky RM. *Why Zebras Don't Get Ulcers: An Updated Guide to Stress, Stress-Related Disease, and Coping.* New York: NY: W.H. Freeman; 1998.

Infectious Respiratory Conditions

Acute Bronchitis

1. Acute bronchitis. American Academy of Family Physicians; 2001. Available at: http://www.familydoctor.org/handouts/677.html. Accessed fall 2001.
2. Bronchitis. Board of Trustees of the University of Illinois; 2001. Available at: http://www.mckinley.uiuc.edu/health-info/dis-cond/cold/bronchit.html. Accessed fall 2001.
3. Qarah S. Bronchitis. eMedicine.com, Inc.; 2001 Available at: http://www.emedicine.com/med/topic247.htm. Accessed fall 2001.
4. Leiner S. Acute bronchitis in adults: Commonly diagnosed, but poorly defined. *Nurse Pract.* 1997. Available at: http://www.springnet.com/ce/j701a.htm. Accessed fall 2001.

Common Cold

1. Common cold statistics. Available at: http://www.cdc.gov/nchs/fastats/colds.htm. Accessed spring 2001.
2. Guidelines for the prevention and treatment of influenza and the common cold. American Lung Association; 2001. Available at: http://www.lungusa.org/diseases/c&fguide/lungcolds_flu.html. Accessed spring 2001.
3. The common cold fact sheet. National Institute of Allergy and Infectious Diseases, National Institutes of Health. Available at: http://www.niaid.nih.gov/factsheets/cold.htm. Accessed spring 2001.
4. Packer-Tursman J. The common cold. *Special to the Washington Post.* November 14, 2000:Z31. Available at: http://www.washingtonpost.com/wp-dyn/articles/A15070-2000Nov14.html. Accessed spring 2001.
5. Understanding colds. Commoncold, Inc.; 1999. Available at: http://www.commoncold.org/sitemap.htm. Accessed spring 2001.

Influenza

1. Is it a cold or the flu? National Institute of Allergy and Infectious Diseases. Available at: http://www.niaid.nih.gov/publications/cold/sick.htm. Accessed spring 2001.
2. Laver WG, Bischofberger N, Webster RG. Disarming flu viruses. *Sci Am.* 1999. Available at: http://www.sciam.com/1999/0199issue/0199laver.html. Accessed spring 2001.

3. Influenza activity—United States, 2000-01 season. Centers for Disease Control; January 26, 2001;50(03):39–40 Available at: http://www.cdc. gov/mmwr//preview/ mmwrhtml/mm5003a2.htm. Accessed spring 2001.

4. Flu-fighting drugs: A way to bounce back quicker. Mayo Foundation for Medical Education and Research; 1995–2000. Available at: http://www.mayohealth.org/mayo/ 9910/htm/ fludrug.htm. Accessed spring 2001.

5. Flu. National Institute of Allergy and Infectious Diseases, National Institutes of Health. Available at: http://www.niaid.nih. gov/factsheets/ flu.htm. Accessed spring 2001.

6. Influenza. Centers for Disease Control. Available at: http://www.cdc.gov/ncidod/ diseases/ hip/pneumonia/1_flu.htm. Accessed spring 2001.

7. Health information: Fight flu and pneumonia. Medicare: The Official U.S. Government Site for Medicare Information. Available at: http://www.medicare.gov/ Health/FluDetails.asp. Accessed spring 2001.

8. Influenza A (H5N1). World Health Organization fact sheet no. 188. WHO/OMS; 1998. Available at: http://www.who.int/ inf-fs/en/ fact188.html. Accessed spring 2001.

Pneumonia

1. Cantu S Jr. Pneumonia, mycoplasma from emergency medicine/pulmonary. eMedicine.com, Inc.; 2001. Available at: http://www.emedicine.com/emerg/topic467 .htm. Accessed spring 2001.

2. Stephen J. Pneumonia, bacterial from emergency medicine/pulmonary. eMedicine.com, Inc.; 2001. Available at: http://www.emedicine. com/EMERG/ topic465.htm. Accessed spring 2001.

3. Pneumonia. National Jewish Medical and Research Center. Available at: http://www. nationaljewish.org/medfacts/pneumonia.ht ml. Accessed spring 2002.

4. Fastats A to Z: Pneumonia. Centers for Disease Control. Available at: http://www. cdc.gov/nchs/fastats/neumonia.htm. Accessed spring 2001.

5. Pneumococcal vaccines: The road to prevention. National Institute for Allergies and Infectious Disease. Available at: http://www.niaid. nih.gov/newsroom/ pneumovaccine.htm. Accessed spring 2001.

Sinusitis

1. Brown E. Treatment updates–A clinical series for physicians. Asthma and sinusitis. *JAMA*. 1997. Available at: http://www.ama-assn.org/ special/asthma/treatmnt/ updates/sinus.htm. Accessed spring 2001.

2. Sinusitis fact sheet. National Institute of Allergy and Infectious Diseases, National Institutes of Health. Available at:

http://www. niaid. nih.gov/factsheets/ sinusitis.htm. Accessed spring 2002.

3. Phalen KF. Treatment of choice. *Special to the Washington Post*. May 23, 2000:Z31. Available at: http://www.washingtonpost. com/wp-dyn/articles/A53771-2000May23. html. Accessed spring 2001.

4. Sinusitis. WellnessWeb; 1995–2001. Available at: http://www.wellnessweb.com/ masterindex/ sinus/about_sinusitis.htm. Accessed spring 2001.

5. Sinusitis. MedicineNet, Inc.; 1996–2001. Available at: http://www.Medicinenet.com. Accessed spring 2001.

6. Tichenor WS. What is sinusitis? WS Tichenor; 1996–2000. Available at: http://www.sinuses. com/. Accessed spring 2001.

Tuberculosis

1. Questions and answers about TB 1994. National Center for HIV, STD and TB Prevention, Division of Tuberculosis Elimination. Available at: http://www.cdc.gov/ nchstp/tb/ faqs/qa.htm. Accessed spring 2001.

2. DOTS: Directly observed treatment short-course. WHO/OMS; 2000. Available at: http://www.who.int/gtb/dots/index.htm. Accessed spring 2001.

3. Ginsberg AM, Sizemore CF, Fauci A. Fighting the white plague. National Institutes of Health press release. National Institute of Allergy and Infectious Diseases. Available at: http://www.nih.gov/news/pr/ mar2001/niaid-24.htm. Accessed spring 2001.

4. World Health Organization fact sheet no. 104. Tuberculosis. WHO/OMS; 2000. Available at: http://www.who.int/inf-fs/ en/fact104.html. Accessed spring 2001.

5. The return of tuberculosis. InteliHealth Inc.; 1996–2001. Available at: http://www. intelihealth.com/IH/ihtIH/WSIHW000/33 1/24290/198334.html?d=dmtContent. Accessed spring 2001.

6. Researchers find key to tuberculosis persistence in the body. Rockefeller University. Available at: http://www.rockefeller.edu/ pubinfo/mckinney081700.nr.html. Accessed spring 2001.

7. Tuberculosis. Fact sheet, National Institute of Allergy and Infectious Diseases, National Institutes of Health. Available at: http://www.niaid. nih.gov/factsheets/ tb.htm. Accessed spring 2001.

8. Tuberculosis summary. WHO/OMS; 2001. Available at: http://www.who.int/gtb/ publications/globrep01/summary.html. Accessed spring 2001.

9. Evaluation of a directly observed therapy short-course strategy for treating tuberculosis—Orel Oblast, Russian federation, 1999—2000. March 23, 2001;50(11): 204–206. Centers for Disease Control & Prevention, National Center for HIV, STD, and TB Prevention. Available at: http://www.cdc.gov/mmwr/preview/

mmwrhtml/mm5011a3.htm. Accessed spring 2001.

Obstructive Pulmonary Diseases

Asthma

1. America Lung Association fact sheet: Asthma in adults. American Lung Association; 2001. Available at: http://www. lungusa.org/ asthma/aduasthmfac99.html. Accessed spring 2001.

2. Packer-Tursman J. Treatment of choice. *Special to the Washington Post*. October 31, 2000:Z19. Available at: http://www. washingtonpost.com/ wp-dyn/articles/ A45856-2000Oct31.html. Accessed spring 2001.

3. Fast facts: Statistics on asthma and allergic diseases. America Academy of Allergy, Asthma and Immunology; 1996–2001. Available at: http:// www.aaaai.org/public/ fastfacts/statistics.stm. Accessed spring 2001.

4. Tichenor WS. Asthma. WS Tichenor; 1998. Available at: http://www.sinuses. com/. Accessed spring 2001.

5. Minerd J. Don't get rid of that cat yet, say asthma researchers. National Institute of Allergy and Infectious Diseases. Available at: http://www.niaid.nih.gov/newsroom/ cats.htm. Accessed spring 2001.

6. Fast facts: Myth vs. reality. American Academy of Allergy, Asthma and Immunology; 1996–2001. Available at: http://www.aaaai. org/ public/fastfacts/mythvsreality.stm. Accessed spring 2001.

7. Asthma self-management. Mayo Foundation for Medical Education and Research; 1995–2000. Available at: http://www. mayohealth.org/mayo/9602/htm/asthma5. htm. Accessed spring 2001.

8. Okie S. Day care may boost immunity to asthma. *Washington Post*. August 24, 2000:A01.

9. Facts about asthma. Centers for Disease Control and Prevention, Office of Communication. Available at: http://www.cdc. gov/od/oc/ media/fact/asthma.htm. Accessed spring 2001.

Chronic Bronchitis (see also, Emphysema)

1. Louie S. Acute bronchitis & acute COPD exacerbation. UC Regents; 1999. Available at: http://medocs.ucdavis.edu/imd/ 420c/syllabus/acutbron.htm. Accessed spring 2001.

2. Bronchitis. Mayo Foundation for Medical Education and Research; 2001. Available at: http://www.mayohealth.org/home?id= DS00031. Accessed spring 2001.

3. Bronchitis. WellnessWeb; 1995–2001. Available at: http://www.wellnessweb. com/masterindex/ breathing/about_bronchitis.htm. Accessed spring 2001.

4. Chronic bronchitis. American Lung Association; 2001. Available at: http://www.

lungusa. org/diseases/lungchronic.html. Accessed spring 2001.

5. Ong S. Acute bronchitis. eMedicine.com, Inc.; 2001. Available at:http://www. emedicine.com/ emerg/topic69.htm. Accessed spring 2001.

Emphysema

1. Around the clock with COPD (chronic obstructive pulmonary disease). American Lung Association; 2001. Available at: http://www.lungusa.org/diseases/copd_clock html. Accessed spring 2001.

2. Chronic obstructive pulmonary disease (COPD): Emphysema and chronic bronchitis. American Lung Association; 2001. Available at: http://www.lungusa.org/pub/minority/copd_00.html. Accessed spring 2001.

3. American Lung Association fact sheet: Chronic obstructive pulmonary disease (COPD). American Lung Association; 2001. Available at: http://www.lungusa.org/diseases/copd_factsheet.html. Accessed spring 2001.

4. Chronic obstructive pulmonary disease. InteliHealth Inc.; 1996–2001. Available at: http://www.intelihealth.com/IH/ihtIH?t=10598&p=~br,IHW|~st,24479|~r, WSIHW000|~b,*|. Accessed spring 2001.

5. Emphysema. InteliHealth Inc.; 1996–2001. Available at: http://www.intelihealth.com/IH/ihtIH?d=dmtContent&c=266753&p=~br,IHW|~st,24479|~r,WSIH W000|~b,*|. Accessed spring 2001.

6. Kleinschmidt P. Chronic obstructive pulmonary disease (COPD). eMedicine.com, Inc.; 2001. Available at: http://www.emedicine.com/ emerg/topic99.htm. Accessed spring 2001.

Other Respiratory Disorders

Lung Cancer

1. Louie S, Lillington G. Bronchogenic carcinoma. UC Regents; 1999. Available at: http://medocs.ucdavis.edu/imd/420c/syllabus/lungCa.htm. Accessed spring 2001.

2. Facts about lung cancer. American Lung Association; 2001. Available at: http://www.lungusa.org/diseases/lungcanc.html. Accessed spring 2001.

3. Lung cancer. A fact sheet of the American Association for Cancer Research. Available at: http://www.aacr.org/5000/5100/5100.html. Accessed spring 2001.

4. Lung cancer. Mayo Foundation for Medical Education and Research; 1998–2000. Available at: http://www.mayohealth.org/home?id= 5.1.1.12.2. Accessed spring 2001.

5. Non-small cell lung cancer (PDQ). National Cancer Institute, National Institutes of Health. Available at: http://cancernet.nci.nih.gov/cgi-bin/srchcgi.exe?DBID=pdq&TYPE= search&SFMT=pdq_statement/1/0/0&Z208=208_00039P. Accessed spring 2001.

6. What you need to know about. . . lung cancer. National Cancer Institute, National Institutes of Health. Available at: http://www.cancer.gov/cancer_information/doc_wyntk.aspx?viewid=4b129348-f3ec4c30-9c65-b342255667eb1. Accessed spring 2001.

7. Prevention of lung cancer (PDQ). National Cancer Institute, National Institutes of Health. Available at: http://cancernet.nci.nih.gov/cgi-bin/srchcgi.exe?DBID=pdq&TYPE= search&SFMT=pdq_statement/1/0/0&Z208=208_04735P. Accessed spring 2001.

8. Small cell lung cancer. National Cancer Institute, National Institutes of Health. Available at: http://cancernet.nci.nih.gov/cgi-bin/srchcgi. exe?DBID=pdq&TYPE= search&SFMT=pdq_statement/1/0/0&Z208=208_00040P. Accessed spring 2001.

9. Small cell lung cancer, an overview. American Heart and Lung Institute, 1996. Available at: http://www.best.com/~gek/smalcel.htm. Accessed spring 2001.

10. Small cell lung cancer (PDQ) treatment–Health professionals. National Cancer Institute, National Institutes of Health. Available at: http://cancernet.nci.nih.gov/cgi-bin/srchcgi.exe?DBID=pdq&TYPE=search&UID=208=00040&ZFILE=professional&SFMT=pdq_treatment/1/0/0. Accessed spring 2001.

11. Porello PT, Peredy T. Bronchogenic carcinoma. eMedicine.com, Inc.; 2001. Available at: http://www.emedicine.com/emerg/topic335.htm. Accessed spring 2001.

Digestive System Conditions

7

CHAPTER OBJECTIVES

After reading this chapter, the reader should be able to . . .

- Name the most dangerous complication of gastroenteritis.
- Name a comfort measure for working with clients who have GERD.
- Know the parts of the alimentary canal that may be affected by Crohn's disease.
- Name the relationship between stress and peptic ulcers.
- Name a risk factor for colorectal cancer.

- Name the difference between diverticulosis and diverticulitis.
- Explain why anemia may be a complication of ulcerative colitis.
- List three complications of cirrhosis.
- Name the primary methods of communicability for hepatitis A, B, and C.
- Explain why statistics for hepatitis C have recently surged upward.

INTRODUCTION

Digestive System Structure and Function

Gastrointestinal Tract

The best way to discuss how the digestive tract works is to follow a piece of food through the system (Fig. 7-1).

When the teeth pulverize a bite of food, it is broken into small pieces so that the digestive enzymes in the saliva and the rest of the gastrointestinal (GI) tract have more access to the nutrients. The food moves from the mouth, down the esophagus, and into a wide place in the tube—the stomach. Here it is further pulverized by powerful muscular contractions of the stomach while being exposed to more chemicals. Accessory organs make their chemical contributions as the former food, now referred to as *chyme*, moves into the small intestine. By now the barrage of digestive enzymes has reduced the meal into its most primitive building blocks: sugars, fats, and proteins. The secretion of digestive enzymes anywhere in the upper GI tract is largely a function of the vagus nerve, the biggest contributor to the parasympathetic nervous system. In this way the efficiency of digestion depends on whether a person is in a sympathetic or parasympathetic state.

The small intestine loops and twirls around the abdomen, secured by sheets of connective tissue membrane called the *mesentery*, a part of the peritoneum. It is lubricated on the outside by other layers of the peritoneum, which allow it to move freely as a person twists, squirms, and changes positions. The inside of a healthy small intestine looks like velvet or velour, with millions of tiny villi, each one supplied with blood and

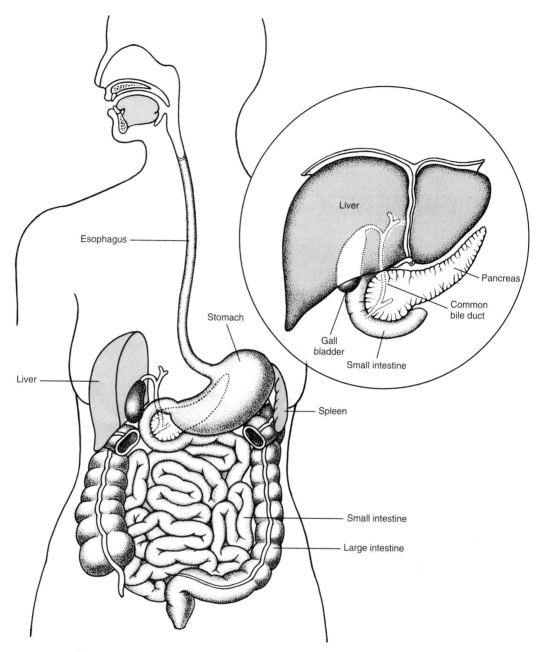

Figure 7-1. Overview of the digestive system

lymph capillaries for the absorption of nutrients and fats; fats are drawn into the lymph system, while the nutrients are drawn into the bloodstream. Rhythmic waves of smooth muscle contraction gently ease the chyme along the tube until, at the distal end of the small intestine, it passes through the ileocecal valve, the entryway to the colon.

The colon is a much shorter and wider section of tubing than the small intestine. It also differs in the absence of villi and the presence of anchoring pieces of connective tissue that bind the colon down at the four flexures, or corners of the abdomen. A healthy colon has segments called *haustra*. In this part of the tube water is squeezed out of the chyme, which is now called a *bolus*. Water is reabsorbed back into the body; this is also the site of vitamin K synthesis. The colon is a kind of trash compactor; everything left of a meal that makes it this far is condensed and excreted.

Accessory Organs

The continuous tube that winds from mouth to anus is only one part of the digestive system; the *accessory organs* contribute to the process of turning food into energy or building blocks as well. These organs include the liver, gallbladder, and pancreas, each of which produces or releases chemicals into the digestive tract. The following is a brief review of each of these organs.

Liver

This is an organ of immense complexity, with literally hundreds of functions. One of the things that make the liver unique is its powers of regeneration; *hepatocytes*, or liver cells are remarkably adaptable. Livers that have been partially removed can recover fully functional size within 1 week of surgery; small pieces of liver that have been transplanted into other hosts can often grow to full function within a similar short period. The liver is also special in that it has twice the blood supply of most other organs. Between the hepatic artery delivering oxygen and the portal vein delivering fresh products of digestion from the small intestine, it is no wonder that this organ is hot and dark red. Although the internal blood pressure is relatively low, cellular activity in the liver is very high.

The liver is the largest gland in the body. It is the destination of the portal system detour, receiving all the vitamins, amino acids, and glucose that are extracted from the small intestine and not immediately needed in the body. By storing glucose as glycogen until it is called for, the liver also acts as a sugar buffer, preventing some of the radical swings in blood glucose levels that would happen if sugar had no intermediate stop. The liver is also the site for much of the most vital protein synthesis in the body. Many of the enzymes that sponsor cellular activity are born here. It is also the origin of blood proteins that regulate intracellular fluid and blood clotting.

Detoxification functions of the liver are well known. The liver alters many drugs into a form that is less toxic or that can be excreted. A functioning liver prevents many substances, including alcohol, from reaching toxic levels. It also processes the poisonous wastes generated by protein digestion, changing them to uric acid to be excreted by the kidneys. In addition to these functions, the specialized leukocytes in the liver called Kupffer cells are constantly watching for any pathogens that they can eradicate. Finally, the liver helps to recycle the heme from dead red blood cells into bilirubin, a major component of *bile*, a substance that is vital for the digestion of fats. The liver produces up to 3 cups of bile each day. Bile leaves the liver via the cystic duct and enters the gallbladder.

Gallbladder

This is a small bright green sack that hangs off the liver about halfway along the costal angle on the right side of the body. Its function is fairly simple: it receives bile from the liver, stores it, and concentrates it. The gallbladder can hold up to 1 cup of bile at a time. On hormonal command it releases the bile into the duodenum via the common bile duct. There the bile helps to emulsify fats: the fats are held in tiny globules to make them easier to digest. The gallbladder and its ducts are susceptible to dysfunction, which can have serious repercussions.

Pancreas

This is a fascinating gland that holds the distinction of being both an exocrine gland, releasing digestive juices into the intestine via the pancreatic duct, and an endocrine gland, releasing hormones directly into the bloodstream. Its exocrine secretions are so alkaline they can be corrosive. Any blockage in the pancreatic duct can lead to very serious tissue damage, as the pancreas is quite capable of digesting itself.

Gastrointestinal Problems and Massage

Most of the GI tract problems that respond well to massage are related to autonomic imbalance. When a person is under stress, digestion becomes a low priority. If this state of affairs goes on for a long time, problems will develop. The most common disorders of this type are spastic or flaccid constipation, indigestion, and gas.

The first concern, however, is to eliminate the possibility of more serious conditions that would contraindicate circulatory massage. Massage practitioners are sometimes put in the position of deciding whether their work is going to help someone get over their stress-related stomachache or put them in the hospital. Symptoms that are a red light for something very serious include severe localized pain, bloody stools, anemia, bloating, and fever. A general rule is that if symptoms have persisted for 3 weeks or more, it is time to visit the doctor.

Problems in the GI tract are impossible to pin down without diagnostic tests, and this is not within the scope of practice of massage therapy. Massage should not be performed when the client has any unexplained or undiagnosed pain. Any relief that a massage provides may delay the client from getting medical assistance for a serious and acute illness. Symptoms of simple, short-term problems are often indistinguishable from very serious illness in the GI tract. Although spastic constipation is not inherently dangerous, colorectal cancer is—and massage therapists are not equipped to tell the difference.

Digestive System Conditions

Disorders of the Stomach and Small Intestine

Gastroenteritis
Crohn's Disease
Gastroesophageal Reflux Disorder
Stomach Cancer
Ulcers

Disorders of the Large Intestine

Appendicitis
Colorectal Cancer
Diverticular Disease
Irritable Bowel Syndrome
Ulcerative Colitis

Disorders of the Accessory Organs

Cirrhosis
Gallstones
Hepatitis
Jaundice

Other Digestive System Conditions

Candidiasis
Peritonitis

Disorders of the Stomach and Small Intestine

GASTROENTERITIS IN BRIEF

What is it?
Gastroenteritis is any form of GI inflammation. This may be due to a viral or bacterial infection, a parasite, fungus, food intolerance, or other cause.

How is it recognized?
The symptoms of gastroenteritis are nausea, vomiting, and diarrhea. Fever, blood in the stools, and other signs may be present, depending on the cause.

Is massage indicated or contraindicated?
Acute gastroenteritis contraindicates massage, especially when it is caused by an infectious agent. Chronic situations may be appropriate for bodywork, as long as the etiology of the problem is clearly understood.

Gastroenteritis

Definition: What Is It?

Gastroenteritis is inflammation of the GI tract, specifically the stomach or small intestine.

Demographics: Who Gets It?

Anyone of any age can get gastroenteritis, although it is most dangerous for the very young, the very old, and people whose immune systems are compromised. Although only about 10% of all affected people seek medical consultation, some estimates suggest that each year some 90 million cases of gastroenteritis occur in the United States. It is responsible for more than 200,000 hospitalizations of children and about 10,000 deaths each year.

Etiology: What Happens?

Gastroenteritis can have several causes. Although each factor may create slightly different symptoms, the basics (nausea, vomiting, diarrhea) are consistent.

- *Viruses.* The most common cause of GI inflammation is an infection with rotavirus or Norwalk virus. Any of the hepatitis viruses can also cause it, as can any member of the enterovirus family. Viral gastroenteritis is highly contagious and can reach epidemic levels in environments such as day care centers where most infants have not yet developed antibodies against infection and the chance of fecal-oral contamination is very high.

- *Bacteria.* Bacterial gastroenteritis is probably at fault when people complain of stomach flu. (Real flu viruses do not attack the GI tract.) Common bacterial pathogens include Salmonella, Shigella, Campylobacter, and *Escherichia coli.* Bacterial gastroenteritis is usually spread through improperly stored or prepared food or contaminated water or ice. Travelers' diarrhea is almost always from the *E. coli* bacterium.

- *Others.* Other causes of gastroenteritis include parasites (i.e., Giardia and cryptosporidium), fungal infections (i.e., *candidiasis*, this chapter), toxins (i.e., poisonous mushrooms or poisonous shellfish), dietary problems (i.e., food allergies), medications (i.e., antibiotics or magnesium-containing laxatives or antacids), or other conditions such as celiac disease, *appendicitis, Crohn's disease, ulcerative colitis, irritable bowel syndrome,* or *diverticulitis* (this chapter).

Once a pathogen, allergen, or toxic substance has gained access to the digestive tract, it can affect the function of the stomach and intestines in several ways. Some pathogens, like Shigella and Campylobacter, directly invade the mucosal lining. Others, like some varieties of *E. coli*, produce wastes that are highly toxic and destroy digestive system cells indirectly. Certain animal and plant poisons are cytotoxic: they kill any intestinal cells to which they are exposed. When the GI tract is damaged or inflamed, absorption of nutrients and water is severely limited. This causes the loss of both water and valuable electrolytes through diarrhea and vomiting.

Signs and Symptoms

Different causative factors of gastroenteritis can lead to various symptoms, but the basic trio of intestinal inflammation includes nausea, vomiting, and diarrhea. These are appropriate responses to infection, as they are efficient methods of clearing out the GI tract, but several of these diseases are spread through oral-fecal contamination, so hygiene becomes critical when dealing with these symptoms.

Other signs that may develop with gastroenteritis include bloating, cramps, gas, and mucus or blood in the stools.

Complications

The most serious complication of gastroenteritis is dehydration from the massive fluid and mineral loss that goes along with diarrhea and vomiting. The loss of critical fluid and electrolytes can be fatal; gastroenteritis is a leading cause of death in many developing nations. In the United States, the people most at risk for this extreme reaction are infants, immune-compromised persons, and the elderly, whose systems are less able to cope with this extreme change in internal environment. Signs of dangerously progressed dehydration include sunken eyes, lack of urination, and skin tenting (i.e., when the skin is pinched it does not immediately contract back to its original position).

Some gastroenteritis factors can cause other complications as well. Campylobacter bacteria have been linked with *Guillain-Barré syndrome* (Chapter 5), and Salmonella can complicate into *meningitis* (Chapter 3) or blood poisoning. Some forms of *E. coli* are highly toxic and can lead to *renal failure* (Chapter 9).

Diagnosis

Diagnosis of gastroenteritis is often a problem. Examining stool samples is the most efficient way to identify infectious agents, but this is a time-consuming and expensive process. On the other hand, treating bacterial infections with the wrong antibiotics can lead to more extreme symptoms and more resistant pathogens. To complicate matters further, it is possible to continue carrying the infectious agents long after symptoms have subsided. This has serious repercussions for food handlers, childcare workers, and health care workers, who are in positions to spread their infection to many other people.

Treatment

Gastroenteritis is usually an acute, self-limiting condition and is not generally treated with anything more sophisticated than rest and fluid and electrolyte replacement. Viruses do not respond to antibiotics, and antibiotics for bacterial infections may make intestinal inflammation worse. The use of anti-diarrhea medications is often discouraged because the body is shedding pathogens; interfering with that process may prolong the infection.

If supplementing fluids by mouth aggravates vomiting, it may be necessary to use intravenous (IV) fluid replacement in a hospital setting.

Gastroenteritis is much easier to prevent than to treat. When gastroenteritis occurs in large outbreaks it is often due to some specific source of contamination (e.g., infected meat, a contaminated well, or shellfish harvested from contaminated water). Since foodstuffs are now shipped quickly over large areas, it is a constant public health challenge to track down the source of infection and to limit its spread among the rest of the population.

Prognosis

Most cases of gastroenteritis resolve within 2 to 3 days without medical intervention. If symptoms persist longer than 2 to 3 weeks it is no longer considered an acute infection, but a chronic condition. This would lead medical professionals to look for an underlying condition such as food allergies, irritable bowel syndrome, diverticulitis, Crohn's disease, ulcerative colitis, or human immunodeficiency virus/acquired immune deficiency syndrome (*HIV/AIDS*, Chapter 5).

Massage?

Acute gastroenteritis contraindicates circulatory massage for several reasons. First, an infection may be present and could be exacerbated. Second, the infection may be communicable. Third, the client is likely to be uncomfortable because he or she will probably be nauseated at the time.

If a client has chronic digestive system irritation that is unrelated to infection, cancer, or other dangerous causes, bodywork could be helpful in creating a parasympathetic state that would improve efficiency and comfort.

CROHN'S DISEASE IN BRIEF

What is it?
Crohn's disease is a progressive inflammatory condition that may affect any part of the GI tract. It involves the development of deep ulcers, blockages, and the formation of abnormal passageways (fistulas) in the small and large intestine.

How is it recognized?
The primary symptom of Crohn's disease is abdominal pain, especially in the lower right quadrant (the distal end of the ileum). Cramping, diarrhea, and pain at the anus may also accompany active flares of this disease.

Is massage indicated or contraindicated?
Massage is appropriate for Crohn's disease patients when their condition is in remission. During flares they may also benefit from non-circulatory work, but abdominal work will be uncomfortable.

Crohn's Disease
Definition: *What Is It?*

Crohn's disease is a progressive inflammatory disorder that can affect any part of the GI tract, from the mouth to the anus. Advanced cases may also involve tissues outside the digestive system.

Crohn's disease and *ulcerative colitis* (this chapter) are often described together under the umbrella term "inflammatory bowel disease" because of the way they affect tissues, but they are etiologically quite different. Although Crohn's disease can and often does affect the large intestine and the upper GI tract, it is discussed in this section to help distinguish it from ulcerative colitis. For more information on how these two conditions are alike and dissimilar, (see *Watch for This: Crohn's Disease and Ulcerative Colitis.*)

Demographics: *Who Gets It?*

Crohn's disease affects about 500,000 Americans; men and women are affected more or less equally. It can develop in young children, but the majority of patients are diagnosed in their 20s or 30s; the average age of onset is 27.

The geographic distribution of this condition is interesting. It is especially common in the United States, Canada, and Scandinavia. It is somewhat less common in the United Kingdom and Western Europe, followed by Australia and South Africa. It is rare in all other countries.

A genetic susceptibility is evidently part of the Crohn's disease profile. Approximately 20% of all patients have a first-degree relative (parent, child, or sibling) who also has an inflammatory bowel disease. Statistically it occurs in higher numbers among Ashkenazi Jews than in other populations. Whites are most at risk for this disorder; it happens among this population 4 times more often than among non-Whites.

Etiology: What Happens?

Crohn's disease involves the development of inflamed areas in the large and small intestine. Many cases begin in the distal portion of the small intestine, the ileum, but this progressive disease can affect upper regions of the GI tract as well as the colon and anus.

One of the distinguishing features of Crohn's disease is that the areas it affects are not continuous; the inflamed regions appear in an unpredictable patchwork anywhere in the GI tract. These lesions may then develop ulcers that affect deep layers of the intestinal wall, even to the point of perforation. Eventually these ulcers can cause accumulations of scar tissue that partially block the intestine, or they can stimulate the development of abnormal connecting tubes from the colon to other organs (i.e., the bladder or even to the surface of the skin). These tubes are called *fistulas*, and they allow intestinal contents to exit the GI tract.

Some specialists classify Crohn's disease into three types:

- *Inflammatory Crohn's disease*, in which the mucosa, submucosa, and deeper layers of the GI tract are affected, leading to chronic diarrhea and the risk of bowel obstruction. This accounts for about 30% of all Crohn's disease patients.

- *Fistulating or perforating Crohn's disease*, in which ulcers burrow so deeply into the walls of the intestine that they perforate it completely, or they stimulate the formation of narrow, delicate tubes of epithelial tissue into nearby hollow organs or even to the skin, where fecal matter may leak. This accounts for about 20% of all Crohn's disease patients.

- *Stenosing Crohn's disease*, in which massive accumulations of scar tissue cause the GI tract to become dangerously narrow. Stenosing Crohn's disease can also lead to the formation of fistulas as the body tries to reroute digestive system contents that have become blocked.

Causes

Crohn's disease is an idiopathic disease. Several theories about its cause are being pursued, but none of them have yet been widely accepted. An inappropriate inflammatory response is part of the picture, but it is unclear whether that response is the *cause* or the *result* of the disease. Some speculation about an initial exposure to a common mycobacterium, *paratuberculosis*, is gaining momentum. The fact that some patients have success with early aggressive doses of antibiotics lends some credence to this approach. Although this condition may be linked to bacterial exposure, it does *not* appear to be contagious. Regardless of the initial trigger, the development of Crohn's disease depends on a genetic susceptibility to this kind of inflammatory response.

Food sensitivities and stress have been seen to exacerbate Crohn's disease symptoms, but they have not been identified as direct causes.

Signs and Symptoms

Crohn's disease occurs in periods of flare and remission, which often implies an autoimmune component. During periods of remission a patient may have no symptoms at all, but during a flare the most common symptoms include abdominal pain, especially at the distal end of the ileum in the lower right quadrant, along with cramping, diarrhea (often with blood), and bloating. Weight loss, fever, joint pain, small ulcers in the mouth and throat, and characteristic lesions on the skin may also accompany acute flares. Many Crohn's disease patients also experience severe pain around the anus, along with anal fissures and localized infections.

Complications

Crohn's disease disrupts normal digestion in several ways. Inflammation in the intestines means a patient has less access to ingested nutrients. When Crohn's disease occurs in young children, this can lead to stunted growth and delayed development. This disease can cause bowel obstruction or perforations, leading to peritonitis. It can cause abscesses to form in the GI tract or around the anus. Additionally, it can cause intestinal hemorrhage if the ulcers erode into blood vessels. If fistulas form into the bladder, leaking fecal material can cause bladder infections. Chronic irritation to epithelial cells in the GI tract also increases the risk of developing colorectal cancer.

Crohn's disease has been linked to problems outside the GI tract as well. It can cause inflammation at the bile duct, leading to *cirrhosis* and *jaundice* (this chapter). It has been linked with acute inflammation affecting the liver, eyes, and joints. It can cause the outbreak of ulcers called *aphthae* in the mouth, and characteristic lesions on the skin as well; these open sores most often appear around the ankles and lower legs.

⚠ WATCH FOR THIS

Crohn's Disease and Ulcerative Colitis

Crohn's disease and ulcerative colitis are two conditions linked under the description *inflammatory bowel disease.* This may create the impression that these two disorders are slightly different manifestations of the same problem, but current research indicates that they are significantly different in etiology, progression, and long-term prognosis. Although differentiating between these conditions has little impact on a massage therapist's decision, it may have big impact on the life of the client.

	CROHN'S DISEASE	ULCERATIVE COLITIS
Area affected	Often begins in the ileum but can spread distally into the colon or proximally into the rest of the small intestine; seldom affects the rectum	Always begins in the rectum; may spread proximally up the colon but never all the way to the small intestine
Pattern of progression	Progression is unpredictable; disconnected patches may appear anywhere along the GI tract	Progresses in a continuous connected series of lesions
Depth of lesions	Ulcers may burrow through the mucosa into the muscular or serous wall of the GI tract; perforation is not uncommon	Ulcers penetrate only the mucosa or submucosa of the colon; they seldom cause perforation
Complications	Can lead to liver problems, skin and mouth ulcers, eye inflammation, peritonitis, bladder infections, and colorectal cancer	Significantly raises the risk of colorectal cancer; other complications include liver inflammation, arthritis, skin rashes, and anemia
Surgery	Surgery can remove affected areas, but it often continues to attack healthy tissue; surgery often needs to be repeated	Surgery to remove the affected area is curative

Treatment

The damage that Crohn's disease can cause to the whole length of the digestive system is significant; thus, it is usually treated aggressively. Treatment during flares usually begins with steroidal anti-inflammatories and immunosuppressant drugs to quell the inflammatory reaction. Many Crohn's disease patients undergo surgery to remove affected sections of intestine, but this surgery is not curative. New patches of inflamed tissue may arise in other places, which then requires further surgery.

Research is being conducted into the role of a bacterial infection as a possible causative factor for Crohn's disease. Promising results with early administration of antibiotics may open new doors to understanding how to treat this disorder (see sidebar).

Crohn's disease patients have to be extraordinarily careful about their diet, especially during flares. High-fiber, bulky foods can exacerbate symptoms and create obstructions if scar tissue has narrowed the passageway. Sometimes high-calorie liquid diets are recommended during these episodes. In extreme cases the patient may take in all nutrients intravenously to give the whole system a break from the stress of digesting food.

Massage?

When this condition is in remission and the digestive tract is not under inflammatory attack, massage is a supportive and appropriate choice for clients with Crohn's disease. Deep abdominal work should probably be avoided, but anything that creates a parasympathetic response for increased efficiency of digestion and nutrient absorption would probably be useful.

During flares a client with Crohn's disease will probably be uncomfortable on the table, and circulatory work may exacerbate symptoms. Other types of bodywork, however, may be welcome and helpful in the effort to reduce pain and distress.

Gastroesophageal Reflux Disease
Definition: What Is It?

GERD is a condition involving damage to the squamous epithelial lining of the esophagus when it is chronically exposed to digestive juices released from the stomach. It is usually associated with weak muscular action at the lower esophageal sphincter.

Demographics: Who Gets It?

Heartburn, the predecessor to GERD, is astonishingly common in the United States. It is estimated that 7 to 10% of all Americans experience heartburn everyday, and up to 40% of all Americans have it at least once a month. GERD is diagnosed

Crohn's Disease History

Throughout the 20th century, Crohn's disease has gone through several incarnations. It has been called *granulomatosis enteritis* for the presence of white blood cell conglomerates called granulomas. It has been called *regional enteritis* for its patchy appearance throughout the small and large intestines. It has also been labeled *terminal ileitis* because it often begins at the distal end of the ileum.

One of the first researchers to document this disorder was a Scottish doctor named Thomas Kennedy Dalziel. In 1913, he noted its similarity to certain inflammatory conditions found among livestock, and he proposed that it might be caused by the same pathogen—mycobacterium *paratuberculosis*.

In 1932 a team of researchers, including Dr. Burrill Crohn (1884–1983), were unable to find significant signs of bacteria in the lesions, and so the theory of bacterial infection was dropped. Instead, the disease was studied as some kind of immune system dysfunction involving inappropriate inflammatory attacks against digestive system tissue.

In 1985 new tests revealed that particles of mycobacterium *paratuberculosis* can indeed be found in Crohn's disease ulcers. Early treatment with the correct antibiotics shows promising results with many Crohn's disease patients, although some of them require these antibiotics for a prolonged period.

Mycobacterium *paratuberculosis* is a common pathogen that most people encounter early in life, when it usually causes a short-term bout of diarrhea. It seems that Crohn's disease patients simply have a genetic susceptibility to creating a life-long inflammatory response to this pathogen that causes significant and extensive damage to the digestive tract.

GASTROESOPHAGEAL REFLUX DISEASE IN BRIEF

What is it?
Gastroesophageal reflux disease (GERD) is a condition involving a weak or impaired esophageal sphincter and the chronic splashing of acidic stomach secretions into the unprotected esophagus.

How is it recognized?
Most people experience occasional heartburn (the sensation of having corrosive gastric juices enter the esophagus). GERD is diagnosed when heartburn symptoms have been present long enough to cause structural changes to the esophageal lining, which could lead to serious complications.

Is massage indicated or contraindicated?
People with GERD often find that lying down exacerbates their symptoms, especially if it is within a couple of hours of eating. Clients may therefore wish to use bolsters that allow them to be in a reclining position, to have the head-end of the table elevated by several inches, or to sit in a massage chair.

when heartburn becomes a chronic ongoing situation, especially in the presence of structural changes to the esophageal lining or to the lower esophageal sphincter. GERD can happen to any person at any age. It has been documented among infants, the elderly, and every age in between.

Etiology: What Happens?

Most cases of GERD are connected to a dysfunctional lower esophageal sphincter. This is the circular muscle that is designed to close off access to the stomach except during swallowing. The sphincter muscle may become stretched, weakened, or overly relaxed. Any one of these problems allows stomach contents, including highly corrosive hydrochloric acid, to enter the esophagus, which lacks the thick layers of mucus that protects the stomach from acid exposure.

Chronic irritation of the esophageal lining can cause several reactions.

- *Respiratory injury* may occur if gastric secretions reach up to the larynx. It is not uncommon for these substances to be aspirated into the lungs, especially by infants and young children.

- *Ulcers* may form in the esophagus. These lesions may become infected or may bleed into the GI tract.

- *A stricture* may form. This is a thickening of the esophageal wall with scar tissue in response to the irritation. Strictures may make it difficult to swallow normally.

- *Barrett's esophagus* may develop. This is a pathologic change in the normal esophageal squamous cells; they mutate into cells that resemble the stomach lining. Barrett's esophagus has been identified as a possible precancerous condition, opening the door to adenocarcinoma, or cancer of the esophagus.

Risk Factors

A number of risk factors for developing GERD have been identified. Some of these are modifiable, which gives most GERD patients some influence over their disease process. Risk factors for GERD include:

- *Pregnancy.* Most pregnant women experience some heartburn, especially when the baby is big enough to put mechanical pressure on the stomach. Some pregnant women go on to develop significant structural changes in the esophagus.

- *Obesity.* Being clinically overweight can cause the abdominal contents to put ongoing mechanical pressure on the diaphragm and esophageal sphincter.

- *Smoking.* Smoking has been seen to weaken and loosen the esophageal sphincter.

- *Diet.* A diet high in fatty or spicy foods, as well as the ingestion of caffeine, alcohol, chocolate, and highly acidic foods, can exacerbate GERD.

- *Connective tissue diseases.* Diseases such as *lupus* (Chapter 5) or *scleroderma* (Chapter 2) may result in inflammation and weakening of the lower esophageal sphincter.

- *Hiatal hernia.* A hiatal hernia (an enlargement of the opening in the diaphragm where the esophagus passes through to the stomach) may catch and irritate the superior part of the stomach. Most people with hiatal hernias experience GERD, although not all GERD patients have hiatal hernias.

- *Delayed stomach emptying.* Some diseases, including *diabetes* (Chapter 9), *ulcers* (this chapter), and *spinal cord injuries* (Chapter 3), cause reduced peristalsis and sluggish movement of substances through the GI tract. When stomach contents linger too long, the accumulation of pressure and gastric juices can cause them to put back-pressure on the esophagus.

- *Other risk factors.* These include exposure to radiation for chest tumors, infection of the esophagus, and certain medications.

Signs and Symptoms

Signs and symptoms of GERD are largely created by the action of gastric juice on the delicate esophageal lining. A bitter taste, a feeling like some food has been regurgitated, gas, indigestion, bloating, and pain in the chest behind the sternum are common symptoms. It is not unusual for the pain of GERD to be mistaken for *heart attack* (Chapter 4) or angina. Symptoms are reliably aggravated by lying down.

Other GERD symptoms that occur less frequently include trouble swallowing, coughing, wheezing, and coughing up blood if ulcers in the esophagus have eroded into a blood vessel.

Diagnosis

Diagnostic tests for GERD reveal very precise information about the nature and location of structural changes to the stomach and esophagus. They include barium x-rays, endoscopy, and possibly a biopsy to examine suspicious-looking cells. About 10,000 GERD patients per year develop Barrett's esophagus, which may be precancerous.

Treatment

Treatment for GERD falls into two categories: managing the problem and repairing the problem. Managing GERD so that it does not get worse includes strategies like losing weight if the patient is overweight; eating smaller portions so the stomach does not get as full; not lying down within 2 hours after a meal; avoiding caffeine, alcohol, and nicotine; raising the bed about 6 inches at the head; and putting a heating pad on the stomach when it is painful.

Medication for GERD can work in a variety of ways. Antacids neutralize stomach acid, but over-the-counter brands may also cause the stomach to expand with gas, putting more pressure on the esophageal valve. Other medications can block receptors in the stomach that stimulate acid production.

Surgery for GERD usually focuses on strengthening the esophageal sphincter and taking pressure off the stomach. If the esophagus is limited by the development of a scar tissue stricture, this may be stretched and dilated. A portion of the stomach may be wrapped around the sphincter to give it external support in a procedure called a *fundoplication*. Of course, if a hiatal hernia is putting pressure on the stomach, surgery may be performed to correct it.

Massage?

Massage usually improves digestive function and efficiency through the parasympathetic response. With GERD patients, however, this may not be a benefit when gastric acid can splash back up into the esophagus. Therefore, it is important to work with clients who have GERD in a way that does not exacerbate symptoms. This may mean not working within 2 hours of the client having eaten, or it may mean working with the client in a massage chair or in a semi-reclined position. It may also mean putting 6-inch blocks under the head-end of the massage table. Although clients with GERD can benefit from bodywork, their special needs may require imaginative accommodations on the part of their massage therapists.

Stomach Cancer

Definition: What Is It?

Stomach cancer is the development of malignant tumors in the stomach that can block the passage of food through the digestive system. It can spread, either through cells flaking off into the peritoneal space or through blood and lymph flow, to other organs.

Demographics: Who Gets It?

Stomach cancer is on a dramatic decline in the United States; it is only one-fourth as common now as it was in 1930. However, in much of the rest of the world, especially in countries in Asia and South America, stomach cancer is one of the leading causes of death by cancer.

In the United States, about 24,000 people are diagnosed with stomach cancer every year. About 14,000 people die of this disease every year. Most stomach cancer patients are in their 60s or 70s. Men with the disease outnumber women by almost 2:1.

Etiology: What Happens?

Although several different types of cancer have been observed to grow from stomach cells, the vast majority of stomach cancer tumors are *adenocarcinomas*, in other words, they arise from epithelial tissue. It is not always clear what triggers the growth of these tumors, but the clear difference in U.S. statistics compared with those of Asia and Latin America have yielded some useful clues about the development of this disease.

Stomach cancer rates in the United States began to decline in the 1930s, about the time that refrigeration became accessible for the majority of Americans. The average diet shifted away from smoked, pickled, and salted foods and toward more fresh meats and fresh, canned, or frozen vegetables. In countries where stomach cancer is very prominent, the consumption of salted, smoked, or pickled foods is significantly higher than it is in the United States.

Studies of the *Helicobacter pylori* bacteria associated with *ulcers* (this chapter) show that these bacteria can convert some of the chemicals in high-risk foods into carcinogens. The majority of stomach cancer patients test positive for *H. pylori*.

As the stomach wall is assaulted with chronic exposure to carcinogenic substances, minute changes in the tissues may develop. These precancerous changes are virtually silent and are almost never detected. Malignant cells can grow into tumors large enough to obstruct the passage of food through the digestive tract, or they can invade and completely permeate the stomach wall, allowing them to spread to nearby abdominal organs.

By the time stomach cancer is detected, it has usually spread into the lymph system. Almost half of all stomach cancer patients experience metastasis in the peritoneum, and about one-third discover cancerous cells in the liver.

Risk Factors

The major risk factors for developing stomach cancer include the following:

- *H. pylori infection.* The majority of stomach cancer patients have *H. pylori* in their digestive tract. These bacteria have been seen to convert certain food products into carcinogens.
- *Diet.* Diets that are high in smoked food, salted fish and meats, and pickled vegetables increase the risk of developing stomach cancer. Nitrates used as food preservatives also contribute to this risk.
- *Tobacco and alcohol use.* These products have been associated with the development of stomach cancer, especially in the proximal portion of the stomach.
- *Other factors.* A wide variety of other factors increase stomach cancer risk, including having had previous stomach surgery, having type A blood, being male, being between 60 and 79 years old, and having the genes that have been associated with *colorectal cancer* (this chapter).

Signs and Symptoms

Signs and symptoms of stomach cancer are mostly related to having a physical obstruction in the digestive tract. They include a feeling of fullness after only a little food, vague abdominal pain above the navel, unintentional weight loss, heartburn and other ulcer symptoms, nausea and vomiting, and the development of *ascites* (the accumulation of excessive fluid in the peritoneal space).

Diagnosis

Because the early changes that occur with stomach cancer are so subtle, it is very seldom identified in the United States before metastasis. In Japan, where it occurs about 5 times more frequently, mass screenings are conducted to try to find the cancer in earlier stages.

Diagnostic techniques for stomach cancer include endoscopy and biopsy, a barium wash of the upper GI tract followed by radiographs, and an endoscopic ultrasound of the stomach wall.

Once the presence of cancerous cells has been determined, the next step is to stage the development of the disease. Staging protocols for stomach cancer are similar to those used for most types of cancer (see *cancer*, Chapter 11).

Treatment

Stomach cancer is treated with the same arsenal of tools used against most cancers: chemotherapy, radiation, and surgery. Because it is not usually found in early stages, many stomach cancer patients will undergo combinations of therapies in an attempt to limit the spread of the cancer through the rest of the body.

Treatment options for stomach cancer statistically have little connection to survival rates. Rather, survival is directly connected to the stage the disease is in when it is detected. Less than 10% of all stomach cancers are found before they have spread beyond the stomach. The 5-year survival rate for this disease is 5 to 15%.

Massage?

If a client has been diagnosed as having stomach cancer, he or she will probably be engaged in a combination of treatments to try to limit the spread of the disease. Cancer treatments can be extraordinarily harsh and taxing for the body to accommodate. Massage has a place in reducing pain, improving sleep, and generally supporting the process for cancer patients, as long as the cautions that accompany various cancer treatment options are respected.

ULCERS IN BRIEF

What are they?
Ulcers are sores that for various reasons do not go through a normal healing process; they remain open and vulnerable to infection. Peptic ulcers occur in the stomach or duodenum (the proximal portion of the small intestine).

How are they recognized?
The symptoms of peptic ulcers include general burning or gnawing abdominal pain between meals that is relieved by taking antacids or eating. Other symptoms can include bloating, burping, gas, and consistent vomiting after meals.

Is massage indicated or contraindicated?
Specific work on the abdomen may exacerbate symptoms of peptic ulcers, so they are at least a local contraindication for mechanical types of bodywork. Other modalities and massage away from the upper abdomen are certainly appropriate for ulcer patients.

Ulcers
Definition: What Is It?

Peptic ulcers of the stomach and duodenum are discussed here, but an ulcer is an ulcer, whether it is in the GI tract or on the skin. An ulcer is the result of tissue damage that, because it is subject to constant irritation and the healing process may be somehow impeded, never gets better. Cells die, are sloughed off, and a crater develops but does not crust over. An ulcer is a perpetually open sore and an invitation to infection (Fig. 7-2). For more information on skin ulcers, see *decubitus ulcers* (Chapter 1).

Demographics: Who Gets It?

Ulcers are a common malady in the United States, although their occurrence has recently begun to decline. It is estimated that about 10% of all Americans will have at least one ulcer in their lifetime. About 25 million Americans have diagnosed ulcers today. Between 350,000 and 500,000 new cases are diagnosed each year, leading to more than 1 million hospitalizations. Men with ulcers outnumber women by about 2:1.

Etiology: What Happens?

Ulcers in the stomach or small intestine are called peptic ulcers, named for the protein-digesting enzyme pepsin that contributes to their development. The general under-

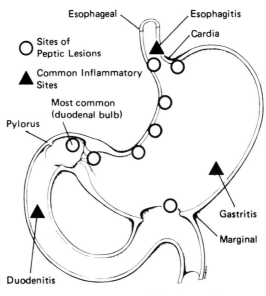

Figure 7-2. Gastric and duodenal ulcers

standing of how ulcers come about has undergone some radical changes in the past several years, and it may be that more changes are on the horizon.

For as long as ulcers have been understood as sores on the stomach or intestinal wall, they have been treated with the assumption that they arise from too much stress and/or spicy food. Ulcer patients have been counseled to eat bland food and avoid getting upset or overly excited. Many found that their ulcers eventually healed, but would recur later; ulcers were essentially a life-long affliction.

Contributing Factors: Stress

It turns out that the link between stress and ulcers is a significant factor, but probably not in the way that had always been assumed. Furthermore, the incidence of ulcers across the population does not follow demographics that are associated with high-stress situations, so some variables in stress coping mechanisms have evidently never been addressed.

The normal environment inside a stomach has features that can be classified as "aggressive" and others that are "defensive." Aggressive features include the production of hydrochloric acid and pepsin, which help to digest proteins. Defensive features include (1) a generous blood supply to the stomach wall, which serves to help damaged cells regenerate quickly and to stimulate the production of mucus; (2) a lining that protects the stomach wall from acid and pepsin; and (3) the production of bicarbonate to neutralize acid. These aggressive and defensive mechanisms work best when they keep each other in balance.

When a person is in a sympathetic state, blood supply to the whole digestive tract is suppressed while blood is rerouted toward skeletal muscle to support the "flight or fight" reaction. Stomach activity is suspended during a sympathetic reaction. Lack of blood flow means that mucus production is slowed, but so is acid and pepsin production; the two mechanisms stay in balance. When the stress is over and a person shifts back into a relaxed, parasympathetic state, stomach secretions are stimulated again. The problem is that the stomach produces acid and pepsin much faster than it rebuilds a thinned, delicate mucous lining. This imbalance between aggressive and defensive features leaves the stomach wall vulnerable to damage. In other words, ulcers seem to be more related to the *relief* of stress than to the presence of stress.[a]

Contributing Factors: *Helicobacter pylori*

Stress is only part of the ulcer picture, however. In 1982 a remarkable discovery revealed an unexpected phenomenon: a bacterium that can survive and thrive in the highly acidic environment of the stomach. This bacterium, called *Helicobacter pylori*, is found in many biopsy specimens of ulcers. It is a spiral-shaped organism that invades the mucous membrane of the stomach when structural weak spots appear. The identification of *H. pylori* led to the conclusion that imbalances in stomach chemistry can initiate tissue damage to the stomach wall, but bacterial infection makes the ulcer a chronic problem (for more information on *H. pylori*, see the sidebar).

The presence of *H. pylori* bacteria in the vast majority of ulcer biopsy specimens led to a new understanding of how peptic ulcers develop and how to treat them. The addition of antibiotics to ulcer treatments leads to a successful, permanent solution for many ulcer patients. This finding was so conclusive that in 1994 the National Institutes of Health issued a statement asserting that up to 90% of all peptic ulcers were related to *H. pylori* infection. A certain population, however, have ulcers that are unrelated to bacteria.

---

[a]This realization often prompts the question, "Shouldn't we just stay in stress all the time then, to avoid ever getting an ulcer?" The answer is that living in chronic low-grade stress opens the door to hosts of other diseases that are far more life-threatening than peptic ulcers.

What is *Helicobacter pylori*?

Helicobacter pylori is a bacterium that is admirably designed to withstand and even thrive in the corrosively acidic environment of the stomach. The bacterium has several anatomic features that allow it to infect the mucous membranes of the stomach wall.

Until 1984 it was never even considered that a bacterium could survive in the stomach. When pioneer researchers Barry Marshall and Robin Warren proposed the possibility, they were all but laughed offstage. However, when biopsy specimens of ulcerous tissue consistently revealed the presence of *H. pylori* bacteria, the laughter quieted. When ulcer patients found that combining appropriate antibiotics with other acid-limiting medications led to a permanent cure for their ulcers—something that was unheard of at the time—the approach to treating this common condition completely changed. In 1994 the National Institutes of Health issued a statement that it was clear that *H. pylori* does indeed cause the majority of peptic ulcers.

What is *H. pylori* and where does it come from? Little is well understood about this pathogen. It is a short, spiral-shaped, microaerophilic gram-negative bacillus. Its presence can be determined easily by a blood test for antibodies. It is sensitive to common antibiotics like tetracycline and amoxicillin. Worldwide, it is estimated that up to two-thirds of all adults have been infected with *H. pylori*. In the United States the majority of infections have been documented among older adults, African-Americans, Hispanics, and people in lower socioeconomic classes.

The discovery of *H. pylori* and its role in peptic ulcers has raised as many questions as it has answered. How is the bacterium communicated? No one knows, but it could be through oral-fecal contamination or through oral-oral contact. How can it be prevented? It is impossible to prevent the spread of *H. pylori* without knowing how it gets from one person to another. If it is sensitive to common antibiotics, why is it not eradicated when a person takes amoxicillin or tetracycline for something else? Antibiotics for *H. pylori* seem to work only when an ulcer has formed. Does the presence of *H. pylori* contribute to general indigestion? It is unclear, but taking antibiotics for indigestion definitely *does not* clear up a *H. pylori* infection or relieve symptoms of dyspepsia.

Finally, some recent research has found conflicting evidence about the frequency of *H. pylori* infections. In a study of several hundred ulcer patients, the bacterium was found in approximately 45% of all ulcer tissue. Given that a certain percentage of patients may have developed ulcers in response to NSAID use, that still leaves a large percentage of people whose ulcers are connected to neither irritating drugs nor infectious bacteria. Their ulcers are idiopathic.[b]

[b]Packer-Tursman J. Treatment of choice. *Special to the Washington Post.* August 22, 2000:Z19. Available at:http://www.washingtonpost.com/wp-dyn/articles/A3292-2000Aug22.html. Accessed spring 2001.

Contributing Factors: NSAIDs

The use of nonsteroidal anti-inflammatory drugs (NSAIDs) for everything from headaches to back pain to heart disease and stroke prevention, has led to some significant disruption of stomach function for many patients. Aspirin, ibuprofen, and naproxen sodium all interfere with the "defensive" aspects of stomach activity. They interfere with blood flow to the mucous membrane, they slow mucus production, and they inhibit the production of bicarbonate. It is estimated that about 10% of all diagnosed peptic ulcers arise from long-term NSAID use instead of from bacterial infection.

Signs and Symptoms

The primary symptom of peptic ulcers is a gnawing, burning pain in the chest or abdomen. It can last anywhere from 30 minutes to 3 hours. When the pain occurs in relation to eating varies greatly from one person to the next (it can depend on the location of the ulcer), but it is generally relieved by antacids or eating more food.

Other signs of ulcers can include nausea, vomiting, loss of appetite, and bleeding into the GI tract.

Complications

Complications of ulcers can be serious. When ulcers erode into capillaries, bleeding occurs, leading to *anemia* (Chapter 4). If the eroded blood vessel is a larger arteriole or artery, hemorrhaging can lead quickly to shock and death if left untreated. Ulcers can also perforate (or eat all the way through) the organ wall, releasing bacteria and partially digested food into the peritoneal space (*peritonitis*, this chapter). Perforation happens about 20 times more often with duodenal than stomach ulcers. Ulcers can create a combination of scar tissue and inflammation that causes the pyloric valve to spasm, thus completely obstructing the digestive tract. If this situation is not quickly resolved it can require surgery to reopen the digestive tract.

Finally, having a peptic ulcer raises the risk of developing *stomach cancer* (this chapter) by 2 to 6 times. Although stomach cancer is on the decline in the United States, it is still the second leading type of cancer worldwide. Another type of cancer, mucosal-associated lymphoid type lymphoma, is also associated with a history of peptic ulcers.

Diagnosis

Blood tests for Helicobacter are a useful tool, but they can reveal false-positive findings. For that reason, ulcers are often diagnosed by having a patient drink a barium preparation, and then taking a series of radiographs of the GI tract. This test reveals not only the presence but also the precise location of the ulcers. Once the presence of an ulcer has been determined, looking for Helicobacter determines whether a bacterial infection is part of the picture.

Treatment

Most ulcer treatments includes antibiotics for *H. pylori*, bismuth (which protects the delicate stomach lining), and medicines that limit acid production. Patients who complete this treatment have up to a 90% chance of permanent recovery.

Ulcers caused by the use of NSAIDs do not respond to antibiotic therapy. The only way to limit them is to suspend the use of the medications that are damaging the stomach lining.

Occasionally, ulcers will not respond to medical therapy or are so far advanced that surgery becomes an important option. Surgeries for ulcers can take one of three forms. A *vagotomy* severs the vagus nerve (the branch of the parasympathetic nervous system that stimulates gastric juice production). Recent advances in neurosurgery mean that just the part of the vagus nerve that controls gastric secretions can be cut. With an *antrectomy* the lower part of the stomach (the *antrum*) is removed. A *pyloroplasty* is a surgery that enlarges the pyloric valve to allow easier flow from the stomach into the duodenum. Antrectomies and pyloroplasties are generally performed in conjunction with vagotomies.

Massage?

Massage is unlikely to make an ulcer worse, unless the therapist is mechanically manipulating the stomach or intestines. The abdomen should be considered a local contraindication for deep specific work. Otherwise, both circulatory and non-circulatory massage can be helpful in reestablishing the autonomic balance that promotes permanent healing.

Disorders of the Large Intestine

Appendicitis
Definition: What Is It?

Appendicitis describes the inflammation, usually with infection, of the vermiform appendix—a structure about the size of a little finger that dangles off the cecum.

Demographics: Who Gets It?

Appendicitis can affect anyone of any age, but it is most common in people between 11 and 20 years of age. The incidence of appendicitis in the United States is about 1 of every 1000 people per year. Approximately 7% of the U.S. population will eventually have appendicitis.

Etiology: What Happens?

In some animals the appendix performs a vital role in digestion and immunity. In humans, however, its function is not completely understood. In fact, it used to be standard procedure to remove the appendix during any abdominal surgery, just in case it

APPENDICITIS IN BRIEF

What is it?
Appendicitis is inflammation of the vermiform appendix. It is usually a result of infection following a blockage at the opening of the appendix. The blockage may be caused by a hardened piece of fecal matter or by lymphatic inflammation.

How is it recognized?
The symptoms of appendicitis are widely variable but include general abdominal pain that gradually settles in the lower right quadrant. Rebound pain is usually severe. Fever, nausea, vomiting, food aversion, constipation, and diarrhea may be present.

Is massage indicated or contraindicated?
Acute appendicitis contraindicates massage. This condition may complicate into peritonitis if it is neglected.

APPENDIX

The Latin root of appendix is *ap-pendo*, which means, "hang something on." This refers to the appendix's location, hanging off the cecum of the large intestine.

should someday cause a problem. More recently it has been recognized that the lymphatic follicles lining the appendix may help to produce some types of immunoglobulins, so the appendix is only taken out when leaving it in poses significant danger.

Inflammation of the appendix is generally precipitated by an obstruction of the opening into the cecum. Many cases are related to the development of *fecaliths* (small hardened stools that block the connection between the appendix and the large intestine). When the appendix cannot drain appropriately, the risk of bacterial infection is very high. Once an infection has begun, the appendix becomes inflamed and may develop internal or external abscesses. Left untreated, the infected appendix may reach the point of perforation or rupture, releasing bacteria and pus into the peritoneum.

Signs and Symptoms

Symptoms of appendicitis are notoriously variable. They cover a wide range of possibilities, and not all patients experience all symptoms. The classic symptoms of appendicitis are a combination of food aversion and general central abdominal pain, which eventually settles into severe pain in the right lower quadrant of the abdomen. However, only about 50% of all appendicitis patients report these symptoms.

Nausea, vomiting, diarrhea, and constipation may be present when the appendix is inflamed. Pain is often aggravated by coughing, sneezing, or abdominal movement. Patients may have a low fever. If the appendix ruptures, the pain may temporarily subside, since the pressure has been relieved and the infection can take a few hours to completely take over the system.

Complications

In a worst-case scenario the appendix may completely rupture, leaking its colonies of bacteria into the peritoneal cavity, and peritonitis is a near certainty. Occasionally, the greater omentum may be positioned to smother a perforated appendix, which can temporarily localize the infection. This generally leads to internal adhesions and abscesses, which without medical intervention, would probably rupture as well.

In some situations the appendix may develop abscesses (small, painful, localized infections). In this case the risk of infection being released by surgery is high, so the abscesses must be drained or resolved by antibiotic therapy before the appendix is removed.

Diagnosis

Although the ability to identify intestinal disorders has taken quantum leaps forward with computed tomography (CT) scans, ultrasounds, and laparoscopes, appendicitis remains extremely difficult to identify. It is especially difficult to diagnose appendicitis correctly in young children, elderly people, and pregnant women.

Appendicitis resembles several other serious conditions including *kidney stones* or *urinary tract infection* (Chapter 8); *Crohn's disease, gastroenteritis, diverticulitis,* or *gallstones* (this chapter); *pelvic inflammatory disease, fibroid tumors,* ectopic *pregnancy,* and *ovarian cysts* (Chapter 10). Several of the tests used to identify appendicitis (white blood cell counts, urinalysis, radiographs, barium enemas, and CT scans) are designed to find the cause of the blockage and to rule out common misdiagnoses.

Ultimately, appendicitis is usually diagnosed through patient history and a physical examination. One fairly dependable sign is rebound pain (i.e., when a person pushes on the lower right side of the abdomen and then lets go suddenly, the pain is worse on the release than with the initial pressure).

Treatment

Once infection in the appendix has been identified, surgery is performed to remove it. This has traditionally been done through an incision close to the site of the appendix, but recent advances have made laparoscopies a viable option. The advantage to this technique is that the wound is much smaller and recovery time is much shorter than for traditional abdominal surgery.

It is best to perform this simple surgery in the early stages of inflammation before tissue death, rupture, or abscesses can create further complications.

In situations in which surgery is impractical, it is occasionally possible to treat appendicitis with antibiotics. However, a large percentage of patients treated this way experience a resurgence of their infections within 1 year.

Massage?

Someone with acute appendicitis needs immediate care, not massage. Even a chronic low-grade infection can flare up quickly, and the risk of rupture and peritonitis is very high. For guidelines about working with someone recovering from an appendectomy, see *postoperative conditions* in Chapter 11.

Colorectal Cancer

Definition: What Is It?

Colorectal cancer is the development of tumors anywhere in the large intestine from the ascending right side to the rectum. Although the two conditions are linked, malignant colon or rectal cancer is not the same thing as the presence of *adenomas*, or colon polyps.

Demographics: Who Gets It?

Statistics on colon and rectal cancers vary, but most suggest that about 140,000 cases of these diseases are diagnosed each year, and they cause about 57,000 deaths each year. This makes colorectal cancer the second leading cause of death by cancer in the United States (only lung cancer is higher).

Although it has traditionally be perceived as a "man's disease," colorectal cancer affects men and women almost evenly. The leading demographic for developing these diseases is age: 90% of all colorectal patients are older than 50 years.

Racial statistics for these diseases show some predictable patterns. Native Alaskans have the highest incidence of colon and rectal cancer among both men and women. African-Americans are diagnosed slightly more often than Whites. Native Americans and Philippinos show the lowest average rates of both colon and rectal cancers.

Etiology: What Happens?

The colon, or bowel, is the last and widest section of the digestive tract. In this 6-foot long piece of tubing the remnants of food are compacted, needed water is reabsorbed into the body, and feces are stored in the rectum until they are expelled. The inner lin-

---

COLORECTAL CANCER IN BRIEF

What is it?
Colorectal cancer is the development of malignant tumors in the colon or rectum. Growths can block the bowel and/or metastasize to other organs, particularly the liver.

How is it recognized?
Colorectal cancer creates different symptoms depending on what part of the bowel is affected. The most dangerous symptoms are extreme changes in bowel habits, including diarrhea or constipation lasting more than 10 days. Other symptoms include blood in the stool, iron-deficiency anemia, and unintentional weight loss.

Is massage indicated or contraindicated?
If a client is diagnosed with colon or rectal cancer in the early stages, some types of massage may be a useful supportive therapy to help deal with the side effects of cancer treatment. Colorectal cancer survivors are good candidates for massage, although the presence of a colostomy bag may require some specialized adjustments.

ing of the colon is composed of epithelium, which, as has been seen in other discussions of cancer, is particularly susceptible to uncontrolled cell growth.

The majority of colorectal cancers begin with the development of adenomas (small polyps in the bowel). Minor chromosome damage is believed to cause the formation of these polyps: the cells in the mucosa of the colon simply multiply without any reason and create these small pile-ups of excess tissue (Fig. 7-3). If the polyps are present for a long period, the chromosome damage may accumulate to the point that these benign growths become malignant. They can invade the deeper layers of the bowel and even erode all the way through it, they can obstruct the movement of fecal matter through the GI tract, and they can metastasize through the lymph system to other places in the body, notably the brain, liver, and lungs. This is the transition from polyps to colorectal cancer, and it generally happens without warning.

Causes

No one knows what prompts common colon polyps, which occur in 30 to 40% of older Americans, to become malignant. Large polyps and ones that have been present for long periods are the most likely to become cancerous, but what actually causes the shift is still a mystery. One theory is that high-fat foods linger in the colon longer than others, and some of their by-products are carcinogenic, or cancer-causing. The presence of these chemicals may contribute to chromosome damage in the polyps, causing them to reproduce at even more abnormal rates. This theory also suggests that diets that are high in fiber cause matter to move through the colon faster and more completely, "scrubbing" the bowel walls of damaging or irritating materials.

Recent research indicates that insoluble fiber itself may not be the major cancer-fighting aspect of eating grains, fruits, and vegetables; it may be the presence of phytochemicals that suppresses the malignant changes in colon polyps.

Regardless of the specific cancer-fighting mechanism, the relationship between diet and colorectal cancer is demonstrable in population studies that show colorectal cancer rates are much higher in cultures that follow a western diet (North America,

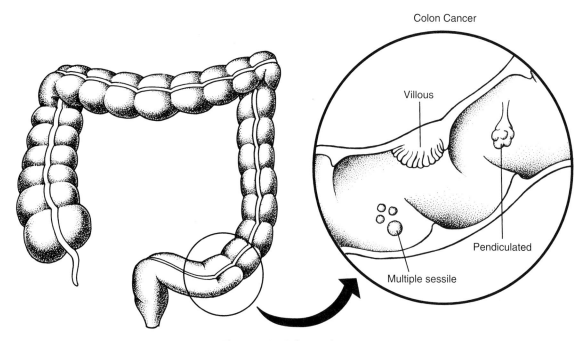

Figure 7-3. Colorectal cancer

Australia, and Europe) than in cultures that do not (South America, Africa, and Asia). Furthermore, colorectal cancer rates are increasing in countries that are moving toward a westernized diet standard. However, when it gets down to individual cases, no specific study has proven that any particular diet prevents or even decreases the chances of developing this disease. This is not to say that no connection exists between diet and colorectal cancer; it is just to point out that no one has yet defined the connection exactly.

Risk Factors

As with many diseases, the risk factors for colorectal cancer include issues that can and cannot be controlled.

- *Obesity.* People who are obese have a statistically higher chance of developing colorectal cancer. The leading theories behind this suggest that excessive fat in the body (especially around the waist in an "apple" shape, as opposed to on the buttocks and thighs in a "pear" shape) changes metabolism and stimulates the growth of new cells in the colon.

- *Family history. Familial adenomatous polyposis* (FAP) and *hereditary nonpolyposis colorectal cancer syndrome* (HNPCC) are two genetic conditions that predispose some people toward the development of colorectal cancer. Although these people have a much greater than average chance of developing the disease, the vast majority of colorectal cancer cases are found in people who are not part of these high-risk groups.

- *Inflammatory bowel disease. Ulcerative colitis* and *Crohn's disease* (this chapter) are very highly connected with colorectal cancer. The younger a person is when diagnosed with either of these problems, the greater his or her chances are of eventually developing colorectal cancer. The risk is so high that for some people preventive surgery to remove the whole colon is suggested before the cancer has a chance to develop.

- *Age.* The chances of having colorectal cancer rise with age; 90% of all colorectal cancer patients are older than 50.

Signs and Symptoms

Like so many other types of cancer, colorectal cancer does not often show distinctive symptoms until it has progressed to dangerous levels. Symptoms also vary according to where tumors are growing. Cancer in the spacious ascending colon is often first manifested as unexplained anemia: tumors can bleed continuously into the colon, making less iron and therefore less oxygen, available to body cells. Iron deficiency anemia, especially among men and postmenopausal women, is a warning sign for colorectal cancer.

Growths in the more constricted descending colon, however, are experienced as extreme constipation or narrowed stools. Other signs of colorectal cancer that a person may or may not be aware of are blood in the stools (sometimes it is obvious and bright red, sometimes it occurs in invisible, microscopic amounts), lower abdominal pain, a feeling that bowel movements are incomplete, and unintentional weight loss.

Diagnosis

Colorectal cancer is not difficult to diagnose, but it requires some simple tests that many people choose to avoid, even though they are not dangerous or painful. Because of this, only 37% of all colorectal cancers are found before the growths have invaded deeply into the colon wall. Nonetheless, aggressive public information campaigns, more consistent early testing, and better treatment options have resulted in a steady decline of colorectal cancer deaths in the past several years.

Basic screening for colorectal cancer begins with a digital rectal examination (DRE). This procedure, which is the same as that for prostate cancer, reveals masses in the rectum. Fecal occult blood tests, special examinations of stool samples that show the presence of microscopic amounts of blood in the stool, are another early screening technique. Although several conditions can involve blood in the stool, this is a serious sign that must be investigated.

If a DRE reveals an abnormality or stool samples are positive for abnormal levels of blood, the next step is usually a barium enema, which shows through radiographs any particular masses in the colon. A sigmoidoscopy may also be used. This is an exploration of the colon via a small tube with a camera attached. This scope looks for polyps that may have become malignant. The sigmoidoscopy is limited to the sigmoid colon. A full colonoscopy can be performed if tumors are suspected higher up in the structure.

If any test reveals the presence of suspicious polyps, tissue samples must be obtained to examine them for cancerous cells. The advantage of sigmoidoscopies and colonoscopies is that tissue biopsies can be performed at the same time as the initial examination. Although barium enemas are cheaper and easier to perform, a positive test always requires surgery to extract a tissue sample.

A new option, an ultra-fast CT scanner, has been applied to colon screenings. This test is much shorter and more comfortable than other screening techniques, but so far it has been imprecise in providing exact information about the location, size, and depth of possible colorectal cancer growths.

All these screening techniques sound to many people almost worse than having the disease itself. However, the statistics that compare survival rates for people who are diagnosed early compared with those who found their cancer later are a convincing reason to follow the basic guidelines for colorectal cancer screening. The National Cancer Institute recommends that all people over 40 years old should have annual DREs and fecal occult blood tests. People older than 50 should have a sigmoidoscopy every 3 to 5 years. Regular colonoscopies are not recommended unless there is reason to suspect the growth of abnormal tissues higher in the colon.[c]

Staging

If a polyp is found to be cancerous, the next step is to determine how far the cancer has progressed. Several staging methods have been developed to identify the progression of colorectal cancer. Many clinicians use a combination of the TNM system (denoting the size of the *t*umor, *n*odal involvement, and extent of *m*etastasis) with the traditional Stage I through Stage IV system used with many other types of cancer.

- *Stage I* colorectal cancer means that the tumor has not invaded deep layers of the bowel wall, nor has it involved any regional lymph nodes or distant metastasis.

---

[c]Colon cancer (PDQ). National Cancer Institute. Available at: http://cancernet.nci.nih.gov/cgi-bin/srchcgi.exe?DBID=pdq&TYPE=search&UID=208+00008&ZFILE=patient&SFMT=pdq_treatment/1/0/0. Accessed spring 2001.

- *Stage II* colorectal cancer means that the tumor or tumors may have invaded into the muscular wall of the bowel, but without affecting lymph nodes or distant metastasis.

- *Stage III* colorectal cancer means the cancer has affected the entirety of the bowel wall, and may have come in direct contact with other pelvic or abdominal organs. Several regional lymph nodes may have been affected.

- *Stage IV* colorectal cancer means that the tumor or tumors have affected all layers of the bowel wall, many regional lymph nodes are positive for cancer cells, and the cancer has affected distant organs.

Treatment

Treatment of colorectal cancer depends on the stage at which it is identified. Stage I or II cancer is generally treated with surgery to remove the affected section of bowel. The remaining bowel may be sewn together if possible, or the healthy section may be connected to a colostomy bag for exterior storage and disposal of wastes. Colorectal cancers that are treated in Stage I or II show a 90% survival rate.

Stage III colorectal cancer requires surgery to remove the affected length of bowel and chemotherapy to reduce the chance of metastasis through the lymph system.

Stage IV colorectal cancer is treated in much the same way as Stage III, but with more aggressive chemotherapy and radiation to limit growths at distant sites. Stage IV colorectal cancer is generally considered to be practically incurable and has a less than 10% 5-year survival rate.

Massage?

Clients who are fighting colorectal cancer need all the support they can get. Massage can be an important and useful addition to therapy to help balance the challenges of surgery, chemotherapy, and radiation, as long as the cautions that accompany those treatments are respected (see *cancer*, Chapter 11).

Colorectal cancer survivors are good candidates for massage. If they use a colostomy bag, special compensations may be needed for comfort and practicality. The best person to consult in this situation is the client.

Diverticular Disease
Definition: What Is It?

Diverticular disease is a condition of the colon in which the mucosa and submucosa layers of the colon bulge through the outer muscular layer to form a small sac or diverticulum. It happens most often in the descending section or sigmoid bend of the colon. These bulges may become infected, leading to diverticulitis.

Demographics: Who Gets It?

Diverticular disease is a common condition. It affects up to half the U.S. population aged 60 to 80 years and two-thirds or more of all people older than 85 years. Men and women are equally affected.

DIVERTICULAR DISEASE IN BRIEF

What is it?
Diverticulosis is the development of small pouches that protrude from the colon. Diverticulitis is the inflammation that happens when these pouches become infected. Collectively these disorders are known as diverticular disease.

How is it recognized?
Diverticulosis is generally silent or symptomless. When inflammation (diverticulitis) is present, lower left side abdominal pain, cramping, bloating, constipation, or diarrhea may occur.

Is massage indicated or contraindicated?
Deep abdominal massage is locally contraindicated if the client knows diverticula have developed. Acute infection of diverticula systemically contraindicates circulatory massage.

DIVERTICULUM

This is a Latin word from *de-verto*, meaning "to turn aside." Diverticula are byroads or detours in the large intestine.

It is most common in countries where diets are based on animal fats and processed grains. Interestingly, it was first documented in the early 1900s, just when new technology had been developed to remove the bran from wheat and the American diet shifted to rely heavily on low-fiber white flour.

Diverticular disease is rare in countries where the diet is built around whole grains, fruits, and vegetables.

Etiology: What Happens?

Diverticula form during a special type of smooth muscle contraction in the large intestine called *segmentation*. These contractions are very strong, but without adequate bulk (supplied by soluble and insoluble fiber) to press against, the pressure causes colon walls to bulge. The mucosa and submucosa of the colon protrude right through the outer muscular layer to form small sacs, or diverticula. These sacs can be filled with fecal matter and bacteria, and the potential for infection is high (Fig. 7-4). About 20% of the people diagnosed with diverticulosis go on to develop diverticulitis, or inflammation of the diverticula.

Most diverticula form in the sigmoid flexure or descending colon, but they have been recorded throughout the alimentary canal, all the way up to the esophagus. They can range from about the size of a kernel of corn to the size of a walnut or even larger.

Signs and Symptoms

Symptoms of diverticulosis may be nonexistent. When infection is present, however, symptoms include nausea, fever, cramping, and severe pain on the lower left side of the abdomen. Diarrhea and/or constipation may also occur. Symptoms of diverticulitis often have a sudden onset and become rapidly worse, but some people experience several days of mild discomfort before severe infection begins.

Complications

Complications of diverticulitis are rare, but they can be serious enough to become life-threatening in a short time. They can include the following:

- *Bleeding.* Sometimes capillaries get stretched over the dome of the protrusion and may tear open and bleed into the colon.

- *Abscesses.* Infected diverticula may develop localized collections of pus and dead white blood cells. If any of these abscesses rupture, their contents may be released into the peritoneum, causing *peritonitis* (this chapter).

- *Perforation.* Diverticula may tear open and release their contents into the peritoneum. This is a medical emergency and requires immediate care.

- *Blockage.* The accumulation of scar tissue where diverticula have formed and become infected may block the colon. A partial blockage requires medical attention but is not an emergency; a total blockage requires immediate intervention.

- *Fistulae.* Areas in the digestive tract that are damaged by inflammation have the potential to become abnormally joined to other abdominal or pelvic organs. Small passageways or *fistulae* may develop between the two organs, allowing the passage of fecal matter into spaces where it does not belong. Diverticula may do this with the urinary bladder, small intestine, or uterus.

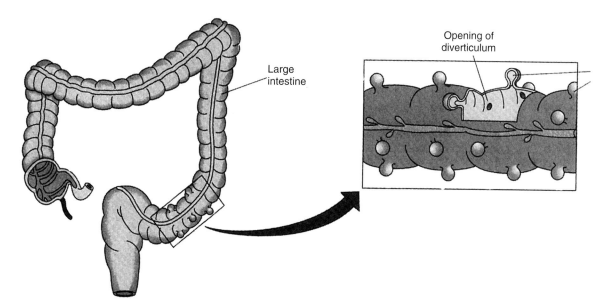

Large intestine

Opening of diverticulum

Figure 7-4. Diverticulosis, diverticulitis

Diverticular disease has not been seen to raise the risk of developing *colorectal cancer*, but this condition can make colorectal cancer more difficult to identify early. Therefore, diverticular disease patients need to take extra care to have regular screenings for colorectal cancer (this chapter).

DIVERTICULOSIS: CASE HISTORY
Cathy, 50 Years Old
"Try warm prune juice."

Cathy is a 50-year-old speech and language pathologist with a number of problems involving a hyperreactive immune system. She suspects she may have rheumatoid arthritis and/or lupus. Although she has never been formally diagnosed for either condition, her blood tests indicate that she is prone to autoimmune dysfunction. In addition to systemic arthritis, Cathy has spondylosis, a degeneration of the articular facets between L5 and S1 resulting in hypermobility of the low back, chronic pain, and a fragile state of balance that is easily disrupted by a minor force such as a cough or sneeze. The following is her story.

My husband's mother had colon cancer. We knew what it was like to have to deal with this disease, so last August we all got checked. I had a colorectal scope that revealed a very large diverticulum—the doctor said it was big enough that he could double up the scope hose into it. I had no pain, and there was no infection. I didn't think much more about it.

For the last 10 years I've had problems with bowel movements, just being regular. I didn't think much of it. I had a hysterectomy 5 years ago and at that time I asked what would be the best way to become regular. I was told to take warm prune juice. I did it, and that took care of the problem for quite a while.

I didn't really know there was anything wrong until last April—Good Friday, as a matter of fact. It was a day worse than most days at work. I didn't have time to eat properly, so I snacked on graham crackers all day. By 2:00 I was just about bent over double—still charting patients, mind you, but bent over double. I just couldn't get any relief.

I continued to work until 6:00, at which point I was just about screaming. (But, of course, not telling anybody.) I went to the after-hours clinic, and they gave me prescription-strength Zantac and an antibiotic. Within half an hour the pain went away—or at least resolved to the point where I could stand myself.

Having had that experience, I decided I better see a gastroenterologist. I had the upper and lower scope—a colonoscopy and endoscopy, and that's when they found the diverticulum again, although there was no longer any infection.

I was diagnosed with diverticulosis along with "chronic inflammatory disease," which may go along with my generally hyperactive immune system.

These days I stick with a low-fat diet, and I drink *lots* of water—64 ounces a day, minimum. I eat small meals. I take Zantac every night, along with Relafen for arthritis pain, and I've never had another episode. I receive massage regularly. Deep psoas work can often help to relieve my lower back pain, but I can't do it every time—some days I'm just too tender.

Treatment

Treatment of diverticulosis alone is not usually necessary, because the symptoms are so mild or do not exist. Although the diverticula are not reversible, further growths can be prevented with changes toward a higher-fiber diet and exercise.

Treatment for diverticulitis starts with antibiotics and a strictly controlled diet. If substantial tissue damage has occurred, including a bowel obstruction, uncontrolled bleeding, perforation, large abscesses, or fistulae, surgery may be performed to resolve the situation.

Massage?

A client probably will not know if he or she has diverticulosis unless the colon has been scanned for some other reason. If the condition has already been diagnosed, deep abdominal work should be conducted with caution; the muscular wall of the colon is already structurally impaired. Acute infection of diverticula, identified by local pain with fever, chills, nausea, and diarrhea or constipation, systemically contraindicates circulatory bodywork.

IRRITABLE BOWEL SYNDROME IN BRIEF

What is it?
Irritable bowel syndrome (IBS) is a collection of signs and symptoms that indicate a functional problem with the digestive system, specifically with the colon. It is aggravated by stress and diet.

How is it recognized?
The symptoms of IBS include alternating bouts of constipation and diarrhea, bloating or abdominal distension, and moderate to severe crampy abdominal pain that is relieved with defecation.

Is massage indicated or contraindicated?
IBS indicates massage, as long as bodywork does not exacerbate symptoms.

Irritable Bowel Syndrome
Definition: What Is It?

IBS is a recently acknowledged and little understood condition involving digestive system dysfunction without structural changes. It has also been known as *spastic colon*, *irritable colon*, *mucus colitis*, and *functional bowel syndrome*.

Demographics: Who Gets It?

IBS statistics vary, but most agree that this is a relatively common condition. Twenty to thirty percent of the U.S. population may have IBS symptoms at some point in their lives. Women are affected about 3 times more often than men. IBS accounts for some 5 million doctor visits each year.

Etiology: What Happens?

In a normal colon, fecal matter is squeezed and compacted while needed water and salts are reabsorbed back into the bloodstream. Material moves back and forth through the colon, but eventually strong contractions move the formed stools into the rectum where they are stored until another bout of strong colon contractions moves them out of the body altogether.

The development of IBS symptoms probably varies by individual, but some general observations have determined that the digestive tract as a whole and the colon in particular are hyperreactive in IBS patients. That is, small stimuli can create major contractions for no discernible reason. In IBS peristalsis, which should be smooth and rhythmic, becomes uncoordinated and irregular.

IBS very often goes hand-in-hand with anxiety and stress. Most people with this condition report flare-ups in conjunction with threatening situations (e.g., job interviews, exams, major life changes). The development of IBS probably has little to do with the presence of stress per se, and more to do with how the individual handles it. While some people lose sleep under stress, IBS patients lose coordinated bowel function.

Signs and Symptoms

IBS can manifest in a variety of ways: cramps, abdominal pain, gas, bloating, constipation and diarrhea (usually in cycles), and a frequent need to defecate, although a feeling of incomplete evacuation is often present. Abdominal pain is usually relieved after bowel movements.

It is important to note that the changes brought about by IBS are purely functional; no structural anomalies develop because of this disorder. For this reason, if a person with IBS develops a fever or has blood in the stool, IBS is *not* the cause, and this is reason for concern.

Diagnosis

IBS can range from being occasionally inconvenient to being severely debilitating, but it is not a life-threatening disease. Its symptoms can mimic several serious digestive system conditions, however. In particular, *colorectal cancer*, *ulcerative colitis*, and *Crohn's disease* (all in this

---

IRRITABLE BOWEL SYNDROME
Debbie, 29 Years Old
"It's just something you ate."

I had my first attack of IBS in January 1991. I woke up out of a dead sleep; I thought I had appendicitis or something. I had diarrhea, I was throwing up, I had never hurt that bad. There was no warning, no build-up, it was just there. I hurt so bad I passed out. My husband called the ambulance and I went to the hospital. In the ambulance they asked about my sunburn—I was completely covered with a red rash. The rash only happened the first time.

At the hospital they gave me something through an IV that was supposed to coat my stomach. They said I probably had food poisoning.

Four months later, it happened again. I woke up out of a dead sleep, and ended up in the hospital. Four months later, there I was again. It was so painful, I was really noisy, but I didn't care. They took a bunch of blood samples, but they didn't show anything. "It's just something you ate," they kept saying. It got to where they would recognize me coming in, and know exactly what to do.

When the attacks started happening more and more frequently, I finally went to see a gastroenterologist. He said, "Write down everything you eat, and call me from the hospital next time it happens." I knew it wasn't anything I was eating—I'd get attacks after a bowl of cereal! And I didn't want another attack to happen. People said it was lactose intolerance, but I have milk all the time—my attacks didn't happen all the time.

The next time was 2 months later. I was in the hospital, and they decided to do a blood gas test—they have to stick the needle into an artery to do that. It is no fun. I couldn't have any medication, I was supposed to lie completely still. Well, they couldn't get the needle in. My gastroenterologist said, "If you can't get the blood gas, I won't see you again." That's when I switched to a different doctor.

I told my new doctor what was happening, and he scheduled me for a colonoscopy right away. He was looking for ulcers or tumors or something, but there was nothing, and he diagnosed me with IBS. He prescribed 25 mg of amitriptyline, a mild anti-depressant, and it cleared right up.

The only problem with the medicine was that I wanted to get pregnant again. I tried to go off it, but found I couldn't go more than one day without another attack.

It was only after all this that I was finally told that IBS is a stress-related disease. I had sort of noticed a pattern: every time I had company, I would have an attack. Whenever my sister came to visit, she would stay with my son while my husband would take me to the hospital. Every time I went on vacation, I'd get so stressed because I didn't know where the hospital was, and sure enough, I'd need to go to one. My doctor said, "Get biofeedback." Well, I'd never even heard of biofeedback, and my insurance company wouldn't cover it. I didn't know what to do.

When I went through a divorce, I stopped taking the amitriptyline, and I didn't have any more major attacks. I went to counseling for a long time to help with other things, and now I'm taking a different anti-depressant. I haven't seen my gastroenterologist in over a year.

These days I will occasionally have a mild episode. Really greasy food tends to aggravate my stomach. I have found that if I can wake up before my stomach-aches get really bad, and if I can make myself breathe slow and deep, I can make them go away—it takes about 20 minutes. But if I get all worked up and I lose control, they just get worse and worse, and I have to go to the hospital. I haven't had to do that for a long time.

chapter) must be eliminated as possibilities. Other GI tract problems that can look like IBS include parasitic infestations (i.e., Giardia), food allergies, and chronic infections.

No definitive test identifies IBS; it is diagnosed in the absence of other conditions that may cause similar symptoms. Fortunately, with the advent of colonoscopes, this is not difficult to do. A colonoscope can confirm that no structural change or damage to the colon has occurred, and it may also show the characteristic uncoordinated contraction of the colon to aid in diagnosis.

Treatment

Treatment of IBS depends on the individual. The first recourse is to consider dietary and stress factors. Nicotine, caffeine, alcohol, and dairy products have been found to be particularly irritating, but no particular food or drink is a definitive trigger for IBS attacks for all patients. Some doctors recommend fiber supplementation; the addition of bulk to the diet can fill the colon more completely and help to limit spasm.

Drug intervention usually involves anti-spasmodics, anti-diarrheals, antacids, and antidepressants. Although these medicines may offer some relief, IBS is generally considered to be a life-long condition, and so patients are encouraged to find their own best ways to cope through dietary changes, therapy, and relaxation techniques.

Massage?

Massage is useful for many IBS patients, if the individual welcomes this kind of stimulus. It is important to treat these clients very conservatively, especially with any mechanical work around the abdomen. Many of them respond well to the autonomic balancing that bodywork provides.

ULCERATIVE COLITIS IN BRIEF

What is it?
Ulcerative colitis is a condition in which the mucosal layer of the colon becomes inflamed and develops shallow ulcers.

How is it recognized?
Symptoms of acute ulcerative colitis include abdominal cramping pain, chronic diarrhea, blood and pus in stools, weight loss, and mild fever.

Is massage indicated or contraindicated?
Acute ulcerative colitis contraindicates circulatory massage at least locally; the presence of fever systemically contraindicates massage. In subacute situations gentle abdominal massage may be helpful, but only within the tolerance of the client.

Ulcerative Colitis
Definition: What Is It?

Ulcerative colitis is a disease of the colon involving progressive inflammation and ulceration. The inflammation is limited to the large intestine, however, which distinguishes it from *Crohn's disease* (this chapter), another condition labeled as an inflammatory bowel disease (see *Watch for This: Crohn's Disease and Ulcerative Colitis*).

Demographics: Who Gets It?

Ulcerative colitis affects men and women about equally. Most patients are diagnosed between 16 and 40 years of age. It is estimated that about 1.5 million people in the United States have ulcerative colitis.

Etiology: What Happens?

The initial cause of ulcerative colitis is a subject of some debate. Although no definitive trigger has been identified, most researchers now agree that it is an autoimmune condition. It occurs in unpredictable flares followed by periods of remission: a pattern similar to other autoimmune conditions like *lupus* (Chapter 5) or *rheumatoid arthritis* Chapter 2).

Ulcerative colitis begins in the rectum when immune system cells attack the most superficial layer of the colon. The resulting inflammation kills tissue and results in the formation of shallow ulcers (open sores that may never fully heal). Colon function is extremely limited, and the patient experiences chronic diarrhea. The sores may become infected, leading to the release of blood and pus in the stools.

Ulcerative colitis is a progressive disease. Although it begins in the rectum, it may spread to affect the whole colon. Lesions are continuous, however, and do not appear in the unpredictable patchy patterns seen with Crohn's disease.

Signs and Symptoms

Symptoms of ulcerative colitis depend largely on how much of the bowel is affected: the greater the extent of inflammation, the worse the symptoms. During flare-ups the primary symptoms include painful, chronic diarrhea with blood and pus in the stools. Abdominal cramping, loss of appetite, and mild fever may also occur during acute episodes.

The inflammatory nature of this disease often affects other systems in the body. A person with ulcerative colitis may also experience liver inflammation (see *hepatitis*, this chapter) *arthritis, osteoporosis* (Chapter 2), *anemia* from blood loss (Chapter 4), and *kidney stones* (Chapter 9) from the disruption in electrolyte balance and chronic dehydration that accompany long-term diarrhea.

Between acute episodes, the ulcerative colitis patient may experience only minimal abdominal pain but must be careful to avoid any triggers of abdominal cramping or discomfort.

Diagnosis

Ulcerative colitis is diagnosed through a variety of tests. Blood tests show signs of anemia and infection, and stool samples reveal whether rectal bleeding is taking place. A colonoscopy shows specific sites of ulcers, which may then be biopsied to examine them for signs of infection or cancer.

It is important to reach a clear diagnosis for ulcerative colitis, because the other two conditions that its symptoms sometimes mimic require different courses of treatment. The two conditions occasionally confused with ulcerative colitis are *irritable bowel syndrome* and *Crohn's disease* (this chapter).

Complications

In addition to the disorders listed among symptoms, patients with ulcerative colitis that involves the whole colon are at significantly more risk of developing *colorectal cancer* (this chapter) than the general population. In some situations the colon may swell up to the point that it is in danger of perforation or rupture. This is called *toxic megacolon* and is a medical emergency.

Treatment

Treatment options for ulcerative colitis begin with a class of medications that lessen the severity of flare-ups and prolong periods of remission. If these do not control the inflammation satisfactorily, corticosteroids may be prescribed for short periods. Immune suppressive drugs and, surprisingly, nicotine patches have also been found to improve symptoms.

If a patient does not get relief with these options, or if inflammation of the colon has progressed to a dangerous degree, surgery is the only permanent solution for ulcerative colitis. Anywhere between 20 and 40% of all ulcerative colitis patients eventually require surgery. Several surgical options have been developed, but all of them involve the removal of the affected section of bowel. External colostomy bags, internal colostomy bags, or the joining of the small intestine to the muscles of the rectum are options for ways to replace the main functions of the colon.

Massage?

Ulcerative colitis contraindicates local mechanical, circulatory massage. Deep abdominal work is inappropriate for a client with ulcerative colitis in any stage; so is any kind of work that reflexively increases blood flow to the pelvic cavity. Massage is systemically contraindicated in the presence of fever. In periods of remission *gentle* massage to the abdomen may be useful, within the client's tolerance, and any other work to balance the autonomic nervous system is highly recommended.

Disorders of the Accessory Organs

CIRRHOSIS IN BRIEF

What is it?
Cirrhosis is a condition in which normal liver cells become disorganized and dysfunctional; many of them are replaced or crowded out by scar tissue. Cirrhosis is often the final stage of chronic or acute liver diseases.

How is it recognized?
Early symptoms of cirrhosis include loss of appetite, nausea, vomiting, and weight loss. Later complications may include muscle wasting, jaundice, ascites, vomiting blood, and mental and personality changes.

Is massage indicated or contraindicated?
Advanced cirrhosis involves difficulties with fluid flow in the body. Bodywork that challenges this ability may not be appropriate. Some cirrhosis patients experience muscle wasting as their ability to metabolize proteins diminishes. Exercise and physical therapy are recommended for these patients for maintenance of strength and function, and massage as part of a health care team may have a role in this process as well.

Cirrhosis
Definition: What Is It?

Cirrhosis is a result of a disease process, rather than a disease itself; it involves the crowding out and replacement of healthy liver cells with non-functioning scar tissue. Cirrhosis can interfere with virtually every function of the liver, with potentially fatal repercussions.

Demographics: Who Gets It?

Cirrhosis and other connected liver diseases affect some 25 million Americans per year, and it kills between 25 and 35 thousand of them. It is the eighth leading cause of death in the United States.

Etiology: What Happens?

The liver is composed of highly organized layers of epithelial hepatocytes: cells that produce myriad vital chemicals for metabolism and survival. Bile is produced here, which helps to metabolize fats; other enzymes that metabolize proteins and carbohydrates are manufactured here as well. Clotting factors, proteins that maintain the proper balance of tissue fluid, and cells that help filter and neutralize toxins and hormones are all produced in the liver.

Under normal circumstances the liver is a remarkably forgiving organ with great powers of regeneration. However, some situations involving chronic, long-term irritation or infection will suppress the regeneration of healthy, organized cells and stimulate the proliferation of extracellular matrix (i.e., collagen and other substances that are meant just to provide structural support for the active hepatocytes). When this happens the tiny channels that are meant to direct fluid flow to the appropriate vessels become blocked and the liver, the largest gland in the body, becomes congested with blood, lymph, bile, and other fluids.

Cirrhotic deposits of scar tissue are interspersed with small nodules of functioning cells, giving the liver a characteristically knobby, bumpy appearance, hence the nickname "hobnailed liver." In the early stages cirrhosis causes the liver to enlarge. As the connective tissue contracts, the liver sometimes returns to a normal size although not to normal function.

Causes

Until recently alcoholism (see *chemical dependency*, Chapter 3) was the leading cause of cirrhosis in the United States. Recently alcoholism was displaced by *hepatitis C* (this chapter) as the leading cause. Cirrhosis can also arise from types B, D, drug-related, and autoimmune hepatitis. Any obstruction of the bile duct can cause cirrhosis, including *gallstones* (this chapter) or pancreatic tumors. Some inherited liver diseases can also cause it. Long-term exposure to environmental toxins can contribute to cirrhosis, as can *congestive heart failure* (Chapter 4).

Signs and Symptoms

Cirrhosis is often a silent disease until it is quite advanced. Early symptoms are vague and can be attributed to any number of other common disorders. They include nausea, vomiting, weight loss, and the development of red patches on the skin of the upper body. At this time blood tests may be normal; no clear signs may point directly to cirrhosis. Later symptoms are usually identified by the complications discussed below.

Complications

As the liver loses more and more function, complications arise according to the parts of the liver affected and the speed of progression. The complications each patient experiences may vary widely; it all depends on which part or parts of the liver are under attack. At the center of several complications is a condition called *portal hypertension*. This happens when the liver becomes so congested that it cannot freely accept blood delivered from the digestive and accessory organs via the portal system, and pressure accumulates in the portal system veins. Other complications arise as the liver simply no longer produces enough vital blood components or adequately filters and neutralizes toxic materials.

- *Splenomegaly (enlarged spleen).* The spleen enlarges because it cannot drain through the portal vein. The danger with splenomegaly is that when fluid backs up in this organ, the risk of rupture and internal hemorrhage is high.

- *Ascites.* When pressure in the portal system increases, plasma seeps out of the veins and lymphatic vessels into the peritoneal space, causing the abdominal distension known as ascites (Fig. 7-5). The bacteria that normally inhabit the GI tract may seep out and set up an infection in this fluid, causing spontaneous bacterial *peritonitis* (this chapter), a life-threatening infection.

- *Internal varices.* Pressure in abdominal veins grows as fluid backs up through the system. This can lead to internal venous distensions and varicosities, especially in the esophagus and stomach. Varicose veins can hemorrhage during vomiting, leading to bloody vomit, shock, or death. Ruptured varices are the second leading cause of death by cirrhosis.

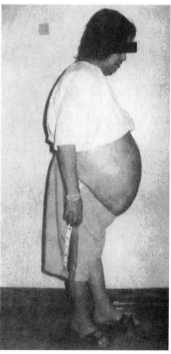

Figure 7-5. Cirrhosis can lead to abdominal distension called ascites

- *Bleeding, bruising.* When the liver no longer produces adequate clotting factors, the ability to heal from minor injury is severely impaired. Cirrhosis patients may bruise extensively and bleed for abnormally long periods.

- *Muscle wasting.* When the enzymes that aid in protein metabolism are in short supply, a cirrhosis patient may experience progressive atrophy or wasting of his or her skeletal muscles. Physical therapy and exercise are often recommended for patients with this problem to minimize permanent loss of bulk and function.

- *Jaundice.* Bilirubin (a by-product of the recycling of dead red blood cells) is produced in the spleen. It is meant to be recycled in the liver to be a component of bile. When cirrhosis interferes with this process, water-soluble components of bilirubin accumulate in the bloodstream. Bilirubin is strongly pigmented, and it can turn the sclera of the eyes and the skin a yellowish color. It can also cause rashes and itching, as some people have an extreme reaction to this unfamiliar chemical in their skin.

- *Systemic edema.* Albumin, one of the critical proteins for maintaining fluid balance in the body, is significantly lowered in advanced cirrhosis. Without albumin, the body cannot maintain proper fluid levels, and edema accumulates systemically in all interstitial spaces (see *edema*, Chapter 5).

- *Hormone disruption.* Men with cirrhosis have livers that no longer inactivate their normal low levels of estrogen; feminizing characteristics such as breast development, loss of chest hair, impotence, and atrophy of the testicles soon follow. For women, hormonal changes include the cessation of periods, infertility, and the growth of body hair. Both men and women with cirrhosis can expect decreased sex drives.

- *Encephalopathy.* When cirrhosis is very advanced, the detoxifying agents in the liver are out of commission. No more protection from the chemicals (ammonia, for instance) that are produced whenever protein is metabolized is provided. Furthermore, the blood–brain barrier that usually keeps the central nervous system safe becomes much less effective with cirrhosis. Metabolic toxins accumulate in the blood and eventually cause brain damage. Symptoms here include somnolence, confusion, tremors, hallucinations, and even coma and death. Up to 70% of all cirrhosis patients experience some level of encephalopathy.

- *Kidney failure.* Advanced cirrhosis can reduce blood flow to the kidneys, resulting in kidney failure. *Hepatorenal syndrome* is an emergency situation that requires a liver transplant for a person to survive.

Treatment

The prognosis for someone in the early stages of cirrhosis caused by alcoholism is excellent *if* the damage can be stopped. That is the main treatment objective: *stop the damage.* Medication is sometimes administered to counteract the complications of the disease: diuretics for edema, antacids for intestinal discomfort, and levulose (an undigestible sugar) to bind with ammonia so that it can be excreted. Vitamins are recommended to guard against malnutrition. Cirrhosis due to hepatitis is treated with interferon as an anti-viral measure. Steroids for inflammation due to autoimmune hepatitis are occasionally prescribed.

New advances with transplant surgery are making it possible to restore normal health to people in end-stage cirrhosis; about 4500 liver transplants are performed yearly in the United States. Transplants are recommended for alcoholic patients only when they have not suffered extensive damage to other organs and when they are in long-term recovery (6 months or more). The rising numbers of hepatitis C patients in end-stage liver failure has resulted in longer waiting lists for liver transplants. About 15% of all people waiting for liver transplants die before they receive an organ.

Massage?

Advanced cirrhosis contraindicates rigorous circulatory massage, because the circulatory system is simply not equipped to handle the changes this work produces. Non-circulatory work may be helpful and supportive, and massage with the goal of helping to maintain muscle health may also be appropriate. Bodywork for cirrhosis patients should be administered as part of an integrated health care effort.

Gallstones

Definition: What Is It?

Gallstones are crystallized deposits of cholesterol and other substances that collect in the gallbladder. They may become lodged in the duct system that connects the accessory organs to the rest of the digestive tract.

Demographics: Who Gets It?

Gallstones are a fairly common condition, affecting some 20 million people in the United States; 1 to 3% of all affected people have symptoms within a given year.

Women are far more prone to developing gallstones than men; they outnumber men by about 2:1. Some races show a predilection for gallstones. Northern Europeans, Native Americans, and Latin Americans all have higher incidences of gallstones than other population groups. Other contributing factors for developing gallstones are discussed shortly.

> ## GALLSTONES IN BRIEF
>
> **What are they?**
> Gallstones are crystallized formations of cholesterol or bile pigments in the gallbladder. They can be as small as grains of sand or as large as a golf ball.
>
> **How are they recognized?**
> Most gallstones do not cause symptoms. When they do, pain that may last several hours develops in the upper right side of the abdomen. Pain may refer to the back between scapula and the right shoulder. Gallstones stuck in the ducts of the biliary system may cause jaundice or pancreatitis.
>
> **Is massage indicated or contraindicated?**
> Silent (symptomless) gallstones have little impact on overall health and function, so massage for these clients is certainly appropriate, although draining strokes over the liver and costal angle are not a good idea. Clients recovering from gallbladder surgery may need some special considerations (see *postoperative conditions,* Chapter 11). A client with a history of gallstones but no present symptoms is a fine candidate for massage.

Etiology: What Happens?

Bile is produced in the liver and delivered to the gallbladder through the hepatic duct and the cystic duct (Fig. 7-6). When a person eats a high-fat meal, hormonal commands cause the gallbladder to release its contents into the cystic duct. The bile then flows into the common bile duct, into the small intestine. Pancreatic secretions also use the common bile duct for entrance to the small intestine.

The purpose of bile is to hold particles of fat in tiny, discreet pieces so that they can be absorbed into the lacteals: lymphatic projections in the intestinal villi. Without bile, fat particles tend to stick together in indigestible clumps. This reduces access to important fat-soluble vitamins and nutrients.

TROUBLE-MAKING CHOLESTEROL

When cholesterol and other substances solidify in the liver or gallbladder, they can block tubes and cause a great deal of trouble. The vocabulary for various cholesterol-stone problems is interesting, but of little impact to the decision-making process for massage therapists:

* The technical term for gallbladder is *cholecyst*, because it is a cyst (holding tank) that collects, among other things, cholesterol.
* The formation of tiny crystals or stones in the gallbladder itself is called *cholelithiasis*
* Inflammation of the gallbladder from having a stone get stuck is called *cholecystitis*.
* When stones become lodged in the common bile duct, the condition is called *choledocholithiasis*.
* Inflammation of any of the ducts in the biliary system (the exocrine ducts of the liver, gallbladder, and pancreas) is called *cholangitis*.

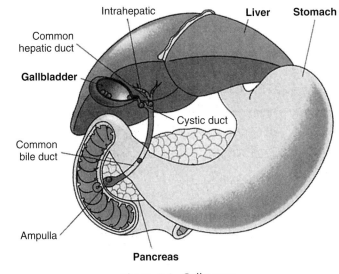

Figure 7-6. Gallstones

Bile is primarily made up of water, bile salts (which help in fat digestion), bilirubin from recycled red blood cells, and cholesterol, which is filtered out of the bloodstream by the liver. When either cholesterol or bilirubin occur in higher than normal concentrations in bile, they can precipitate out of the liquid to become tiny granules called "bile sludge" or larger stones.

Most gallstones (80 to 90%) are composed of cholesterol. The others are made of bilirubin, the coloring agent for feces. Bilirubin stones are also called pigment stones. They are usually a sign of some type of blood dysfunction that causes premature destruction of red blood cells, resulting in abnormally high levels of bilirubin in the blood and in the liver.

Contributing Factors:

Cholesterol stones are the most common type of gallstones. Several factors can increase the risk of developing cholesterol stones, including the following:

* *Obesity.* Obesity reduces the amount of bile salts in bile, resulting in high levels of cholesterol.

* *Estrogen.* Estrogen tends to increase the amount of cholesterol in bile while decreasing gallbladder activity, which allows the cholesterol to crystallize. Estrogen levels may be related to pregnancy, birth control pills, or hormone replacement therapy.

* *Race.* Northern Europeans, Native Americans, and Latin Americans have the highest incidence of gallstones of any specific racial group.

* *Gender.* Women with gallstones outnumber men by about 2:1.

* *Age.* The incidence of gallstones rises with age; most gallstone patients are older than 60 years.

* *Cholesterol-lowering drugs.* Drugs that are designed to lower blood cholesterol help to concentrate cholesterol in the gallbladder, increasing the risk of forming stones.

* *Diabetes.* Diabetics have higher levels of triglycerides, which raises the risk for gallstones.

* *Rapid weight loss.* Rapid weight loss causes the liver to metabolize fat for fuel, resulting in higher levels of cholesterol in the bile.

- *Fasting*. Fasting reduces gallbladder emptying, so bile becomes concentrated and cholesterol precipitates out into stones.

Signs and Symptoms

It is estimated that up to 80% of all people who have gallstones experience no symptoms. The only reason a person *would* have symptoms would be if a stone got lodged in the hepatic duct, the cystic duct, or lower down in the common bile duct. In this situation the pain is excruciating and is referred to as "biliary colic." ("Colic" is the spasmodic contraction of involuntary muscle, in this case in the common bile duct.) This extreme local pain often lasts for hours, building to a peak and then gradually subsiding when the stone moves either back into the gallbladder sack or into the duodenum. The pain may be intense enough to induce nausea and vomiting. If the stone gets immovably stuck, the patient may require hospitalization to have it surgically removed.

The gallbladder refers pain between the shoulder blades and over the right shoulder. Although most patients experience pain in the upper right-hand quadrant of the abdomen, some may feel it primarily in the back where, mysteriously, the most gifted massage in the world will not relieve it.

Lose the Gallbladder, Keep the Fat

Bile, manufactured in the liver and stored in the gallbladder, suspends and separates consumed fats in tiny pieces so the body can absorb them in the small intestine. If the gallbladder is removed, then the person has less access to incoming fat. Thus, less fat is absorbed.

Why then do gallbladder surgery patients *not* lose a lot of weight after surgery? (We know they *don't* because if they did, having one's gallbladder taken out would probably beat liposuction as the most popular form of elective surgery!)

It turns out that to *burn* fat that is stored in the body's lipid cells, humans need to *consume* certain kinds of fats that help to soften those lipid cells' membranes. When the gallbladder is removed and a person loses access to incoming nutrition in the form of fats, it actually becomes *harder* to lose weight. This is because the body retains whatever fat is in the lipid cells much more tenaciously. Obesity is a leading risk factor for the formation of gallstones, and gallbladder removal makes it doubly hard to resolve problems with being overweight.

Complications

Gallstones in themselves are not a serious threat, but they can create some unpleasant or even life-threatening complications. The most obvious is an obstruction of the cystic or hepatic duct, which can lead to *jaundice* (this chapter). If the clog is distal to where the pancreas adds its secretions to the common bile duct, the pancreas can also sustain damage from a back-up of its highly corrosive digestive juices; this is acute pancreatitis, and gallstones are the leading cause of this disorder. The pooling of stagnant bile can also lead to infection of the gallbladder, or cholecystitis. It is possible for an infected gallbladder to rupture, releasing its contents and causing *peritonitis* (this chapter).

Treatment

Surgery is the most common intervention to deal with gallstones. The whole gallbladder is removed, thereby preventing the formation of future gallstones. Recent advances in laparoscopic surgery have made it possible to remove the gallbladder using a series of very small incisions instead of through open surgery. This minimizes general trauma to the body and radically reduces recovery time. About half a million gallbladder surgeries are performed every year; 80% are by laparoscopy.

If the gallbladder is removed, the body still produces bile, which drips into the duodenum in a steady trickle rather than being saved for high-fat meals. The only real concern is that the patient may lose some access to important fat-soluble vitamins. Fortunately, digestive supplements can aid in the digestion of fats.

Massage?

Acute biliary colic (a gallbladder attack) contraindicates massage, especially if signs of an infection (fever, chills, sweating) are present. If a client *knows* that he or she has gallstones but they are silent, the costal angle on the right side should be considered a local caution. Otherwise, people with gallstones or people with a history of gallstones or gallbladder surgery are fine candidates for massage.

Hepatitis

Definition: What Is It?

Hepat-itis means *inflamed liver*. It can be caused by drug reactions or exposure to certain toxins, but it is most often one of a variety of viral infections that can mildly or severely impair liver function. Seven types of viral hepatitis have been identified: hepatitis A through G. Hepatitis A, B, and C cause about 90% of all U.S. cases and are the focus of this discussion.

Etiology: What Happens?

Hepatitis A, B, and C all involve viral attacks against liver cells. Each type of virus is unique, however. Exposure to one type of hepatitis does *not* impart immunity to any other type of hepatitis.

Methods of transmission and communicability of each type of virus are discussed in individual sections. Once the virus has gained access to the body, however, it attacks liver cells and stimulates an immune system response. Hepatitis can be identified and diagnosed by the presence of specific antibodies in the blood and also by the presence of specific enzymes that indicate liver damage.

The viral attack on liver cells leads to the characteristic signs and symptoms of liver dysfunction: malaise, fatigue, nausea, and for many patients, *jaundice* (the result of a backup of bilirubin because the liver cannot send it to the gallbladder as usual) (this chapter). Hepatitis infections may be acute or chronic. The severity of symptoms varies widely from one person to another, depending on the phase of the infection, the general health of the patient, and the type of virus involved.

Hepatitis A
What Is it?

This used to be called infectious hepatitis. It is a short, acute infection and usually causes no lasting damage. It creates life-long immunity.

Demographics: Who Gets It?

Hepatitis A occurs among all age groups. Estimates suggest that about 180,000 people in the United States are infected every year. Up to 30% of Americans have antibodies to hepatitis A, showing that they have been exposed to this virus.

Risk groups for hepatitis A include travelers to places where water contamination is likely, day care workers, IV drug users, and people who have unprotected sex with hepatitis A patients.

Communicability

Hepatitis A virus concentrates in the feces of an infected person; therefore, it is most easily transmitted through oral-fecal contact, often through contaminated food or water.

Hepatitis A is the reason for those huge signs about hand washing in restaurant bathrooms. Raw or undercooked shellfish grown in contaminated water can spread the disease to humans.

Oral-fecal contact is the most common transmission route for hepatitis A. It can also be carried in the blood and body fluids, so shared drug needles or unprotected sex with hepatitis A patients can also spread the infection.

Signs and Symptoms

Symptoms of hepatitis A are similar to those of the rest of the hepatitis family, but they tend to be the most severe and the shortest in duration. They include weakness, nausea, fever, anorexia, and possible jaundice that is accompanied by dark urine and pale stools. This virus incubates for 2 to 6 weeks before symptoms appear, but it is contagious during this period. Once symptoms appear the virus is present in the system for another 2 to 3 weeks, although a person may not feel fully restored to health for up to 6 months.

Treatment

Treatment of hepatitis A is a combination of rest, fluids, and good sense. About 99% of hepatitis A patients recover without medical intervention. In some cases gamma globulin shots are recommended to provide short-term protection when a specific source of infection has been identified, such as a contaminated restaurant. A vaccine against this infection is available for people traveling, working, or living in places where the virus is prevalent.

Massage?

Acute hepatitis contraindicates circulatory massage. The liver is a keystone for fluid management in the body. To push more fluid through a system that is not functioning well could lead to some serious repercussions. Non-circulatory techniques, however, may be welcome and very supportive during a long recuperation.

Hepatitis B
What Is It?

The hepatitis B virus works very differently from hepatitis A. It causes long-term chronic infections with much subtler symptoms. Hepatitis B carries risks and possible complications that are much more serious than those associated with hepatitis A.

Most people who are exposed to hepatitis B recover fully with immunity and no serious problems. About 5% of those exposed develop chronic infections and may be long-term carriers of the virus. Within that group of patients, the risk of developing other liver diseases later in life is higher than that of the general population.

Demographics: Who Gets It?

High-risk groups for hepatitis B include any person who comes in contact with someone else's body fluids. This includes people who live or work with hepatitis B patients, anyone who has unprotected sex with a hepatitis B patient, infants born to hepatitis-B–positive mothers, immigrants from countries where hepatitis B is prevalent, and IV drug users.

Statistics vary, but estimates for hepatitis B infections range from 150,000 to 200,000 new cases per year in the United States. Most new cases are among people between 15 and 39 years old, and the vast majority of those are among newly sexually active teenagers. Between 1 and 1.25 million Americans currently carry the hepatitis B virus in a chronic infection; all these people are capable of spreading the virus to others.

Communicability

Hepatitis B is communicable primarily through body fluids. It does *not* appear to spread through the digestive system, like hepatitis A. Hepatitis B virus is most densely found in blood, semen, and vaginal fluid, but viral particles may also be found in saliva.

Unlike many pathogens, this virus is quite sturdy and can remain viable for up to 7 days outside a human body. Very little exposure may spread the infection; 500 million viral particles can be found in a teaspoon of blood from a person with an active hepatitis B virus infection. In the same amount of blood from a person with a late-stage HIV infection, only 15 to 20 million HIV particles will be found. For this reason, it is especially important to sterilize any instruments that come in contact with human blood; tattoo needles, body piercing equipment, acupuncture needles, and professional medical and dental tools all fall into this category.

Infants born to mothers with hepatitis B are at particularly high risk for infection; 90% of all such infants become infected. If they are not treated immediately, most infants with hepatitis B will develop chronic liver disease early in life.

Signs and Symptoms

Symptoms of hepatitis B are basically the same as those of hepatitis A, but the onset is slower and they last for a much longer time. The incubation period is 2 to 6 months in this case (it is contagious during all that time), and it can stay in the system for months or years. The severity and duration of the viral attack is largely determined by the general health of the infected person. Long-term carriers of hepatitis B may have no symptoms at all.

Complications

About 5% of the people who get hepatitis B develop chronic infections. Chronic liver inflammation can lead to the development of varicose veins on the stomach and esophagus, which may rupture and bleed. *Cirrhosis* (this chapter) is another possibility. Statistically, people with chronic hepatitis B infections also have higher risks of developing liver cancer.

Treatment

Hepatitis B treatments are only sporadically successful. Interferon is effective slightly more than half the time, but it carries many unpleasant and even dangerous side effects. Another anti-viral agent, lamivudine, is better tolerated by most patients but tends to be less effective against viral activity.

Prevention

A vaccine series against hepatitis B has been developed. People who work in hospitals, prisons, and long-term care facilities are often required to get it. People traveling to high-risk areas or people living with an infected person are also targeted. The hepatitis B vaccine series is now considered by some to be part of routine pediatric care to guard against the spread of the disease when children become sexually active.

Massage?

Hepatitis B contraindicates circulatory massage in the acute stage, when the liver is already overtaxed with cellular damage. If a client has a chronic version of the disease, the decision about circulatory massage must be determined based on that person's overall health and resiliency. The benefits include improved immune system activity, restoration of autonomic balance, and so on, but the risks could involve stressing a weak system that is incapable of adapting to the changes circulatory massage brings about. Non-circulatory massage may provide many of the benefits while minimizing the possible risks.

Clients who have recovered from hepatitis B infections with no other problems are fine candidates for massage.

Hepatitis C
What is it?

Before hepatitis viruses D, E, F, and G were discovered, this disorder was called hepatitis non-A non-B. Although it had been investigated since the late 1970s, the causative virus was not identified until 1989.

Like hepatitis B, hepatitis C causes long-term chronic infections. Unlike hepatitis B, however, the percentage of hepatitis C patients who develop long-term problems is very high. Only 5 to 25% recover spontaneously; the other 75 to 85% of hepatitis C patients experience a chronic infection. Of those with chronic hepatitis C, about 15% will develop cirrhosis within 10 to 20 years, and the risk of liver cancer is much higher than that for the general population. The presence of other illnesses, specifically HIV or alcoholism, raises the risk of complications from long-term hepatitis C infections.

Hepatitis C is estimated to cause about 8,000 to 10,000 deaths per year.

Demographics: Who Gets It?

Hepatitis C is something of a silent epidemic. Although many people have never heard of it, this virus is the most common blood-borne infection in the United States. It is carried by close to 4 million Americans today.

The primary risk group for new hepatitis C infections is IV drug users. An estimated 38,000 new infections occur among this group every year. Happily, that number is on the decline; statistics in the early 1990s were much more severe.

Another risk group for hepatitis C infections is people who received transfusions of blood or blood clotting factors before 1987. Since then, improved screening techniques have made the public blood supply much safer.

Communicability

Blood-to-blood contact is the most reliable way to transmit hepatitis C, although in about 30% of all cases the mode of transmission is unclear. Blood-to-blood contact can come about in the form of shared drug needles, accidental needle sticks in medical settings, or contaminated medical, tattoo, or body-piercing instruments.

Signs and Symptoms

Symptoms of hepatitis C are weakness, fever, nausea, and possible jaundice, but they are generally milder than those seen with hepatitis A or B. Many people may never know that they have been infected with the hepatitis C virus.

Treatment

Treatment of hepatitis C is good sense (rest, fluids, and good nutrition) and close monitoring to watch for signs of complications. No vaccine has been developed against this virus. Interferon and ribavirin may be prescribed separately or together to try to control the severity of the viral attack. Almost half of all liver transplants performed in the United States every year are to correct the damage brought about by hepatitis C infections.

Massage?

As with other hepatitis infections, the presence of acute disease contraindicates massage. When the infection is chronic, judgments must be made based on the overall health and circulatory resiliency of the client.

Other Types of Hepatitis

Hepatitis may be caused by factors other than viruses A, B, and C. Hepatitis D is an incomplete virus that can only work in the presence of hepatitis B. Hepatitis E, F, and G are rare viruses that are uncommon in the United States.

It is also possible for other viruses to cause liver inflammation, often as a complication of a different primary infection. Epstein–Barr virus (see *mononucleosis*, Chapter 5) and cytomegalovirus are two examples.

Nonviral hepatitis has been seen as a reaction to certain medications or as an autoimmune disease launched against hepatocytes.

Massage?

The same rules apply here as for other types of hepatitis: acute infection contraindicates circulatory massage, although energetic work may be supportive and helpful. Chronic situations must be determined by the overall health of the client and his or her ability to adapt to changes brought about by massage.

JAUNDICE IN BRIEF

What is it?
Jaundice is a symptom of liver dysfunction involving the presence of excess bilirubin in the blood. The bilirubin is then distributed and dissolved in subcutaneous fat, mucous membranes, and the sclera of the eyes.

How is it recognized?
Jaundice gives the skin, eyes, and mucous membranes a yellowish cast.

Is massage indicated or contraindicated?
The presence of jaundice is not enough information on which to base a decision about bodywork. The underlying cause for the jaundice must be understood before a decision can be made, based on the comparative risks and benefits of bodywork in the context of that condition.

Jaundice

Definition: What Is It?

Jaundice, from the French *jaune* (yellow), is not a disease in itself, but a symptom of some underlying liver or gallbladder pathology leading to the accumulation of bilirubin in the blood.

Etiology: What Happens?

One of the functions of the liver is to accept the by-products of dead red blood cells, including bilirubin, delivered from the spleen through the portal system. It synthesizes the bilirubin into bile. Bile drips from the liver into a storage tank: the gallbladder. Bile is used for the digestion and absorption of fats and fat-soluble vitamins. Eventually all the bilirubin gets into the digestive tract and is a coloring agent for feces, which makes it a useful diagnostic tool.

When bile cannot leave the liver for a variety of reasons, it stays in the bloodstream. Eventually levels of bilirubin can rise enough to visibly stain the skin, mucous membranes, and the sclera of the eyes.

Several types of jaundice have been identified, and each one is categorized by the pathology that created the problem. Jaundice is treated according to the underlying causes.

- *Neonatal jaundice.* This is a fairly common condition for newborns. Their livers are not yet mature and cannot keep up with the turnover of fetal red blood cells. It takes a few days to process this extra load to catch up. Treatment is usually exposure to "bili-lights."

- *Hemolytic jaundice.* This is a rare condition that is specifically related to hemolytic anemia. In this situation red blood cells die too fast. Although the liver may be functioning at normal levels, it cannot keep up with the volume. Therefore, bilirubin backs up into the system (see *anemia*, Chapter 4). Hemolytic anemia and jaundice may be caused by infection or incompatible blood transfusions.

- *Hepatic jaundice.* This covers any jaundice caused by other liver dysfunction: *cirrhosis*, *hepatitis* (this chapter), malaria, or more rarely a congenital malfunction of liver enzyme systems. In any case, the liver is compromised by scar tissue or inflammation, and it is incapable of processing the bilirubin delivered from the portal system.

- *Extrahepatic jaundice.* This is jaundice caused by a mechanical obstruction somewhere outside the liver; gallstones, pancreatic tumors, or colon tumors may be responsible. Advanced pregnancy can also constrict the gallbladder in a way that prevents the drainage of bile. The pooling of fluid because of blockage can lead to infection and permanent liver damage. Extrahepatic jaundice not caused by pregnancy may require surgery to excise the obstruction.

Signs and Symptoms

Jaundice indicates that bilirubin is backing up into the bloodstream and is being distributed throughout the body, instead of passing from the liver into the duodenum. Skin, mucous membranes, and eyeballs take on a characteristic yellow color, and urine gets unusually dark as the kidneys excrete excessive bilirubin. Fecal matter, no longer colored by bilirubin, gets lighter instead of darker. One of the symptoms of jaundice is light or clay-colored stools.

Complications

Although jaundice is simply a signal of some other problem, it can itself create some difficulties. Without adequate secretion of bile, little or no absorption of fats is possible, so access for important fat-soluble vitamins is limited. One of the most serious short-term consequences of this problem are bleeding disorders caused by a shortage of vitamin K.

Massage?

Jaundice does not occur in a vacuum; it always accompanies some other kind of liver dysfunction, which may range from being very mild to being life-threatening. An episode of jaundice would indicate, however, that even chronic situations are in a severe state, so circulatory massage may not be an appropriate choice.

When a massage therapist understands the underlying factors contributing to a client's jaundice, he or she will be in a better position to make an informed choice about which modalities will offer maximum benefits with minimum risk.

Other Digestive System Conditions

Candidiasis

Definition: What Is It?

Candida albicans are one type of many yeast-like fungi that inhabit the digestive tract, often from the mouth to the anus. They are usually beneficial organisms that live in balance with other flora and fauna of the GI tract (Fig. 7-7). Under certain circumstances that balance can be upset, and candida can replicate too easily, leading to a variety of problems. This condition of having normal levels of candida fungi grow out of control is called candidiasis.

Demographics: Who Gets It?

Candidiasis affects different people in different ways, and its incidence as a health problem is largely a matter of opinion. Some experts only recognize an imbalance in people who are very extremely affected. These include groups whose immune systems are generally weaker than normal such as infants, AIDS patients, diabetics, organ transplant recipients, and the elderly.

Other experts suggest that candidiasis affects a much broader population in a much more subtle way, and that the symptoms of an imbalance are either too subtle to identify or attributed to other problems such as allergies, chronic fatigue syndrome, chronic yeast infections, hypothyroidism, and other disorders.

Etiology: What Happens?

Under normal circumstances, a balanced environment of flora (plant-like organisms) and fauna (animal-like organisms) peacefully coexist in the GI tract. The flora keep the fauna from replicating too much, and the fauna do likewise for the flora. These organisms live in symbiosis, a mutually beneficial relationship with their human hosts.

When something happens that disrupts the balance in the GI tract, either plants or animals can begin to take precedence. When bacteria are suppressed, candida in the GI tract

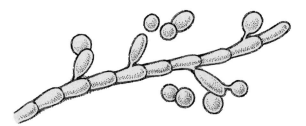

Figure 7-7. *Candida albicans,* the yeast that causes candidiasis

change their form from being benign, helpful yeast-like organisms to more aggressive fungi. In the absence of balancing bacteria, the fungi gain unlimited capacity to reproduce and spread. Because candida live in virtually every human digestive tract, the exact delineation between colonization and infestation is not always clear. Opinions vary about how extensive a candida colonization has to be before it causes symptoms (see sidebar).

Candidiasis Triggers

The trigger for intestinal imbalance is often the prescription of antibiotics (medications designed to kill harmful bacteria that also kill beneficial bacteria). This is why many health care providers recommend supplementing lactobacilli along with antibiotic prescriptions. Other well-accepted causes of candidiasis include disorders involving genetic immune system dysfunctions, thymus tumors, and hormonal imbalances.

Some experts propose that candida overgrowth can also be a result of taking birth control pills or steroidal anti-inflammatories, and having a diet that is high in simple sugars, wheat, and alcohol (all favorite foods for the growing fungi).

Signs and Symptoms

- *Mouth lesions.* Severe candida infections can take several forms. Thrush, an outbreak of whitish, usually painless lesions in the mouth, is one form that is commonly seen in infants and immune-suppressed people. Candidiasis may also create red, sore areas in the mouth and on the tongue.

- *Anal lesions.* Babies with candida can develop painful and persistent "diaper rash." In this case, it is not irritation caused by exposure to the ammonia in urine, but a skin reaction to the fungi colonizing the rectum and anus.

- *Other skin lesions.* Systemic candidiasis may affect finger and toenails, causing them to become thickened and discolored, often with edema around the cuticles. Lesions sometimes occur on the scalp, leading to baldness.

- *Systemic symptoms (acute infection).* Fever and chills that do not respond to antibiotics may indicate *invasive candidiasis*, in which the organisms have directly entered the bloodstream through compromised capillaries in the intestines. Invasive candidiasis can be a very serious problem, as the organisms can affect and impair function in virtually any organ. The rise of invasive candidiasis has been cause for concern, since the introduction of powerful antibiotics and other immunosuppressants have made many people, especially those with compromised immune systems, susceptible to candida overgrowth.

- *Systemic symptoms (chronic infection).* If a person has an imbalance of fungi in the GI tract, he or she may experience any combination of the following: food and chemical sensitivities, headaches (including migraines), chronic yeast and urinary tract infections, fatigue, reduced resistance to infection, acne, and many others.

Is it Candidiasis?

Two schools of thought dominate the discussion of candidiasis. The more conservative allopathic approach generally assumes that the overgrowth of candida is not a problem until very severe symptoms occur, which may involve the skin, mucous membranes, or invasive candidiasis, a systemic infection of the blood.

Many naturopathic and holistic practitioners propose that milder overgrowths of candida can also cause many chronic, low-grade symptoms. The fungi may grow and spread throughout the intestines, sinking root-like structures into the walls. They produce waste products that can be highly irritating to the host. Invasion of the intestinal wall may also allow substances to enter into the bloodstream, where immune system responses launched against incompletely digested material may be extreme. Between losing access to nutrition because the fungi get it first, dealing with fungal metabolic wastes, and immune system responses against digestive contents, a person with chronic, low-grade candidiasis could develop a number of subtle or severe symptoms.

The practitioners who deal with candidiasis as a contributor to many other chronic conditions often report success when helping their patients change their diets and lifestyles in ways that restore balance to intestinal flora and fauna. This clinical evidence has yet to be reproduced in a formal research setting, however, which leads to resistance to the acceptance of candidiasis as a common, chronic disorder responsible for symptoms that range from fatigue to menstrual pain to food allergies.

Diagnosis

The sheer number and variety of symptoms that a candida imbalance can induce makes this condition a challenge to identify and treat. Many clinicians do not recognize that many common and persistent signs and symptoms may be fungi-related, and many patients may read about candida symptoms and assume (rightly or wrongly) that this is the source of all their problems. For all but the most extreme versions of the condition, it may be difficult to get an accurate diagnosis or successful treatment.

Diagnosis for extreme versions of candidiasis involves skin biopsies to examine obvious lesions for signs of fungal infection. For chronic cases of this condition, a stool sample is often examined to look for signs of intestinal imbalance. Not many facilities exist that test for this kind of subtle problem, however, and the process can be time-consuming and expensive.

Treatment

Various topical anti-fungal medications may be recommended for severe versions of candidiasis, along with treatment for whatever underlying conditions may be contributing to the disorder.

For subtler versions of the disorder, internal antifungals are sometimes recommended, although these can take a long time to work and some people have very severe reactions to them. Reestablishing internal bacteria to balance out the fungi is a high priority. Research is being conducted into how to inhibit the transformation of the relatively passive yeast form of the organism into the more aggressive fungal form.

Massage?

A person with a severe candidiasis infection is likely to be under medical care for any of a variety of immune-compromising conditions. Massage in this situation depends on the health of the skin and whatever underlying disorders might be present.

Massage for someone who may be trying to conquer a less severe, chronic infestation of candida is appropriate and may aid in the attempt to rid the body of yeast-related toxins.

Peritonitis

Definition: What Is It?

Peritonitis is an infection that has become established in the peritoneal space, where it is dark, moist, and just about 100°F—a perfect growth medium. Bacteria may also thrive in the peritoneal space because some key immune devices are absent. White blood cells have no direct access, nor do any corrosive fluids such as digestive juices that might impede bacterial expansion (Fig. 7-8).

Etiology: What Happens?

The bacteria that cause peritonitis can gain access to the peritoneal space through a variety of sources:

* *Rupture* of an organ is one possibility. This is a complication of *appendicitis*, perforated *ulcers*, and *diverticulitis* (all in this chapter).

PERITONITIS IN BRIEF

What is it?
Peritonitis is inflammation, usually due to bacterial infection, of the peritoneal lining of the abdomen.

How is it recognized?
Acute peritonitis shows the signs of systemic infection: fever and chills along with abdominal pain, distension, nausea, and vomiting.

Is massage indicated or contraindicated?
Acute peritonitis is a medical emergency and contraindicates massage.

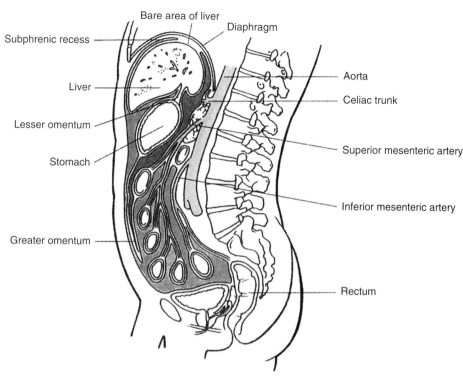

Figure 7-8. Peritonitis is an infection in the peritoneal space

PERITONEUM
This is a Latin word derived from a Greek root. *Periteino* means "to stretch over," which is an apt description of the peritoneum, which stretches over all the abdominal contents.

- *Pelvic or abdominal abscesses* such as those seen with *ulcerative colitis* (this chapter) or *pelvic inflammatory disease* (Chapter 10) can release bacteria into the peritoneal space, leading to systemic infection.

- *Mechanical perforation* of the abdomen can introduce bacteria from the outside (e.g., a knife wound). This is an occasional complication of intestinal or colon surgery, and the possibility of peritonitis is the reason behind the heavy doses of antibiotics that are prescribed before such surgeries take place.

- *Spontaneous peritonitis* is an occasional complication of advanced *cirrhosis* (this chapter) and other liver diseases, where ascites (the seepage of plasma into the abdomen) may carry intestinal bacteria along with it.

- *Peritoneal dialysis* is a method of kidney dialysis for people with advanced kidney failure. It uses the peritoneal membrane as a filter to clean the blood. One of the risks of peritoneal dialysis is the contamination of the tubing that connects to the peritoneum. This contamination can cause peritonitis.

Signs and Symptoms

The symptoms of peritonitis vary, depending on the original cause. Abdominal pain is always part of the picture. It usually begins as diffuse pain, but it eventually localizes at the original site of infection. Nausea and vomiting are usually present, and if the infection is untreated, severe dehydration may result. Many patients experience reduced urine output and difficulty passing gas or bowel movements. After 2 or 3 hours the abdomen will swell and pain may subside, but this is not a sign of improvement; rather, it is an indication that the intestines have gone into paralysis. At this point death is not far away unless the patient gets immediate hospital care.

Treatment

Treatment for peritonitis varies according to cause and severity. At the very least, antibiotics are needed. Emergency situations require abdominal surgery to remove or repair the ruptured organ and to wash out the peritoneal cavity as fully as possible. When peritonitis is caught early, it usually responds well to treatment. If it is left untreated too long, it can be deadly.

Massage?

Any form of acute peritonitis systemically contraindicates massage until all signs of infection have passed.

Chapter Review Questions: Digestive System Conditions

1. Describe how ongoing stress can contribute to digestive system problems.

2. Why is the appendix no longer routinely removed in the course of other abdominal surgery?

3. What is ascites? How can liver dysfunction cause it?

4. Why might someone with ulcerative colitis be at a higher risk of developing colorectal cancer than the general population?

5. Describe the leading theory behind the development of colorectal cancer.

6. What is the difference between diverticula and colon polyps?

7. Most people with gallstones never have symptoms. What finally causes symptoms to occur?

8. Why are oral antibiotics often ineffective for dealing with a bacterial infection of the gastrointestinal tract?

9. What is a possible cause of ulcers that does not involve the *Helicobacter pylori* bacterium?

10. A client is recovering from a bout with hepatitis A. His skin has a yellowish tone and the sclerae of his eyes are yellow too. What condition is probably present? Is this client a good candidate for circulatory massage? Why?

Bibliography, Digestive System Conditions

General References, Digestive System

1. de Dominico G, Wood E. *Beard's Massage.* Philadelphia, PA: WB Saunders; 1997

2. Damjanou I. *Pathology for the Health-Related Professions.* Philadelphia, PA: WB Saunders; 1996.

3. Travell J, Simons DG. *Myofascial Pain and Dysfunction: The Trigger Point Manual.* Baltimore, MD: Williams & Wilkins; 1983.

4. Clemente CD. *Anatomy: A Regional Atlas of the Human Body.* 3rd ed. Baltimore, MD: Urban & Schwarzenburg; 1987.

5. Tortora GJ, Anagnostakos NP. *Principles of Anatomy and Physiology.* 6th ed. New York, NY: Harper & Row; 1990.

6. *Taber's Cyclopedic Dictionary.* 14th ed. Philadelphia, PA: FA Davis; 1981.

7. *Stedman's Medical Dictionary.* 26th ed. Baltimore, MD: Williams & Wilkins; 1995.

8. Memmler RL, Wood DL. *The Human Body in Health and Disease.* 5th ed. Philadelphia, PA: JB Lippincott; 1983.

9. Juhan D. *Job's Body: A Handbook for Bodywork.* Barrytown, NY: Station Hill Press; 1987.

10. Mulvihill ML. *Human Diseases: A Systemic Approach.* 2nd ed. Norwalk, CT: Appleton & Lange; 1987.

11. Kunz JRM, Finkel AJ, eds. *The American Medical Association Family Medical Guide.* New York, NY: Random House; 1987.

12. Marieb EM. *Human Anatomy and Physiology.* Redwood City, CA: Benjamin/ Cummings; 1989.

13. Sapolsky RM. *Why Zebras Don't Get Ulcers: An Updated Guide to Stress, Stress-Related*

Disease, and Coping. New York, NY: W.H. Freeman; 1998, NYC.

Disorders of the Upper Gastrointestinal Tract

Gastroenteritis

1. VanGilder T, Steiner TS, Thielman NM, et al. Practice guidelines for the management of infectious diarrhea. *Clin Infect Dis.* 2001;32:331–351. Available at: http://www.journals.uchicago.edu/ CID/journal/ issues/v32n3/001387/001387.html. Accessed spring 2001.
2. The Norwalk virus family. U.S. Food & Drug Administration Center for Food Safety & Applied Nutrition Foodborne Pathogenic Microorganisms and Natural Toxins Handbook. Available at: http://vm.cfsan.fda.gov/~mow/ chap34.html. Accessed spring 2001.
3. Gastritis. National Digestive Diseases Information Clearinghouse. National Institute of Diabetes and Digestive and Kidney Diseases. NIH publication no. 00-4764. Available at: http://www.niddk.nih.gov/ health/digest/summary/gastritis/gastritis. htm. Accessed spring 2001.
4. Diskin A. Gastroenteritis. In *Emergency Medicine/Gastrointestinal.* eMedicine.com, Inc.; 2001. Available at: http://www. emedicine.com/ emerg/topic213.htm. Accessed spring 2001.
5. Diarrhea. National Digestive Diseases Information Clearinghouse. National Institute of Diabetes and Digestive and Kidney Diseases. NIH publication no. 01-2749. Available at: http://www.niddk.nih.gov/ health/digest/pubs/diarrhea/diarrhea.htm. Accessed spring 2001.

Crohn's Disease

1. Crohn's disease. American Society of Colon and Rectal Surgeons. Available at: http://www. fascrs. org/brochures/ crohn'ss-disease.html. Accessed spring 2001.
2. Crohn's disease. Available at: http://www. hopkins-gi.org/subspecialties/crohn's/ overview.htm. Accessed spring 2001.
3. Crohn's disease FAQ. Crohn's Disease Web Site; 2000. Available at: http://www. angelfire. com/ga/crohns/faq.html. Accessed spring 2001.
4. Shafran I. History of Mycobacterium paratuberculosis. Available at: http://www.shafran.net/ crohns/ history_of_m__para_.htm. Accessed spring 2001.
5. Shapiro W. Inflammatory bowel disease. In *Emergency Medicine/Gastrointestinal.* eMedicine.com, Inc.; 2001. Available at: http://www.emedicine.com/emerg/ topic106.htm. Accessed spring 2001.
6. Crohn's disease. National Digestive Diseases Information Clearinghouse. National Institute of Diabetes and Digestive and Kidney Diseases. NIH publication no. 98-3410. Available at: http://www. niddk.nih.gov/health/digest/pubs/crohn'ss/ crohn'ss.htm. Accessed spring 2001.

Gastroesophageal Reflux Disorder

1. Levin H. Acid indigestion, sour stomach, heartburn. In *Consumer Treatment Guidelines/Stomach, Bowel and Rectal Problems.* eMedicine.com, Inc.; 2001. Available at: http://www.emedicine. com/general/topic1. htm. Accessed spring 2001.
2. Sweeney L. Esophagitis. In *Emergency Medicine/Gastrointestinal.* eMedicine.com, Inc.; 2001. Available at: http://www. emedicine.com/ emerg/topic175.htm. Accessed spring 2001.
3. Gastro-esophageal reflux disease. diagnosishealth.com; 1999–2002. Available at: http://www.diagnosishealth.com/gerd.htm. Accessed spring 2001.
4. Heartburn. Mayo Foundation for Medical Education and Research; 1998–2000. Available at: http://www.mayoclinic.com/ home?id=5.1.1.8.7. Accessed spring 2001.
5. Gastroesophageal reflux disease (hiatal hernia and heartburn). National Digestive Diseases Information Clearinghouse. National Institute of Diabetes and Digestive and Kidney Diseases. NIH publication no.94-882. Available at: http://www.niddk. nih.gov/health/digest/pubs/heartbrn/ heartbrn.htm. Accessed spring, 2001.

Stomach Cancer

1. What is stomach cancer? American Cancer Society. Available at: http://www3.cancer. org/cancerinfo/load_cont.asp?st=wi&ct= 40&language=english Accessed spring 2001.
2. Epidemiology of stomach cancer. Trustees of the University of Pennsylvania; 1994–2001. Available at: http://cancer.med. upenn.edu/disease/gastric/gastric_review. html. Accessed spring 2001.
3. Stomach cancer. MedicineNet, Inc.; 1996–2001. Available at: http://www. aboutdigestion.com/script/main/ Art.asp?li=DIG&ArticleKey=486&page= 1. Accessed spring 2001.
4. NCI/PDQ patient statement: Gastric cancer—Updated 11/2000. National Cancer Institute. http://cancer.med.upenn.edu/ pdq_html/2/engl/200025.html. Accessed spring 2001.
5. What you need to know about stomach cancer. National Cancer Institute. Available at: http://cancer.gov/cancer_information/ doc_wyntk.aspx?viewid=606874d8-bc0d-410c-8d80-38d6438db916. Accessed spring 2002.

Ulcers

1. *Helicobacter pylori* and peptic ulcer disease. Centers for Disease Control and Prevention. National Center for Infectious Diseases. Division of Bacterial and Mycotic Diseases. Available at: http://www.cdc. gov/ulcer/md.htm. Accessed spring 2001.
2. NSAIDs and peptic ulcers. National Digestive Diseases Information Clearinghouse. National Institute of Diabetes and Digestive and Kidney Diseases. NIH publication no. 99-4644. Available at: http://www.niddk.nih.gov/health/ digest/summary/nsaids/index.htm. Accessed spring 2001.
3. Shayne P. Gastritis and peptic ulcer disease. In *Emergency Medicine/Gastrointestinal.* eMedicine.com, Inc.; 2001. Available at: http://www.emedicine.com/EMERG/ topic820.htm. Accessed spring 2001.
4. Packer-Tursman J. Treatment of choice. *Special to the Washington Post.* August 22, 2000:Z19. Available at: http://www. washingtonpost.com/ wp-dyn/articles/ A3292-2000Aug22.html. Accessed spring 2001.
5. H. Pylori and peptic ulcer. National Digestive Diseases Information Clearinghouse. National Institute of Diabetes and Digestive and Kidney Diseases. NIH publication no. 97-4225. Available at: http://www. niddk.nih.gov/health/digest/pubs/hpylori/ hpylori.htm. Accessed spring 2001.

Disorders of the Large Intestine

Appendicitis

1. Appendicitis. National Digestive Diseases Information Clearinghouse. National Institute of Diabetes and Digestive and Kidney Diseases. NIH publication no. 99-4547. Available at: http://www.niddk.nih. gov/health/digest/summary/append/index. htm. Accessed spring 2001.
2. Appendicitis. MedicineNet, Inc.; 1996–2001. Available at: MedicineNet.com. Accessed spring 2001.
3. Craig S. Appendicitis. In *Emergency Medicine/Gastrointestinal.* eMedicine.com, Inc.; 2001. Available at: http://www.emedicine. com/ emerg/topic41.htm. Accessed spring 2001.

Colorectal Cancer

1. Colorectal cancer: ©1996–2002. Intelihealth Inc. Available at http://www.intelihealth.com/IH/ihtIH/WSIHWOOO/ 24560/3168.html. Accessed spring 2002.
2. Colorectal cancer: What is it? American Cancer Society; 2000. Available at: http:// www3.cancer.org/cancerinfo/load_cont.asp? st=wi&ct=10. Accessed spring 2001.
3. Cancer of the colon and rectum. National Cancer Institute. NIH Publication No. 99–1552. Available at: http://cancernet.nci. nih.gov. Accessed spring 2002.
4. Colon and rectum cancer statistics. Available at: http://www.cancer.

org/statistics/cff2000/selectedcancers. html#colon. Accessed spring 2001.

5. Colon cancer (PDQ). National Cancer Institute. Available at: http://cancernet. nci.nih. gov/cgi-bin/srchcgi.exe?DBID= pdq&TYPE= search&UID=208= 00008&ZFILE=patient& SFM=pdq_treatment/1/0/0. Accessed spring 2001.

6. Mansell DE. Colon polyps and colon cancer. DE Mansell; 1996. Available at: http://www. maxinet.com/mansell/ polyp.htm. Accessed spring 2001.

Diverticulosis/Diverticulitis

1. Kazzi AA. Diverticular disease. In *Emergency Medicine/Gastrointestinal.* eMedicine.com, Inc.; 2001. Available at: http://www.emedicine.com/ emerg/ topic152.htm. Accessed spring 2001.

2. Diverticulitis. Mayo Foundation for Medical Education and Research; 1998–2000. Available at: http://www.mayoclinic.com/ home?id= DS00070. Accessed spring 2001.

3. SSAT patient care guidelines 2000. Surgical treatment of diverticulitis. SSAT, Inc.; 1996–2000. Revised January 2000. Available at: http://www.ssat.com/guidelines/ divert.htm. Accessed spring 2001.

4. Diverticular disease. National Digestive Diseases Information Clearinghouse. National Institute of Diabetes and Digestive and Kidney Diseases. NIH publication no. 97-1163. Available at: http://www.niddk. nih.gov/health/digest/pubs/divert/divert. htm. Accessed spring 2001.

Irritable Bowel Syndrome

1. Stephens E. Irritable bowel syndrome. In *AAEM Emergency Medical and Family Health Guide/Digestive Tract.* eMedicine.com, Inc.; 2001 Available at: http://www.emedicine.com/ aaem/ topic274.htm. Accessed spring 2001.

2. Irritable bowel syndrome. American Society of Colon and Rectal Surgeons. Available at: http:// www.fascrs.org/brochures/ irritable-bowel.html. Accessed spring 2001.

3. Irritable bowel syndrome. American Gastroenterological Association; 2001. Available at: http://www.gastro.org/ public/ibs.html. Accessed spring 2001.

4. Irritable bowel syndrome. Mayo Foundation for Medical Education and Research; 2000. Available at: http://www. mayohealth.org/mayo/ 9812/htm/irs.htm. Accessed spring 2001.

5. Irritable bowel syndrome. National Digestive Diseases Information Clearinghouse. National Institute of Diabetes and Digestive and Kidney Diseases. NIH publication no. 97-693. Available at: http://www.niddk. nih.gov/health/digest/pubs/irrbowel/ irrbowel.htm. Accessed spring 2001.

Ulcerative Colitis

1. Ulcerative colitis. National Institute of Diabetes and Digestive and Kidney Diseases.

NIH publication no. 95-1597. Accessed spring 2001.

2. Shapiro W. Inflammatory bowel disease. In *Emergency Medicine/Gastrointestinal.* eMedicine.com, Inc.; 2001. Available at: http:// www.emedicine.com/emerg/topic106.htm. Accessed spring 2001.

Disorders of the Accessory Organs

Cirrhosis

1. Wolf DC. Cirrhosis. In *Medicine, Ob/Gyn, Psychiatry, and Surgery/Gastroenterology.* eMedicine.com, Inc.; 2001. Available at: http://www. emedicine.com/med/ topic3183.htm. Accessed spring 2001.

2. Cirrhosis. National Institute of Diabetes and Digestive and Kidney Diseases. NIH publication no. 00-1134. Available at: http://www. niddk.nih.gov/health/ digest/pubs/cirrhosi/cirrhosi.htm. Accessed spring, 2001.

3. The liver and exocrine pancreas. State University of New York at Stony Brook. Available at: http://www.path.sunysb.edu/. courses/hbp310/liver_and_pancreas.htm. Accessed spring 2001.

Gallstones

1. The liver and exocrine pancreas. State University of New York at Stony Brook. Available at: http://www.path.sunysb.edu/ courses/hbp310/liver_and_pancreas.htm. Accessed spring 2001.

2. Santen S. Gallstones. In *Emergency Medicine/Gastrointestinal.* eMedicine.com, Inc.; 2001. Available at: http://www.emedicine. com/ EMERG/topic98.htm. Accessed spring 2001.

3. Gallstones (cholelithiasis). Colorado State University. Available at: http://arbl.cvmbs. colostate.edu/hbooks/pathphys/digestion/ liver/gallstones.html. Accessed spring 2001.

4. Gallstones. National Institute of Diabetes and Digestive and Kidney Diseases. NIH publication no. 99-2897. Available at: http://www. niddk.nih.gov/health/digest/ pubs/gallstns/gallstns.htm. Accessed spring 2001.

Hepatitis

1. The liver and exocrine pancreas. State University of New York at Stony Brook. Available at: http://www.path.sunysb.edu/ courses/hbp310/liver_and_pancreas.htm. Accessed spring 2002.

2. Diagnosis and treatment. Hepatitis Foundation International. Available at: http://www.hepinfo.org/pages/liv_ diagnosis.html. Accessed spring 2002.

3. Viral hepatitis A to E and beyond. National Institute of Diabetes and Digestive and Kidney Diseases. NIH publication no. 00-4762. Available at: http://www.niddk.nih. gov/health/digest/pubs/hep/hepa-e/hepa-e.htm. Accessed spring 2001.

4. The ABC's of Hepatitis. Hepatitis Foundation International; 2002. Available at: http//www.hepinfo.org/pages/liv_abc.html. Accessed spring 2002.

5. Buggs AM. Hepatitis. In *Emergency Medicine/Gastrointestinal.* eMedicine.com, Inc.; 2001. Available at: http://www.emedicine. com/emerg/topic244.htm. Accessed spring 2001.

6. Hepatitis statistics. Hepatitis Foundation International. Available at: http://www.hepfi.org/ stats.htm. Accessed spring 2001.

7. Fact sheet. Hepatitis Foundation International. Available at: http://www.hepfi. org/Hepinfo/ FACT%203-99.htm. Accessed spring 2001.

8. Thomas DL. Report from the 7th CROI: Hepatitis C emerging. The Johns Hopkins University; 1997–2001. Available at: http://www. hopkins-aids.edu/ publications/report/ mar00_5.html. Accessed spring 2001.

9. Facts about hepatitis C. Centers for Disease Control and Prevention. Available at: http:// www.cdc.gov/od/oc/media/fact/ hepcqa.htm. Accessed spring 2001.

10. Chronic hepatitis C: Current disease management. National Institute of Diabetes and Digestive and Kidney Diseases. NIH publication no. http://www.niddk.nih. gov/health/digest/ pubs/chrnhepc/ chrnhepc.htm. Accessed spring 2001.

11. What Is hepatitis? The National Hemophilia Foundation. Available at: http://www. hemophilia.org/hepatitis/ Accessed spring 2001.

12. Worman HJ. Autoimmune hepatitis. Columbia University Division of Gastroenterology; 1995. Available at: http://home.iatronet.net/papers/ autoimmune.html. Accessed spring 2001.

Jaundice

1. The liver and exocrine pancreas. State University of New York at Stony Brook. Available at: http://www.path.sunysb.edu/ courses/hbp310/liver_and_pancreas.htm. Accessed spring 2002.

2. Santen S. Gallstones. In *Emergency Medicine/Gastrointestinal.* eMedicine.com, Inc.; 2001. Available at: http://www.emedicine. com/ EMERG/topic98.htm. Accessed spring 2001.

Other Digestive System Conditions

Candidiasis

1. Scully C. Candidiasis. In *Emergency Medicine/Gastrointestinal.* eMedicine.com, Inc.; 2001. Available at: http://www.emedicine.com/ derm/topic68.htm. Accessed spring 2001.

2. Invasive candidiasis (infections in the bloodstream and organs). Centers for Dis-

ease Control and Prevention. Available at: http://www.cdc.gov/ncidod/dbmd/disease-info/candidiasis_inv_g.htm. Accessed spring 2001.

3. The Candida albicans mystery. SB Edelson; 1998. Available at: http://www.ephca.com/ca_mys.htm. Accessed spring 2001.

4. Chronic candidiasis. Doctor Fungus; 2000. Available at:http://www.doctorfungus.org/fungi_action/human/candida/Chronic_Candidiasis.htm. Accessed spring 2001.

5. Candidiasis: Overview and full index. Doc-

tor Fungus; 2000. Available at: http://www.doctorfungus.org/fungi_action/human/candida/Candida_index.htm. Accessed spring 2001.

Peritonitis

1. Bandy SM. Spontaneous bacterial peritonitis. In *Emergency Medicine/Infectious Diseases*. eMedicine.com, Inc.; 2001. Available at: http://www.emedicine.com/emerg/topic882.htm. Accessed spring 2001.

Endocrine System Conditions

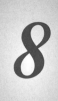

CHAPTER OBJECTIVES

After reading this chapter, the reader should be able to . . .

- List three hormones secreted by the pituitary gland and the tissues they affect.
- Name two hormones associated with changing levels of bone density.
- List two risks for working with clients who have acromegaly.
- Name the difference between type 1 and type 2 diabetes.

- Name three possible complications of inadequately treated type 2 diabetes.
- Name three signs or symptoms of hyperthyroidism.
- Name the major risk for hyperthyroidism treatment.
- Describe the hormone shifts that lead to hypoglycemia.
- Name three signs or symptoms of hypothyroidism.
- Name the visible sign that is common to both hyperthyroidism and hypothyroidism.

INTRODUCTION

Endocrine System Introduction

The endocrine system is a collection of glands that secrete hormones, which are chemical messengers that instruct or stimulate other glands and tissues in the body to function in a variety of ways. Whereas the nervous system exerts electrical control over body functions, the endocrine system exerts chemical control. Interestingly, the control center for both systems is the same structure—the hypothalamus.

The hypothalamus is a mass of tissue deep in the middle of the brain. It has a generous blood supply, which allows it to monitor functions of the body. The hypothalamus is primarily responsible for maintaining homeostasis (a stable internal environment). It does so through electrical transmission to the brainstem to manage heart rate, blood pressure, temperature, and other functions and also through chemical transmission to the pituitary gland. The hypothalamus is located directly above and behind the pituitary, and it actually controls what the pituitary secretes, sometimes sending out some of its own hormones (via a stalk called the infundibulum) to be released into the blood by the pituitary gland.

Chemicals released by the hypothalamus and pituitary glands travel to their target glands through the blood. They stimulate those glands to release *their* hormones. When those secretions reach appropriate levels in the blood, the hypothalamus and pituitary stop sending out their signals. The endocrine system is an excellent example of a negative feedback system.

The cycle of hormone stimulation and suppression usually works best when it occurs in gentle, rhythmic fluctuation. For example, when a person's blood glucose levels get

liberal

low, two things happen. The person perceives that he or she is hungry, and the pancreas secretes a hormone called glucagon that stimulates the liver to release stored glucose. The person eats in response to hunger, the digestive tract absorbs sugar from the meal, and the blood glucose level rises. This stimulates the pancreas to release insulin to carry the sugar out of the blood and into cells, lowering blood glucose. When levels are low enough, the person gets hungry again and eats, beginning the cycle all over. The blood glucose/insulin cycle takes place several times a day; it only takes a few hours to move from one state to another. Other endocrine cycles move on a roughly 24-hour rotation (these are called circadian rhythms). The menstrual cycle also depends on rhythmic fluctuation, but this one takes about 4 weeks to complete. Other cycles, specifically those related to stress and perceived threat, depend on external circumstances to determine their frequency and duration.

Endocrine system glands secrete more than 50 different chemicals, each of which has specific target tissues and functions. Endocrine effects may also be determined by the frequency with which they are released into the bloodstream and the balance between each hormone and its antagonists.

Hormones fall into three chemical classes:

- *Peptides.* Peptides are the most common types of hormones. They are made of chains of amino acids and are stored in various cellular holding tanks. Growth hormone, erythropoietin, and parathyroid hormone are types of peptide hormones.

- *Amines.* Amines are derived from a specific amino acid, *tyrosine*. They are also stored in cellular holding tanks. Adrenaline and thyroxine are examples of amine hormones.

- *Steroids.* Steroids are lipids and are not stored; steroid levels are maintained by constant production and replacement. Cortisol and testosterone are steroid hormones.

It is useful for massage therapists to be able to recognize the names of most hormones and their actions, since this is a key feature of physiology. A few hormones are so strongly implicated in basic health issues that massage therapists may benefit from more than just passing familiarity.

- *Growth hormone.* Growth hormone is released from the pituitary gland and stimulates the conversion of fuel into new cells. Infants, children, and teenagers secrete massive amounts of growth hormone; adults secrete less. When a person has finished growing, the primary purpose of growth hormone is to stimulate the regeneration and repair of damaged tissue (in other words, healing). Growth hormone is secreted primarily in stage IV sleep. *Sleep disorders* can lead to a shortage of this important chemical (see Chapter 3).

- *Adrenaline.* Also called epinephrine, this steroid hormone comes from the adrenal gland medulla, along with a very similar hormone, noradrenaline (norepinephrine). It is associated with short-term, high-grade stress and acts to reinforce all the reactions initiated by the sympathetic nervous system. A slow connection between the pituitary gland and the adrenal glands can cause a sluggish stress response system; this is discussed in *depression* (Chapter 3).

- *Cortisol.* This steroid hormone is one of a group of *glucocorticoids* secreted by the adrenal cortex, and it influences the metabolism of proteins. It is the hormone secreted under long-term, low-grade stress and is measurable in the saliva. Cortisol is important for several reasons. It is a very powerful anti-inflammatory and is sometimes used systemically or locally for that purpose; it is very hard on connective tissues—people with systemically high levels of cortisol are more prone to musculoskeletal injury and osteoporosis; and it suppresses immune system response to disease and infection.

- *Mineralocorticoids.* These adrenal cortex secretions help to regulate electrolyte balance and they control fluid retention. *Aldosterone* is a major mineralocorticoid.

- *Insulin/glucagon.* These hormones work together to regulate blood glucose; insulin decreases it, and glucagon increases it. Both these hormones are manufactured and released by the pancreas. Their relationship to endocrine pathology is discussed in the sections on *diabetes mellitus* and *hypoglycemia* in this chapter.

- *Thyroxine, triiodothyronine.* These hormones are secreted by the thyroid gland. They stimulate the metabolism of fuel into energy. Thyroid pathologies have to do with overproduction or underproduction of thyroid hormones.

- *Calcitonin.* This thyroid secretion stimulates osteoblasts to extract calcium from the blood and add to bone density. In other words, it decreases blood calcium.

- *Parathyroid hormone.* This hormone comes from the tiny parathyroid glands located deep to the thyroid gland. It is the antagonist of calcitonin, stimulating osteoclast activity and pulling calcium off the bones to raise blood calcium.

- *Testosterone, estrogens, progesterone.* These steroid hormones are released mainly by the gonads (testicles for men, ovaries for women) and have to do with secondary sexual characteristics, menstrual cycle, maintaining pregnancy, and several other issues including bone density, skin function, and cardiovascular health. Testosterone and its synthetic forms have both androgenic (sexual) and anabolic (promoting protein production) effects. Some athletes use anabolic steroids (testosterone or one of its derivatives) for their anabolic or muscle-building effects. However, the androgenic effects cannot be eliminated. Use of such substances by athletes is often associated with unforeseen and dangerous results.

  The negative feedback loops in these hormone relationships seem to be especially precarious, possibly because environmental exposures to various types of hormones (in medications, dairy products, meat, plastics, pesticides, and other environmental toxins) overbalance the scales. A phenomenon called "estrogen dominance" is now being considered in the identification and treatment of symptoms relating to *premenstrual syndrome, menopause,* and other women's health issues. These are discussed further in Chapter 10.

- *Other hormones.* Other hormones have less implication for massage but big impact on how well the body works. One is *erythropoietin* (EPO), which is secreted by the kidneys. EPO stimulates the production of red blood cells. It can be artificially supplemented to increase oxygen carrying capacity of the blood, which may also increase the risk of blood clots. *Thymosin* is a hormone from the thymus; it is involved with the maturation of T-cells. *Melatonin* comes from the pineal gland and helps to create wake/sleep cycles. *Prostaglandins* are hormone-like substances produced by almost any kind of cell for local action. Prostaglandins create myriad effects in the body, including smooth muscle contraction and increased pain sensitivity.

Endocrine glands release their secretions (often under direction of the pituitary/hypothalamus unit) directly into the blood. This distinguishes them from exocrine glands, which send their secretions into ducts for release in specific areas. Some glands, such as the liver, pancreas, and stomach, produce both endocrine and exocrine secretions. The hormones circulate systemically through the body but attach to specific receptor sites on their target tissues. Then they stimulate the target tissue to perform some function, such as making red blood cells (EPO from the kidneys acting on bone marrow) or pulling calcium off the bones (parathyroid hormone acting on osteoclasts).

Endocrine system disorders usually involve imbalances in the hormones being produced. Autoimmune attacks or tumors often stimulate or suppress certain glands, leading to problems with creating an efficient negative feedback loop. When too much or too little of any hormone is present in the blood, symptoms can be felt throughout the body. Other endocrine disruptions occur when circulating hormone levels are normal but target tissues have built up resistance to their action.

Existing methods to measure and evaluate hormone balance are as accurate as scientists can make them, but it is likely that subtle dysfunctions are often missed in diagnosis, leading to chronic low-grade symptoms that may never successfully be resolved. Fortunately, most extreme endocrine problems are fairly rare and not negatively affected by massage. Most clients with endocrine disorders can receive great benefits from bodywork.

Endocrine System Disorders

Endocrine System Disorders
  Acromegaly
  Diabetes Mellitus
  Hyperthyroidism
  Hypoglycemia
  Hypothyroidism

Endocrine System Disorders

Acromegaly
Definition: What Is It?

Acromegaly is a disorder of the pituitary gland, usually related to the development of a slow-growing tumor. It involves abnormal growth (*mego* is from the Greek for "large") of many different body parts, especially the hands and feet (*acro* refers to extremities).

Etiology: What Happens?

Among the many functions of the pituitary gland is the secretion of growth hormone, under the command of the hypothalamus. Growth hormone stimulates the metabolism of fuel into new cells for growth (in young people) and for repair (in older people). The secretion of growth hormone in turn stimulates the release of another hormone from the liver—somatomedin C, also known as insulin-like growth factor I (IGF-I). IGF-I suppresses further secretion of growth hormone. Thus, these two chemicals keep each other in check.

When a tumor grows on the pituitary gland, excessive amounts of growth hormone are released, leading to an excessive secretion of IGF-I. This stimulates the production of new tissues, resulting in bone enlargement, which often leads to joint distortion and pain, and a terrible burden on the cardiovascular system to supply nutrition to new tissues.

Imbalances in the types of growth hormones that are secreted leads to hyperglycemia (i.e., abnormally high blood glucose levels). This can cause *hypertension* and accelerate the development of *atherosclerosis*, both of which can also contribute to *congestive heart failure* (Chapter 4).

In addition, the tumor itself can cause abnormal secretion of other pituitary hormones, or it can exert mechanical pressure in the central nervous system, causing problems unrelated to hormonal disruption. The type of tumor associated with acromegaly is usually benign, but it is dangerous because of endocrine symptoms it causes.

Signs and Symptoms

Excessive growth hormone secretion in adulthood leads to enlargement of the hands and feet as well as facial changes including enlarged mandibles and spaces between teeth. Joint pain, fatigue, excessive sweatiness, and *sleep apnea* (see *sleep disorders*, Chapter 3) are frequent problems. If a tumor grows to a significant size, central nervous system symptoms may occur, including debilitating headaches, vision problems, or cranial nerve damage.

Complications

Because the sudden growth of new tissues late in life puts a significant stress on the heart, many of the most serious complications of acromegaly are related to cardiovascular stress. High blood pressure is a common complication, along with a pathologic enlargement of the heart. Eventually, many acromegaly patients experience congestive heart failure.

Some acromegaly patients develop diabetes mellitus (this chapter). Some research indicates a higher incidence of certain types of cancer, especially *colon cancer* (Chapter 7) among acromegaly patients.

Diagnosis

Acromegaly is diagnosed when abnormal growth is detected, and when both growth hormone and IGF-I levels are elevated.

Pituitary tumors often grow slowly, so the symptoms of acromegaly develop over a prolonged period. More than 90% of all diagnoses are made when the tumor is larger than 1 cm, which makes surgical removal more difficult.

Treatment

Surgery for acromegaly is most successful when the pituitary tumor is smaller than 1 cm, but only a minority of cases are diagnosed at this stage. Other therapies focus on restoring the balance between growth hormone and IGF-I that is lost when the pituitary gland becomes hyperactive. Classes of medications have been developed that mimic the action of hormones to inhibit growth hormone secretion. If an acromegaly patient can begin treatment with these medications before developing circulatory problems, the disease can be manageable and not necessarily a life-shortening condition.

Massage?

High blood pressure, enlargement of the heart, and congestive heart failure are key complications of acromegaly. Swedish massage, sports massage, or other modalities that focus on pushing fluid through the system may not be appropriate for these clients.

Joint pain and arthritis are other common complications of acromegaly. Although bodywork cannot reverse these changes, it may be able to alleviate some of the musculoskeletal pain that they cause.

A massage therapist working with an client who has acromegaly should be part of a well-informed health care team.

Diabetes Mellitus

Definition: What Is It?

Diabetes is not a single disease but rather a group of related disorders that all result in hyperglycemia, or elevated levels of glucose in the bloodstream. The glucose is then excreted in the urine. Two main varieties of the disease are examined here: type 1 and type 2. These account for about 98% of all diabetes diagnoses.

Demographics: Who Gets It?

Diabetes is the seventh leading cause of death in the United States, causing about 200,000 deaths per year. An estimated 16 million Americans have diabetes, but 5 million do not know it yet. Rates of diabetes have risen by 600% in the past 4 decades. Researchers credit higher numbers of obese people coupled with sedentary lifestyles for this alarming increase.

Diabetes, a largely treatable and even preventable disease, costs approximately $98 billion a year in direct medical costs and indirect costs of disability, lost wages, and premature mortality. It accounts for approximately one dollar out of every seven spent on health care.

Type 2 diabetes occurs among all races but is most common among Native Americans and Alaskans, African-Americans, Pacific Islanders, and Hispanic populations. Until recently type 2 diabetes was a mature adult's disease; now half of all new diagnoses are among children between 9 and 19 years old. About 7 million people in the United States live with type 2 diabetes today; about 3 million of them experience some level of disability.

Etiology: What Happens?

Insulin is required to escort glucose into cells where it can be consumed to produce energy; insulin also aids in the removal of fat from the blood into storage lipid cells. In diabetes, glucose and fats build up in the blood because insulin is in short supply, because insulin receptors on cells have developed resistance, or both. In the absence of insulin, the body cannot burn glucose, a remarkably clean fuel source, and must resort first to stored fat reserves and then finally to proteins. Eventually, in the absence of any other fuel source, the body will burn its own muscle tissue. These fuel sources do not burn cleanly. They leave behind a large amount toxic debris, which is largely responsible for the complications associated with diabetes.

DIABETES MELLITUS IN BRIEF

What is it?
Diabetes is a group of metabolic disorders characterized by glucose intolerance and disturbances in carbohydrate, fat, and protein metabolism.

How is it recognized?
Early symptoms of diabetes include frequent urination, chronic thirst, and increased appetite along with weight loss, nausea, and vomiting. These symptoms are often so subtle that the first signs of disease are the complications it can cause: peripheral neuropathy, impaired vision, kidney dysfunction, or other problems.

Is massage indicated or contraindicated?
Diabetes indicates massage as long as tissues are healthy and circulation is unimpaired. Many people with advanced or poorly treated diabetes experience numbness, cardiovascular problems, and/or kidney failure. Circulatory massage in these situations is not appropriate.

DIABETES MELLITUS

Diabetes comes from the Greek for "a siphon" or "to pass through," referring to the tendency for diabetics to urinate frequently. *Mellitus* is from Latin for "sweetened with honey." Diabetes mellitus essentially means "sweet pee."

Several types of diabetes mellitus have been identified. The two most common varieties are considered in the following sections.

Type 1 Diabetes

Type I diabetes is an autoimmune disorder. It can be brought about by a number of different factors, including exposure to certain drugs and chemicals, or as a complication of some kinds of infections. Killer T-cells of people with type 1 diabetes attack parts of the beta cells in the pancreas where insulin is produced. The destruction of these cells leads to a lifelong deficiency in insulin.

Type 1 diabetes usually shows up in the teen years, almost always before age 20. It is the rarer and more serious of the two basic types of diabetes. About 300,000 people in the United States have type 1 diabetes, and about 30,000 new cases are diagnosed each year. It accounts for 5 to 10% of all diabetes in this country. Because type 1 diabetes requires self-administered doses of insulin to take the place of the constant steady production provided by a healthy pancreas, type 1 diabetics can experience extreme fluctuations in blood sugar levels—from very, very high, which can cause ketoacidosis and diabetic coma, to dangerously low, which can lead to dangerously severe hypoglycemia.

Type 2 Diabetes

Type 2 diabetes is more common in women than men. Approximately 80% of people with type 2 diabetes are overweight. It is especially prevalent in African-Americans, Hispanics, Pacific Islanders, and Native American populations. Type 2 diabetes is usually controllable with diet, exercise, and possibly some anti-diabetes drugs, depending on how advanced it is when treatment begins. Some patients will eventually have to use self-administered insulin to control their disease.

The exact cause of type 2 diabetes is uncertain and is probably different for different people. For some it seems clear that a lifelong habit of a high carbohydrate diet simply wears out the pancreas and makes the insulin-producing cells less efficient. In others the insulin production may be at normal levels, but the incoming flood of sugar is too much to deal with. For still others insulin production may be normal or even above normal, but for some reason the target cells have fewer receptor sites to receive the insulin. In any case the results are the same: frequent urination, excessive thirst, and excessive hunger, along with the possibility of dangerous accumulations of atherosclerotic plaques and other serious complications.

Other Types of Diabetes

Other types of diabetes include *gestational diabetes* (see *pregnancy*, Chapter 10) in which a woman develops a transient case during pregnancy. Somewhere between 2 to 5% of all pregnancies involve gestational diabetes. This condition can cause birth defects in the child as well as routing massive amounts of blood glucose to the developing baby, resulting in very high birthweights and a high incidence of Cesarean section surgeries. Women who have gestational diabetes also have a 50% chance of developing type 2 diabetes later in life. *Secondary diabetes* may develop with damage or trauma to the pancreas, or as a symptom of some other endocrine disorder such as *acromegaly* (see this chapter) or Cushing Syndrome (hyperactive adrenal glands).

Signs and Symptoms

Three defining "polys" are common to all types of diabetes. *Polyuria*, or frequent urination results from elevated blood sugar, which acts as a diuretic. It pulls water from the cells in the body, and then excess water is expelled in the urine. *Polydipsia* means excessive thirst, which accompanies the loss of water with polyuria. *Polyphagia* refers to increased appetite, since cells are starved for glucose; this triggers the sensation of hunger. Other symptoms of diabetes include fatigue, weight loss, nausea, and vomiting.

Signs of diabetes are often missed until the disease has caused permanent damage to other organs in the body. These problems are discussed in *complications*.

Diabetic Emergencies

People with diabetes are vulnerable to two specific medical emergencies, both of which can be fatal if not treated promptly.

- *Ketoacidosis* involves a critical *shortage* of insulin and lack of glucose in the cells. It occurs most often in type 1 diabetics. In this situation the body will partially metabolize fats for fuel, and the acidic by-products of that metabolism (ketones) dangerously change the pH balance of the blood. Ketoacidosis is identifiable by a characteristic sweet or fruity odor to the breath. Ketoacidosis can be triggered by stress, infection, or trauma and can lead to shock, coma, and death.

- *Severe hypoglycemia* or "insulin shock" is an emergency at the other end of the scale. In this case *too much* insulin is circulating, either because too much has been administered or because a skipped meal, sudden exertion, stress, infection, or trauma has resulted in the consumption of all available blood sugar. The consequence of having too much available insulin is a dangerously low blood sugar level. Symptoms of severe hypoglycemia include hunger, irritability, dizziness, sweating, confusion, weakness, irregular heart beat, and tremors. It too can lead to coma and death if not treated (with juice, candy, or non-diet soda to replace blood glucose) quickly.

Complications

Complications of diabetes are many and serious.

- *Cardiovascular disease*. Diabetics are especially prone to these problems because residue left from the metabolism of fats and proteins (which contributes to high serum triglyceride and low-density lipoprotein levels), along with chronic hyperglycemia, lead to the aggressive development of *atherosclerosis* (Chapter 4). Unlike many atherosclerosis patients, diabetics do not just accumulate plaque on coronary arterial walls, they accumulate it systemically throughout the body. Diabetes also increases the risk of *stroke* (Chapter 3), *hypertension*, and *aneurysm*. (Chapter 4). Some degree of cardiovascular disease is present in 75% of all diabetes-related deaths. About 65% of people with diabetes have high blood pressure.

- *Edema*. This condition develops in the extremities because of sluggish blood return. Edema can also give rise to stasis dermatitis (see *dermatitis*, Chapter 1).

- *Ulcers, necrosis, amputations*. Imagine what would happen if *all* the body's blood vessels were caked with plaque. Absence of blood flow carrying nutrients and white blood cells would make it difficult or impossible to heal from even minor skin lesions. Furthermore, reduced sensation in the extremities makes it easier for small lesions to go unnoticed. Ingrown toenails and blisters can become life-threatening for diabetics; instead of healing they become necrotic. The tissue either dies of starvation or is infected with pathogens that are impossible to fight, forming characteristic diabetic ulcers, usually on the feet (Fig. 8-1, Color Plate 39). Diabetes leads to about 60,000 lower extremity amputations every year.

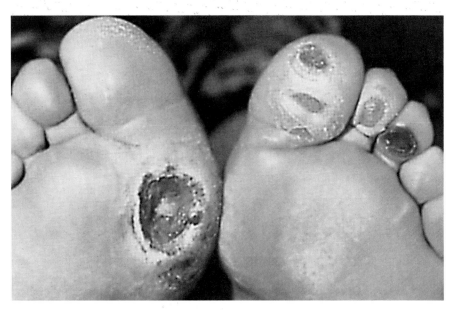

Figure 8-1. Diabetic ulcers

- *Kidney disease.* Renal vessels become clogged with plaques very readily, since they are one of the first diversions from the descending aorta. Excess blood glucose, which acts as a powerful diuretic, is also hard on the kidneys. Not surprisingly then, diabetes is the leading cause of renal failure and of the need for kidney transplants; about 10,000 diabetes patients experience kidney failure and the need for dialysis or transplantation every year (see *renal failure*, Chapter 9).

  Renal failure is the leading cause of death for people with diabetes. Research indicates that frequent monitoring and adjustments of blood sugar levels (meaning 4 to 6 times per day, as opposed to the more usual 1 to 2 times) can significantly reduce the amount of glomerular build-up in diabetic kidneys, thus reducing the risk of secondary hypertension by about 50%.

- *Impaired vision.* The capillaries of the eyes of diabetic persons can become abnormally thickened, depriving eye cells of nutrition. Diseased capillaries leak blood and proteins into the retina. Microaneurysms can form that also cut off circulation. All these contribute to diabetic *retinopathy.* Excess glucose also binds with special proteins in the lens causing first cataracts, then blindness. This disease is the leading cause of new blindness in the United States; it causes up to 24,000 cases per year.

  About half of all diabetes patients will experience some level of visual impairment within 10 years of being diagnosed. Close to 80% will have some vision loss within 15 years.

- *Peripheral neuropathy.* Lack of capillary circulation and excess glucose in the blood both contribute to nerve damage. Symptoms of diabetic neuropathy include tingling or pain and eventual numbness. It often affects the spinal nerves but can damage autonomic cranial nerves as well. Autonomic nerve damage can cause low blood pressure, diarrhea, constipation, or sexual impotency. Peripheral neuropathy generally appears about 10 to 20 years after diabetes is diagnosed. It is estimated that up to 25% of all diabetes patients will experience some degree of neuropathy (see *neuritis*, Chapter 3).

- *Others.* Diabetes affects just about every body system in some way. It is linked to *urinary tract infections* (Chapter 9), *candidiasis* (Chapter 7), birth defects, and higher than normal rates of gum disease and tooth loss.

Treatment

Before the development of insulin in 1921, the diagnosis of diabetes was considered a death sentence. Most people lived only a few years after the disease was identified. Nowadays the goal with insulin treatment is to keep blood sugar levels as stable as possible. Type 1 diabetes is treated primarily with a synthetic form of human insulin. New techniques of administering insulin more frequently have been developed to minimize the dangerous roller coaster ride of too much or too little blood glucose that these people experience.

Type 2 diabetes is first addressed with changes in diet and exercise. It has been found that exercise improves insulin uptake in resistant target cells, and a sedentary lifestyle may be more responsible for the rising statistics in type 2 diabetes in the United States and all developed nations than diets high in saturated fats and simple carbohydrates. About 35% of type 2 diabetes patients are treated with insulin supplementation. Hypoglycemic agents may also be prescribed.

Many diabetes patients eventually develop renal insufficiency. Their kidneys will simply be incapable of keeping up with their needs. Hemodialysis is a therapy that involves rerouting the blood through a "kidney machine" that removes excess water and waste products before returning the blood to the body. Dialysis is usually a stop-gap measure while a person waits for a kidney to become available for transplant.

Massage?

Massage may be appropriate for people with diabetes under the right circumstances. The main condition is that the client must have healthy, responsive tissue with good blood supply. For clients with advanced diabetes, kidney failure, and atherosclerosis, circulatory massage is not a good choice, but energetic techniques are certainly appropriate. A combination of poor circulation and renal dysfunction raises the risk of pitting *edema*—a red flag for massage therapy (see Chapter 5). Therapists must be aware that diabetic neuropathy can involve lack of sensation. Someone with type 2 diabetes may be completely unaware of the condition until someone points out ulcers, which often occur on the feet.

MAUREEN, AGE 43

Maureen had experienced gestational diabetes while pregnant with two of her three children. One year ago she began experiencing chronic yeast infections, unintentional weight loss, blurred vision, and unusual thirstiness. When she went for her annual check-up she was not happy, but also not surprised to be diagnosed with type 2 diabetes.

At first Maureen was intimidated by the glucose-testing equipment she had to use, and she was terrified by the long-term complications that often develop with diabetes. As she did more research, she came to the conclusion that diabetes is very much a "do-it-yourself" project. She found that proper control can be achieved through education, hard work, and stress reduction.

She tests her blood frequently, and sees immediate relationships between her glucose levels and how much stress she has and how much exercise she gets. Since her diagnosis, Maureen's diabetes medication has been cut in half, and she is able to maintain reasonable glucose levels by being proactive about her health. Although she is still upset about her disease, she is thankful that she was diagnosed early enough to take control of her situation and change it for the better.

Hyperthyroidism

Definition: What Is It?

Hyperthyroidism is a condition in which the thyroid gland produces excessive amounts of two forms of thyroxine, a hormone that stimulates metabolism of fuel into energy. Most cases of hyperthyroidism are related to autoimmune attacks against the whole thyroid gland. In these cases it may also be called *Graves disease* or *diffuse toxic thyroid*. More rarely, thyroid hyperactivity may be confined to one or more localized nodes, or it may be due to thyroid infection.

Demographics: Who Gets It?

Hyperthyroidism is a common disorder, affecting between 1 and 2% of all people in the United States at some time in their lives. About 500,000 new cases are diagnosed each year. Women are affected more often than men, by a margin of about 3–4 to 1. Most cases are diagnosed between the ages of 20 and 40.

A strong genetic link has been established in Graves disease. If one person has this disorder, it is likely that some form of thyroid dysfunction will be present in another first- or second-degree relative. Studies of identical twins show that if one twin develops Graves disease, the other twin probably will as well, although the leading signs and symptoms could be significantly different.

Etiology: What Happens?

Hyperthyroidism is usually caused by one of three things: a thyroid infection, a nodule or group of nodules that become hyperactive for unknown reasons (this is called *toxic nodular* or *multinodular goiter*), or an autoimmune attack against the thyroid gland that causes it to secrete excessive amounts of metabolic hormones. A tumor on the pituitary that stimulates excessive secretion of thyroid-stimulating hormone, or a tumor on the thyroid itself may also cause hyperthyroidism, but these are rarer situations.

Autoimmune hyperthyroidism, or Graves disease, is by far the most common variety of this disorder, accounting for some 70 to 80% of all cases. In this situation, antibodies called *thyroid-stimulating immunoglobulins* (TSIs) mistakenly attack the thyroid gland, causing it to grow to huge dimensions. The visible and palpable mass on the thyroid gland is called a goiter.

Under normal circumstances pituitary secretions of thyroid-stimulating hormone (TSH) tell the thyroid when and how much to metabolize fuel into energy. When the thyroid is under attack from TSIs, it behaves as though it were being bombarded with TSH. Consequently, it releases abnormally high levels of both thyroid hormones, thyroxine (T_4) and triiodothyronine (T_3). The result is that the conversion of fuel into energy increases by 60 to 100%.

Although genetics clearly plays a major part in Graves disease, its onset often seems to be connected to a stressful situation like a death in the family or a job change. Other risk factors for developing this disorder include exposure of the thyroid to x-rays or antiviral medications like interferon or interleukin.

Graves disease is named after an Irish physician, Robert J. Graves (1796–1853) who first documented the relationship between an enlarged thyroid gland (goiter) and the symptoms it produces (bulging eyes and excessive production of energy from fuel).

Signs and Symptoms

The primary symptom of Graves disease is the development of a goiter: the gland becomes enlarged enough to create a visible, painless swelling in the neck. Other signs and symptoms are mostly related to the secretion of thyroxine. They include anxiety, irritability, insomnia, rapid heartbeat, tremor, increased perspiration, sensitivity to heat, and unintentional weight loss. Skeletal muscles, especially in the arms, often become weak. Other symptoms may include a lighter than normal flow during menstrual periods, dry skin and brittle nails, and problems specifically with the skin and eyes, discussed below.

Complications

Hyperthyroidism can affect the eyes in a variety of ways. One fairly common situation involves the elevation of eyelids; this makes the eyes appear to bulge. Another eye problem related to Graves disease is a disorder called *Graves ophthalmopathy*. This causes the eyeball to protrude beyond its protective orbit because of edema in the orbit combined with weak extra-orbital muscles. The front surface of the eye can dry out, causing light sensitivity, double vision, decreased freedom of movement within the orbit, pain, and excessive production of tears. Protrusion of the eyes is known as *exophthalmos* or *proptosis* (Fig. 8-2).

Some Graves disease patients develop red raised patches of skin on their shins and feet. These rashes are called *pretibial myxedema* and are generally not painful or dangerous.

In addition to eye and skin problems, some Graves disease patients experience occasional episodes of especially high metabolism called *thyroid storms*. In these episodes symptoms become suddenly acute and may include rapid heartbeat, fever without infection, intolerance to heat, confusion, agitation, and finally shock. Thyroid storms can be medical emergencies and require immediate intervention to slow the heart and bring down the fever. They are relatively rare, however, and occur mainly in patients who undertreat their disorder or who are experiencing other stressful situations like cardiovascular disease, dialysis, or infection.

Diagnosis

Graves disease is usually diagnosed through a physical examination, a blood test, and an examination of the way the thyroid takes up radioactive iodine.

The physical examination concentrates on issues like goiter, temperature, heart rate, muscle weakness, and tremor. Blood tests look for low levels of TSH combined with high levels of TSIs, along with abnormally high levels of thyroxine. The ingestion of radioactive iodine shows how quickly the thyroid absorbs iodine (a primary component of thyroxine), along with which parts of the thyroid appear to be hyperactive. This test helps to delineate between Graves disease and nodular hyperthyroidism.

Treatment

Hyperthyroidism can be treated in a number of ways, depending on the underlying causes and the severity of the symptoms.

- *Radioactive iodine*. Although this is also a diagnostic tool, radioactive iodine can be used to gradually kill off a portion of the hyperactive thyroid to bring levels of thyroxine to within safe and normal standards. Many Graves disease patients find that their symptoms are relieved with only one or two doses of radioactive iodine, although the majority of them develop signs of hypothyroidism (this chapter) in

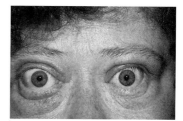

Figure 8-2. Hyperthyroidism: exophthalmos

later months or years. Hypothyroidism is easier to manage than hyperthyroidism and is therefore considered the lesser of the two evils.

- *Antithyroid medications.* Several classes of medications have been developed that prevent the thyroid from producing too much thyroxine or that prevent thyroxine from having a major impact on the body. Sometimes these medications are used to prepare a patient for surgery or radioactive iodine treatment, but occasionally they are successful by themselves.

- *Surgery.* Patients who cannot take antithyroid drugs or radioactive iodine may consider a thyroidectomy, a surgery in which most of the thyroid is removed. This is a risky procedure, however, because the parathyroids (which control calcium metabolism) can be damaged in the process, along with the vocal cords and laryngeal nerves. Surgery for hyperthyroidism is generally avoided if at all possible.

Massage?

As long as the person's skin is healthy and intact, massage of all kinds may be beneficial to clients with hyperactive thyroid glands. The calm, relaxed response that massage creates may provide a welcome change to the symptoms of hyperthyroidism. Care must be taken, however, not to massage or directly stimulate the thyroid gland itself, as this could possibly stimulate a sudden release of T_3 and T_4, leading to the possibility of a thyroid storm. Therefore, any work in the anterior triangle of the neck is locally contraindicated.

HYPOGLYCEMIA IN BRIEF

What is it?
Hypoglycemia is the condition of having abnormally low levels of blood glucose, so cells have no access to important fuel.

What does it look like?
Signs and symptoms of a hypoglycemic episode include dizziness, confusion, chills and sweating, hunger, headache, and pallor. Symptoms pass when a person eats or drinks something with quickly available glucose.

Is massage indicated or contraindicated?
A person in a hypoglycemic episode needs to replace glucose first, get a massage second. Once the symptoms have passed, bodywork is a fine choice. If a person experiences ongoing hypoglycemic symptoms or frequent acute episodes, he or she should find out why.

Hypoglycemia
Definition: What Is It?

Hypoglycemia is the condition of having an inadequate amount of glucose circulating in the blood to fuel all the body's needs. It is usually a complication of other problems, especially *diabetes mellitus* (this chapter), but it occasionally stands alone as a primary disorder.

Demographics: Who Gets It?

Many people experience occasional hypoglycemic episodes when they have been stressed, have not eaten enough, or eat large meals separated by long periods (a schedule that does not allow for gentle fluctuations of blood glucose levels). However, outside the context of diabetes, hypoglycemia is a relatively unusual problem for someone to have in an ongoing, chronic context. It can happen with fasting and some rare genetic diseases that interfere with glucose digestion.

Etiology: What Happens?

The cyclic nature of blood glucose levels is an excellent example of an efficient negative feedback loop. The pancreas secretes two hormones: insulin and glucagon. Insulin *lowers* blood sugar levels by escorting glucose into hungry cells. Glucagon *raises* blood sugar levels by stimulating the liver to release stored glucose into the blood. When blood sugar levels are slightly higher than usual (e.g., after a meal), the pancreas releases insulin to lower them. When they are too low, the pancreas releases glucagon to raise them.

Hypoglycemia occurs when blood glucose levels are abnormally low. The normal range is 60 to 120 mg/dL of blood; hypoglycemia is suspected when the blood glucose level drops below 45 mg/dL. Although the pancreas may release glucagon in an attempt to raise blood glucose levels, the liver may simply not be able to comply or it may comply too slowly. The body is in need of fuel and cannot function normally. Extreme episodes of hypoglycemia can lead to loss of consciousness or even coma.

Hypoglycemia is an occasional reaction to fasting, infection, or stressful situations. When it occurs in diabetes patients, it is in reaction to a dose of insulin that has not been matched by adequate nutrition (see *diabetes*, this chapter).

Signs and Symptoms

Signs and symptoms of hypoglycemia are created by cells that are starving for glucose. They include dizziness, hunger, headache, confusion, blurred vision, and a decreased ability to concentrate. Sweating and chills, pallor, shakiness, increased heart rate, and nausea may also occur. If a person in a hypoglycemic episode does not eat something soon, he or she may lapse into unconsciousness or coma.

Massage?

As stated previously, many people experience occasional episodes of hypoglycemia due to stress, infection, or temporary undereating. Clients experiencing a hypoglycemic attack are better off drinking some juice or eating something high in carbohydrates than they are receiving a massage. When the symptoms have subsided, massage is a perfectly appropriate choice.

If a client reports repeated hypoglycemic episodes, that person would be well advised to pursue the reasons with a nutritional expert. It may be that his or her ability to regulate blood glucose levels is failing, and the early stages of diabetes are present. It may be that the person is showing signs of a hereditary disorder. It could also be that a change in eating habits is in order so that the body can experience less stress in the ongoing job of supplying cells with fuel.

Hypothyroidism
Definition: What Is It?

Hypothyroidism is a condition in which circulating levels of thyroid hormones are abnormally low. This interferes with the body's ability to generate energy from fuel.

Demographics: Who Gets It?

Hypothyroidism is a fairly common condition, affecting about one-tenth of one percent of the population overall. Women are five times more likely to develop hypothyroidism than men. Statistics rise with age; in women older than 65 the incidence of this disorder may be as high as 10%.

Etiology: What Happens?

The thyroid gland produces two different thyroid hormones that influence the metabolism of fuel into energy: triiodothyro-

---

HYPOTHYROIDISM IN BRIEF

What is it?
Hypothyroidism is a condition in which the thyroid gland produces an inadequate supply of the hormones that regulate metabolism of fuel into energy. Some cases of hypothyroidism are the result of an autoimmune attack on the thyroid gland, but others are related to the long-term complications of treatment for *hyperthyroidism* (this chapter) or other factors.

What does it look like?
Symptoms of hypothyroidism are subtle and often missed. They include fatigue, weight gain, depression, intolerance of cold, and for women, heavy menstrual periods.

Is massage indicated or contraindicated?
One of the complications of hypothyroidism, especially in elderly patients, is the accelerated development of *atherosclerosis* (Chapter 4). As long as this condition is recognized and respected, massage can be a supportive and positive experience for hypothyroidism patients.

nine (T_3) and thyroxine (T_4). It does this under the direction of the pituitary gland, which releases thyroid-stimulating hormone (TSH). When adequate amounts of T_3 and T_4 are circulating in the blood, secretion of TSH is suppressed. Thus, the thyroid and the pituitary glands keep each other in balance.

The purpose of thyroid hormones is to stimulate the conversion of fuel (oxygen and calories) into energy. In hypothyroidism, inadequate amounts of thyroid hormones are produced, so incoming fuel is simply stored and never used.

Several different contributing factors of hypothyroidism have been identified.

- *Hashimoto's disease.* This is an autoimmune attack against the thyroid gland that results in the suppression of thyroid secretions (as opposed to the autoimmune attack that stimulates excessive thyroid secretions seen with *Graves disease*, this chapter).

- *Complication of treatment for hyperthyroidism.* Up to 90% of hyperthyroidism patients who use radioactive iodine to suppress thyroid activity eventually develop hypothyroidism.[a]

- *Congenital birth defect.* Some babies are born with abnormally small thyroid glands or no thyroid gland at all. If these children are not treated, they experience stunted growth and mental retardation.

- *Medications.* Some medications, specifically lithium (used to treat bipolar depression) or iodides (used as a form of iodine), can suppress thyroid function.

- *Exposure to radiation.* Persons who have been exposed to radiation in the neck for cancer treatment or in more general ways have a high risk of developing hypothyroidism. Overexposure to radiation and subsequent hypothyroidism has been an issue for survivors of the Chernobyl nuclear plant accident.

- *Idiopathic.* Some cases of hypothyroidism do not seem to be related to any specific underlying disorder, but simply arise without known cause. This situation seems to be especially prevalent among middle-aged women. This type of hypothyroidism is often linked with other chronic conditions including *chronic fatigue syndrome* (Chapter 5) and *fibromyalgia syndrome* (Chapter 2).

Whatever the cause for hypothyroidism, the net result is that a person has difficulty turning fuel into energy. The body tends to absorb nutrition and store it indefinitely, either as fat in lipid cells or as cholesterol in atherosclerotic plaques (see *atherosclerosis*, Chapter 4).

Signs and Symptoms

Signs and symptoms of hypothyroidism are often subtle but steadily progressive. A person may not realize the extent of the problem until it is pointed out by someone else. The result of not being able to convert fuel into energy means that a person gains weight, feels fatigued and depressed, and has a sluggish digestive system with chronic constipation. She has poor tolerance of cold, and her skin is puffy but dry. She may have many symptoms of fibromyalgia syndrome, *depression* (Chapter 3), or chronic fatigue syndrome. Her hair will be flat and brittle and may even fall out. Menstrual periods tend to be heavy and long lasting. Some hypothyroidism patients will develop goiter, a painless enlargement of the thyroid that is also seen with hyperthyroidism.

[a]The overactive thyroid: Hyperthyroidism caused by Graves' disease (diffuse toxic goiter). Thyroid Foundation of America; 1998. Available at: http://www.tsh.org/ Accessed spring 2001.

It is common for hypothyroid patients to develop atherosclerosis, as liver function to produce the chemicals that expel cholesterol from the body is sluggish. High cholesterol levels from hypothyroidism do not respond to cholesterol-lowering medications. Fluid retention in the arms and wrists raises the risk of *carpal tunnel syndrome* (Chapter 3); fluid retention in the neck along with goiter may cause chronic hoarseness. Severe cases may cause a patient to become so cold and drowsy that she becomes unconscious. This is called *myxedema coma* and it is a significant cause of death among elderly hypothyroidism patients.

Diagnosis

Physical examinations for hypothyroidism look for goiter along with a significantly slowed heart rate. Reflexes are often slower in hypothyroid patients.

Blood tests may be conducted to look for elevated levels of antithyroid antibodies, which would point to a diagnosis of Hashimoto's disease. TSH levels may also be evaluated. If the thyroid is underactive, the pituitary may pour more of this chemical into the bloodstream.

It is especially important for pregnant women to be tested for thyroid function. Pregnancy can hide some symptoms of hypothyroidism, which can create serious repercussions for the unborn child. Most newborns are tested for thyroid function as a matter of course; early intervention in the rare cases when thyroid function is subnormal can prevent stunted growth and mental retardation.

Controversy is developing over what is considered "normal" levels of circulating thyroid hormones. The standards now employed may not reflect the true needs of many people who live with hypothyroidism at levels that are too subtle to be detected by current tests. As research continues into this condition, new ranges of normal levels may be developed to meet the needs of individuals more accurately than do current standards.

Treatment

The treatment of hypothyroidism is to supplement thyroid hormones. In the early days of understanding this disease, desiccated thyroid glands of a variety of animals were prescribed to treat hypothyroidism. The doses were difficult to regulate, since potency could vary widely. Nowadays thyroxine is replaced with synthetic versions of the hormone. Hypothyroidism is a progressive disease, and medications must be monitored carefully to ensure that a patient is getting the correct dose.

Massage?

Outside the risk of atherosclerosis (which is a risk for many mature clients regardless of thyroid function), massage is a perfectly appropriate choice for hypothyroidism clients. Although it is unlikely to stimulate normal production of thyroxine, massage can certainly improve the quality of life of people who feel chronically drained and lethargic.

Chapter Review Questions: Endocrine System Conditions

1. Describe the negative feedback loop between insulin and glucagon.

2. What structure controls both the autonomic nervous system and the endocrine system?

3. Describe two ways in which acromegaly can contribute to congestive heart failure.

4. How can diabetes contribute to heart disease? Kidney disease? Blindness?

5. What are three symptoms of abnormally low levels of thyroid hormones?

6. What are three symptoms of abnormally high levels of thyroid hormones?

7. How can hyperthyroidism eventually lead to hypothyroidism?

8. Describe the signs and symptoms of a person experiencing a hypoglycemic attack.

9. Your client has type 2 diabetes. Her tissues are warm, elastic, and responsive. She exercises regularly and eats carefully to control her disease. What are some concerns or cautions for Swedish massage?

10. Your client has type 2 diabetes. Her legs are cool and clammy and have red patches of stasis dermatitis. Her feet show no open ulcers, but an ingrown toenail looks inflamed and painful; she is unaware that it is there. What are some concerns or cautions for Swedish massage?

Bibliography, Endocrine System Conditions

General References, Digestive System

1. de Dominico G, Wood E. *Beard's Massage.* Philadelphia, PA: WB Saunders; 1997

2. Damjanou I. *Pathology for the Health-Related Professions.* Philadelphia, PA: WB Saunders; 1996.

3. Travell J, Simons DG. *Myofascial Pain and Dysfunction: The Trigger Point Manual.* Baltimore, MD: Williams & Wilkins; 1983.

4. Clemente CD. *Anatomy: A Regional Atlas of the Human Body.* 3rd ed. Baltimore, MD: Urban & Schwarzenburg; 1987.

5. Tortora GJ, Anagnostakos NP. *Principles of Anatomy and Physiology.* 6th ed. New York, NY: Harper & Row; 1990.

6. *Taber's Cyclopedic Dictionary.* 14th ed. Philadelphia, PA: FA Davis; 1981.

7. *Stedman's Medical Dictionary.* 26th ed. Baltimore, MD: Williams & Wilkins; 1995.

8. Memmler RL, Wood DL. *The Human Body in Health and Disease.* 5th ed. Philadelphia, PA: JB Lippincott; 1983.

9. Juhan D. *Job's Body: A Handbook for Bodywork.* Barrytown, NY: Station Hill Press; 1987.

10. Mulvihill ML. *Human Diseases: A Systemic Approach.* 2nd ed. Norwalk, CT: Appleton & Lange; 1987.

11. Kunz JRM, Finkel AJ, eds. *The American Medical Association Family Medical Guide.* New York, NY: Random House; 1987.

12. Marieb EM. *Human Anatomy and Physiology.* Redwood City, CA: Benjamin/Cummings; 1989.

13. Sapolsky RM. *Why Zebras Don't Get Ulcers: An Updated Guide to Stress, Stress-Related Disease, and Coping.* New York, NY: W.H. Freeman; 1998.

14. Endocrinology and hormone rhythms. Endocrine Society; 2001. Available at: http://216.205.53.178/endo/pubrelations/patientInfo/hormone.htm. Accessed spring 2001.

15. The endocrine system. M.J. Farabee; 1992, 1994, 1997, 1998, 2000. Available at: http://gened.emc.maricopa.edu/bio/bio181/BIOBK/BioBookENDOCR.html#Hormones. Accessed spring 2001.

16. Mulinda JR. Goiter. In *Medicine, Ob/Gyn, Psychiatry, and Surgery/Endocrinology.* eMedicine. com, Inc.; 2001. Available at: http://www.emedicine.com/med/topic916.htm. Accessed spring 2001.

17. Tuck J. Cortisol. Available at: http://www.science.mcmaster.ca/Biology/4S03/cortisol.html. Accessed spring 2001.

Acromegaly

1. Katznelson L. Acromegaly: Complications and therapeutic update. *Neuroendocrine Center Bulletin.* 1997;4(1). Available at: http://neurosurgery.mgh.harvard.edu/NCBV4I1.htm#Acromeg. Accessed spring 2001.

2. Khandwala HM. Acromegaly. In *Medicine, Ob/Gyn, Psychiatry, and Surgery/Endocrinol-* *ogy.* eMedicine.com, Inc.; 2001. Available at: http://www.emedicine.com/med/topic27.htm. Accessed spring 2001.

3. Somavert (Pegvisomant) blocks excessive growth hormone in acromegaly. Available at: http://www.docguide.com/dgc.nsf/news/3447F2DE54084450852568C700468953?OpenDocument&id=1BC2BB3D41D43C10852568C90015700D&c=Endocrinology%20Other&count=10. Accessed spring 2001.

Diabetes Mellitus

1. Diabetes emergencies. Mayo Foundation for Medical Education and Research; 2000. Available at: http://www.mayohealth.org/mayo/9805/htm/dia_sb5.htm. Accessed spring 2001.

2. Endocrinology and type 1 diabetes—insulin dependent diabetes mellitus (IDDM). The Endocrine Society; 2001. Available at: http://216.205.53.178/endo/pubrelations/patientInfo/diabetes1.htm. Accessed spring 2001.

3. Endocrinology and type II diabetes. The Endocrine Society; 2001. Available at: http://216.205.53.178/endo/pubrelations/patientInfo/diabetes2.htm. Accessed spring 2001.

4. Diabetes: A serious public health problem AT-A-GLANCE 2000. Centers for Disease Control and Prevention. National Center

for Chronic Disease Prevention and Health Promotion. Available at: http://www.cdc.gov/diabetes/pubs/glance.htm. Accessed spring 2001.

5. Tuomilehto J, Lindstrom J, Eriksson JG, Valle TT, et al. Prevention of type 2 diabetes mellitus by changes in lifestyle among subjects with impaired glucose tolerance. *N Engl J Med.* 2001;344(18). Available at: http://www.docguide.com/news/content.nsf/PaperFrameSet?OpenForm&id=1BC2BB3D41D43C10852568C90015700D&newsid=8525697700573E1885256A41004A6139&u=http://www.nejm.org/content/2001/0344/0018/1343.asp&ref=/news/content.nsf/news/8525697700573E1885256A41004A6139?OpenDocument&id=1BC2BB3D41D43C10852568C90015700D&c=&count=10. Accessed spring 2001.

6. NINDS diabetic neuropathy information page. National Institute of Diabetes and Digestive and Kidney Diseases, The National Institute of Neurological Disorders and Stroke, National Institutes of Health. Available at: http://www.ninds.nih.gov/health_and_medical/disorders/diabetic_doc.htm. Accessed spring 2001.

7. Peritoneal dialysis. The University of Kansas Medical Center. Available at: http://www.kumc.edu/SAH/resp_care/cybercas/franperi.html. Accessed spring 2001.

8. Lindner L. Type 2 diabetes hits kids. *Special to The Washington Post.* December 5, 2000:Z10. Available at: http://www.washingtonpost.com/wp-dyn/articles/A25424-2000Dec5.html. Accessed spring 2001.

9. What is type 1 diabetes? American Diabetes Association; 1999. Available at: http://www.diabetes.org/ada/Type1.asp. Accessed spring 2001.

10. What is type 2 diabetes? American Diabetes Association; 1999. Available at: http://www.diabetes.org/ada/type2.asp. Accessed spring 2001.

Hyperthyroidism

1. Grave's disease. Mayo Foundation for Medical Education and Research; 2001. Available at: http://www.mayoclinic.com/home?id=5.1.1.7.7. Accessed spring 2001.

2. The overactive thyroid: Hyperthyroidism caused by Graves' disease (diffuse toxic goiter). Thyroid Foundation of America; 1998. Available at: http://www.tsh.org/. Accessed spring 2001.

3. Hyperthyroidism. American Thyroid Association; 1996. Available at: http://www.thyroid.org/patient/brochur4.htm. Accessed spring 2001.

4. Manifold CA. Hyperthyroidism, thyroid storm and Graves' disease. In *Emergency Medicine/Endocrine and Metabolic*. eMedicine.com, Inc.; 2001. Available at: http://www.emedicine.com/emerg/topic269.htm. Accessed spring 2001.

5. Shomon M. Thyroid disease 101: Basic information on hypothyroidism, hyperthyroidism, nodules, goiter, and thyroid cancer. http://www.about.com/library/weekly/aa042100a.htm. Accessed spring 2002.

6. Schlichtmann J, Graber MA. Hematologic, electrolyte, and metabolic disorders: Thyroid storm. Department of Family Medicine, University of Iowa; 1992–2001. Available at: http://www.vh.org/Providers/ClinRef/FPHandbook/Chapter05/13-5.html . Accessed spring 2001.

Hypoglycemia

1. Hypoglycemia. National Institute of Diabetes and Digestive and Kidney Diseases (NIDDK). NIH publication no. 95-3926. Available at: http://www.niddk.nih.gov/health/diabetes/pubs/hypo/hypo.htm. Accessed spring 2001.

Hypothyroidism

1. What tests will confirm the diagnosis of hypothyroidism? WebMD Corporation; 1996–2001. Available at: http://my.webmd.com/content/article/1680.51479. Accessed spring 2001.

2. Hypothyroidism: The underactive thyroid. The Thyroid Foundation of America; 1998. Available at: http://www.tsh.org/ptinfo/hypobroc.html. Accessed spring 2001.

3. Manifold CA. Hypothyroidism and myxedema coma. In *Emergency Medicine/Endocrine and Metabolic*. eMedicine.com, Inc.; 2001. Available at: http://www.emedicine.com/emerg/topic280.htm. Accessed spring 2001.

Urinary System Conditions

CHAPTER OBJECTIVES

After reading this chapter, the reader should be able to . . .

- Name four major structures that comprise the urinary system.
- Name a hormone produced by the kidneys and its function.
- Name the primary causative factor for most kidney stones.
- Name the causative agent in most cases of pyelonephritis.
- Name two types of renal failure.

- Name two contributing factors for acute renal failure.
- Name the most commonly recognized factor in the development of bladder cancer in industrialized countries.
- Explain why women get urinary tract infections more often than men.
- Explain why if a man gets a urinary tract infection it could indicate a serious problem.
- Name the difference between interstitial cystitis and a bladder infection.

INTRODUCTION

Urinary System Introduction
Function and Structure

The urinary system is a relatively small system in the body, composed of the kidneys, the ureters, the bladder, and the urethra.

The huge renal artery comes directly off the aorta and enters the kidneys. It rapidly decreases in diameter to form thousands of capillaries. Each of these is entangled with another type of epithelial tube: the nephron, which surrounds the knot-like capillary glomerulus with the Bowman's capsule and winds a complicated pathway all around the capillary loop (Fig. 9-1). The constant force of blood pressure from the renal artery forces movement of fluids from circulatory capillaries into the nephrons. Chemical exchanges are made back and forth at this point. Waste products and water are squeezed out of the capillaries and into the nephrons, and then later in the loop the capillaries reabsorb whatever water and salts are needed to keep the blood properly diluted. The nephron then takes its load of wastes and excess water to the renal pelvis where it delivers everything that the body needs to expel. The renal pelvis empties into the ureters; they lead to the bladder, which acts as a holding tank. When enough urine has accumulated, it is expelled through the urethra.

The cleansed blood, now relieved of excess water, nitrogenous wastes, uric acid, and other debris, exits the kidney through the renal vein.

The kidneys have another function that is not directly involved in the filtering of waste products from the blood. *Erythropoietin* (EPO), a hormone that stimulates red blood cell production, is produced in the kidneys. Damage to these delicate organs can therefore sometimes be identified by changes in red blood cell production.

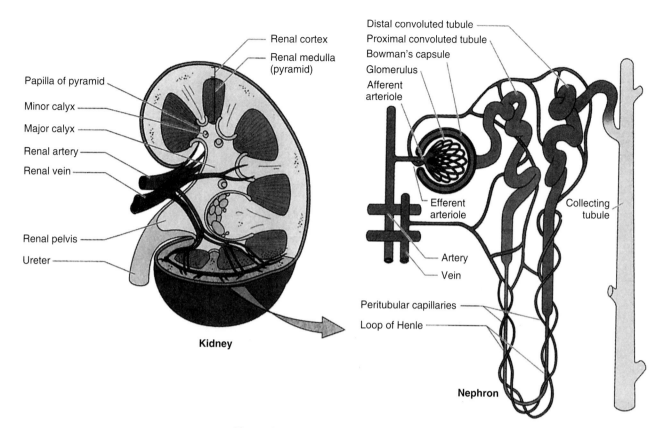

Figure 9-1. Overview of the urinary system

Kidneys are constructed primarily of epithelial tissue, which makes them vulnerable to injury. This is why tapotement along the inferior edge of the rib cage is not recommended; it is unlikely, but possible to injure the kidneys here. When the kidneys have been damaged, red blood cells leak from capillaries into the nephrons. This shows as blood in the urine (*hematuria*) and is evidence of trauma, infection, or other potentially dangerous situations in the kidneys.

Filtration, the movement of substances through a membrane by external mechanical pressure (in this case the blood pressure), is the mechanism by which most substances are exchanged between the circulatory system and the urinary system. It is clear how carefully intertwined blood pressure and kidney health must be. If blood pressure is consistently high (see *hypertension*, Chapter 4), then the kidneys will sustain damage and become less efficient. Conversely, if the kidneys are not functioning adequately, the body accumulates excess fluid, which forces blood pressure to rise. Some of the conditions discussed in this chapter have to do with the complicated relationship between the urinary and circulatory systems. Other conditions considered here will be related to the vulnerability of the urinary system organs to infection.

Urinary System Conditions

Kidney Disorders
Glomerulonephritis
Kidney Stones
Pyelonephritis
Renal Failure

Bladder and Urinary Tract Disorders
Bladder Cancer
Interstitial Cystitis
Urinary Tract Infection

Kidney Disorders

Glomerulonephritis

Definition: What Is It?

Glomerulonephritis is a relatively rare but serious situation involving inflammation and scarring of the glomeruli (microscopic knots of epithelial tissue that are surrounded by capsules). This is where fluids expressed from the circulatory system enter the nephron. Several types of glomerulonephritis have been classified. Many of them have no known cause, some are related to other specific diseases, and some are complications of or autoimmune reactions to other infections in the body.

Demographics: Who Gets It?

Different age groups are at risk for different types of glomerulonephritis. Children may experience this disease as a complication of a streptococcal infection. Adults may experience glomerulonephritis as a spontaneous event or as a part of an autoimmune disorder, an allergy, or a reaction to toxic exposure.

Etiology: What Happens?

The semipermeable membranes that separate the circulatory capillaries from the nephrons act as filters to keep vital blood components in the bloodstream while allowing water and wastes to exit into the urinary system. An acute or chronic inflammatory reaction in these filters can compromise their effectiveness and allow important substances to leave the body through the urine. Glomerulonephritis is defined by an inflammatory reaction, usually in association with immune system dysfunction. The chronic inflammation leads to an accumulation of scar tissue where only soft, pliable epithelium should be; this means the kidneys become progressively less able to manage fluids in the body, and it may lead to chronic *renal failure* (this chapter).

When the body launches a specific immune system attack against an invader, a variety of things can happen. One mechanism involves the formation of "immune complexes": sticky bits of pathogens and their antibodies, often accompanied by *complement* (a series of immune system chemicals that are meant to aid in the destruction of invading pathogens). Under normal circumstances, these clumps of material would be consumed by macrophages. Occasionally they can develop in or get caught by the glomeruli, leading to a localized inflammatory reaction. This seems to be the case in most types of glomerulonephritis.

It is not always clear what leads to the development of immune complexes in the kidneys. For some people this is connected to autoimmune dysfunction; glomerulonephritis is a common complication of *lupus* (Chapter 5) or other autoimmune diseases. It can also be related to a delayed reaction against certain kinds of streptococcal infections, especially when this is seen in young children. Many people who have glomerulonephritis have also been exposed to environmental toxins (notably hydrocarbons, silicon, mercury, and lithium), which opens the possibility that this disorder may arise as a kind of hypersensitivity reaction.

GLOMERULONEPHRITIS IN BRIEF

What is it?
Glomerulonephritis is a condition in which the glomeruli (small structures that are part of the nephron-capillary unit) become inflamed and cease to function efficiently.

How is it recognized?
Early symptoms of glomerulonephritis include dark or rust-colored urine, foamy urine, or blood in the urine. Later symptoms indicate chronic renal failure and include systemic edema, fatigue, headaches, decreased urine output, rashes and discoloration of the skin, and general malaise.

Is massage indicated or contraindicated?
Symptomatic glomerulonephritis systemically contraindicates circulatory massage. This is an inflammatory condition that impairs the body's ability to manage fluid exchanges. Bodywork that does not significantly impact circulation may be appropriate.

GLOMERULUS
This is the diminutive form of the Latin word *glomus*, for "ball of yarn," which is an excellent description of the tufts of capillary loops that allow for diffusion and filtration in the kidneys.

Prognosis

Depending on the cause, glomerulonephritis can be a short-term acute infection with complete recovery (this is usually the case when it accompanies a streptococcal infection), or a long-term progressive condition in which the kidneys are slowly destroyed, leading to end-stage renal failure and dependence on dialysis. No preventive or curative measures have been developed. Some varieties of this disease have been known to recur even after the kidneys have been replaced.

Signs and Symptoms

When the kidneys function inefficiently, the repercussions are felt throughout the rest of the body. However, it may take a long time to see the results. Early symptoms of glomerulonephritis are abnormalities in the urine such as high protein levels or red blood cells. *Hematuria,* or blood in the urine, can be observed as dark or rust-colored urine or as urine that looks pink or foamy. The location of the bleeding determines the color. Occasionally, no observable signs develop. Glomerulonephritis is sometimes found only when a routine analysis reveals higher-than-normal levels of protein or blood in the urine.

Another indicator of glomerulonephritis is *hypertension* (Chapter 4). This is both a symptom and a complication of most chronic kidney disorders, since a disruption in urine output will cause fluid retention and external pressure on all blood vessels. Hypertension that does not respond to normal interventions can sometimes lead to a diagnosis of glomerulonephritis.

Later symptoms of glomerulonephritis are indicators of renal failure, including general malaise, skin discoloration, itching, fatigue, low urine output, systemic edema, and, in very severe cases, lethargy, confusion, and coma.

Treatment

The treatment for this disease depends entirely on the cause and is generally geared toward symptom abatement. Controlling high blood pressure is the first priority. If glomerulonephritis is a complication of a general infection, antibiotics may lead to a complete recovery. If it is an autoimmune or other inflammatory problem, corticosteroids may be used to limit damage to the nephrons. Cytotoxic drugs are also used to inhibit the damaging effects of an immune system attack against the kidneys.

Massage?

This is a condition in which the kidneys are inflamed from a pathogen, an autoimmune reaction, or some unknown reason. The result is a person who may have an infection, who probably has high blood pressure, and who is incapable of processing fluids under normal conditions, much less under the increased volume that massage may produce. Glomerulonephritis systemically contraindicates circulatory massage, although many non-circulatory techniques can yield important benefits without challenging fluid flow.

Kidney Stones
Definition: What Are They?

Also called *renal calculi,* or *nephrolithiases,* kidney stones are crystals that sometimes develop in the renal pelvis. The size of kidney stones varies widely, depending on how long they have been developing and what comprises them. Some stones even grow into the cortex of the kidney, forming what is called a *staghorn calculus* (Fig. 9-2).

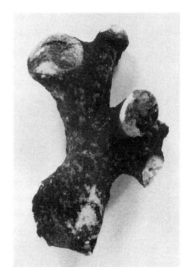

Figure 9-2. Staghorn calculus

KIDNEY STONES IN BRIEF

What are they?
A kidney stone is a solid deposit of crystalline substances inside the kidney.

How are they recognized?
Small stones may create no symptoms at all, but when larger stones enter the ureters, they can cause extreme pain called renal colic. Renal colic may be accompanied by nausea and vomiting. Fever and chills indicate that infection is part of the problem. Pain may refer from the back into the groin.

Is massage indicated or contraindicated?
Acute renal colic contraindicates massage, although any kind of bodywork is appropriate for people with a history of stones but no current symptoms.

Small stones may pass through the urinary tract with no symptoms, but larger ones may get stuck in the ureters. The technical name for them in this location is *ureterolithiasis*.

Demographics: Who Gets Them?

Kidney stones usually form in the absence of adequate fluids. Thus, they are very common in tropical environments where people tend to lose more liquid through sweat than they replace. Peak months for the diagnosis of kidney stones in the United States are June through August, for the same reason. The incidence of kidney stones in the United States is rising, particularly in the southeast. This has given rise to the term "stone belt" for this part of the country.

Four of five people diagnosed with kidney stones are men. Kidney stones happen more frequently among Whites than among other races. Every year about 1 million people in the United States pass a stone; this accounts for almost half a million emergency room visits per year. It is predicted that about 10% of all Americans will pass a stone at some time. Most people who are susceptible to kidney stones get their first one between 20 and 30 years old, and 75% of them will experience at least one repeat stone sometime in their life.

Etiology: What Happens?

Kidney stones can be composed of several different substances, each one indicative of a different type of metabolic problem.

- *Calcium oxalate or calcium phosphate stones.* These account for the largest majority of kidney stones, from 75 to 85%. They are associated with parathyroid dysfunction (too much calcium is pulled off the bones into the bloodstream), too much vitamin D, abnormally high rates of calcium absorption in the gastrointestinal tract, abnormal leakage of calcium or phosphate into the nephrons, or other problems.

- *Struvite stones.* These stones are associated with chronic *urinary tract infection* (this chapter). Approximately 15% of all kidney stones are struvite stones.

- *Uric acid stones.* These stones form in the kidneys of people whose blood is abnormally acidic. Accounting for about 6% of all kidney stones, uric acid stones are associated with a diet high in meat and purines. People who have uric acid kidney stones are also at high risk for *gout* (Chapter 2).

- *Cystine stones.* These stones are relatively rare, comprising only 2% of all kidney stones. They are directly related to a genetic dysfunction with the metabolism of cystine, an amino acid.

- *Other stones.* A tiny percentage of all kidney stones falls outside the four main categories. Genetic problems with metabolism or the use of protease inhibitors (see *HIV/AIDS*, Chapter 5) are usually the causes of these stones.

Signs and Symptoms

The vast majority of kidney stones are completely silent: 85% or more of them pass through the ureters without pain. When they get stuck or when they are large enough to scrape the delicate lining of the urinary tract, however, kidney stones cause a typical extreme "grabbing pain." The ureters contract in irritation, causing *renal colic*. The pain has a sudden onset, comes and goes in waves, and can be so severe that it causes nausea and vomiting as a sympathetic reaction. The pain often refers into the groin area. Occasionally the stone may be caused by or may lead to an infection in the kidneys; in these instances, fever and chills accompany the severe pain.

Complications

Most kidney stones that are big enough to cause problems are excruciatingly painful, but they do eventually pass into the bladder and out in the urine without causing long-lasting damage to the urinary system. Occasionally, however, a stone can grow to be of a size to seriously disrupt kidney function. This may lead to chronic or acute *renal failure* (this chapter).

Diagnosis

The large majority of all kidney stones are too small to cause any pain or symptoms, although they may be discovered during routine radiographs for other problems. When they are big enough to get lodged in some spot in the urinary tract, the typical flank pain is often accompanied by signs of blood in the urine. The precise size and location of the stones can be determined by use of radiography or sonography.

Treatment

The pain of kidney stones is so intense that long ago people operated on them without anesthesia; "cutting for stone" was considered worth living through, just to get rid of them. Nowadays several other options are available, and only a small percentage of kidney stone patients have to go through major surgery. Three main interventions for kidney stones have been developed. Which one is appropriate is determined by the stones' size, location, and the general health of the patient.

- *Percutaneous nephrolithotomy* is a surgery conducted through a tiny tunnel in the back leading to the offending stone. When the stone is reached, it is either extracted or subjected to sonic waves that reduce its size.

- *Uteroscopic stone removal* uses a flexible tube that is inserted into the urethra and snakes up to where the stone is lodged to remove it from the ureters.

- *Extracorporeal shockwave lithotripsy* is the use of sound waves to break up stones into a size that can be passed through the ureters with minimal risk for getting stuck. This procedure can leave the patient feeling bruised and battered from the extremity of the shock waves that are required to break up stones, but it can treat larger deposits than either of the other two options.

Preventive treatments for persons susceptible to kidney stones depend on what comprises the stones. This is why it is necessary for patients to catch their stones as they pass with the urine. The stones are then analyzed, as is the urine passed, within a 24-hour period after the stone passes. A treatment program is developed based on these findings.

Some interventions include surgery to remove the parathyroid glands, medication to regulate metabolism, dietary adjustments, and most importantly adequate hydration. Kidney stone patients need to drink up to 1 gallon of water every day to keep stones moving through the system before they become big enough to cause problems.

Massage?

Massage for people with a history of kidney stones but no present symptoms is perfectly appropriate. However, a person with or without a history of kidney stones who is experiencing *any* symptoms of renal colic is not a good candidate for massage.

CASE HISTORY: KIDNEY STONES
Walter B, Age 77
"Once you've had a kidney stone, you never forget it."

I've had kidney stone attacks since 1939, then in 1944, and so on and so forth. The first time I was 19 years old. I'd been horseback riding the day before, so when the pain started we figured I had just thrown my back out somehow. The director of the hospital finally detected what it really was.

In 1944 I had an attack at night, in bed. Once you've had a kidney stone attack, you never forget what it feels like. I knew immediately what was happening and they rushed me via command car to the military hospital, 20 miles away from the Battle of the Bulge. The renal surgeon authorized an attempt to remove the stone with an uteroscopic tube. Back in those days the tube was metal, not flexible—hence the discomfort, which I've never forgotten. The procedure was unsuccessful because somehow I had already passed the stone.

The doctor said that I had "anomalous kidneys."

"What the hell does that mean?" I asked.

"It just means they're unlike any kidneys I've ever seen," he said.

After these two incidents I wasn't given any further treatment or medication. I was just told to drink plenty of liquids.

I had another attack in the 1960s. I was visiting a friend in Swampscott and had to try to drive 25 miles into Boston without killing myself or anyone else—quite an ordeal. But I never passed a whole stone; they all turned to gravel.

Then in the Blizzard of '78, I had my last attack. Boston was digging out from a huge snowstorm. No one was allowed to drive; the streets had to be clear for ambulances and fire trucks. The pain was God-awful, just unbearable. They always say it's like having a baby—you just wouldn't believe it. I couldn't get to the hospital right away, so the doctor told me to drink some whiskey to dull the pain. Finally, I was given special dispensation to take a taxicab to the hospital.

In the hospital they put a tube up the urethra to try to "basket" the stone. That was the only one they ever got. I remember, I was laying on my side with the sheet like a big tent draped over me. I just had a local anesthetic, and when the doctor finally got the stone, he dropped it on my sheet—it sounded just like a pebble dropping.

When the stone was basketed at the hospital it was sent to the kidney stone lab, where it was identified as a calcium stone. The medication consisted of Allopurinol tablets and hydrochlorothiazide pills taken daily. There's been no sign of an attack since then.

About 4 years ago I had another uteroscopic procedure as part of a regular examination. The urologist used a new flexible tube (not like the metal one from 1944!). The whole thing took about 4 minutes and involved a minimum of discomfort. Several of my friends, though, have had attacks within the past year or two, and their treatment and recovery seemed to be much more painful and prolonged than mine, in spite of all the new techniques available.

PYELONEPHRITIS IN BRIEF

What is it?
Pyelonephritis is an infection of the kidney and/or renal pelvis.

How is it recognized?
Symptoms of acute pyelonephritis include burning pain with urination, back pain, fever, chills, nausea, and vomiting. Chronic infections may show no symptoms.

Is massage indicated or contraindicated?
Kidney infections systemically contraindicate circulatory massage until the infection has been completely eradicated.

Pyelonephritis
Definition: What Is It?

As the name implies, pyelonephritis is an infection of the nephrons in the kidney, although the renal pelvis may also be involved. Infections may be acute and severe, or chronic with few or no symptoms, but damage to the kidneys progresses nonetheless.

Etiology: What Happens?

Most kidney infections are a complication of an *Escherichia coli* infection in the urinary tract that travels up the ureters to set up an infection in the kidneys themselves (see *urinary tract infection*, this chapter). Other kidney infections can develop from more obscure pathogens. They can also be related to *diabetes* (Chapter 8) or pregnancy, they can arise from a neurogenic bladder (a bladder that has no motor control and so empties passively into a bag), or they can come from surgical or medical instrumentation such as catheters or cystoscopes. Some kidney infections can be a complication of a *kidney stone* (this chapter) or a tumor that blocks the ureters.

Signs and Symptoms

Acute pyelonephritis usually involves the rapid onset of symptoms that begin with a urinary tract infection and move deeper into the body. They include fever, burning and frequency of urination, cloudy urine, extreme back pain, fatigue, nausea, and vomiting.

Chronic pyelonephritis is often a situation in which an acute infection has been incompletely treated, and so bacterial invasion of the kidney continues but in a quieter fashion. Therefore, many chronic kidney infections are silent; they create no symptoms, but damage accumulates in the kidney.

Complications

Regardless of whether the situation is chronic or acute, if pyelonephritis is recurrent it can cause scarring and long-lasting kidney damage. Insufficient kidney activity leads to *hypertension* (Chapter 4) and *renal failure* (this chapter). Another possible complication of a very acute infection is sepsis (blood poisoning from the infection leaking into capillaries). This is a life-threatening situation that can lead rapidly to dangerously *low* blood pressure and death.

Diagnosis

Urinalysis to look for signs of infection, combined with symptoms that describe pain higher and more extreme than found with a typical urinary tract infection, is usually enough information for a diagnosis of kidney infection. If the infectious agent is something unusual, more tests may be needed. Computed tomography (CT) scans or intravenous pyelograms are sometimes used to look for kidney stones or tumors that might be causing problems or abscesses on the kidneys that can create similar symptoms.

Treatment

Most kidney infections clear up satisfactorily with antibiotic therapy. If the infection is very extreme, the patient may need to be hospitalized to monitor how well he or she is processing fluids.

Prevention

Acute pyelonephritis is almost always related to bacteria that enter the body at the urethral opening. Let this be a lesson, ladies: always wipe front to back.

Massage?

Acute kidney infections contraindicate circulatory bodywork. The risk of making the situation worse is matched only by the patient's inability to lie still, since the pain is so extreme. Chronic kidney infections are less dramatic, but the kidneys are still vulnerable to damage. The safest course is to avoid any circulatory work until all signs of infection have been eradicated.

RENAL FAILURE IN BRIEF

What is it?
Renal failure is a situation in which the kidneys are incapable of functioning at normal levels. It may be an acute or a chronic problem, but it is often life-threatening.

How is it recognized?
Symptoms of acute and chronic renal failure differ in severity and type of onset, but some things they have in common are reduced urine output, systemic edema, and changes in mental state brought about by the accumulation of toxins in the blood.

Is massage indicated or contraindicated?
Acute and chronic renal failure systemically contraindicate circulatory massage.

Renal Failure
Definition: What Is It?

Renal failure means that for various reasons the kidneys are not functioning adequately. If the kidneys slow down suddenly (e.g., in response to shock or systemic infection), this is referred to as *acute renal failure*. If they sustain cumulative damage over the course of many years, this is called *chronic renal failure*. In either case, although the name implies that they have ceased functioning altogether, the truth is that the kidneys are still working but they are simply unable to keep up with the body's demands.

Demographics: Who Gets It?

Statistics for renal failure vary according to whether it is an acute or chronic problem. Risk factors for developing chronic renal failure are having chronic *hypertension* (Chapter 4) and/or *diabetes* (Chapter 8). Some incidence of renal failure is determined by geographical distribution, suggesting the influence of environmental toxins. Race is also a determining factor: African-Americans are far more likely to experience both chronic high blood pressure and chronic renal failure than are Whites. This is a phenomenon that is currently being researched.

Etiology: What Happens?

Although the kidneys are able to heal from most short-term abuse, any chronic or severe recurrent problems may eventually cause permanent damage to the delicate tissues, thereby interfering with kidney function. Fortunately, the human body is equipped with about twice as much kidney as it really needs, so people can tolerate a large amount of damage before they have problems.

Kidneys have several important functions: they produce EPO, the hormone that stimulates blood cell production; they manage electrolyte levels in the blood; they concentrate urine; and they manage overall fluid levels by taking water and wastes out of the blood and then putting whatever water the body still needs back in. When kidney function is measured, it is often in terms of *glomerular filtration rate*, that is, how efficiently fluid moves from the glomeruli into the nephrons. Kidney failure is classified as acute or chronic.

Causes of Acute Renal Failure

Acute renal failure is identified when the glomerular filtration rate suddenly drops to 50% or less of normal levels; this may take place over several hours or days. Causes of acute renal failure usually fall into one of three categories.

- *Prerenal problems.* This means something is preventing blood flow into the kidneys, which means the glomeruli and nephrons essentially collapse from lack of fluid volume. Prerenal problems can include reduced blood volume, low blood pressure from septicemia or traumatic shock, extreme dehydration, or an embolism that blocks the renal artery.

- *Intrarenal problems.* These are pathologies that arise within the kidneys themselves, including *glomerulonephritis* (this chapter), an embolism caught inside the kidney, an *E. coli* infection that produces tissue-damaging toxins (this is also called *hemolytic uremic syndrome),* drug reactions, and other problems.

- *Postrenal problems.* When fluid is prevented from leaving the kidneys, damage to the delicate nephrons can accumulate to dangerous levels. *Kidney stones* (this chapter), *enlarged prostate* (Chapter 10), or tumors can create this kind of problem.

Acute renal failure is generally a short-term problem that may become life-threatening. Its high mortality rate is usually connected to the general health and resiliency of the patient. It may last for days or weeks, but if the contributing factors are controllable, kidney function may be restored. Some patients, however, go on to have chronic renal failure.

Causes of Chronic Renal Failure

Chronic renal failure is an impairment in kidney function that may persist for years before it gets serious or causes any symptoms. It is usually diagnosed when glomerular filtration rate drops below 20% of normal levels. Chronic renal failure occurs in three stages.

- *Diminished renal reserve.* This is the first stage of chronic renal failure. During this stage scar tissue gradually replaces nephrons injured in recurrent infections, from recurring stones, or from chronic high blood pressure, often related to *diabetes* (Chapter 8). Up to 75% of the nephrons may be lost before any symptoms of this stage appear.

- *Renal insufficiency.* This is the second stage of chronic renal failure. At this point the kidneys are functioning at about 25% of normal levels. Blood levels of nitrogenous wastes, uric acid, and creatinine are increasing. Tests for protein in the urine are positive at this time, although no other specific symptoms may be observable.

- *End-stage kidney failure.* This is the last stage of the disease. In this situation up to 90% of the nephrons have been lost. Patients must rely on hemodialysis to process wastes out of the blood. They are candidates for a kidney transplant if they are strong enough to withstand the surgery.

Signs and Symptoms

Because the kidneys have so many functions, symptoms of renal failure affect virtually every major organ system of the body. Symptoms include decreased urine output, systemic *edema* from salt and water retention (Chapter 5), arrhythmia from potassium retention, *anemia* from the lack of EPO (Chapter 4), and osteomalacia (bone thinning) from the lack of vitamin D (which is necessary for calcium metabolism). Rashes and skin discoloration arise from the retention of toxic pigments in the blood. Other symptoms include lethargy, fatigue, headaches, loss of sensation in the hands and feet, tremors, seizures, easy bruising and bleeding, muscle cramps, and changes in mental and emotional states as the accumulation of wastes in the blood affects the brain.

Treatment

Treatment for acute and chronic renal failure is determined by whatever underlying pathologies caused the damage. Treatment goals are to control the symptoms, prevent further complications, and slow the progress of the disease. This often means controlling blood pressure and blood sugar levels (if diabetes is part of the picture). Medication to control potassium levels in the blood is important to avoid heart problems. Fluid and salt intake may be restricted until kidney function can keep up with the body's demands. Diuretics are sometimes prescribed to help the kidneys process fluids.

If a patient's kidneys are simply incompetent regardless of these interventions, dialysis may become necessary. This routes the blood through a machine or through the peritoneum to extract wastes from the blood. Approximately 200,000 people in the United States use kidney dialysis to stay alive.

Kidney transplants replace a damaged organ with a healthy kidney from an appropriate donor. They can be successful if the new tissue is not rejected. Unfortunately, the shortage of suitable donated organs means that among the 27,000 people waiting for kidney transplants today, only 11,000 operations will be performed.

Massage?

Any stage of renal failure contraindicates circulatory massage, although energy work may be supportive and helpful. If a client has a history of renal failure, the massage therapist should inform the health care team that the client wishes to receive massage.

Bladder and Urinary Tract Disorders

BLADDER CANCER IN BRIEF

What is it?
Bladder cancer is the growth of malignant cells in the urinary bladder. Most bladder cancer starts in the superficial layer of transitional epithelium.

How is it recognized?
The earliest sign of bladder cancer is the appearance of blood in the urine, which may be red or rust colored. Bladder cancer is painless at this point. In later stages the bladder may become irritable. Painful urination, reduced urination, or increased urinary frequency may all occur.

Is massage indicated or contraindicated?
As with most varieties of cancer, massage with its parasympathetic effects and immune system support has a place in the recovery process. Bladder cancer has a high recurrence rate and most patients undergo surgery at some point. As long as these issues are respected and the massage therapist works as part of a well-informed health care team, bodywork may be appropriate for these patients.

Bladder Cancer

Definition: What Is It?

Bladder cancer is the development of malignant cells in the urinary bladder.

Demographics: Who Gets It?

Bladder cancer is a relatively common disease. It is the fourth leading cancer among men (following prostate, lung, and colorectal cancers), and the eighth leading cancer among women. About 54,000 new cases are diagnosed each year, and it causes about 12,000 deaths each year in the United States.

Bladder cancer occurs in men about 3 times more often than in women. It affects White men more than any other group, but women and African-American men usually have poorer survival rates than White men. It is usually a disease of older people; the average age at diagnosis is 68 years.

Etiology: What Happens?

Like most types of cancer, most cases of bladder cancer involve epithelial cells, in this case, the transitional epithelium that lines the urinary bladder. Constant, repetitive damage to this epithelium causes the mature cells to die. This stimulates rapid replication in the basal layer, and soon new colonies of immature cells migrate to the surface. These new cells are easily disrupted by genetic mutations and may become malignant growths that cause bleeding into the bladder.

Causes of bladder cancer vary according to medical history and geographic region. Persons who have undergone pelvic radiation for other problems are at an increased risk for developing bladder cancer, as are people who have had chronic infections, bladder stones, or catheter use. In Africa, Asia, and South America, bladder cancer is associated with a specific parasitic infestation, *Schistosoma haematobium*. In the United States and developing countries, most cases of bladder cancer are directly related to more controllable factors.

The transitional epithelium of the bladder seems to be particularly susceptible to damage from environmental toxins. Several genetic mutations that limit the body's ability to inhibit tumor growth or invasion have been linked to bladder cancer. These mutations are frequently triggered by exposure to carcinogenic substances. Approximately half of all bladder cancer cases are believed to be related to cigarette smoking. Other contributing factors include exposure to aromatic amines (chemicals used in dry cleaning fluid, hairdressing chemicals, and textile and rubber industries). The relationship between bladder cancer and carcinogenic substances is one of the most clearly demonstrable links between environmental exposures and cancer. The good news is that bladder cancer is probably a completely preventable disease, if exposure to the carcinogenic substances is limited or eradicated.

Signs and Symptoms

The earliest and most dependable sign of bladder cancer is *hematuria*, or blood in the urine. The urine of a bladder cancer patient is often visibly reddened or rust colored, although the patient experiences no particular pain in the early stages of the disease. If the tumors continue to grow and invade deeper layers of the bladder, secondary symptoms may develop that are related to mechanical pressure, including bladder irritability (painful urination, increased urinary frequency, reduced urine output) and compression on the rectum, pelvic lymph nodes, and any other structures that happen to be in the way.

Diagnosis

If a person in his 60s or 70s has no pain but his urine is bright red or rusty, the immediate conclusion most doctors will come to is that he has bladder cancer. Urine samples may be tested to look for shedding cancer cells, and a digital rectal examination (or pelvic examination if the patient is a woman) will provide information about tumors. Other diagnostic techniques include using dye to stain the urine and make the bladder easy to radiograph; using a cystoscope, with which a physician visually examines the bladder through a tube inserted through the urethra; and performing local biopsies to examine abnormal tissue for signs of metastasis.

Staging

A variety of criteria have been developed to stage bladder cancer. As with all cancers, the earlier it is caught, the better the chances for long-term survival. Although each individual's course of development is different, the progression of bladder cancer is staged as follows:

- *Stage 0: In situ.* This is cancer found very early in its development; it is limited to the most superficial layers of the transitional epithelium.

- *Stage 1:* Cancer cells have invaded deeper layers of the bladder lining but are still within the epithelial boundary.

- *Stage 2:* Cancer cells have invaded the edge of the smooth muscle layer of the bladder.
- *Stage 3A:* Cancer cells have invaded deep into the muscle layer of the bladder.
- *Stage 3B:* Cancer cells have penetrated through the muscle layer and into the connective tissue covering of the bladder.
- *Stage 4A:* Cancer cells are present in the pelvic cavity and the pelvic lymph nodes.
- *Stage 4B:* Cancer cells are present throughout the abdominal cavity and may be found in organs above the diaphragm. The liver, the lungs, and the central nervous system are frequent sites of metastasis.

Treatment

Bladder cancer treatment depends on what stage it is in when it is diagnosed. Surgeons can use a small wire loop on the end of a cystoscope to remove abnormal tissue, or another tool may be used to burn the tumor away with electricity. More invasive surgeries may remove part or all of the bladder, and if signs of pelvic metastasis are present, other tissues as well. Men may lose the prostate gland; women may lose the uterus, ovaries, and parts of the vaginal wall. Pelvic lymph nodes are also removed, leading to the risk of lymphedema in the legs. Urine flow may be routed out of the body through a stoma, or a variety of surgeries have been developed to form artificial bladders from parts of the large or small intestines.

In addition to surgery, radiation and chemotherapy may be used to battle bladder cancer. Chemotherapy may be administered intravenously, orally with pills, or through a site-specific bladder wash to distribute the medication directly to the target tissues.

Prognosis

A huge majority of bladder cancer cases are diagnosed before the cells have moved out of the bladder. This is excellent news, of course, because the survival rate for cancers caught early is much better than for cancers caught in Stage 3 or later. Nevertheless, bladder cancer has an unusual habit of growing in several places at the same time, so although it may be possible to catch one or two tumors, the invisible third, fourth, and fifth tumors may not become symptomatic for another several months. This means that the recurrence rate for bladder cancer is surprisingly high: up to 80% of all patients have at least one recurrence of their cancer during their lifetime.

Overall, the 5-year survival rate for bladder cancer is 76% for Whites and 55% for African-Americans. All bladder cancer patients must follow up their treatment with life-long regular examinations to guard against recurrence.

Massage?

The main issues of concern in working with bladder cancer patients are the high rates of recurrence and the frequency with which surgery is an early treatment intervention. The rules for massage and bladder cancer are the same as the rules for massage and any kind of cancer. While the benefits that bodywork has to offer in the way of immune system strengthening, pain reduction, anxiety reduction, and general support are powerful, massage therapists need to be working as part of a team, sharing information and concerns with the rest of the client's health care staff.

Interstitial Cystitis

Definition: What Is It?

IC is a condition in which the urinary bladder becomes small and inelastic. It is not to be confused with ordinary cystitis, which is a complication of a *urinary tract infection* (this chapter).

Demographics: Who Gets It?

Statistics on IC have been difficult to gather, but it is estimated that somewhere between 450,000 and 1 million Americans have it. Of those, 90% are women, 10% are men. IC is rare in children. The population group most at risk is women between 20 and 50 years of age; the average age at onset is 40.

Etiology: What Happens?

The bladder, a hollow organ, is designed to shrink when it is empty and expand when it is full. A healthy bladder can hold about 1 to 1.5 cups of urine. The average adult passes about 1 to 1.5 quarts of urine every day, depending on how much liquid has been consumed and a number of other factors.

Normal urine is composed of water, excess salts extracted from the blood, nitrogenous wastes like urea and uric acid, and other debris. It should not contain any living microorganisms. Fragments of white blood cells or pathogens indicate an infection somewhere in the urinary system. The bladder itself is shielded from the acidity of urine by a lining of protective mucous.

IC occurs when the inner lining of the bladder no longer protects the organ from urine. Most IC patients develop tiny bleeding areas called pinpoint hemorrhages in the bladder wall. A small number of patients develop a particular kind of star-shaped lesion called a Hunner's ulcer inside the bladder. As the problem progresses, the muscular walls of the bladder become fibrotic and inelastic. Patients find that they have little capacity for storing urine; it is not unusual for them to have to use the bathroom about every 20 minutes.

The cause of IC is a mystery. Leading theorists are looking at the problem as a syndrome, a collection of related signs and symptoms, rather than as a single disease. Many IC patients have symptoms of other chronic pain syndromes, including *fibromyalgia syndrome* (Chapter 2) and *irritable bowel syndrome* (Chapter 7). Further research may eventually reveal that what is now called "interstitial cystitis" is in fact several different disorders that all lead to the same condition: increased frequency, urgency, painful urination, and a bladder the size of a walnut.

One theory at the forefront of IC research is that this may be an autoimmune disease or allergy that weakens the protective mucous membrane in the bladder's epithelium. In this way, irritating chemicals from urine can infiltrate and damage the bladder wall. The presence of abnormal numbers of mast cells in some IC patients supports this theory. Other researchers are considering the possibility that the causative agent for IC may be some pathologic agent that has yet to be identified. IC does not respond to antibiotic therapy, so it is clear that no known strain of bacteria causes this problem.

INTERSTITIAL CYSTITIS IN BRIEF

What is it?
Interstitial cystitis (IC) is a chronic inflammation of the bladder involving scar tissue, stiffening, decreased capacity, pinpoint hemorrhages, and sometimes ulcers in the bladder walls.

How is it recognized?
Symptoms of IC are very much like those of urinary tract infections: burning, increased frequency, and urgency of urination; decreased capacity of the bladder; and pain, pressure, and tenderness.

Is massage indicated or contraindicated?
IC is a poorly understood condition that seems to be exacerbated by stress. Bodywork may be a helpful and supportive choice for IC patients, although it probably will not do anything to reverse the situation.

Signs and Symptoms

Symptoms of IC include pain and burning on urination, increased frequency, urgency, and painful intercourse. Symptoms tend to progressively worsen for about 5 years and then stabilize. Some patients find that symptoms occur in periods of flare and remission; others find that their daily experiences are all about the same.

Diagnosis

IC is diagnosed by the process of exclusion. Conditions that must be ruled out for a positive diagnosis include urinary tract infections, vaginitis, *bladder cancer, kidney stones* (this chapter), *endometriosis* for women, and prostatitis for men. Once these have been ruled out, a cystoscopic examination may be conducted to look for ulcers or bleeding spots, which can only be seen when the bladder is fully distended.

Treatment

Because this is a disease without a known cause, it is also without a known cure. IC treatment is generally aimed at symptomatic relief and the development of coping skills. Often the diagnostic tool of bladder distension can give relief, as can a "distillation" or bladder wash. This is done with dimethyl sulfoxide (DMSO), which can pass into the bladder wall to act as an anti-inflammatory and block pain sensation. Aspirin and other painkillers may be recommended, as are exercise, smoking cessation, and dietary changes. No single intervention is successful for all patients, however, and nothing has yet provided a permanent solution. IC may recur after months or even years of remission.

Some patients have such severe problems that surgery becomes an option. They may have a new bladder constructed from a segment of the colon, or they may have the bladder removed altogether and replaced with a stoma and external bag.

Massage?

Among the interventions IC patients may need to explore are options to reduce the stress and anxiety that accompany chronic, painful conditions. Acupuncture, hypnotherapy, biofeedback, and other therapies are often recommended. Massage can be a useful tool in this effort too, as long as the client's need for frequent urination can be met.

Urinary Tract Infection
Definition: What Is It?

UTIs are infections that may occur anywhere in the urinary system, from the kidneys to the bladder to the urethra. Because kidney infections are discussed elsewhere (see *pyelonephritis*, this chapter), this section focuses on infections of the lower urinary tract: the urethra (urethritis) and the bladder (cystitis).

Demographics: Who Gets It?

UTIs are the cause of about 7 million visits to the doctor every year. Estimates vary, but somewhere between 20 and 50% of all women will have a UTI at least once. It is almost always a women's disorder, because the female urethra is so short and located close to the anus where bacteria that are harmless in the digestive tract can cause havoc if they gain access to the urinary tract.

Although women, particularly sexually active young women, are most at risk for UTIs, other populations may also have this problem. It is certainly possible for men to have a UTI; this is sometimes the warning sign of something potentially serious, like prostate problems (see *prostate cancer* and *benign prostatic hyperplasia*, Chapter 10). People who must drain their bladder with a catheter are virtually assured of eventually having a UTI; their chances rise an estimated 5% per day of catheter use.

Etiology: What Happens?

Under normal circumstances the environment in the bladder is sterile. The urine contains waste products to be expelled from the body, but no living microorganisms should be in it. Furthermore, the bladder is lined with a protective mucus-producing layer of cells that works to prevent infectious or noxious agents from harming the bladder walls.

Sometimes, however, foreign microorganisms are introduced into the urethra. If the circumstances are right, they can set up an infection that may stay localized or may travel further into the urinary system.

URINARY TRACT INFECTION IN BRIEF

What is it?
A urinary tract infection (UTI) is an infection of the urinary tract, usually from bacteria that live in the digestive tract.

How is it recognized?
Symptoms of UTIs include pain and burning sensations during urination, increased urinary frequency, urgency, and cloudy or blood-tinged urine. In the acute stage, fever and general malaise may be present.

Is massage indicated or contraindicated?
Acute UTIs contraindicate circulatory massage, as do all acute infections. Massage may be appropriate in the subacute stage, although deep work on the abdomen is still locally cautioned until all signs of infection are gone.

Causes

E. coli is the causative agent behind close to 90% of all UTIs. These strains of bacteria live normally and harmlessly in the digestive tract. Certain varieties of staphylococcus cause a small percentage of UTIs, and other agents including Klebsiella, chlamydia, and mycoplasma are behind a tiny minority of infections. It is important to identify the correct causative agent, because not all of them respond to the same antibiotics.

Chronic irritation can also contribute to the development of UTIs. "Honeymoon cystitis" refers to inflammation and subsequent infection brought about by repeated irritation of the urethra from sexual activity.

The relationship between stress and UTIs has much anecdotal support. Living in a sympathetic state may reduce blood flow to the bladder, which in turn may make it more susceptible to infection. However, clinical evidence shows that although stress may aggravate symptoms of UTIs, it has not been proven to cause them.

Risk Factors

Some women have been found to be more susceptible to UTIs than others, although the reasons for this are not completely clear. Some factors, however, are reliable predictors of who will develop a UTI:

- *Blood types.* Some blood types are more prone to this disorder than others; slight differences in internal chemistry seem to make it easier for invading bacteria to cling to the bladder walls.

- *Spermicides.* Spermicide foams and jellies used with diaphragms or alone have been shown to raise the risk of UTIs in some women.

- *Diaphragm use.* Women who use diaphragms show statistically higher rates of UTIs than women who do not.

- *Pregnancy.* Pregnant women do not necessarily get more UTIs than women who are not pregnant, but the risk of having a simple infection complicate into a more dangerous one is higher for these patients.

- *Diabetes.* Elevated sugar levels in the urine make a hospitable environment for bacteria to grow in the bladder.

- *Neurogenic bladder.* If a bladder has lost motor function, it does not empty as completely as a normal one. This raises the potential for infection, as does the presence of catheter tubes, which are used for people with limited bladder function.

Signs and Symptoms

The symptoms of UTIs are painful, burning urination; a frequent need to urinate; reduced bladder capacity; urgency; and blood-tinged or cloudy urine. Men with UTIs may also experience pain in the penis or scrotum. If back pain and fever develop, a kidney infection should be suspected.

Complications

Bacteria that live in the digestive tract cause almost all UTIs. If the bacteria are able to travel up the system, they may set up an infection in the bladder (cystitis). (This is not to be confused with *interstitial cystitis*, this chapter). If the infection remains unchecked it may move all the way up the ureters and into the kidneys, causing a kidney infection. Untreated kidney infections can lead to the release of infectious bacteria in the blood (life-threatening septicemia).

Unfortunately not all UTIs show symptoms, so they may be neglected. It is possible for some people to experience extreme complications of this type of infection that can easily lead to permanent kidney damage or even to death.

Treatment

The first step in self-treatment of a UTI is to drown it: radically increasing fluid intake gives the body the much needed opportunity to fully and frequently empty the bladder—not only of urine but of bacteria as well. Drinking highly acidic liquids like blueberry or cranberry juice is helpful for many women, as an acidic environment inhibits bacterial growth. These berries also contain chemicals that limit the ability of bacteria to cling to bladder walls. It is important, however, to avoid *sweetened* juice; the amount of sugar it takes to make cranberry juice sweet may actually make the bladder a more hospitable environment for infection. In subacute situations, hydrotherapy in the form of hot and cold sitz baths may be recommended.

UTIs usually respond well to a short course of antibiotics. In this case, 3 to 5 days' worth of medication is more appropriate than 2 weeks' worth because the body concentrates antibiotics in the urine. With bladder infections, as with all types of bacterial infections, it is especially important to take the *full* prescription of antibiotics. Stopping too soon often results in recurrent infections with more highly resistant bacteria.

People who experience low-grade chronic UTIs that do not clear up with normal treatments are sometimes successfully treated with long-term low doses of antibiotics. Structural problems with the way urine drains from the bladder may contribute to chronic infections; surgery may be recommended to correct these problems.

Prevention

Some basic precautions can help prevent UTIs, especially for women who are especially vulnerable to them. These include drinking *lots* of water and acidic juices; urinating whenever necessary rather than holding it for a more convenient time; wiping from front to back after a bowel movement to prevent the introduction of digestive bacteria into the urethra; taking showers rather than baths; emptying the bladder after sex; and avoiding feminine hygiene sprays and douches that can aggravate the urethra.

Massage?

Acute UTIs are sometimes accompanied by *fever* (Chapter 5), a systemic contraindication. A small but significant risk of spreading the infection to the kidneys should also be considered. Even in the post-acute stage (after signs of acute infection have subsided), the lower abdomen is a local contraindication for massage until all signs of infection have been eradicated.

Chapter Review Questions: Urinary System Conditions

1. Describe how high blood pressure can lead to kidney dysfunction.

2. Describe how kidney dysfunction can lead to high blood pressure.

3. Why do people get kidney stones more often in hot environments than in other places?

4. Why are women more likely to get urinary tract infections than men?

5. How can renal failure lead to disconnected symptoms like itching or mental incapacitation?

6. Describe the relationship between long-term stress and urinary tract infections.

7. A client complains of transient extreme pain on one side of her mid-back. Her muscles are not particularly tender, and she shows no signs of infection. What condition is likely to be present?

8. A client who is an elderly man mentions that he has been passing blood in his urine. What condition is likely to be present?

Bibliography, Urinary System Conditions

General References, Urinary System

1. de Dominico G, Wood E. *Beard's Massage.* Philadelphia, PA: WB Saunders; 1997.

2. Damjanou I. *Pathology for the Health-Related Professions.* Philadelphia, PA: WB Saunders; 1996.

3. Travell J, Simons DG. *Myofascial Pain and Dysfunction: The Trigger Point Manual.* Baltimore, MD: Williams & Wilkins; 1983.

4. Clemente CD. *Anatomy: A Regional Atlas of the Human Body.* 3rd ed. Baltimore, MD: Urban & Schwarzenburg; 1987.

5. Tortora GJ, Anagnostakos NP. *Principles of Anatomy and Physiology.* 6th ed. New York, NY: Harper & Row; 1990.

6. *Taber's Cyclopedic Dictionary.* 14th ed. Philadelphia, PA: FA Davis; 1981.

7. *Stedman's Medical Dictionary.* 26th ed. Baltimore, MD: Williams & Wilkins; 1995.

8. Memmler RL, Wood DL. *The Human Body in Health and Disease.* 5th ed. Philadelphia, PA: JB Lippincott; 1983.

9. Juhan D. *Job's Body: A Handbook for Bodywork.* Barrytown, NY: Station Hill Press; 1987.

10. Mulvihill ML. *Human Diseases: A Systemic Approach.* 2nd ed. Norwalk, CT: Appleton & Lange; 1987.

11. Kunz JRM, Finkel AJ, eds. *The American Medical Association Family Medical Guide.* New York, NY: Random House; 1987.

12. Marieb EM. *Human Anatomy and Physiology.* Redwood City, CA: Benjamin/ Cummings; 1989.

13. Sapolsky RM. *Why Zebras Don't Get Ulcers: An Updated Guide to Stress, Stress-Related Disease, and Coping.* New York, NY: W.H. Freeman; 1998.

14. Glomerular diseases. The National Kidney and Urologic Diseases Information Clearinghouse. NIH publication no. 99-4358.

Available at http://www.niddk.nih. gov/health/kidney/pubs/glomer/glomer. htm. Accessed spring 2001.

15. High blood pressure and kidney disease. The National Kidney and Urologic Diseases Information Clearinghouse. NIH publication no. 99-4572. Available at http://www.niddk.nih.gov/health/kidney/ summary/hypotens/hypotens.htm. Accessed spring 2001.

Kidney Disorders

Glomerulonephritis

1. Ravnskov U. Glomerulonephritis. U. Ravnskov; Available at: http://www. ravnskov.nu/index.htm. Accessed spring 2001.

2. Glomerulonephritis. National Kidney and Urologic Diseases Information Clearinghouse. Available at: http://www.niddk.nih. gov/health/kidney/summary/glomneph/ glomneph.htm. Accessed spring 2001.

3. Kazzi AA. Glomerulonephritis, acute. In *Emergency Medicine/Genitourinary.* eMedicine.com, Inc.; 2001. Available at: http://www.emedicine. com/emerg/ topic219.htm. Accessed spring 2001.

Kidney Stones

1. Ask the Mayo physician, 6.21.99. Category: Kidney & urinary tract. Mayo Foundation for Medical Education and Research; 2000. Available at: http://www.mayohealth. org/mayo/ askphys/qa990621.htm. Accessed spring 2001.

2. Saelinger L. Nephrolithiasis. University of Chicago. Available at: http://pcg.uchicago. edu/pcgauthored/Nephrology/nephro. html. Accessed spring 2001.

3. Craig S. Renal calculi. In *Emergency Medicine/Genitourinary.* eMedicine.com, Inc.; 2001. Available at: http://www. emedicine.com/emerg/topic499.htm. Accessed spring 2001.

4. Kidney stones in adults. The National Kidney and Urologic Diseases Information Clearinghouse. NIH publication no. 00-2495. Available at: http://www.niddk.nih. gov/health/kidney/pubs/stonadul/stonadul. htm. Accessed spring 2001.

Pyelonephritis

1. Kidney infection, chronic. Rxmed, inc. Available at: http://www.rxmed.com/ illnesses/kidney_infection,_chronic.html. Accessed spring 2001.

2. Kidney infection, acute. Rxmed, inc. Available at: http://www.rxmed.com/illnesses/ kidney_infection,_acute.html. Accessed spring 2001.

3. Pyelonephritis (kidney infection) in adults. The National Kidney and Urologic Diseases Information Clearinghouse. NIH publication no. 99-4628. Available at: http://www.niddk.nih.gov/health/kidney/ summary/pyelonep/pyelonep.htm. Accessed spring 2001.

Renal Failure

1. Krause RS. Renal failure, chronic dialysis complications. In *Emergency.* eMedicine.com, Inc.; 2001. Available at: http://www.emedicine.com/emerg/ topic501.htm. Accessed spring 2001.

2. Acute renal failure. U.S. National Library of Medicine. Available at: http://www.nlm. nih.gov/medlineplus/ency/article/000501. htm. Accessed spring 2001.

3. Siner R. Renal failure, acute. In *Emergency Medicine, Genitourinary.* eMedicine.com, Inc.; 2001. Available at: http://www. emedicine.com/emerg/topic500.htm. Accessed spring 2001.

4. End-stage renal disease: Choosing a treatment that's right for you. National Kidney and Urologic Diseases Information Clearinghouse. NIH publication no. 94-2412. Available at: http://www.niddk.nih.gov/ health/kidney/pubs/esrd/esrd.htm. Accessed spring 2001.

Bladder and Urinary Tract Disorders

Bladder Cancer

1. Steinberg GD. Bladder cancer. *eMedicine Journal.* 2001;2(5). Available at: http://www.emedicine. com/med/ topic2344.htm. Accessed spring 2001.

2. Introduction to bladder cancer. Trustees of the University of Pennsylvania; 1994–2001. Available at: http://www.oncolink.upenn. edu/disease/bladder/intro_bladder.html. Accessed spring 2001.

3. Bladder cancer. InteliHealth Inc.; 1996–2001. Available at: http://www. intelihealth.com/ IH/ihtIH?t= 24408&p=~br,IHW1~st,24479l ~r,WSIHW0001~b,*1. Accessed spring 2001.

4. Bladder cancer (PDQ) treatment— Patients. National Cancer Institute. Available at: http://cancernet.nci.nih.gov/cgi-bin/ srchcgi.exe?DBID=pdq&TYPE=search&

UID=208=01206&ZFILE=patient& SFMT=pdq_treatment/1/0/0. Accessed spring 2001.

5. NCI/PDQ patient statement: Bladder cancer–Updated 11/2000. Available at: http://www. oncolink.upenn.edu/ pdq_html/2/engl/201206.html. Accessed spring 2001.

Interstitial Cystitis

1. Interstitial cystitis. urologychannel.com.; 1998–2001. Available at: http://www. urologychannel.com/interstitialcystitis/ index.shtml. Accessed spring 2001.

2. Zamula E. Interstitial cystitis progress against disabling bladder condition. U.S. Food and Drug Administration. Available at: http://www.fda.gov//fdac/features/ 995_cystitis.html. Accessed spring 2001.

3. What is interstitial cystitis? Interstitial Cystitis Association. Available at: http://www. ichelp.org/whatisic/AnIntroductionToIC. html. Accessed spring 2001.

4. Interstitial cystitis. The National Kidney and Urologic Diseases Information Clearinghouse. NIH publication no. 99-3220. Available at: http://www.niddk.nih. gov/health/urolog/pubs/cystitis/cystitis. htm. Accessed spring 2001.

Urinary Tract Infection

1. Orenstein R. Urinary tract infections in adults. American Academy of Family Physicians; 1999. Available at: http://www.aafp.org/afp/990301ap/ 1225.html. Accessed spring 2001.

2. Urinary tract infections in women. Board of Trustees of the University of Illinois, 1998. Available at: http://www.mckinley. uiuc. edu/health-info/womenhlt/ utiwomen.html. Accessed spring 2001.

3. Urinary tract infections. urologychannel.com; 1998–2001. Available at: http://www.urologychannel.com/ index.shtml. Accessed spring 2001.

4. Urinary tract infections in adults. National Kidney and Urologic Diseases Information Clearinghouse. NIH publication no. 01-2097. Available at: http://www.niddk. nih.gov/health/ urolog/pubs/utiadult/ utiadult.htm. Accessed spring 2001.

Reproductive System Conditions

CHAPTER OBJECTIVES

After reading this chapter, the reader should be able to . . .

- Name the causative agent for most cases of cervical cancer.
- Name three possible causes of secondary dysmenorrhea.
- Explain the connections between endometriosis and anemia, dysmenorrhea, and infertility.
- Name the lifetime chance of a woman having breast cancer in the United States.
- Name the challenges with identifying ovarian cancer in the early stages.

- Name three signs or symptoms of benign prostatic hypertrophy.
- Explain why low back pain or pain into the groin and legs may accompany prostate cancer.
- Name the difference between perimenopause and menopause.
- Name the most frequent and serious sexually transmitted disease (excluding human immunodeficiency virus).
- Name three possible complications associated with pregnancy.

INTRODUCTION

Introduction

This chapter is mostly devoted to women's health problems, except for benign prostate hyperplasia and prostate cancer. Therefore, the only anatomic review will be of the female reproductive system, with an eye on where these conditions occur (Fig. 10-1).

Terminology for structures in the reproductive system can sometimes be confusing. Many researchers have recently moved toward labeling structures by their location or function rather than by their traditional names, which often refer to the physicians or anatomists who first recorded them. Thus, fallopian tubes, named for 16th century anatomist Gabriele Fallopio, may now be called oviducts or uterine tubes, which is more descriptive. Traditional names are still in common use, however. In this chapter structures are referred to by both traditional and functional/locational names, so that practitioners trained in either terminology will feel at home.

Function and Structure

Low in the female pelvis are two small structures called the *ovaries*. They are attached via the ovarian ligament to the uterus. The ovaries produce hormones, which are released into the bloodstream, and they produce eggs (usually one each month during ovulation), which are released into the peritoneal space. The fimbriae of the fallopian (uterine) tubes gently caress the ovaries, coaxing the egg toward them. Once inside tubes, the eggs make the 5-day journey to the uterus itself. If an egg is going to be fertilized, it generally happens inside the uterine tube.

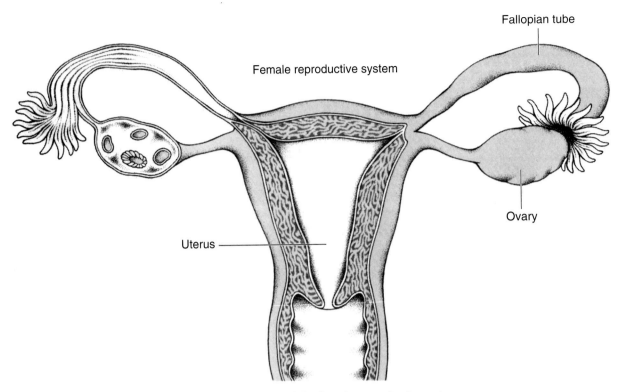

Figure 10-1. Overview of the female reproductive system

What Is This Thing Called Estrogen?

Estrogen is not a single hormone, but a group of closely related chemicals that includes *estradiol, estriol,* and *estrone.* These chemicals are synthesized from cholesterol primarily in the ovaries during a woman's fertile years. After menopause, they continue to be manufactured in peripheral tissues in much smaller amounts, using root chemicals secreted by the adrenal cortex.

Estrogens are received by target tissues all over the body. They are not only associated with sex organ function; they influence the growth, health, and activity of many organs, including bones and the heart. They influence cell production and differentiation. Estrogens are also associated with mood swings and emotional responsiveness.

The liver makes estrogens chemically able to stimulate biological activity in their target cells. This metabolism can occur in a variety of ways, all of which have great implications for long-term health. Some "bad" estrogen metabolites are associated with tissue proliferation (i.e., cancer) of the breast, uterus, cervix, ovaries, and thyroid. "Good" estrogen metabolites are associated with healthy bone maintenance and cardiovascular protection.

What determines which estrogen metabolites will be present in a woman's body? Two main factors are at work here—diet and estrogen exposure.

Diet

High-fat, low-fiber diets do several things to estrogen production. By providing excessive cholesterol, they allow the body to manufacture more estrogens. By providing a minimum of fiber, they prevent the binding of excessive estrogens to the molecules that would inactivate them. By disrupting the healthy balance of bacteria in the intestines, poor diets allow some estrogens to reenter the circulation.

Estrogen Exposure

People are exposed to estrogen from internal production (endogenous estrogens) and external sources (exogenous estrogens). Endogenous estrogens have already been discussed as a function of diet and estrogen metabolism. Endogenous estrogen exposure is also increased by obesity; all body fat cells can contribute to estrogen production. Exogenous estrogen exposure is an issue that has only recently begun to be discussed. Oral birth control pills, hormone replacement therapy, and supplements found in meat and dairy products, as well as environmental chemicals like pesticides, herbicides, plastics, and industrial solvents, all contribute to cumulative endogenous estrogen exposure.

Excessive estrogen exposure and the metabolism of "bad" estrogens have been identified as contributing factors in several cancers of hormone-dependent tissues.[a] In addition, estrogen dominance is being investigated as an issue in other reproductive system disorders, including premenstrual syndrome, endometriosis, uterine fibroids, and menopause. The good news is that estrogen exposure and metabolism can be influenced by diet and nutrition. Estrogen receptor sites in target tissues can bind with several different estrogen-like substances (*phytoestrogens,* including soy, legumes, and other sources), and some nutritional supplements can help disable free estrogen metabolites before they influence cell proliferation or differentiation.

Ultimately these reproductive system disorders may be treated or even prevented by having patients take greater control over how much estrogen they are exposed to and how their bodies put that estrogen to use.

[a]Hall DC. Nutritional influences on estrogen metabolism. *Appl Nutr Sci Rep.* 2001;1–8.

When the egg reaches the uterus it finds itself inside a hollow organ that is built of criss-crossed layers of muscle. The inside surface of the uterus, the *endometrium*, is made of delicate epithelial tissue that holds vast billowy supplies of blood to provide a nest for a fertilized egg. If an egg is not fertilized, the uterus sheds the blood and egg with it in the menses. Then it begins the process of building a new nest for next month's candidate.

The timing of the ripening and release of eggs from the ovaries and the building and shedding of the endometrial nest is under the control of the endocrine system. Hormones secreted from the ovaries themselves as well as the pituitary gland determine when and how these various events happen. Birth control pills work because they introduce artificial hormones into the blood. These trick the pituitary into believing that the woman is always pregnant, and so she never ovulates.

The relationship between the reproductive system and the endocrine system is extremely tight; the reproductive cycle is determined by hormone secretions. Several conditions discussed in this chapter could be considered endocrine system disorders, but the tissue changes occur in reproductive system organs, so they are discussed here (see sidebar).

Reproductive conditions that have significance for massage therapists generally have to do with growths or local tenderness deep in the abdomen. Although working deeply in the vicinity of the uterus or ovaries is not generally practiced, sometimes these conditions can displace internal organs, making them vulnerable in places they would not ordinarily be found.

Reproductive System Conditions

Disorders of the Uterus
   Abortion, Spontaneous and Elective
   Cervical Cancer
   Dysmenorrhea
   Endometriosis
   Fibroid Tumors

Disorders of Other Reproductive Structures
   Breast Cancer
   Ovarian Cancer
   Ovarian Cysts

Disorders of the Male Reproductive System
   Benign Prostatic Hypertrophy
   Prostate Cancer

Other Reproductive System Conditions
   Menopause
   Pelvic Inflammatory Disease
   Pregnancy
   Premenstrual Syndrome

Disorders of the Uterus

Abortion, Spontaneous and Elective
Definition: What Are They?

An elective abortion is the intentional termination of a pregnancy. A spontaneous abortion is an unintentional termination.

Etiology of Elective Abortion: What Happens?

A pregnancy can be terminated in different ways, depending on the stage. If it happens within the first 12 weeks, an elective abortion will probably be accomplished by a vac-

ABORTION, SPONTANEOUS AND ELECTIVE IN BRIEF

What are they?
Spontaneous and elective abortions are pregnancies that are ended, unintentionally or intentionally, before the fetus is born naturally.

How are they recognized?
Generalized or pelvic pain may be present, along with vaginal bleeding. Often, however, no outward signs may show that a woman is recovering from a spontaneous or elective abortion.

Is massage indicated or contraindicated?
Massage is locally contraindicated (no deep abdominal work) for a woman recovering from a recent spontaneous or elective abortion until her bleeding has stopped and she is free of any signs of infection. Bodywork elsewhere can be supportive and helpful.

uum suction. The walls of the cervix are dilated to allow a flexible tube into the uterus, which removes the fetal tissue. In the 13th to 15th weeks, *dilatation and curettage* (D&C) may be performed. This is a more complicated procedure and requires more anesthetic and sometimes a hospital stay. Later terminations are conducted by inducing premature labor. They can be very difficult and always require hospitalization.

Etiology of Spontaneous Abortion: What Happens?

Several factors may contribute to the disruption of a pregnancy. In many cases it can be hard to discover exactly what causes a fetus to die, but many issues have been identified, some of which are controllable, but many of which are not.

Controllable factors that may raise the risk of spontaneous abortion or miscarriage include smoking, untreated infections of the reproductive tract (see *pelvic inflammatory disease*, this chapter), untreated *diabetes* or *thyroid disorders* (Chapter 8), exposure to toxic chemicals (especially solvents), and progesterone deficiency in the early weeks of pregnancy before the placenta has begun to secrete its own supply of this hormone that supports fetal implantation. An immune system response that causes blood in fetal vessels to clot can be controlled with low doses of aspirin or other blood thinners.

Factors that a woman has no control over include structural problems in the uterus like *fibroid tumors* (this chapter) or a weak cervix, the fertilization of multiple eggs, age, autoimmune disease (especially *scleroderma*, Chapter 2), an immune system rejection of fetal tissue, failure of the fetus to implant into the endometrium, or what is perhaps the most common cause of miscarriage: the fetus is simply missing key genetic information that would allow it to continue to develop. When the moment comes that the missing genes are needed, the fetus dies.

Miscarriages usually happen in the first 14 weeks of pregnancy, although the risk of miscarriage goes way down after the 8th week. If the fetus dies after the 20th week it is no longer called a miscarriage or spontaneous abortion—it is called a stillbirth, but the principles are the same.

The frequency of spontaneous abortions is a subject of debate. It is estimated that up to 50% of all fertilized eggs are expelled from the body for one reason or another before a woman may know that she is pregnant at all. Of recognized pregnancies, anywhere from 25 to 30% of all fetuses are spontaneously aborted.

Signs and Symptoms

When the endometrial lining of the uterus is disrupted in any way but a normal menses, what is left is a large surface area of raw, bleeding epithelium. This is true for elective and spontaneous abortions and also for childbirth. Symptoms of this trauma can include pain (local and referred), bleeding, and cramping. These are generally self-limiting; that is, the symptoms resolve themselves with time, unless complications develop.

Complications

Complications of abortions or miscarriages can include infection from incomplete shedding of the uterine lining and possible hemorrhaging. *Depression* (Chapter 3) is also a frequent complication of these events.

Treatment

The best treatment for a woman recovering from an elective abortion, a miscarriage, or successful childbirth is tender loving care. If any infection develops, or if uterine lining has not been shed completely, a D&C and antibiotics may be needed.

Massage?

Deep abdominal massage is locally contraindicated for women recovering from spontaneous and elective abortions and postpartum situations, at least until the bleeding has stopped. Massage elsewhere is a good idea, although the risk of blood clotting for pregnant women is quite high, so it is wisest to stick with non-circulatory modalities (see *pregnancy*, this chapter).

Cervical Cancer

Definition: What Is It?

Cervical cancer is the growth of malignant cells in the lining of the cervix. Whereas some types of abnormal cells grow slowly and do not present a serious threat, other types are aggressive and invasive.

Demographics: Who Gets It?

Cervical cancer accounts for about 6% of all malignancies experienced by women. Approximately 16,000 women in the United States are diagnosed with invasive cervical cancer per year; estimates suggest that 4 times that many are diagnosed with noninvasive abnormal cervical cells. Cervical cancer kills about 5,000 American women each year.

The average age at which a woman may be diagnosed with precancerous changes in her cervix is 28 years. Nevertheless, cervical cancer can develop at any age, from the beginning of sexual activity to long after menopause.

Etiology: What Happens?

Cervical cancer is an example of a malignancy brought about directly by a viral infection, in this case with some of the 80 known varieties of human papilloma virus (HPV) family. Around 30 of these viruses are associated with genital warts, although not all types of HPV cause visible growths.

HPV is a sexually transmitted disease, transferred by direct skin-to-skin touching. It is *not* preventable by the use of condoms, since other parts of the genitals still come in contact during sex. Statistics on the incidence of HPV infection in the United States vary. Some say about 6 million women are currently infected; others suggest that up to 40 million Ameri-

CERVICAL CANCER IN BRIEF

What is it?
Cervical cancer is the development of cancerous cells in the lining of the cervix. These may spread to affect the whole cervix, the rest of the uterus, and other pelvic organs.

How is it recognized?
Early stages of cervical cancer are virtually silent. This disease is detected by Pap tests before symptoms develop. Later signs and symptoms include bleeding or spotting outside a normal menstrual period, vaginal discharge, and pelvic pain.

Is massage indicated or contraindicated?
Most cases of cervical cancer are caught and eradicated before the woman is in serious danger of metastasis. These patients are good candidates for any kind of bodywork. For a woman dealing with advanced stages of cervical cancer, the massage therapist must make adjustments for the radiation, chemotherapy, or surgical procedures that may be part of her experience.

Cervical Cancer: History of a Disease

In the early part of the 20th century, cervical cancer was one of the leading causes of death by cancer for women in the United States. This disease is virtually silent, creating no symptoms until it has spread throughout the pelvic cavity and into the lymph system—by which time it is practically impossible for the patient to survive.

From 1955 to 1992 a remarkable phenomenon occurred: rates of death by cervical cancer took a huge downswing, dropping by some 74%.

What made the difference? A simple examination: the Pap test, which makes it possible to detect precancerous cells in the cervix before they spread. Because of the Pap test women could have abnormal cells detected and removed before they had a chance to become malignant, and they could find and remove malignancies before they had a chance to spread throughout the pelvic cavity. Consequently, the 5-year survival rate for cervical cancer is now close to 100% for preinvasive cells, 91% for early invasive cells, and 70% overall.

Today the recommended protocol for cervical cancer detection is to receive a Pap test once a year. If a woman has three consecutive years without any sign of dysplasia, her doctor may recommend that she can have Pap tests less frequently. Higher mortality rates among non-White women and women of low socioeconomic status point to the fact that up to 30% of at-risk women still do not have access to this inexpensive and highly useful test.

Cervical cancer has been largely controlled in the United States, but it is still a leading cause of death by cancer in countries where women do not have access to Pap tests. Although currently no vaccine against dangerous types of HPV has been approved for humans, several are in development, and the future promises that one day cervical cancer may become a completely preventable disease.

cans are HPV carriers. Being infected with HPV is not a dependable indicator of cervical cancer, however. Many of the viruses in this family are *not* associated with aggressive or invasive cancers.

When a woman is infected with HPV, the virus may trigger cellular changes in the lining of her cervix. Precancerous changes are called *dysplasia* and can be stimulated by both low-risk and high-risk types of HPV. At this point it is difficult to predict whether a woman's abnormal cells put her at risk for invasive cervical cancer, but tests to clarify this question are in development.

If a woman happens to be infected with a low-risk type of virus, her abnormal cells may spontaneously resolve, and she may never know anything had happened. However, if she is infected with an aggressive form of HPV, cancerous cells grow in the lining of the cervix and then may spread throughout the uterus, the vagina, and into the pelvic cavity, affecting the bladder, colon, and inguinal lymph nodes. Ultimately the cancer may travel to distant parts of the body.

Exposure to HPV is the central risk factor for developing cervical cancer. However, other factors may contribute to the likelihood of having abnormal cells become malignant. Smoking raises this risk by close to 100%. Immune system suppression also increases the risk of developing cervical cancer. Finally, socioeconomic standing is a major factor, as this often determines whether a woman has adequate access to early detection and care.

Signs and Symptoms

Early stages of cervical cancer have no symptoms to speak of. The cancer must be significantly advanced before any signs appear. These usually include bleeding or spotting between menstrual periods or after menopause, vaginal discharge, and pelvic or abdominal pain.

Diagnosis

The Pap test is the current standard for early cervical cancer detection. In this test a small scraping of cells and mucus from the cervix is withdrawn and analyzed. If abnormal cells are found, a follow-up test that visually examines the cervix for suspicious changes (a *colposcopy*) may be conducted. A biopsy removes the affected part of the cervix; if more suspicious cells are found, further tests may be conducted to stage the cancer and determine the best possible treatment options.

Pap tests are fast, cost-effective, and only mildly painful, but if the tissue sample happens to miss some abnormal cells, false-negative results may be returned. Fortunately, most types of cervical cancer grow slowly, and yearly examinations are usually adequate to ensure protection from having dysplasia become cervical cancer.

Staging

Cervical cancer is staged in much the same way as several other cancers, in levels 0 through IV.

- *Stage 0.* Also called *in situ*, this means that dysplasia has only affected the most superficial layers of the cervical epithelium.

- *Stage I.* Cancerous cells are still localized in the cervix.
  - *IA:* The cells are not yet visible.
  - *IB*

The cells have formed visible clumps.

- *Stage II.* Cancerous cells are elsewhere in the pelvis.
  - *IIA:* The upper two-thirds of the vagina may be affected.
  - *IIB:* The tissue around the cervix and into the uterus may be affected.
- *Stage III.* Cancerous cells are found throughout the pelvis, vagina, and may be pressing on the bladder and ureters.
- *Stage IV.* The cancer has spread to other parts of the body.
  - *IVA:* Cancerous cells are found on the bladder and rectum as well as in the inguinal lymph nodes.
  - *IVB:* Cancerous cells are found on the other side of the diaphragm, notably in the lungs.

Treatment

Treatment for cervical cancer depends entirely on the stage in which it is diagnosed. Most cases are found in Stage 0 or Stage I, which means treatment can be limited to removing the abnormal cells and watching carefully for further changes. Surgical interventions to remove cervical dysplasia include cryotherapy, in which cells are frozen off; loop electrosurgical excision procedure (LEEP), in which electricity is passed through a loop of thin wire to slice off the suspicious tissue; laser surgery; and a cone biopsy.

Surgical procedures for cancer caught in later stages may range from full or partial hysterectomies to full pelvic exenteration, in which virtually all the pelvic organs are removed.

Radiation and chemotherapy may also be utilized with advanced cases of cervical cancer.

Massage?

Massage for a client who has cervical dysplasia is certainly fine, especially if she is receiving appropriate care. Clients who are dealing with advanced cases of cancer must cope not only with the disease process, but with the many complex and extremely unpleasant complications those treatments may involve. Carefully conducted bodywork that respects the many challenges of surgery, radiation, and chemotherapy can offer all the benefits of massage while minimizing any possible risks. See more on this topic in *Cancer*, Chapter 11.

Dysmenorrhea
Definition: What Is It?

Dysmenorrhea is a technical term for painful menstrual periods. Generally a woman is said to have dysmenorrhea if she has to limit her regular activities or requires medication to function for 1 day or more every month.

DYSMENORRHEA IN BRIEF

What is it?
Dysmenorrhea is the technical term for menstrual pain that is severe enough to interfere with and limit the activities of women of childbearing age. It may be a primary problem or secondary to some other pelvic pathology.

How is it recognized?
The symptoms of dysmenorrhea are dull aching or sharp severe lower abdominal pain preceding and/or during menstruation. Nausea and vomiting may accompany very severe symptoms. Secondary dysmenorrhea may create pelvic pain outside normal periods as well.

Is massage indicated or contraindicated?
Massage is appropriate for primary dysmenorrhea, although the abdomen locally contraindicates deep work during days of heavy menstrual flow. The appropriateness of bodywork for secondary dysmenorrhea depends on the type of pathology involved, along with stage, severity, and other variables.

Demographics: Who Gets It?

Most women have severe menstrual pain at least once in their life. It is estimated that 40% of all women experience regular painful periods in the United States, and about 10% of all women are incapacitated for 1 to 3 days each month. Dysmenorrhea is the leading cause of lost time from school or work for women of child-bearing age. Primary dysmenorrhea usually affects women in their late teens or early 20s and subsides as a woman grows older. It is generally not changed by childbearing.

Etiology: What Happens?

Dysmenorrhea can be primary, that is, it starts within the first 3 years of menstruation in an otherwise healthy woman. It can also be secondary to some underlying pathology.

Causes of Primary Dysmenorrhea:

Several different factors can contribute to primary dysmenorrhea.

- *Prostaglandins.* These are chemicals produced all over the body and especially in the uterus. They cause smooth muscle contractions, but they also sensitize the body to pain. Prostaglandins are found in higher concentrations in women who have menstrual pain than in women who do not. Progesterone, a hormone involved in the menstrual cycle, inhibits the action of prostaglandins. Just before menstruation begins, however, progesterone levels plummet, leaving the prostaglandins to do their work unchecked.

- *Pain-spasm cycle.* When the uterus is in sustained contraction, oxygen cannot easily supply the muscle. Ischemia causes pain, which reinforces the spasm, and so on.

- *Ligament irritation.* The uterine ligament, which anchors the uterus to the pelvic wall, can be pulled and irritated when the uterus is in spasm.

It is easy to see how physical or emotional stress fits into the picture of menstrual pain. Sympathetic reactions in the body exacerbate uterine ischemia, leading to pain, which causes more spasm. The emotional state of dreading the pain and discomfort of menstrual periods can then become a self-fulfilling prophecy—the stress of anticipating an unpleasant event works to make that event even more unpleasant.

Causes of Secondary Dysmenorrhea

Secondary dysmenorrhea is a complication of some other pelvic disorder. Some of the most common problems that cause menstrual pain include *pelvic inflammatory disease, fibroid tumors,* and *endometriosis* (all in this chapter). Pelvic adhesions (deposits of scar tissue from previous surgeries or trauma) may also contribute to menstrual pain.

Signs and Symptoms

Symptoms of dysmenorrhea vary. They can include dull aches in the abdomen and low back, or sharp pains and cramping in the pelvis and abdomen. These usually happen early in menstruation, but some women have symptoms during their whole period. Headaches, nausea, vomiting, diarrhea, and constipation are all possibilities, along with a frequent need to urinate. If dysmenorrhea is related to underlying pathology, pelvic pain may not be limited to the menstrual cycle; it can happen at any time.

Diagnosis

Ongoing debilitating menstrual pain is important to investigate because it could be indicative of serious underlying problems. Diagnosis often involves a laparoscopy to check for endometriosis, which is a leading cause of secondary dysmenorrhea. Ultrasounds to look for fibroid tumors may be performed. Cultures of vaginal secretions may also be examined to look for signs of pelvic inflammatory disease, chlamydia, syphilis, or gonorrhea. In the absence of these conditions, painful periods can be treated without fear of ignoring some important underlying causes.

Treatment

For most cases of dysmenorrhea, painkillers such as ibuprofen and naproxen work by inhibiting the secretion of prostaglandins. A thorough nutritional analysis may also reveal strategies for dealing with menstrual pain; this is a useful course for many women, but no specific nutritional supplements have been found to alleviate all cases of dysmenorrhea. Certain exercises and stretches can also relieve the pain caused by the irritated uterine ligament, which is tugged on by a uterus in spasm.

For more serious situations where painkillers, heat, and stretching do not affect the pain, more aggressive interventions may be considered. Low-dose birth control pills prohibit ovulation, which in turn prohibits the secretion of prostaglandins in the uterus. If a structural issue like fibroid tumors is at the root of the problem, surgery may be an option. Medications or laparoscopic surgery for endometriosis may alleviate symptoms.

Massage?

A woman who is in the middle of a painful period will probably not respond well to deep abdominal massage, but nurturing touch elsewhere is highly called for and beneficial. A woman who regularly has painful periods but who has no known pelvic pathologies is a good candidate for abdominal massage when she is *not* menstruating. It may help to relieve tension, take stress off the uterine ligament, and even minimize abdominal adhesions that may contribute to pain.

Endometriosis
Definition: What Is It?

Endometriosis is a condition in which cells from the endometrium, the inner lining of the uterus, become implanted elsewhere in the body. They usually begin in the pelvic cavity, but may spread further into the abdomen, and even above the diaphragm.

Demographics: Who Gets It?

Endometriosis is probably fairly common. It is estimated more than 5 million American women deal with this problem, but statistics are difficult to gather since it cannot be diagnosed without surgery. It affects females as young as 9 years old and postmenopausal women, but most patients are diagnosed between ages 20 and 45. Most endometriosis pa-

ENDOMETRIOSIS IN BRIEF

What is it?
Endometriosis is the implantation and growth of endometrial cells in the peritoneal cavity (and possibly elsewhere) that swell and decay with the menstrual cycle.

How is it recognized?
Endometriosis may have no symptoms. When it does, they generally include pelvic and abdominal pain, difficulties with urination or defecation, painful intercourse, and other problems, depending on which tissues have been affected. Symptoms worsen during menstruation. Infertility is a frequent complication of endometriosis.

Is massage indicated or contraindicated?
If a client knows she has endometriosis, deep abdominal or pelvic work may be painful, especially when it is close to her menstrual cycle. The supportive effects of massage, however, can be an important part of the coping mechanisms women with this disorder must develop.

tients are women who have heavy, long-lasting menstrual periods, whose cycles occur in less than 28 days, and who have never had children. Women of Asian descent have statistically higher rates of endometriosis than other populations. Until recently it has been assumed that non-White and non-Asian women had lower rates of endometriosis, but that observation may be influenced more by the accessibility of health care than by any racial or genetic predisposition.

Etiology: What Happens?

Endometriosis involves the implantation and growth of endometrial cells anywhere outside the uterus. It was first described in 1921 by Dr. James Sampson, who noted these growths in the peritoneal cavities of women undergoing abdominal surgery. He hypothesized that the endometrial cells got out of the uterus via retrograde backflow through the uterine tubes, or through circulatory or lymphatic dissemination. Seventy years later, these theories are still the basis for understanding the etiology of this disorder.

Having endometrial cells find their way out of the uterus is not uncommon. In fact, up to 90% of all menstruating women have some loose cells in the pelvic cavity. Not all these women experience what happens when those cells successfully colonize a pelvic organ, however. The differences in cellular activity between women who have endometriosis and women who do not yield some clues about how this disease develops.

Women who have endometriosis have some immune system anomalies that are not seen with other women. These include low levels of the killer T-cells and natural killer (NK) cells that would normally eradicate stray endothelial cells in the pelvic cavity. They have higher than normal levels of suppressor T-cells, which serve to quell an appropriate immune system response. Women with endometriosis have a high number of macrophages around their growths, but instead of phagocytizing the new material, these macrophages secrete chemicals that inhibit T-cell and NK cell activity, while stimulating the growth of new blood vessels and the production of scar tissue. The activated B-cells of women with endometriosis do produce antibodies to attack the new tissue, but they do not seem to work very well outside the uterus. Unfortunately, these antibodies *do* work *inside* the uterus, which can increase symptoms and make the implantation of a fertilized egg difficult. Finally, women with endometriosis secrete unusually high levels of prostaglandins, which contribute to severe cramping and pain sensitization.

Endometrial growths usually become established on the outside of the uterus, on the uterine tubes, the broad ligaments, the ovaries, the bladder, or the colon (Fig. 10-2). Growths have been found as far away from the uterus as the lungs and even the brain. Wherever they land, they stimulate the growth of supplying blood vessels, and they proliferate in accordance with the hormonal commands in the body. However, these growths cannot be shed with normal menstruation. Instead, they decay and accumulate in local areas, stimulating an inflammatory response. The body attempts to isolate them by surrounding the deposits with fibrous connective tissue. Eventually multitudes of fibrous "blood blisters" accumulate on whatever surfaces the endometrium can find.

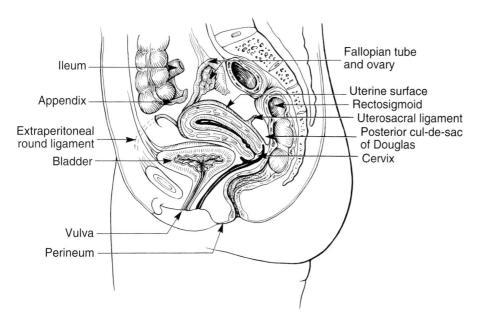

Figure 10-2. Sites of endometriosis

Endometrial growths that are found early look like clear vesicles on whatever structures they have colonized. Later these vesicles become bright red. Over a course of 10 or more years they will appear thick, black, and scarred.

Causes

Backflow through the uterine tubes or capillary and lymphatic dissemination of endometrial cells are still considered the leading initiators of endometriosis, but it is unclear why some women develop permanent growths and others do not. A genetic potential clearly exists, because women with mothers or sisters who have been diagnosed with endometriosis have a much higher chance of being diagnosed themselves. However, these statistics do not reflect variables such as the likelihood that these women will seek medical care, or whether their disease is brought about by genetic problems or by shared environmental factors. One such environmental factor is exposure to dioxins (chemicals produced by the manufacture and use of pesticides, paper pulp, and the burning of hazardous waste). Endometriosis has been observed in monkeys exposed to these toxins, and the longer the exposure, the more advanced the disease became.[b]

Signs and Symptoms

Infertility is very often the symptom that brings a woman with endometriosis to a physician for a diagnosis. Other symptoms of endometriosis are often nonexistent, at least in the early stages, but premenstrual spotting, a sensation of urinary urgency with painful urination, and diarrhea and rectal bleeding during menstruation may occur. Some cases may show severe *dysmenorrhea* (this chapter) before, during, and *after* periods. Interestingly, the amount of pain a woman experiences has little to do with the size of her endometrial growths; many women with microscopic growths report more pain that women with advanced deposits.

[b]Causes of endometriosis. Inlet Medical Inc.; 2000. Available at: http://www.dyspareunia.org/html/endometriosis_causes.htm. Accessed summer 2001.

Symptoms of endometriosis are cyclical and reach a peak during menstruation. This feature has probably prevented many women from seeking medical help, since traditionally it has been assumed that painful menstruation is a normal and expected part of the having "the curse." As women have become more proactive about health care, they have discovered that painful menstruation is *not* a given and have become more willing to explore the causes and possible solutions to their pain.

Complications

Accumulations of bloody deposits and fibrous connective tissue can cause a great deal of damage in the pelvic cavity. Scar tissue deposits can create adhesions in or on the uterine tubes and ovaries, which cause infertility or *ectopic pregnancy* (this chapter). The collecting of blood in these extra, unintentional deposits routes blood away from where it can be useful, resulting in *anemia* (Chapter 4). Uterine hyperplasia is a condition that occasionally accompanies endometriosis; the normal endometrial lining becomes pathologically thickened, leading to excessive bleeding and further difficulties with fertility.

Diagnosis

Only one definitive diagnostic test for endometriosis works every time: laparoscopic surgery. Although patients may describe characteristic symptoms that become progressively worse and peak during menstruation, only a laparoscopy will specifically identify the lesions.

Treatment

Treatment for endometriosis depends on what outcome the woman desires. No permanent solution for this disorder has yet been developed. Even a complete hysterectomy will not protect a patient from endometriosis if any microscopic deposits remain that may be stimulated with hormone replacement therapy.

Because many women wish to treat endometriosis so that they can become pregnant, treatment options are often geared toward limiting symptoms and progression long enough to allow fertilization to take place. Symptoms disappear during pregnancy, because no estrogen is secreted to stimulate the menstrual cycle, but they usually recur after a baby is born.

Four main goals are at the center of medical intervention for endometriosis. These are to relieve pain, to stop the progression of established growths, to prevent the establishment of any new growths, and to maintain or restore fertility, if that is the patient's wish. Nonsteroidal anti-inflammatory drugs (NSAIDs) or other analgesics may be adequate for pain relief. Hormone therapy that disrupts the secretion of estrogen may be used to limit growths. These may be used alone or as a preparation for surgery. Surgical interventions can include the use of lasers or electrocauterization to ablate (remove the top layer of tissue) or cut out visible growths, and to reduce adhesions between pelvic organs.

Massage?

Endometriosis is one of those reproductive system disorders that can cause the pelvic organs to become displaced, as they are distorted with abnormal deposits and scar tissue. Consequently, deep abdominal massage is not appropriate for clients who know they have endometriosis, especially for those who are menstruating. The presence of inflammation and the threat that cells may break free and settle elsewhere in the pelvic cavity both make doing deep abdominal work problematic.

However, many women with endometriosis also live in a state of anxiety, stress, and frustration with their own bodies that may exacerbate their most painful symptoms. Massage therapy along with other relaxation techniques is frequently recommended for women who must learn to cope with the long-term consequences of a disorder that has no permanent solution.

Fibroid Tumors

Definition: What Are They?

Fibroid tumors, or *leiomyomas*, are benign tumors that grow in or around the uterus. They can grow within the smooth muscle walls or, more rarely, can be suspended from a stalk into the pelvic cavity or into the uterus. Some can even hang down into the vagina (Fig. 10-3). Fibroids vary in size from being microscopic to weighing several pounds and completely filling the uterus.

Demographics: Who Gets Them?

Approximately 20 to 30% of premenopausal women older than 35 have fibroids. This number is largely postulation because they are mostly symptomless and therefore go unreported. Growth of fibroids seems to be stimulated by estrogen; after menopause they tend to shrink and ultimately disappear. Fibroids are far more common in African-American women than they are in other populations.

FIBROID TUMORS IN BRIEF

What are they?
Fibroid tumors are benign growths in the muscle or connective tissue of the uterus.

How are they recognized?
Fibroid tumors are often asymptomatic. Some, however, cause heavy menstrual bleeding or may put mechanical pressure on other structures in the pelvis.

Is massage indicated or contraindicated?
Large, diagnosed fibroid tumors contraindicate deep abdominal massage. However, most fibroids are quite small and virtually symptomless, and massage will not affect them. In these cases massage can benefit the client, although it will not change the state of her fibroid tumors.

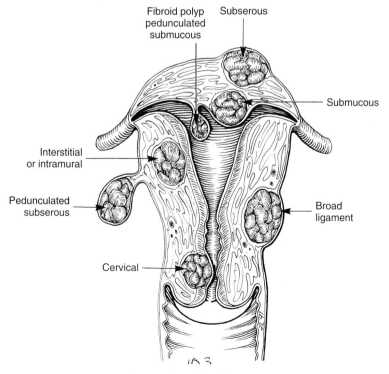

Figure 10-3. Fibroid tumors

Signs and Symptoms

Fibroids usually do not create symptoms. In very extreme cases the fibroid may grow large enough to put pressure on the sensory nerves inside the uterus or press on nearby structures like the bladder (which can cause urinary frequency) or the rectum (which can cause difficulties with defecation). If they press on the fallopian (uterine) tubes they may interfere with pregnancies. They can also cause heavy menstrual bleeding and occasionally bleeding between menstrual periods.

Complications

Fibroids are very seldom a serious condition, but they can lead to some troubling consequences. The heavy periods they cause sometimes lead to *anemia* (Chapter 4) from excessive blood loss. They can cause infertility by obstructing fallopian tubes or interfering with the implantation of a fertilized ovum. They can also interfere in pregnancies brought to term. If a fibroid is large enough, it can crowd the growing fetus or block the exit through the cervix. These problems can lead to premature births and cesarean sections.

Pedunculate fibroids, the type that dangle into the uterus or vagina, have been known to twist on their stalks, which causes extreme pain and requires surgery to remove. It is also possible for very large fibroids to outgrow their blood supply. This leads to a process called *degeneration*, in which tissue that is deprived of oxygen dies. The necrotic mass will usually be slowly reabsorbed by the body, but can be painful in the process; more often, surgery is required to remove the fibroid.

Diagnosis

Fibroids are generally found during pelvic examinations when it is noted that the uterus is enlarged or irregularly shaped. The diagnosis can usually be confirmed by ultrasound or magnetic resonance imaging (MRI), but occasionally it can be difficult to tell whether it is the uterus that is distended or if a cyst or tumor is growing on the ovaries—a potentially much more dangerous situation. If it is not clear what kind of growth is present, a computed tomography (CT) scan or laparoscopy may be called for to rule out *ovarian cancer* (this chapter).

Fibroids typically grow slowly, but occasionally they can grow fast, doubling their size within a few months. In this situation a biopsy is recommended to rule out the possibility of a uterine malignancy.

HYSTERECTOMY
This comes from the Greek root *hystera*, which means womb or uterus. The word hysteria comes from the same root. In the early days of medicine, hysteria was assumed to be a woman's complaint, associated with womb-related disturbances.

Treatment

Fibroids seldom require treatment unless they cause pain and excessive bleeding, or if they interfere with pregnancy.

Hormone therapy can shrink them, but they grow back when medication is stopped. Treatment with the "morning after pill" (RU-486) yields consistently good results. Surgical options range from minimally invasive procedures to shrink the growths with liquid nitrogen (*cryomyolysis*), to blocking off the supplying arteries (*uterine artery embolization*), to laser surgery, to partial hysterectomies, to full hysterectomies. Fibroid tumors lead to an estimated 200,000 hysterectomies in the United States every year.

Massage?

Diagnosed fibroids locally contraindicate deep abdominal work. Undiagnosed fibroids (which are probably present in about 20% of all women) are not affected by massage to speak of, and so indicate massage for the benefit of the client, if not for the improvement of her condition.

Disorders of Other Reproductive Structures

Breast Cancer

Definition: What Is It?

Breast cancer is the development of tumors in the epithelial or connective tissue of the breast. These growths may start out as nonmalignant, but may become invasive if neglected for a prolonged period.

Demographics: Who Gets It?

The American Cancer Society estimates that about 184,000 new cases of breast cancer will be diagnosed in women and about 1,000 cases in men this year in the United States. Most women with breast cancer are mature; 75% of them are older than 50 years when diagnosed.[c]

Before 1980 the lifetime risk of contracting breast cancer was 1 in 11. Now it is 1 in 8, but some factors may be falsely driving that number up, including women's increasing longevity (the chance of getting breast cancer increases significantly just with age) and the fact that breast cancer is being found and diagnosed earlier than ever before.

Breast cancer accounts for 29% of all cancers in women; only skin cancer is diagnosed more frequently. It is the leading cause of death by cancer in women younger than 54 years old and the second most common cause of death by cancer for women older than 54 (lung cancer is the first). It is responsible for the deaths of some 41,000 women and about 300 men each year.

Etiology: What Happens?

Breasts are constructed of lobes (where milk is produced in lactating women), ducts (where milk is delivered to the nipple), and stroma (collagen, elastin, and fat cells that provide support and the bulk of breast tissue). The lobes and ducts are made of epithelial cells; the stroma is connective tissue. Although cancer can grow in any of these tissues, the lobes and ducts are by far the most likely to develop malignant cells.

- *Ductal carcinoma.* This is the most common type of breast cancer, accounting for between 70 and 80% of all diagnoses. It can occur in situ, in which cells only affect the epithelial lining of the ducts, or it can become invasive. Ductal carcinoma

---

BREAST CANCER IN BRIEF

What is it?

Breast cancer is the growth of malignant tumor cells in breast tissue; these cells can invade skin and nearby muscles and bones. If they invade lymph nodes, they can metastasize to the rest of the body.

How is it recognized?

The first sign of breast cancer is a small painless lump or thickening in the breast tissue or near the axilla. The lump may be too small to palpate, but may show on a mammogram. Later the skin may change texture, the nipple may change shape, and discharge from the nipple may be present.

Is massage indicated or contraindicated?

Many breast cancer patients undergo treatment options that are extremely taxing on general health and physical and emotional well-being. As long as bodywork choices are made that respect these challenges, massage can be a wonderful, supportive, important coping mechanism for many breast cancer patients.

---

[c]Fast facts. American Cancer Society; 2000. Available at: http://www.cancer.org/NBCAM_fastfacts.html. Accessed summer 2001.

in situ (DCIS) is associated with the development of small calcified deposits in the breasts.

- *Lobular carcinoma.* This is less common than ductal carcinoma, accounting for 5 to 10% of all tumors. It can be limited to the epithelial lining of the lobes (lobular carcinoma in situ, or LCIS), but this condition carries a high risk of becoming invasive. Lobular carcinoma also has a higher incidence of appearing in both breasts than ductal carcinoma.

- *Other types of breast cancer.* Several other types of breast cancer may develop, but collectively they account for only 10 to 15% of all diagnoses. Inflammatory breast cancer is associated with edema, redness, and heat in the breast; this occurs because the tumors block lymphatic return. Inflammatory breast cancer usually has a poor prognosis. Paget's disease of the breast specifically affects the nipple and presents with specific eczema-like changes in the skin. Medullary breast cancer is a rare malignancy of the connective tissues in the breast.

Many types of breast cancer begin as in situ growths, which eventually develop malignant characteristics. It can take a long time for a tumor to become large enough to notice; it is estimated that it takes about 9 years for a growth to reach a diameter of 1 cm.

As tumors grow, the risk of having some cells invade the circulatory or lymphatic system increases. The proximity of the axillary lymph nodes makes these a common site for the spread of malignant cells. Between 30 and 40% of all breast cancers have spread to the axillary nodes by the time the tumors are palpable.

Tumors are usually composed of several different types of cells. Some of them may be vulnerable to chemotherapeutic drugs; others are not. Unfortunately, when medications kill off the vulnerable tumor cells, they may then be replaced with drug-resistant cells.

Breast cancer usually metastasizes to nearby lymph nodes in the axilla and thoracic cavity first; invasion of chest muscles, bones, and skin then follow. Finally distant metastatic sites include the liver, lung, and brain. If the cancer is not successfully treated, several complications may develop, including spinal cord pressure, bone fractures, pleural effusion, or bronchial obstruction.

Staging

Although the progression of cancer from stage to stage has been categorized for the sake of convenience, it is impossible to predict accurately and exactly how this disease will progress in each person. Every person with breast cancer undergoes a unique disease process, unlike anybody else's.

- *Stage O.* This is in situ cancer, in which cells are limited to the lining of the ducts or lobes. In situ cancer has the risk of becoming invasive in later stages.

- *Stage I.* Tumors are smaller than 2 cm and are confined to the breast.

- *Stage II.*

  - *II-A:* The tumor is smaller than 2 cm but has spread to the axillary lymph nodes, or the tumor may be up to 5 cm but has not spread to the axillary nodes.

  - *II-B:* The tumor is between 2 and 5 cm across with spreading into the axillary nodes, or a tumor larger than 5 cm is present with no spreading to the axillary nodes.

- *Stage III.*

  - *III-A*: The tumor is smaller than 5 cm and has spread to the axillary nodes; the nodes are attached to each other or to other structures, *or* the tumor is larger than 5 cm and has spread to axillary nodes.

  - *III-B*: The cancer has spread to areas near the breast (the skin, muscles, and bones of the thoracic cavity), *or* the cancer has spread to the mediastinal lymph nodes.

- *Stage IV.* The cancer has spread to other organs. The bones, liver, lungs, or brain are the most frequently affected.

- *Recurrent breast cancer:* This is a cancerous growth that appears after all treatment for previous cancer.

Risk Factors

One of the most frustrating things about this disease is that no dependable profile of the women most likely to get it has ever been developed. Some cancers, like lung, colon, and skin cancer, can be directly linked to diet or environmental factors; breast cancer cannot. Although some risk factors have been identified as increasing the chance that a woman may develop breast cancer, the majority of women with these risk factors (outside of genetic predisposition) never develop the disease, and the majority of breast cancer patients do not carry most of these risk factors.

Statistically, women who started having menstrual periods early in life, who had children after age 30 or not at all, who have late onset of menopause, and who are obese, especially after menopause, are at greater risk than the general population. Women who have more than two alcoholic drinks every day or who have a history of proliferative breast disease (a type of nonmalignant breast change) are also at a slightly increased risk of breast cancer.

The only risk factor for breast cancer that reliably predicts the development of the disease is the presence of two abnormal "breast cancer genes," BRCA 1 and BRCA 2. About 80% of all women carrying these genes develop breast cancer, but they account for only 5 to 10% of all diagnosed patients. For the other 90% the only dependable risk factor is age.

Signs and Symptoms

Early symptoms of breast cancer are subtle. Breast tissue is soft; tumors have ample room to grow without causing pain. Sometimes self-examination will find hard spots or lumps before a mammogram may show them, and sometimes a mammogram reveals thickenings or minute calcifications that are too subtle to feel. Advanced cases of breast cancer show asymmetrical breast growth, inverted nipples that may have discharge, and sometimes a characteristic "orange peel" texture of the skin on the breast. Advanced cases may also create symptoms in other parts of the body that are damaged by the growth of invasive tumors: bone pain, weight loss, spinal cord compression, and swelling in the arms may be the result of tumors far from the original site of the cancer.

Diagnosis

Breast cancer is usually detected first by self-exam and then confirmed by mammogram (Fig. 10-4), ultrasound, and tissue biopsy. These procedures will rule out nonmalignant breast changes (see sidebar).

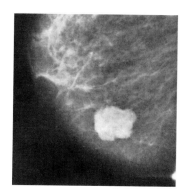

Figure 10-4. Mammogram of breast cancer (note the irregular shape and borders of the growth)

Biopsy procedures are becoming more sophisticated. Several different techniques have been developed to offer the best chance of an accurate diagnosis while doing the least amount of damage to the body.

If breast cancer is identified, it is then staged according to the criteria listed above. If lymph node involvement is suspected, a search for the "sentinel node" may be conducted. This means that a radioisotope is injected near the breast, and clinicians examine where the substance is taken up; the majority usually flows into a single lymph node before moving on to other nodes. This first stop is the sentinel node. If this lymph node is clear of cancer cells, the likelihood is that all the lymph nodes will be clear.

Prevention and Early Detection:

Breast cancer is currently not a preventable disease. The two most dependable risk factors, age and genetics, are not controllable. Therefore, efforts toward prevention are targeted at early detection, which significantly increases the life expectancy of the breast cancer patient. The three main courses for early detection are self-exam, breast exam by a professional, and mammograms, which use radiation to look for unusually dense masses in the breast tissue.

Opinions vary over how frequently mammograms should be performed. This stems from the fact that the breast tissue of many women is too dense to yield dependable results before the age of 40 or even older. However, most health care agencies now recommend that women 40 and older should have yearly professional breast exams and mammograms, and all women should perform monthly self-exams.

It is important to understand that a mammogram is not a definitive test for breast cancer. Mammogram interpretations can vary widely, and mammograms may miss the subtle changes in breast tissue that only women who perform monthly self-exams may notice. Therefore an "all clear" from a mammogram does not rule out the possibility of breast cancer.

Treatment

Breast cancer treatment depends entirely on what stage the disease is in when it is found. Whatever treatment strategy is followed, every cancer patient should have access to support groups that will benefit her healing process.

Four main options for treatment are often used in combinations for best results.

- *Surgery.* Lumpectomies, partial mastectomies, total mastectomies, and modified mastectomies are surgical options for removing tumors and nearby lymph nodes. Lymph nodes are then examined for signs of further metastasis.

- *Radiation.* Radiation is aimed at tumors to slow or stop growth or to shrink tumors to make them easier to remove surgically. Radiation may be applied externally or internally with radioactive pellets that are surgically placed around the tumors and later removed.

- *Chemotherapy.* Chemotherapy is the treatment of cancer with highly toxic drugs that may slow or stop the growth of tumors.

- *Hormone therapy.* Some breast cancer tumors have been found to be sensitive to estrogen; they need access to this hormone to grow. A medication called *tamoxifen* binds up the estrogen receptors on tumors, which then prevents them from growing.

Treatment Complications

Cancer is a life-threatening disease that aggressively invades the body. Options to deal with cancer are similarly aggressive and often create serious side effects, which, although not as deadly as the disease itself, can be debilitating.

Surgery that removes part of the breast tissue and lymph nodes can also injure brachial plexus nerves, resulting in chronic pain in the shoulder and arm. If enough lymph nodes are removed, *lymphedema*, the accumulation of interstitial fluid in the arm, can be a serious problem. A variety of pumps and drainage devices have been developed, but all have limited success. Lymph drainage techniques can deal with this problem, but this is a very different approach than Swedish massage and is not appropriate to practice without rigorous training. Fortunately, as diagnosticians are refining their skills, fewer lymph nodes are generally taken for analysis than in the past. This means that the incidence of lymphedema as a complication of breast cancer is declining.

Radiation therapy can cause skin problems from drying and itchiness to burns and localized ulcerations.

Chemotherapy introduces highly toxic drugs into the body. These drugs can kill cancer cells, but they also cause hair loss, nausea, mouth sores, and immune suppression. Extremely high doses of chemotherapy can be successful for treating advanced cases of cancer but must be followed by bone marrow transplants to replace damaged tissue there as well.

Tamoxifen is effective at keeping hormone-sensitive tumors under control but is associated with several side effects, including menopause-like symptoms, an increased chance of uterine cancer, and, for some women, a tendency to form blood clots leading to *deep vein thrombosis*, *pulmonary embolism* (Chapter 4), or *stroke* (Chapter 3).

Prognosis

If breast cancer is caught and removed before it spreads into the axillary lymph nodes, patients have a 97% chance to live 5 years or more. Overall, the 5-year survival rate is 83%, the 10-year survival rate is 65%, and the 15-year survival rate is 56%. Not surprisingly, women in whom cancer cells have been found in the lymph nodes have a much higher recurrence rate.

Breast cancer is not the kind of disease in which a person can ever say, "I'll never have to worry about that again." Because it can take many years for tumors to grow to palpable size and because metastasis may occur before this point, even a radical mastectomy may miss far-flung cells that invade distant tissues. Breast cancer patients are obliged to be forever vigilant against the possibility of new growths.

Massage?

For many years it was assumed that because Swedish massage increases circulation and lymph flow, it could contribute to cancer metastasis. Although conducting research to

Nonmalignant Breast Growths

Not all breast growths are malignant. The vast majority of growths in breast tissue are cysts or benign tumors; many fall into the classification of what used to be called *fibrocystic breast disease*. It turns out these are so common (more than 50% of all autopsied women show signs of fibrocystic breast growths) that this condition is no longer even called a disease; it is now referred to as *fibrocystic breast changes*. Some of these growths carry a risk of eventually becoming malignant, but they are, for the most part, not serious conditions and can easily be distinguished from malignancies with testing procedures that include mammograms, fine needle aspiration (FNA), ultrasound, or biopsy.

- *Gross cysts*. In this situation "gross" means large, not ugly. Gross cysts are large enough to create a visible distortion of the breast. They grow most often in women in their 40s and can be reduced with FNA. They may recur, however, with the menstrual cycle.

- *Fibroadenomas*. These are smaller cysts that may grow in clusters. They are most common in women in their 30s and 40s. Fibroadenomas are sensitive to estrogen. They tend to become enlarged and tender in the days that precede a menstrual period, and then they subside until the following month.

- *Atypical hyperplasia*. This is also called *proliferative breast disease*. It involves changes in the epithelial lining of both ducts and lobes. When it grows in the ducts it can be difficult to differentiate from in situ ductal carcinoma. Of all the noncancerous breast changes, this one carries the highest risk for malignancy: about 13% of all patients with atypical hyperplasia go on to develop invasive breast cancer.

- *Fibrosis*. Sometimes the connective tissue framework for breast tissue, sometimes called the *stroma*, becomes thick and dense with excessive connective tissue. These areas of fibrosis have a characteristic hard, rubbery texture. They are firm and painless.

- *Phyllodes tumors*. These are relatively rare growths of both epithelium and connective tissue. Most are benign, but Phyllodes tumors carry a 10% risk of becoming cancerous.

- *Papillomas*. These are tiny warts, each less than 1 cm in diameter, which may grow inside the ductal tissue.

- *Other breast pathologies*. Breasts can also be affected by infection (called *mastitis* if a woman is lactating or *ductal ectasia* if she is not). Injury from trauma, surgery, or radiation may cause *fat necrosis*, a condition in which the fat cells that make up the bulk of breast tissue degenerate and die. Breast infections and fat necrosis can be serious situations that require medical intervention for the best outcomes.

BREAST CANCER: CASE HISTORY
Carol E, 60 Years Old
"When you have had breast cancer, the thought of possible recurrence is always with you. It makes you look at what is really important in life."

It was in July, right before my 57th birthday, when I found a lump in my left breast while doing a breast exam in the shower. We were just getting ready to leave on a vacation with friends, so I did not say anything. My annual mammogram was already scheduled in about 3 weeks.

When I went in for my mammogram, I told the doctor about the lump. He said he couldn't feel a lump. The mammogram was normal. A subsequent ultrasound did not reveal anything, and the technician also could not feel what I felt. So, even though I knew better, because of a medical background, this gave me a sense of security that all was well.

Until January. I could still feel the lump and by now my husband could also—so I was not imagining it. I talked with our daughter, an RN involved in risk management. She said, "You could have a normal mammogram and ultrasound and still have breast cancer. You have to go by what you know is normal for you." So, I made an appointment with a surgeon for the week I returned from a previously planned trip to Florida.

I returned on Valentine's Day, and my appointment was on February 16th. The surgeon not only felt what I had felt (which was a thickening, more than a lump), but in checking my previous mammogram, he found pinpoints of calcium in the right breast, which are sometimes indicators of cancer. Three days later I had bilateral biopsies.

During the biopsies, a frozen section was done on the thickening on the left side, which meant the pathologist could tell right away whether the tissue was malignant. (The tissue from the right breast biopsy went through routine pathology, and I had to wait for several days for those results). So there I was, in the recovery room, when the doctor came in and told me that the left breast biopsy was malignant. Then he left to talk to my husband and I was by myself. The greatest feeling I had was just incredible sadness. I don't know why I wasn't angry or anything else; I was just so sad. After a few minutes I was able to join my husband and we both cried.

When something like this happens to you, you begin by wondering, how bad is it? Are you going to die soon? Then you go home and do the waiting game again—for the results of the other biopsy—and this was absolutely, incredibly stressful. You are already facing surgery on one breast, and now you are wondering if you will lose both breasts. After 3 days, the call came saying the second biopsy was not malignant. By that time I was thankful that only one breast had a malignancy. Strange thing for which to be thankful.

My diagnosis was a Stage 1 infiltrated ductal carcinoma, upper medial quadrant, left breast. After getting a second opinion, surgery was scheduled for the following Monday. Before that, I had to have chest x-rays, bone scan, and a radiation oncology consult as I had opted to have conservative surgery (a lumpectomy followed by 6 weeks of radiation).

The surgeon performed a lumpectomy and also did an axillary dissection—removal of some lymph nodes in the armpit. It is during this surgery that a nerve in the armpit is either severed or damaged. This produces numbness in the underarm and inner upper arm that can be permanent. The lymph nodes removed (16 in my case) were tested for malignancy, and later I learned that they showed no cancer. Chances were that the cancer had been confined to the breast tissue. Good news indeed!

However, the next Thursday, the surgeon called and said that the margins of the tissue removed were not clean—meaning that there were still some cancer cells in the breast. So, back to surgery the next Monday for a re-resection of the breast. My surgeon did not usually do this, but he felt that there was very little cancer left, and a mastectomy could still be avoided.

After a few days of recuperation, I returned home after being out to find my husband in bed with a bad headache. This was very rare, so I didn't bother him. The telephone rang and it was my surgeon again, saying (in a very upset and sad tone) that the margins on the last tissue sample still were not clean. He had spoken with the radiation oncologist and she felt she could kill the remaining cancer cells with radiation. However, the surgeon felt he could give me even better odds by performing a total mastectomy. Of course, I opted for the better odds against recurrence, and the following Monday again found me in surgery having a total mastectomy. Three major surgeries in 3 weeks with general anesthetic each time are a lot to cope with, but you do what you have to do.

Because I had a mastectomy, I did not have to have any radiation, and because my lymph nodes were negative for cancer cells, I also did not have to have chemotherapy. A big relief!

I do take tamoxifen, an anti-breast cancer drug used in certain circumstances to guard against recurrence. The standard commitment to this is 5 years. I also take amitriptyline, a mild anti-depressant, to help break the cycle of chronic nerve pain that I have had in my left arm—an unusual and difficult complication. About 8 months ago I also started on Neurontin, an anti-seizure drug which can also work on nerve pain, and in my case it has really helped. So, after almost 2 years, the pain in my arm is under control. I have no lymphedema (swelling of the arm due to a compromised lymph system). However, this could happen at any time.

I do not feel that the doctors emphasize enough how vulnerable the affected arm is. Infections can develop very easily and I have to be really careful, especially working in the garden. It seems that little burns and scratches take forever to heal. I should not lift more than 10 pounds with the affected arm and should not have any needle sticks or have blood pressure taken on that arm. Once I awoke after minor surgery to find a blood pressure cuff on my left arm, and was I upset! I thought that I had taken enough precautions that this should not have happened. The prescription for post-surgery medication had been clipped over the warning note! The next time I had an anesthetic, I wrote on my left arm with a surgical pen, and that did not come off!

When you have had breast cancer, the thought of possible recurrence is always with you. Breast cancer does not follow the 5-year rule; it can come back at any time. It is a lifelong commitment to always be on the watch and take really good care

Continued

BREAST CANCER: CASE HISTORY—continued
Carol E, 60 Years Old

of yourself. This makes you look at what is really important in life. You try not to put off things that you want to say or do. Life is precious and I am glad to still have it!

As a part of her recovery process, Carol became active in several breast cancer support groups. One of the groups of "Bosom Buddies" that she helped to co-facilitate still meets every month to have fun and draw support from each other. Through "Reach to Recovery," Carol does hospital and home visits to new breast cancer patients, teaching them about their options, telling them what they might expect, and giving them guidance in getting more information. She would like to see women become their own advocates as they deal with the complexities of this disease.

---

specifically explore this idea is ethically impractical, a closer look reveals some basic problems with this assumption. Firstly, it takes years for tumors to reach palpable size; any tumor that is found after a massage has been in the making for a long time. Secondly, exactly how much massage increases blood and lymph movement and for how long are variables that have never been fully quantified. Does doing a 60-minute full-body Swedish massage move as much lymph or blood as taking a long, hot shower? How does it compare to a vigorous half-hour walk?

Obviously, a massage therapist needs to locally avoid tumor sites, especially if they are close to the surface of the skin, but most of the other cautions that surround massage and breast cancer have to do with respecting the challenges brought about by the treatment these clients must deal with, more than with the disease itself. Massage therapists can gauge their choices to provide the maximum benefit for cancer patients (anxiety and pain reduction, immune system strengthening, better appetite and sleep quality, along with general support and informed, nurturing touch) while minimizing the risks of overchallenging a client who is already struggling to keep up with the demands of surgery, chemotherapy, radiation, or a combination of all three.

If a decision is made to include massage as part of a treatment program for a cancer patient, certain cautions must be observed. Radiation and tumor sites are local contraindications. Chemotherapy compromises immune system reactions, making the client vulnerable to a variety of infections that may contraindicate massage. Changes in the health of the tissues may make clients susceptible to blood clots, bruising, or other damage that healthy people would not sustain. Because the severity of cancer treatment symptoms vary widely, it is impossible to predict what is appropriate for all clients. Rather, the therapist should work as part of a well-informed health care team to provide the best care and support possible.

Regardless of whether massage therapists choose to work with women who have breast cancer, one thing they *can* do is encourage their women clients to perform monthly self-exams. It is not within the scope of practice to do this for clients, or even to teach them how, but stressing the importance of self-exams is a meaningful way that all massage therapists can support their clients.

Ovarian Cancer

Definition: What Is It?

Ovarian cancer is the growth of malignant tumors on the ovaries. Several varieties of ovarian cancer have been identified, but most of them begin in the epithelial lining of these organs. The tumors may take a long time to become established, but once they do, some types may grow quickly and metastasize readily to other organs in the abdomen.

OVARIAN CANCER IN BRIEF

What is it?
Ovarian cancer is the development of malignant tumors on the ovaries that may metastasize to other structures in the pelvic or abdominal cavity.

How is it recognized?
Symptoms of ovarian cancer are generally extremely subtle until the disease has progressed to life-threatening levels. Early symptoms include a feeling of heaviness in the pelvis, vague abdominal discomfort, occasional vaginal bleeding, and weight gain or loss.

Is massage indicated or contraindicated?
As with all cancers, the appropriateness of massage depends on what treatment measures the client is going through. Massage therapists working with clients who have ovarian cancer should be part of a fully informed health care team.

Demographics: Who Gets It?

Ovarian cancer mostly strikes women who live in industrialized areas. Whites are the highest risk group for this disease. It can occur at any age, but is most common in women who are 60 years old or older. Ovarian cancer affects about 23,000 women each year; that means about 1 of every 55 women in the United States will have this disease. Although the incidence of this disease is low compared to other cancers, its mortality rate is high; ovarian cancer kills about 14,000 women every year. It is the second leading cause of death by gynecologic cancer (breast cancer is the first).

Etiology: What Happens?

Three specific types of tumors have been found to grow on ovaries: tumors of germ cells, tumors of stromal cells, and tumors of epithelial cells. As with most types of cancers, epithelial tumors are the most common and often the most invasive. Epithelial tumors, or *adenocarcinomas*, comprise about 90% of all ovarian cancers.

Epithelial tumors of the ovaries fall into several different categories, each with different growth patterns and prognoses. Some of these tumors are slow-growing and may never become malignant. Early identification and removal of these growths may leave the reproductive system intact if the woman wishes to have more children. Many types of epithelial ovarian tumors aggressively invade not only the ovaries, but other pelvic and abdominal organs as well. These tumors are life threatening, not only because they are so prone to metastasis, but because they create few (if any) noticeable symptoms in their early stages. Usually by the time a woman is concerned enough to consult a doctor, ovarian cancer has progressed into advanced stages that are difficult or impossible to treat.

Risk Factors

Although the specific triggers for the formation of tumors on the ovaries are unknown, some of the most important risk factors for developing the disease have been identified.

- *Familial history.* Perhaps the greatest risk factor for ovarian cancer is having it in the family. Women who have a first-degree relative (mother, sister, daughter) with ovarian cancer could have up to a 50% chance of developing the cancer themselves. Having a second-degree relative (grandmother, aunt, half-sister) with ovarian cancer also increases the chance of developing the disease. Families with a history of *breast cancer* (this chapter) also have statistically higher rates of ovarian cancer than the general population.

- *Reproductive history.* Any woman who has never had a child or taken birth control pills, or who has experienced multiple miscarriages, is at increased risk for ovarian cancer. In addition, women who have taken fertility drugs without conceiving and bearing a child may also be at increased risk, although the statistics for these women have been inconsistent.

- *Health history.* Women who have a history of breast or colon cancer themselves have approximately twice the chance of developing ovarian cancer as the rest of the population. Women who carry the breast cancer genes BRCA 1 and BRCA 2 are at especially high risk.

- *Estrogen replacement therapy.* Women who have utilized estrogen replacement therapy against *osteoporosis* (Chapter 2) for more than 4 years have a higher chance of developing ovarian cancer than others.

- *Other.* Other risks involve exposure to radiation or asbestos, the use of talcum powder on the genitals, a high-fat diet, and age. The chance of developing ovarian cancer goes up considerably between ages 40 and 60.

Signs and Symptoms

The thing that makes ovarian cancer such a dangerous disease is that early symptoms are practically nonexistent or so subtle that they are easily passed over. Then when the cancer is finally identified, it has often metastasized beyond the point of control.

Early symptoms of ovarian cancer include a feeling of heaviness in the pelvis; vague abdominal discomfort including bloating, nausea, diarrhea, and constipation; vaginal bleeding; a change in menstrual cycles; and weight gain or loss. Later symptoms can include a palpable abdominal mass, increased girth around the abdomen, and ascites (the accumulation of fluid in the peritoneum).

Diagnosis

Ovarian cancer is difficult to diagnose early. A pelvic examination may reveal unusual abdominal masses, but only one-fourth of these turn out to be cancerous. Other tests that may be conducted include ultrasound tests conducted through the vagina, CT scans, and MRIs. Barium enemas and pyelograms (a process that stains urine in the kidneys to see how it moves down the ureters into the bladder) may be conducted to look for structures that may be pressing on other abdominal organs. A blood test called CA-125 looks for a particular tumor marker in the bloodstream. This has been useful in confirming a diagnosis, but it occasionally yields false-positive and false-negative results, so it is not a definitive test. Ultimately, a laparotomy or laparoscopy must be conducted to take a tissue sample from the ovaries for analysis.

Staging

If the test results from a biopsy are positive, further abdominal exploration is conducted to see how far (if at all) the cancer has progressed. Samples from nearby lymph nodes, the diaphragm, and peritoneal fluid are examined to look for signs of metastasis. Ovarian cancer is staged similarly to other types of cancer, on a scale of I to IV.

- *Stage I.* Tumor cells are confined to the ovary.
  - *I-A:* One ovary is affected, the tumor is completely contained, and no ascites is present.
  - *I-B:* Two ovaries are affected.

- *I-C*: One or two ovaries are affected; the outer surface of the tumor is ruptured; ascites is present; and malignant cells are found in the fluid.
  - *Stage II*. Other pelvic organs are affected.
    - *II-A*: The uterus and/or uterine tubes are affected.
    - *II-B*: The bladder and/or rectum are affected.
    - *II-C*: The outer surfaces of tumors are ruptured, ascites is present, and malignant cells are found in the fluid.
  - *Stage III*. Tumors are found in the peritoneum and pelvic lymph nodes.
    - *III-A*: Tumors are visible on the ovaries but not anywhere else, although they have begun to form.
    - *III-B*: Tumors in the peritoneum/and or lymph nodes are visible but are smaller than 2 cm.
    - *III-C*: Tumors are larger than 2 cm.
  - *Stage IV*. Tumors have metastasized to distant organs, usually the lungs and liver.

Ovarian cancer is found in Stage I or II only 25% of the time. Most diagnoses come when the cancer has advanced to Stage III or IV, when the chances for survival fall drastically. The overall 5-year survival rate for ovarian cancer is 50%, but those women who find their disease in Stage I have close to a 100% chance of reaching that goal.

Treatment

Ovarian cancer is generally treated with surgery and chemotherapy. Surgery is done to remove the ovaries (oophorectomy) and sometimes the uterine tubes and uterus as well. Chemotherapy can be conducted orally at home or intravenously in a hospital. One method delivers the cytotoxic drugs directly into the peritoneum where it can have immediate access to malignant tumors.

Radiation therapy is not usually used for ovarian cancer.

Massage?

As with any kind of cancer, the appropriateness of massage for ovarian cancer is a matter of personal choice. A client who is recovering from ovarian cancer may find that massage can ameliorate the challenges of surgery and chemotherapy. If a client wishes to include massage in her treatment program, she and her massage therapist should consult with her oncologist and other health care team members for the best and safest results.

Ovarian Cysts
Definition: What Are They?

A variety of cysts may grow on the ovaries. They may be related to *endometriosis* (these are called "chocolate cysts" because they are filled with brownish endometrial deposits), or they may be varieties of precancerous growths that may develop into *ovarian cancer* (this chapter). The cysts discussed here, however, are *functional cysts*, that is, they arise from normal ovaries, usually as a result of hormonal imbalance or dysfunction.

Demographics: Who Gets Them?

Ovarian cysts have been found in females of all ages, from pre-natal babies to elderly women. The majority of functional cysts are found in women between the onset of menstruation (menarche) and the onset of menopause. In other words, women who ovulate are at greatest risk for functional ovarian cysts.

Functional cysts are very common among fertile women. Up to 30% of all women with regular menstrual cycles develop an ovarian cyst at least once; up to 50% of women with irregular cycles develop at least one ovarian cyst.

When ovarian cysts are found in premenarchal girls or post-menopausal women, the chances of malignancy are much higher than among other patients. Abnormal growths among these populations are treated much more aggressively than among women of childbearing age.

Etiology: What Happens?

A follicle is a small sac or cavity that produces a secretion. Every month a fertile woman develops several follicles on one of her ovaries. As her cycle progresses, a single follicle becomes dominant, while the other ones recede. At the appropriate hormonal signal, the follicle ruptures, releasing a mature egg, or oocyte, into the pelvic cavity, where it is drawn into the uterine tubes for the journey toward the uterus.

Each follicle that develops is a potential cyst. Sometimes the follicle does not rupture completely, and a blister forms on the ovary. Sometimes the ruptured follicle (now called the *corpus luteum*) forms a kind of blood blister that may eventually break and bleed into the pelvic cavity. Some other cysts arise in conjunction with abnormal pregnancies or as a result of hormonal imbalances that may begin in the pituitary gland.

Most ovarian cysts are not dangerous, but they have the potential to become large and painful and may develop dangerous complications.

Types of Cysts

Several types of cysts can form on the ovaries. Three of the most common kinds are discussed here:

- *Follicular cysts.* When a follicle that holds a mature egg does not rupture completely, a blister forms at the site. Follicular cysts rarely get bigger than 2 to 3 inches across, and they usually spontaneously recede within two menstrual cycles (Fig. 10-5). Follicular cysts are the most common of all ovarian cysts.

- *Corpus luteum cysts.* Blisters can form over the corpus luteum, which then changes the balance of hormones being secreted from the ovaries. Corpus luteum cysts will delay subsequent ovulations and produce pregnancy-like symptoms (nausea, vomiting, breast tenderness) until they spontaneously resolve, usually within a month or two. Corpus luteum cysts are less common than follicular cysts, but they can be more serious, as they may create bleeding into the peritoneal space.

- *Polycystic ovaries.* Also called *Stein-Leventhal syndrome*, this condition involves enlarged ovaries with multiple small cysts. The interference in hormone secretion

---

OVARIAN CYSTS IN BRIEF

What are they?
Most ovarian cysts are fluid-filled growths on the ovaries. Some types of cysts are associated with ovarian cancer or other reproductive disorders, but the cysts discussed here are benign.

How are they recognized?
The symptoms of ovarian cysts may be nonexistent or may cause a disruption in the menstrual cycle. Constant or intermittent pain in the pelvis, pain with intercourse, or symptoms similar to early pregnancy may arise from different types of ovarian cysts.

Is massage indicated or contraindicated?
Ovarian cysts that have been diagnosed locally contraindicate massage.

MITTELSCHMERZ
This is a term derived from German for "middle pain." This refers to the sensation some women have when the leading follicle on an ovary ruptures and the egg is released into the pelvic cavity. It is called "middle" because it occurs precisely in the middle (about day 14) of the menstrual cycle.

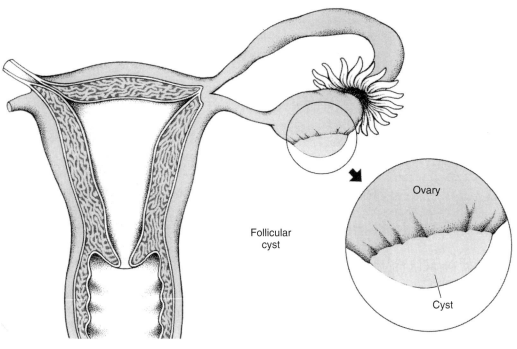

Figure 10-5. Ovarian cyst

that this condition creates may cause obesity, loss of menstrual cycle, *acne* (Chapter 1), and increased body hair.

Other cysts that can grow on the ovaries may be part of endometriosis, cystadenomas (usually benign tumors but can occasionally become cancerous), and dermoid cysts or *teratomas*. In these cysts some primitive cells have been isolated from the rest of the body and have developed into different types of tissues. Dermoid cysts have been found that contain teeth, hairs, bone fragments, and other types of tissue. They are usually harmless in women. Men can develop them too, but for males teratomas are a much more serious condition that may involve testicular cancer.

Signs and Symptoms

Most ovarian cysts have no symptoms until the cyst is injured in some way. Some women, however, experience a constant dull ache in the lower abdomen on the affected side. A firm, painless swelling may develop in the pelvis, and occasionally an ovarian cyst causes pain with intercourse. Large cysts may create low back pain, or, through pressure on the lumbar plexus, pain into the legs. Corpus luteum cysts and polycystic ovaries have special symptoms of their own, which are described above. In the absence of these signs, a person would never know a cyst was present unless it grew big enough to interfere with other functions or if it ruptured.

Complications

Size is the major factor that determines whether ovarian cysts are going to cause any trouble. They can grow big enough to interfere with blood flow; they may also rest on the bladder. In rare cases they can grow to incredible dimensions. An ovarian cyst that hangs from a stalk may sometimes get twisted. If that happens, acute abdominal pain, nausea, and fever will develop; medical intervention is necessary, as the tissue may die and become necrotic. Similar symptoms will be present if the cyst ruptures. The risk of *peritonitis* (Chapter 7) is high in this situation.

Perhaps the most serious complicating factor of ovarian cysts is that their early symptoms, subtle as they may be, mimic an *advanced* case of *ovarian cancer* (this chapter). This is a highly dangerous cancer that has few early symptoms. By the time a person can feel a firm painless swelling in her pelvis, the disease will be dangerously advanced. Therefore, if a client displays any of these symptoms but has not been examined, urge her to get checked out as soon as possible.

Diagnosis

Ovarian cysts are frequently found as a swelling or mass during a routine pelvic examination. Ultrasound pictures will generally confirm the diagnosis. If the patient is at high risk for cancer, or if the cyst looks to have a solid rather than liquid core, a laparoscopy may be performed to take a tissue sample for analysis. It is important to follow up on cyst-like symptoms that last for more than 60 days, since follicular and corpus luteum cysts, the two most common and benign varieties, will usually have been resolved within this period.

Treatment

Follicular and corpus luteum cysts are often treated with oral contraceptives. Birth control pills alter hormonal secretions and allow the cysts to recede completely or to shrink to a size that is easily removed. Ovarian cysts that do not spontaneously resolve may be aspirated, but more often surgery is performed to remove them. The affected ovary is usually taken too. In some cases a complete removal of the ovaries and uterus is recommended because some types of cysts tend to recur and can develop into cancer.

Massage?

Ovarian cysts locally contraindicate massage. Be aware that ovarian cysts can also displace the pelvic contents, so deep abdominal work done where it would be safe on a woman without cysts may lead to bruising of the ovaries or even rupture of the cyst on someone who has this condition. Massage elsewhere on the body is appropriate.

Disorders of the Male Reproductive System

Benign Prostatic Hyperplasia
Definition: What Is It?

Benign Prostatic Hyperplasia (BPH) is a condition in which the prostate gland of mature men becomes enlarged. This growth late in life is not related to *prostate cancer* (this chapter), hence the name "benign."

Demographics: Who Gets It?

The single greatest risk factors for developing BPH are simply being a male and being mature. Although not all men with BPH experience symptoms, its incidence is remarkably high. Nearly 50% of all men older than 60 years have some level of BPH; 70% of men over 70 have it; 80% of men over 80 have it, and so on.

Etiology: What Happens?

The prostate gland of a preadolescent male is very small. As a boy enters puberty this pea-sized gland that wraps around the urethra just below the bladder grows approximately to the size of a walnut. It stays that size until a man is around 40 years old, and then some prostates begin to grow again.

It is unclear why some prostate glands grow and others do not. Theories about triggers for late prostate growth involve hormonal changes with maturity. One possible factor may be the formation of dihydrotestosterone (DHT). This hormone is a form of testosterone that has been seen to increase prostate size. Another theory is that as men age they produce less testosterone to balance out their normal levels of estrogen; this may lead to hyperplasia, as estrogen is also associated with prostate growth.

Regardless of the cause of prostate growth, BPH may result in pressure on the urethra, which can interfere with normal urination. The extent of growth does not always correspond with the amount of pressure on the urethra. Some men have advanced BPH with no urinary symptoms at all, whereas others have minimal amounts of prostate growth and severe urethral constriction.

Mechanical pressure on the urethra makes it difficult to expel urine from the body. Long-term consequences can lead to pathologic changes in the bladder, which can become stiff, inelastic, and irritable. The risk of *urinary tract infections, pyelonephritis* (see Chapter 9), and bladder stones is much higher in men who cannot urinate easily; these are common complications of BPH.

Signs and Symptoms

Signs and symptoms of BPH, when any develop at all, involve difficulties with urination. Weak flow, interrupted flow, increased frequency, and a feeling that the bladder is never completely emptied are often reported. Leaking or dribbling urine between visits to the bathroom is common. Some men find it difficult to initiate urination and must strain or push to start their flow. Other men find that they need to urinate more frequently, especially at night.

One rare but serious symptom of BPH is an abrupt obstruction of the urethra, called *acute urinary retention*. In this situation the urethra is suddenly completely obstructed and urine has no way to get out of the body. This is a medical emergency and must be treated in a hospital.

Diagnosis

BPH is diagnosed in a number of ways, to identify exactly where and how seriously the urethra is obstructed. Tests may measure the speed and completeness of urination, pressure in the bladder, or how much urine is left in the bladder after urination.

BPH has no relation to prostate cancer, although the symptoms may be similar. Therefore, part of any screening for BPH includes a digital rectal examination (DRE) and a prostate-specific antigen (PSA) blood test to look for signs of prostate cancer.

WATCH FOR THIS

Prostate Cancer Versus Benign Prostatic Hyperplasia Versus Prostatitis

When the prostate gland becomes enlarged, symptoms are predictable: restriction of urinary flow, bladder irritation, and a high probability of kidney infection. The causes of prostate enlargement, however, are not so consistent. Benign prostatic hyperplasia is difficult to delineate from prostate cancer, and a third disorder, prostatitis, may further confuse the diagnostic picture. Because prostate cancer is second only to skin cancer in cancer rates among men, and because as men age they have higher probabilities of BPH, it is useful to be familiar with some of the key features of each of these disorders.

	PROSTATE CANCER	BENIGN PROSTATIC HYPERPLASIA	PROSTATITIS
Who gets it?	Usually this is a disease of men older than 50 years, although certain populations may have an earlier onset	The incidence of this condition increases with age; the older a man is, the more likely it is that he will have some level of BPH	This enlargement of the prostate may occur in males of any age
Signs and symptoms	Symptoms include restricted urinary flow, bladder irritation, and possibly pain related to pressure put on other pelvic structures; blood may appear in the urine if tumors have eroded into the urethral canal	Symptoms include restricted urinary flow and bladder irritation	Symptoms include frequency and restricted urinary flow, but depending on underlying causes they may also include fever, inflamed lymph nodes, impotence, premature ejaculation, burning or painful urination, and the presence of white blood cells in urine or semen
Diagnosis	Prostate cancer is usually diagnosed through DRE, PSA test, and ultrasound imaging	BPH is usually diagnosed through DRE, PSA test (to rule out prostate cancer), and tests to measure the force of urinary flow	Diagnosis is centered on identifying what the contributing causes are; semen and urine tests for bacteria and other tests are conducted to rule out BPH and prostate cancer
Treatment	Treatment of prostate cancer is determined by the age of the patient and the aggressiveness and the stage of his disease; options include radiation, surgery, hormone therapy, or chemotherapy	Medications that limit prostate growth may be prescribed; surgery to enlarge the urethral passageway is sometimes performed	Treatment is determined by the cause of the inflammation; infections are treated with antibiotics. Non-infectious inflammation may be treated with medication, hydrotherapy, or other methods
Implications for massage	Although prostate cancer does not rule out massage, therapists need to adjust their modality to accommodate for whatever treatment program the client is undergoing	BPH indicates massage, as long as the client is comfortable on the table and no signs of bladder or kidney infection are present	Prostatitis indicates massage if the risk of acute infection has been ruled out; clients who exhibit signs of prostate enlargement or inflammation should be encouraged to find out why

Treatment

BPH is treated according to severity. If it does not seriously affect a man's ability to urinate, it may be left untreated but closely monitored for signs of further growth. A number of options have been developed to limit prostate growth, including medications and a variety of surgeries.

Medications for BPH include drugs designed to lower levels of DHT, the testosterone derivative believed to stimulate prostate growth, and alpha-blockers, a group of medications that help the prostate and bladder to relax. The side effects of these medications can be severe, however, including the inability to achieve erection, lowered sex drive, lowered sperm counts, and others. Several herbal preparations may be recommended to prevent or limit prostate growth. Saw palmetto has been seen in clinical trials to be as effective as some medications, while creating fewer side effects. The challenge with this option is finding a source in which potency and dosage is consistent.

Surgical options for BPH include a variety of techniques that cut away, vaporize, burn, or otherwise remove small sections of the prostate gland to relieve pressure on the urethra. This field is rapidly expanding since the American population is aging and it is estimated that 25 to 30% of all American men may need surgical intervention to help with BPH symptoms at some time. Tissue removed with prostate surgery is routinely examined for signs of cancer. About 15% of all men who undergo surgery for BPH have developed early signs of prostate cancer.

Massage?

Massage can have little (if any) impact on prostate growth, and the prostate itself is located in an area that most bodyworkers never access. Although massage will not improve this situation, it can certainly improve the quality of life of the patient; therefore, BPH indicates massage systemically, if not locally. If a client reports any symptoms of a urinary tract or kidney infection, however, it is important that he get appropriate care as soon as possible.

PROSTATE CANCER IN BRIEF

What is it?
Prostate cancer is the growth of malignant cells in the prostate gland, which may then metastasize, usually to nearby bones or into inguinal lymph nodes.

How is it recognized?
The symptoms of prostate cancer include problems with urination: weak stream, increased frequency, urgency, nocturia, and other problems arising from constriction of the urethra.

Is massage indicated or contraindicated?
Prostate cancer patients may face any combination of surgery, radiation, chemotherapy, and hormonal therapy to deal with their disease. Bodywork that accommodates for these challenges while minimizing risks can be helpful and supportive, as long as the massage therapist is working as part of a fully informed health care team.

Prostate Cancer
Definition: What Is It?

Prostate cancer is the growth of malignant tumor cells in the prostate gland. This cancer often grows slowly but can metastasize to other parts of the body, most often the bladder, rectum, and bones of the pelvis.

Demographics: Who Gets It?

Between 180,000 and 200,000 cases of prostate cancer are diagnosed in the United States every year. Approximately 32,000 men die of this disease every year. Prostate cancer is rarely found in men younger than 40 years of age, but microscopic precancerous changes are found in about 30% of men older than 50. The incidence of prostate cancer rises with increasing age. The average age at diagnosis is 65 years. The lifetime risk of developing prostate cancer for all males is about 10%. For men older than 50 years, it is about 25%. For men older than 80 years, it is about 50%. Prostate cancer is the second most commonly diagnosed cancer in men (skin cancer is first) and the second leading cause of death by cancer in men (lung cancer is first).

African-American men are about twice as likely to develop prostate cancer as Whites. They are also about twice as likely to die of this disease.

Etiology: What Happens?

The prostate is a donut-shaped gland that lies inferior to the bladder and encircles the male urethra (Fig. 10-6). It produces the fluid that allows for the motility and viability of sperm. The prostate also controls release of the urine from the bladder. Some enlargement of the prostate in later years is almost a guarantee for men. Simple enlargement with no malignant cells is called *benign prostatic hyperplasia* (this chapter). Sometimes the growth and thickening of the prostate gland is not benign; it indicates prostate cancer.

When cancerous cells begin to form a tumor in the prostate, they can exert direct pressure on the urethra. This can lead to a number of different problems, from difficulty in urinating to urgency, increased frequency, nocturia (the need to urinate frequently during the night), and bladder infections. Because the symptoms of prostate cancer are so similar to those of BPH, these signs may be ignored until the urethra is seriously restricted. Prostate cancer grows slowly. It can stay silent for long enough for cells to metastasize before it is detected.

Causes

The precise causes of prostate cancer are unknown. It has been observed, however, that for tumors to grow they must have access to testosterone from fully functional testes. This disease is unknown in men who have been castrated, and castration has also been shown to shrink cancerous tumors.

Men with prostate cancer in their immediate family are more likely than others to develop this disease; heredity is estimated to account for about 10% of all prostate cancer cases. Men whose diets are high in animal fats have higher rates of prostate cancer than others. As discussed previously, advanced age and being African-American are two other risk factors for this disease. It is important to point out however, that risk factors are only

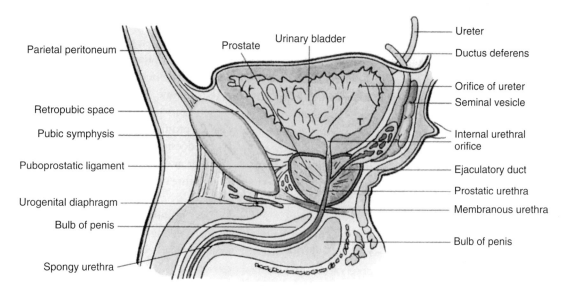

Figure 10-6. Benign prostatic hyperplasia; when the prostate enlarges, it can restrict urinary flow.

general tendencies. As with many other types of cancers, many prostate cancer patients do *not* fit the profile, and being free from these identified risk factors does not mean a person is necessarily going to avoid this problem.

Signs and Symptoms

Symptoms of prostate cancer are exactly the same as those for BPH: an enlarged, hard prostate, obstruction of the urethra with resulting difficulty in urination, and susceptibility to *urinary tract* and *kidney infections* (Chapter 9). In addition, men with prostate cancer may also experience pain while urinating, blood in the urine, and the inability to maintain an erection. Low back pain and pain that refers into the upper thighs may follow as the growths become large enough to put mechanical pressure on pelvic nerves.

Diagnosis

Historically, prostate cancer has been difficult to diagnose in the early stages because its only signs and symptoms are so close to BPH, a disorder experienced by a majority of elderly men. The advent of some early detection tests has made prostate cancer much easier to find before it has spread beyond the prostate.

A digital rectal exam (DRE) is the first step in prostate cancer detection. A blood test to look for prostate-specific antigen (PSA) is another early detection device. Its usefulness is somewhat debatable since many variables may cause PSA levels to rise or fall, but when levels are higher than normal, this blood test can serve as a warning sign to consider the possibility of prostate cancer. The American Cancer society recommends that most men have a yearly DRE and PSA test after age 50, and that Black men and men with other family members who have prostate cancer should start by age 40 or 45.[d]

If the DRE and/or PSA turn up any specific concerns, further exploration may be conducted through a transrectal ultrasound and the biopsy of suspicious tissue.

Prostate cancer is staged by advancement and by the aggressiveness of the growths. Early detection methods have made it possible to find close to 80% of all cases before the cancer has spread beyond the prostate. The 5-year survival rate for these patients approaches 100%.

Treatment

Treatment options for prostate cancer include radiation from internal or external sources, surgery to remove part or all of the prostate or the testes, and hormone therapy (estrogen counteracts elevated levels of testosterone). Chemotherapy is generally reserved for very advanced cases. Most treatment options for prostate cancer involve serious complications including incontinence, impotence, and the development of feminine characteristics. Elderly men with slow-growing tumors may simply opt not to treat their disease because their quality of life would be so seriously affected.

Massage?

Most massage therapists who have elderly men as part of their clientele have some clients who live with the threat of prostate cancer. It is important to know how the client keeps his condition under observation and what treatment options he uses. Massage therapists working as part of a health care team can certainly improve the quality

---

[d]What is it? American Cancer Society; 2000. Available at: http://www3.cancer.org/cancerinfo/load_cont.asp?ct=36&st=wi. Accessed summer 2001.

of these clients' lives by providing supportive, informed touch during a time of great stress and challenge.

Other Reproductive System Conditions

Menopause

Definition: What Is It?

Menopause refers to a specific event: the moment the ovaries permanently stop secreting enough hormones to initiate a menstrual cycle. The time leading up to this event is called *perimenopause*, and many of the symptoms associated with declining hormone secretion occur during this period. Menopause itself is not absolutely identified until menstruation has completely stopped for a full year.

Demographics: Who Gets It?

All women who live long enough will experience a decline in ovarian function. In 1900 the average female life expectancy was 51, and menopause was not a significant health care issue. In 2000, the average female life expectancy was close to 80. Women today can expect to live one-third to one-half of their lives after menopause.

The average age for the onset of perimenopausal symptoms is 47.5 years; the average age at which the transition is final is 51.4 years. These average ages have not changed since records on menopause have been kept, but some factors like cigarette smoking or genetic predisposition appear to be associated with an earlier onset of perimenopausal symptoms.

As the U.S. population ages, increasing numbers of women now live with the consequences of menopause. Today approximately 40 million women are postmenopausal. It is estimated that by 2020, 46 million living American women will have gone through menopause.

Etiology: What Happens?

In addition to ripening several eggs each month and releasing at least one for the possibility of fertilization, the ovaries have the job of secreting a variety of chemicals into the bloodstream. Estrogen and its chemical predecessor progesterone are two of these. It is somewhat misleading to refer to estrogen and progesterone as only two hormones; both of these substances are produced in various chemical formats, each of which are metabolized and used in numerous different ways.

Estrogens and progesterones work on sex organs to either support a pregnancy or to shed the endometrial lining of the uterus. When the ovaries lose function, either as a normal part of aging or because their function has been interrupted by surgery, radiation, or

---

MENOPAUSE IN BRIEF

What is it?
Menopause refers to the moment when functioning ovaries become nonfunctioning ovaries. Although this usually happens as a normal part of aging, menopause can be induced through surgery, radiation, or medication.

How is it recognized?
The symptoms associated with a decline in ovarian function ("perimenopause") include night sweats, hot flashes, insomnia, mood swings, decreased sex drive, vaginal itchiness or dryness, and poor concentration and memory. Longer-term symptoms include an increased risk for osteoporosis and cardiovascular disease.

Is massage indicated or contraindicated?
Bodywork is highly appropriate for a woman who is going through the transition of losing ovarian function. While for some women this is a liberating, exciting time, for others it involves radical and not always welcome changes in self-definition and self-perception. Massage gives powerful positive feedback about physical experience and can help to ameliorate some of the psychological and physical disruptions that menopause can trigger.

What are all these *men* doing in women's health issues? The root word is *mēn*, which is Greek for "month."

Menarche is "*mēn*" plus "*arche*," or "beginning."

Menstruation is "*mēn*" plus "*atus*," meaning "to be menstruant."

Menses is the plural for "*mēn*", meaning many months.

Menopause is "*mēn*" plus "*pausis*," or "cessation."

drugs (this is called "induced menopause") these processes stop. A woman no longer ovulates, she no longer grows an endothelial lining in her uterus, and she no longer sheds that lining during menstruation—she is infertile. However, these ovarian hormones also work on many other tissues in the body, in ways that are only just beginning to be explored.

- *Bone density.* The role of estrogens and progesterones in maintaining bone density is complex. It seems clear that estrogen inhibits osteoclast activity, that is, it helps to prevent the thinning of bone tissue. Some forms of progesterone are involved in maintaining bone density as well; this class of chemicals appears to stimulate osteoblast activity. In other words, estrogen prevents bone from being dissolved, while progesterone helps it to build up (see more in *osteoporosis*, Chapter 2).

- *Cardiovascular health.* When women go through menopause one of the many changes that occurs is in the types of cholesterol that are present in the blood. It has been dependably observed that postmenopausal women have higher levels of low-density lipoproteins and triglycerides (the "bad" types of cholesterol) than premenopausal women. It has been assumed that since estrogens influence the metabolism of fats, lowering estrogen levels could be reflected in these pathologic changes, but the precise chain of events has not been thoroughly explored. The high incidence of cardiovascular disease among postmenopausal women, and the fact that women who supplement estrogen during and after menopause have a lower chance of dying of heart disease than others, point to a central role for some type of estrogen in this process (see more in *atherosclerosis*, Chapter 4).

- *Protection from some types of cancer.* This is an extremely complex issue that reflects just how little is understood about the effects of different types of estrogens and progesterones on different types of tissues. High levels of some types of estrogen have a statistical link with lower rates of colon cancer but higher rates of some other types of cancer, including breast and ovarian cancers. Ultimately it may be found that whether hormone levels are dangerous or protective depends on the chemical variation of the hormone, where it comes from, how it is metabolized, where it is used, and other variables that have not even been considered yet.

- *Central nervous system functions.* Estrogen seems linked in ways that are not clearly understood to mood, depression, and basic cognitive function. Supplementing low doses of estrogen has been seen to be effective for dealing with the mild depression, insomnia, and short-term memory loss that may accompany menopause, but it is not effective for more severe depressive disorders (see *depression*, Chapter 3).

When the ovaries have decreased the levels of hormones they produce, a woman becomes dependent on other tissues to secrete enough estrogens and progesterones to provide for her daily function. Some fat cells and other tissues continue to produce these hormones after the ovaries atrophy, but at a fraction of previous levels. In addition, although a postmenopausal woman may have to get by on 30 to 40% of her previous estrogen levels, her progesterone may fall to as low as $1/20$ of her premenopausal levels. This has implications for general health, because estrogens and progesterones are designed to balance each other in their effects on a variety of tissues. Add the fact that environmental estrogens can enter the body through hormone-supplemented meats and exposure to many common toxins (see sidebar that accompanies the introduction to this chapter), and it is easy to see how precarious is the balance of hormones in a postmenopausal woman.

Historically, much of the common wisdom about the effects of hormones on the body is based on conclusions drawn from observing what happens when those hormones are in short supply. This is a fairly clumsy way to try to understand such a complex subject. As our ability to trace the subtle interplay of hormone subtypes, metabolic pathways, and target tissues improves, our general concepts about menopause as a potential threat to health may also change.

Signs and Symptoms

Menopause itself is simply the event in which ovaries permanently cease to secrete hormones or to produce eggs. Menopause is not identified until a full year after a woman has stopped having menstrual cycles. It can take several years for ovaries to slow down, during which time their function becomes irregular but does not entirely cease. This time leading up to menopause is referred to as perimenopause, and the symptoms women experience during this time have to do with sudden changes in hormone secretion. Symptoms generally subside when hormone levels stabilize.

The signs and symptoms of perimenopause vary with each individual, but some of the most common ones are hot flashes, night sweats, insomnia, mood swings, decreased sex drive, vaginal dryness or itchiness, confusion, short-term memory loss, and poor concentration. Some of these symptoms may be interrelated, for instance, insomnia may have to do with night sweats and hot flashes; depression and decreased sex drive may have to do with a change in self-perception as a woman enters a time in her life when she is no longer fertile. For some women the symptoms of perimenopause are directly linked to hormonal disruption, and taking steps to smooth out the hormonal shifts can alleviate a great deal of discomfort.

The long-term consequences of menopause include pathologic thinning of bones and decreased resistance to heart disease. These phenomena are discussed in the etiology section.

Treatment

Treatment options for the symptoms of perimenopause and the long-term consequences of reduced estrogen/progesterone secretion are many and varied. Estrogen replacement therapy (ERT) provides supplements of various types of estrogens. This seems to be adequate for some women, but it does not address the lost balance between estrogens and progesterones that are implicated in many health issues. Hormone replacement therapy (HRT) supplements both estrogen and progesterone in varying levels and in varying forms. It is a good option, especially for women with a high risk of cardiovascular disease, but HRT is also associated with increased risk of stroke and some types of cancer. Many studies have been conducted and are ongoing to try to decipher how to get the best out of hormone supplementation while reducing possible risks.

It is also possible to supplement hormones in the form of a topical cream, which allows access to the bloodstream without processing in the liver. Many women successfully treat their perimenopausal symptoms with these applications, although they must also be used with care, as the potency from one brand to another may vary.

Massage?

Bodywork is a perfectly wonderful idea for a woman who is experiencing symptoms of perimenopause. This condition is not a disease; it is a natural process. Although many women feel that entering this phase of life is a liberating, exciting time, others may feel that their role in life must change so fundamentally that they lose touch with their own self-definition. Massage, because it involves supportive, nurturing, informed touch, can reinforce the positive aspects of a woman's physical experience and help her through what can be a difficult time.

PELVIC INFLAMMATORY DISEASE IN BRIEF

What is it?
Pelvic inflammatory disease (PID) is an infection of female reproductive organs. It starts at the cervix and can move up to infect the uterus, fallopian (uterine) tubes, ovaries, and entire pelvic cavity.

How is it recognized?
The symptoms of acute PID include abdominal pain, fever, chills, headache, nausea, and vomiting. Chronic PID may produce no symptoms or may involve chronic pain, lassitude, and pain during urination and intercourse.

Is massage indicated or contraindicated?
Acute PID systemically contraindicates massage until all signs of infection have subsided. Chronic PID may be appropriate for massage if the woman is aware of her condition and is treating it appropriately. Deep work in the lower abdomen and/or pelvis is not appropriate for women with PID.

Pelvic Inflammatory Disease

Definition: What Is It?

PID refers to infections anywhere in the upper reproductive tract of women. Infection of the uterus (*endometritis*), infection of the uterine tubes (*salpingitis*), or abscesses on the ovaries can all fall under the umbrella term of PID.

Demographics: Who Gets It?

PID is usually a disorder of young women. It is most common among women between 16 and 25 years old who have had multiple sexual partners; it is rare in women older than 35. More than 1 million cases of PID are reported in the United States every year; it accounts for 250,000 hospitalizations, and between $4 and $7 billion in medical costs in the United States every year. Excluding HIV, PID is considered the most frequent and most serious sexually transmitted infection affecting women today.

Etiology: What Happens?

PID is usually the result of a bacterial infection that begins in the vagina. The infectious agents are almost always chlamydia or gonorrhea, but irritation from an intrauterine device (IUD) or incomplete elective or spontaneous abortions can also be precipitators for PID. Although it usually begins in the vagina, the infection may spread to the uterus, the fallopian tubes, the ovaries, and into the pelvic cavity.

Other agents that have been found in PID infections include mycoplasma, some anaerobic bacteria, and some forms of bacteria that occur naturally in the lower reproductive tract. It is not clear how or why these bacteria change their character to cause these serious infections.

Signs and Symptoms

PID may be an acute or chronic infection. Acute PID, as its name implies, is a serious and severe condition. Its symptoms include abdominal pain, low back pain, fever, chills, nausea, vomiting, painful intercourse, heavy irregular periods, and heavy, pus-laden vaginal discharge. Chronic PID has low-grade, long-term symptoms that seldom flare up into an acute situation but can ultimately cause the same kind of internal damage as acute PID. Its symptoms include mild abdominal pain, backache, heavy menstrual periods, painful intercourse, and general lethargy.

Complications

If an infection backs up from the vagina to the uterus to the fallopian tubes, it can start growing in the open pelvic cavity. This is *peritonitis* (see Chapter 7), and it can be a life-threatening situation.

More common complications of PID include infertility, ectopic pregnancy, and chronic pelvic pain. Infertility arises from the accumulation of scar tissue that may block fallopian tubes (women with a history of three PID infections have a 40% chance of becoming infertile). Women with a history of PID have ectopic pregnancies approximately

6 times more frequently than women who have not; these pregnancies can result in severe internal bleeding and always involve the loss of the fetus (see more in *pregnancy*, this chapter). About 18% of all women diagnosed with PID go on to experience chronic pelvic pain that may outlast their infection by many years.

Diagnosis

Diagnosis of this disorder is based on several different signs: abdominal tenderness and pain at the uterine cervix, ovaries, and fallopian tubes. These are palpated during a standard pelvic examination. In addition to these symptoms a high white blood cell count will be present, pelvic abscesses may develop, and an analysis of vaginal or cervical secretions will show signs of infection. A laparoscopy may be performed to look for abscesses and internal adhesions that may interfere with reproductive function.

Treatment

Most of the time PID is a fairly simple bacterial infection. Caught early, it responds well to antibiotics and bed rest, although some 20 to 40% of women require hospitalization and intravenous antibiotics. Sexual activity needs to be curtailed for several weeks, and the woman's sexual partner(s) should also be treated for gonorrhea or chlamydia, if those are involved in the infection.

Massage?

PID is a potentially dangerous infection that can complicate into peritonitis. Acute cases systemically contraindicate massage until the client has completed a course of antibiotics and has been cleared by her doctor. Chronic PID patients also need to be under a doctor's care and treating their infection appropriately before receiving massage.

Pregnancy
Definition: What Is It?

Pregnancy, obviously, is the condition a woman is in when she is carrying a fetus. Most of the general information about pregnancy will be skipped in this discussion, but it is worthwhile to look at some of the aspects of this condition in the context of massage.

Signs and Symptoms

Pregnancy creates a wide array of symptoms, and some of them have specific implications for massage. The following are some of the symptomatic complaints of pregnant women that bodyworkers can influence:

- *Loose ligaments.* One of the hormones secreted during pregnancy is *relaxin*. Its job is to loosen the ligaments so that the pelvis will be elastic enough to allow the baby to emerge. Relaxin starts working very early in pregnancy, making all the ligaments in the body looser and more mobile. This can cause numerous problems from unstable vertebrae to asymmetrical sacroiliac joints. Muscles then tighten up to stabilize the joints, causing *spasm* (Chapter 2) and pain.

PREGNANCY IN BRIEF

What is it?
Pregnancy is the state of carrying a fetus.

How is it recognized?
The symptoms of advanced pregnancy are obvious, but symptoms that specifically pertain to massage include loose ligaments, muscle spasms, clumsiness, and fatigue.

Is massage indicated or contraindicated?
All stages of uncomplicated pregnancy indicate massage, with specific cautions relating to each trimester.

- *Fatigue.* Pregnant women carry around a lot of extra weight. The baby itself is only a tiny part of the whole load, which includes the placenta, amniotic fluid, 40% more blood, and any extra body fat cells she may accumulate during her pregnancy. In addition to carrying extra weight, a pregnant woman secretes hormones that require her to get a great deal of rest. This is a command that many pregnant women do not have the luxury of obeying, at least while they are trying to hold down a job and grow a baby at the same time.

- *Shifting proprioception.* Pregnant women change their size every day. This is especially true in the last trimester, when the baby grows at an astounding rate. The result is that a pregnant woman never knows exactly how much room she takes up. Her sense of where in space her body ends and the rest of the world begins is very shaky. This tends to make a pregnant woman clumsy and prone to injury. Massage provides an extraordinary sense of where bodies are in space. It can improve proprioceptive senses by giving continuous and positive feedback about boundaries.

Complications

In the vast range of things that could possibly go wrong in a pregnancy, three conditions are especially important for massage therapists to consider: *gestational diabetes, pregnancy-induced hypertension*, and *ectopic pregnancy*.

- *Gestational diabetes.* Pregnancy-related diabetes develops in about 3% of all pregnancies. It is diagnosed through a glucose tolerance test, in which the woman drinks a sweet beverage after fasting, and then her plasma is examined for elevated levels of glucose. Gestational diabetes is usually identified in the fifth or sixth month of pregnancy (between 24 and 26 weeks of gestation).

  If diabetes develops because of pregnancy, risks to the baby and mother are serious. The incidence of birth defects (especially spina bifida and Down syndrome) and stillbirths with diabetic mothers is 3 times greater than with non-diabetic mothers. The rerouting of nutrients in the blood can cause babies to grow abnormally large, requiring a cesarean section. A woman who develops prenatal diabetes *must* be under a doctor's care and get clearance before receiving circulatory massage; her blood pressure may be higher than is otherwise healthy.

- *Pregnancy-induced hypertension (PIH).* This is a condition that generally starts mildly but can quickly become life-threatening both for the baby and the mother. It occurs in three categories: hypertension alone, *preeclampsia* (which is hypertension along with elevated proteins in the urine and possible systemic edema), and *eclampsia* (which is the same situation as preeclampsia but it also involves convulsions).

  The exact causes of PIH are unknown. Some postulate that it may be an autoimmune problem, or even an allergic reaction to the baby. Others suggest that in processing waste products for two people the mother's system is simply overloaded. In any case, increased blood pressure drastically reduces the efficiency of the placenta to deliver nutrients to the baby. PIH tends to affect women in their first pregnancy, especially those with a personal or family history of hypertension. Treatment includes medication to bring down the blood pressure, strict bedrest, and when appropriate, cesarean section.

  Complications of PIH for mothers include renal failure, cerebral hemorrhage, liver damage, and blindness. Risks to the baby include reduced growth from circulatory impairment and *placenta abruptio*, a condition in which the placenta prematurely separates from the uterus.

- *Ectopic pregnancy.* An ectopic pregnancy is any fertilized egg that implants outside the uterus. Most ectopic pregnancies develop in the fallopian tubes; others may implant in the peritoneum, on the ovaries, or on the cervix. Risk factors include IUD use and a history of *pelvic inflammatory disease, endometriosis* (both in this chapter), and adhesions from previous abdominal surgeries. Ectopic pregnancies cannot come to term; the fallopian tube eventually ruptures, killing the fetus and endangering the life of the mother. Ectopic pregnancies that are recognized early (usually by ultrasound) may be terminated by laparoscopic surgery, preserving fertility for the chance of another successful pregnancy.

Massage?

For pregnancies that are *not* complicated by diabetes, hypertension, or other disorders, massage is a wonderful gift for someone whose body does not quite belong to herself for a while.

Special training is available to learn pregnancy and prenatal massage, but for more general purposes, the following are some guidelines and cautions to preserve the pregnant client's comfort and safety:

- *First trimester:* From the moment a woman knows she is pregnant to several days after she has delivered the baby, her condition contraindicates deep abdominal work. The first and last trimesters are the times when the fetal attachment is most fragile, and massage therapists must respect that fragility. Practitioners of Eastern techniques would add that other cautions for massage in the first trimester include deep specific point work on the heels and Achilles tendons (reflexology abortion points) and on the *hoku* point in the web of the thumb.

- *Second trimester:* This is the safest, easiest part of the pregnancy. Very often a woman's energy levels will be up while her nausea levels will be down. She probably has not yet gained enough weight to be very uncomfortable, *but* connective tissue changes begin to show during this time. Ligaments begin to loosen, and muscles may go into spasm in response. Massage at this stage centers on making sure the client is comfortable. Somewhere in this trimester, often around week 22, the client will no longer want to be face down. The therapist is then limited to doing work from the side or supine, unless bolsters or support cushions are used.

- *Third trimester:* A midwife once said, "God invented the third trimester of pregnancy to make labor look like a pretty good deal." Massage therapists are more limited in what they do in this trimester than any other, but their work is more important than ever. Prone work is out of the question at this point, and supine work probably needs to be limited or modified, according to the mother's comfort. Being fully reclined allows the fetus to rest directly on the big abdominal blood vessels, which may either limit blood flow to the legs, leading to cramping in the gastrocnemius, or limit blood flow up the vena cava, leading to dizziness and unconsciousness (Fig. 10-7). It may be best to do a lot of side work unless the client can be in a semi-reclined position.

    Another caution for this stage is limited blood return from the legs, leading to edema. Watch for varicose veins as well, which, combined with long-standing edema and the increased number of red blood cells that is a normal part of being pregnant, can be ideal environments for clot formation. Some people suggest that to be completely safe, the medial calf and thigh (in other words, the area around the great saphenous vein) should be a local contraindication for massage during the third trimester regardless of whether edema or varices are present.

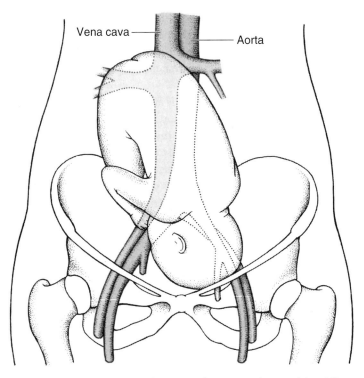

Figure 10-7. Pregnancy; a late-term fetus can obstruct blood flow

If *pitting* edema coupled with fever, dizziness, headache, and nausea are present, the client may have pre-eclampsia and needs immediate medical referral. This situation contraindicates massage until she has medical clearance.

PREMENSTRUAL SYNDROME IN BRIEF

What is it?
Premenstrual syndrome (PMS) is a collection of many signs and symptoms that occur in the time between ovulation and menstruation, and then subside after menstruation begins. It may have several different causes and triggers.

How is it recognized?
Signs and symptoms of PMS are often divided into physical and emotional features. Physical symptoms include breast tenderness, bloating, digestive upset, fatigue, changes in appetite, backache, and many others. Emotional signs include irritability, anxiety, depression, mood swings, and other possible problems.

Is massage indicated or contraindicated?
Although the specific causes of PMS are not clearly understood, it is clear that this condition is not related to infection, structural problems, or neoplasm. Therefore, PMS indicates bodywork, which may help to reestablish balance in the endocrine and nervous systems.

Premenstrual Syndrome
Definition: What Is It?

PMS is a collection of signs and symptoms that combine to interfere with a woman's ability to function normally during the luteal phase of the menstrual cycle (i.e., the time between ovulation and menstruation).

Demographics: Who Gets It?

Up to 85% of all women between the onset of menarche and menopause report some symptoms of PMS. About 20 to 40% of those women feel their symptoms create a problem, but only 5 to 10% of them are significantly affected by PMS.

Whereas symptoms of PMS have been seen to be more severe among women who have high-fat diets, no other particular risk factors or target populations have been identified.

Etiology: What Happens?

PMS is one of the most common and least well-understood conditions that women experience. It has been described since ancient times. It was recognized as a specific pattern in 1931 and finally named in 1953. Nonetheless, the etiology of this condition remains mysterious. Several different factors seem to contribute to this problem, and each woman's experience is unique. This makes it difficult to predict or treat, as no single approach is universally successful.

Some of the theories for the causes or triggers of PMS include the following:

- *Hormonal imbalance.* During the luteal phase of the menstrual cycle, the body prepares to shed the endometrial lining that has accumulated for the implantation of a fertilized egg. Estrogen and progesterone levels rise as the lining thickens, and then just before menstruation begins, these hormones suddenly and rapidly drop in production. One theory behind PMS is that this precipitous drop in hormones is difficult to accommodate, and that exposure to environmental estrogens (in animal fats and toxic exposures) may cause the endometrial lining to become overactive, thus requiring an even more extreme fluctuation in hormonal levels. In addition to problems with estrogen and progesterone levels, some women with PMS report problems with adrenal function as well.

- *Nutritional deficiencies.* Some women with PMS are deficient in specific areas, notably calcium, vitamin B_6, and some essential fatty acids.

- *Neurotransmitter imbalance.* Plunging estrogen and progesterone has been seen to suppress the secretion of serotonin, a neurotransmitter that is strongly related to mood swings and depression. Opioid peptides are other brain chemicals that appear to be adversely affected by hormone disruption. These chemicals also help to determine mood.

- *Other factors.* Some factors that may contribute to PMS are more vague but are definitely a part of the picture for many women. Genetic predisposition may be a factor, but no genetic mutation has been isolated for PMS. It is unclear whether the condition is passed on through heredity, or the likelihood to seek help for the condition is passed on through environmental influence. Cultural expectations, general stress, and a number of unrelated disorders may also contribute to signs and symptoms of PMS.

Signs and Symptoms

More than 150 different signs and symptoms have been documented among PMS patients. These have been categorized into physical and emotional indicators of this disorder.

- *Physical symptoms.* The most common physical symptoms associated with PMS include bloating, breast tenderness, acne, salt and sugar cravings (along with binge eating), headaches, backaches, insomnia, and digestive upset (diarrhea and/or constipation). Less common physical symptoms can include sinus problems, heart palpitations, dizziness, asthma, and seizures.

- *Emotional symptoms.* These include confusion, depression, anxiety, panic attacks, mood swings, and general irritability.

Diagnosis

It seems clear that PMS has several different causes and creates a different experience for every woman who has it. The one constant in this condition is that symptoms appear after ovulation and subside when menstruation begins. The most important diagnostic test for PMS is a diary in which a woman records her experiences and finds that this pattern is consistent with her menstrual cycle.

Several other conditions create overlapping symptoms with PMS, including *diabetes* or *hypothyroidism* (Chapter 8), *eating disorders* or *depression* (Chapter 3), *chronic fatigue syndrome*

(Chapter 5), *irritable bowel syndrome* (Chapter 7), or any combination of these disorders. Only PMS shows a cessation of symptoms during and after menstruation, however.

Treatment

Since PMS is not understood as a distinct disease process, it is treated symptomatically. Women who consult allopathic physicians for this disorder may be prescribed low-dose birth control pills to control estrogen and progesterone levels, diuretics to control water retention, or antidepressants to address serotonin levels. Most women are also strongly recommended to make sure that they get the best quality sleep they can muster during their difficult time and to exercise regularly.

Health professionals who focus on nutritional aspects of this disorder often recommend that patients follow a low-fat vegetarian diet to avoid excessive estrogen exposure and that they avoid salt, sugar, caffeine (specifically in soda, coffee, tea, and chocolate), and alcohol. Many herbal remedies have been reputed to help PMS; few of them have been accepted by the medical mainstream. Some of the more common herbal recommendations include borage or evening primrose (for essential fatty acids), black cohash, and dong quai.

Ultimately, PMS is a condition that can usually be managed successfully so that a woman does not have to lose function for 10 days every month, but it seldom spontaneously disappears until the onset of menopause.

Massage?

PMS is a condition in which symptoms are not related to circulatory dysfunction, neoplasm, structural problems, infection, or any other situation that might make bodywork impractical. PMS definitely indicates massage and other kinds of bodywork, which have been shown to reduce depression and anxiety and to help ameliorate some of the fluid retention that makes PMS so physically uncomfortable.[c]

Chapter Review Questions: Reproductive System Conditions

1. Why is the incidence of advanced cervical cancer a fraction of what it was in the first half of the 20th century?

2. Is the risk factor profile a very useful guideline for breast cancer? Why or why not?

3. What are prostaglandins, and how are they involved in dysmenorrhea?

4. Describe how stress can exacerbate menstrual pain.

5. Under what circumstances can fibroid tumors cause symptoms?

6. How can endometriosis or pelvic inflammatory disease lead to sterility?

7. An elderly client has been diagnosed with prostate cancer. He has opted not to treat it. Is he a good candidate for bodywork? What modalities are most appropriate, and why?

8. Discuss the relationship between certain hormonal changes that occur in pregnancy and muscle spasm.

9. Why may it be uncomfortable to work with a late-term pregnant woman in a fully supine position?

10. A client has been diagnosed with endometriosis but has no particular symptoms at the time of her appointment. To help with her low back pain her massage therapist works deeply on the psoas. Within a few hours the client has sharp shooting pains low in her abdomen and cannot stand up straight. What may have happened?

[c]Field T. *Touch Therapy.* London: Churchill, Livingstone; 2000:78.

Bibliography, Reproductive System Conditions

General References, Reproductive System

1. de Dominico G, Wood E. *Beard's Massage.* Philadelphia, PA: WB Saunders; 1997
2. Damjanou I. *Pathology for the Health-Related Professions.* Philadelphia, PA: WB Saunders; 1996.
3. Travell J, Simons DG. *Myofascial Pain and Dysfunction: The Trigger Point Manual.* Baltimore, MD: Williams & Wilkins; 1983.
4. Clemente CD. *Anatomy: A Regional Atlas of the Human Body.* 3rd ed. Baltimore, MD: Urban & Schwarzenburg; 1987.
5. Tortora GJ, Anagnostakos NP. *Principles of Anatomy and Physiology.* 6th ed. New York, NY: Harper & Row; 1990.
6. *Taber's Cyclopedic Dictionary.* 14th ed. Philadelphia, PA: FA Davis; 1981.
7. *Stedman's Medical Dictionary.* 26th ed. Baltimore, MD: Williams & Wilkins; 1995.
8. Memmler RL, Wood DL. *The Human Body in Health and Disease.* 5th ed. Philadelphia, PA: JB Lippincott; 1983.
9. Juhan D. *Job's Body: A Handbook for Bodywork.* Barrytown, NY: Station Hill Press; 1987.
10. Mulvihill ML. *Human Diseases: A Systemic Approach.* 2nd ed. Norwalk, CT: Appleton & Lange; 1987.
11. Kunz JRM, Finkel AJ, eds. *The American Medical Association Family Medical Guide.* New York, NY: Random House; 1987.
12. Marieb EM. *Human Anatomy and Physiology.* Redwood City, CA: Benjamin/Cummings; 1989.
13. Field T. *Touch Therapy.* London: Churchill, Livingstone; 2000.
14. Sapolsky RM. *Why Zebras Don't Get Ulcers: An Updated Guide to Stress, Stress-Related Disease, and Coping.* New York, NY: W.H. Freeman; 1998, NYC.
15. Hall DC. Nutritional influences on estrogen metabolism. *Appl Nutr Sci Rep,* 2001.

Abortion, Spontaneous and Elective

1. Miscarriage. Women's Health, UK. Available at: http://www.womens-health.co.uk/miscarr.htm. Accessed summer 2001.
2. Trafford A. Second opinion: The "morning after pill" comes home. *The Washington Post.* May 15, 2001:HE04. Available at: http://www.washingtonpost.com/wp-dyn/health/columns/secondopinion/A26692-2001May14.html. Accessed summer 2001.
3. Repeated miscarriage. WebMD Corporation; 1996–2001. Available at: http://my.webmd.com/content/dmk/dmk_article_5461667. Accessed summer 2001.

Cervical Cancer

1. Cervical cancer—Overview. American Cancer Society; 2000. Available at: http://www3.cancer.org/cancerinfo/load_cont.asp?ct=8&doc525&Language=English. Accessed summer 2001.
2. Cervical cancer (PDQ) treatment–Patients. National Cancer Institute. Available at: http://www.nci.nih.gov/cancer_information/doc_pdq.aspx?version=patient&viewid=862ac265-8ff9-4bc5-8b68-1458c603458d. Accessed summer 2002.
3. Human papillomavirus (HPV). American Cancer Society; 2000. Available at: http://www3.cancer.org/cancerinfo/load_cont.asp?ct=8&doc=84&Language=English. Accessed summer 2001.
4. NCI fact sheet: Human papillomaviruses and cancer—Updated 06/1998. National Cancer Institute. Available at: http://oncolink.upenn.edu/pdq_html/6/engl/600320.html. Accessed summer 2001.
5. NCI/PDQ physician statement: Cervical cancer—Updated 11/2000. National Cancer Institute. Available at: http://oncolink.upenn.edu/pdq_html/1/engl/100103-1.html#General_information. Accessed summer 2001.
6. Scientists testing cancer vaccine. The Associated Press; 2001. Available at: http://www.intelihealth.com/IH/ihtIH/WSIHW000/333/24524/312065.html?d=dmtICNNews&k=ThisjustinFR408. Accessed summer 2001.
7. Uterine cervix. American Cancer Society; 2000. Available at: http://www.cancer.org/statistics/cff2000/selectedcancers.html#colon. Accessed summer 2001.

Dysmenorrhea

1. Menstrual cramps (dysmenorrhea). The Board of Trustees of the University of Illinois, 1999. Available at: http://www.mckinley.uiuc.edu/health-info/womenhlt/mencramp.html. Accessed summer 2001.
2. Barnard ND. Nutritional factors in menstrual pain and premenstrual syndrome. Physician's Committee for Responsible Medicine. Available at: http://wwwpcrm.org/research/menstrual.html. Accessed summer 2001.

Endometriosis

1. Causes of endometriosis. Inlet Medical Inc.; 2000. Available at: http://www.dyspareunia.org/html/endometriosis_causes.htm. Accessed summer 2001.
2. Corwin EJ. Endometriosis: Pathophysiology, diagnosis, and treatment. *Nurse Pract.* 1997. Available at: http://www.springnet.com/ce/j710a.htm. Accessed summer 2001.
3. Endometriosis. Available at: http://www.ahcpr.gov/consumer/uterine1.htm#sec5. Accessed summer 2001.
4. Endometriosis–Treatment. Inlet Medical Inc.; 2000. Available at: http://www.dyspareunia.org/html/endometriosis_treatments.htm. Accessed summer 2001.
5. What is endometriosis? IVF.com; 2000. Available at: http://www.ivf.com/endoass.html. Accessed summer 2001.
6. What is endometriosis? Inlet Medical Inc.; 2000. Available at: http://www.dyspareunia.org/html/endometriosis.htm. Accessed summer 2001.
7. What is endometriosis? Endometriosis Association; 2001. Available at: http://www.endo-online.org/endo.html. Accessed summer 2001.

Fibroid Tumors

1. Fibroids. Available at: http://www.ahcpr.gov/consumer/uterine1.htm#sec4. Accessed summer 2001.
2. Phalen KF. Treatment of choice. *Special to the Washington Post.* October 24, 2000:Z23. Available at: http://www.washingtonpost.com/wp-dyn/articles/A62965-2000Oct23.html. Accessed summer 2001.

Breast Cancer

1. Fast facts. American Cancer Society; 2000. Available at: http://www.cancer.org/NBCAM_fastfacts.html. Accessed summer 2001.
2. Benign breast conditions. American Cancer Society; 2000. Available at: http://www3.cancer.org/cancerinfo/load_cont.asp?ct=5&doc=16&Language=English. Accessed summer 2001.
3. Wolberg WH. Benign breast disease and breast cancer tutorial. Available at: http://www.surgery.wisc.edu/wolberg/breast.html. Accessed summer 2001.
4. Liu L. Breast cancer overview. The Trustees of the University of Pennsylvania; 1994–2001. Available at: http://cancer.med.upenn.edu/disease/breast/general/breast_intro.html. Accessed summer 2001.
5. New technique quickly distinguishes breast cancer types, offering better treatment. Associated Press; 2001. Available at: http://www.intelihealth.com/IH/ihtIH/WSIHW000/333/8012/312134.html. Accessed summer 2001.
6. Liu L. Histologic classification of breast cancer. The Trustees of the University of Pennsylvania; 1994–2001.Available at: http://cancer.med.upenn.edu/disease/breast/screen/breast_type.html. Accessed summer 2001.
7. Kotz D. A "Pap smear" for breast cancer? *The Washington Post.* September 5, 2000:Z06. Accessed summer 2001.
8. About male breast cancer. Available at: http://interact.withus.com/interact/mbc/about.htm. Accessed summer 2001.
9. NCI fact sheet: Lifetime probability of breast cancer in American women—Updated 03/2000. National Cancer Institute. Available at: http://oncolink.upenn.edu/pdq_html/6/engl/600056.html. Accessed summer 2001.
10. NCI fact sheet: Breast cancer prevention studies—Updated 08/1999. National Cancer Institute. Available at: http://oncolink.

upenn.edu/ pdq_html/6/engl/600418.html. Accessed summer 2001.

11. NCI/PDQ patient statement: Breast cancer—Updated 02/2001. National Cancer Institute. Available at: http://cancer.med. upenn.edu/ pdq_html/2/engl/200013.html. Accessed summer 2001.

Ovarian Cancer

1. Green A. Borderline ovarian cancer. eMedicine.com, Inc.; 2001. Available at: http://www. emedicine.com/med/ topic3233.htm. Accessed summer 2001.
2. Okie S. Estrogen, ovarian cancer linked. *The Washington Post.* March 21, 2001:A01. Available at: http://www. washingtonpost.com/wp-dyn/health/ women/news/A33884-2001Mar20.html. Accessed summer 2001.
3. Okie S. Estrogen, ovarian cancer link expanded. *The Washington Post.* March 26, 2001:A06. Available at: http://www. washingtonpost.com/wp-dyn/health/ women/ news/A56737-2001Mar25.html. Accessed summer 2001.
4. NCI fact sheets questions and answers about ovarian cancer—Updated 10/1999. National Cancer Institute. Available at: http://oncolink. upenn.edu/pdq_html/ 6/engl/600633.html. Accessed summer 2001.
5. Ovarian cancer—Overview. American Cancer Society; 2000. Available at: http://www3.cancer.org/cancerinfo/load_ cont.asp?ct=33&doc=37&Language= English. Accessed summer 2001.
6. Cancer statistics. American Cancer Society; 2000. Available at: http://www.cancer.org/ statistics/cff2000/selectedcancers. html#colon. Accessed summer 2001.
7. What is ovarian cancer? National Ovarian Cancer Coalition. Available at: http://www. ovarian.org/ Accessed summer 2001.
8. What is ovarian cancer? Gilda Radner Familial Ovarian Cancer Registry. Available at: http://www.ovariancancer.com/grwp. html. Accessed summer 2001.
9. What is ovarian cancer? Ovarian Cancer National Alliance. Available at: http://www. ovariancancer.org/index.html. Accessed summer 2002.

Ovarian Cysts

1. Helm CW. Ovarian cysts. eMedicine.com, Inc.; 2001. Available at: http://www. emedicine.com/ med/topic1699.htm. Accessed summer 2001.
2. Rich W. What is an ovarian cyst? Available at: http://www.personal.u-net.com/~njh/ cyst.html. Accessed summer 2001.

Benign Prostatic Hypertrophy

1. Benign prostate disease. National Kidney Foundation; 2001. Available at: http://www. kidney.org/general/news/benprostate.cfm. Accessed summer 2001.
2. Prostate BPH. urologychannel.com; 1998–2001. Available at: http://www.

urologychannel.com/prostate/bph/index.sht ml. Accessed summer 2001.
3. Benign prostatic hyperplasia. Mayo Foundation for Medical Education and Research; 2000. Available at: http://www. mayohealth.org/ mayo/9811/htm/bph.htm. Accessed summer 2001.
4. Prostate enlargement: Benign prostatic hyperplasia. The National Kidney and Urologic Diseases Information Clearinghouse, National Institute of Diabetes and Digestive and Kidney Diseases. NIH publication no. 98-301. Available at: http://www. niddk.nih.gov/health/urolog/pubs/prostate/ index.htm. Accessed summer 2001.
5. What is prostate gland enlargement? Mayo Foundation for Medical Education and Research; 1998–2000. Available at: http://www.mayohealth.org/home?id= DS00027. Accessed summer 2001.
6. Henderson SO. Prostatitis. eMedicine.com, Inc.; 2001. Available at: http://www. emedicine.com/EMERG/topic488.htm. Accessed fall 2001.
7. Causes of prostatitis. The Prostatitis Foundation; 2000. Available at: http://www.pro-statitis. org/causes.html. Accessed fall 2001.
8. Prostatitis. National Kidney and Urologic Diseases Information Clearinghouse. NIH publication no. 00-4553. Available at: http://www. niddk.nih.gov/health/ urolog/summary/prostat/prostat.htm. Accessed fall 2001.

Prostate Cancer

1. What is it? American Cancer Society; 2000. Available at: http://www3.cancer.org/ cancerinfo/load_cont.asp?ct=36&st=wi. Accessed summer 2001.
2. NCI fact sheet: Prostate cancer among different races and ethnic groups—Updated 03/1996. National Cancer Institute. Available at: http://oncolink.upenn.edu/ pdq_html/6/engl/600624.html. Accessed summer 2001.
3. Andriote J-M. No-wait prostate test results. *The Washington Post.* February 6, 2001:HE06. Available at: http://www. washingtonpost.com/ ac2/wp-dyn/ A20578-2001Feb2?language= printer. Accessed summer 2001.
4. Prostate cancer—Earlier detection, better outcomes. Mayo Foundation for Medical Education and Research; 1998–2000. Available at: http://www.mayohealth.org/ home?id=HQ01271. Accessed summer 2001.
5. Cancer statistics. American Cancer Society; 2000. Available at: http://www.cancer.org/ statistics/cff2000/selectedcancers. html#colon. Accessed summer 2001.
6. Prostate cancer–Overview. American Cancer Society; 2000. Available at: http://www3.cancer.org/cancerinfo/ load_cont.asp?ct=36&doc=38&Language= English. Accessed summer 2001.
7. Prostate cancer. urologychannel.com; 1998–2001. Available at: http://www. urologychannel.com/prostate/cancer/. Accessed summer 2001.

8. NCI fact sheet: Questions and answers about early prostate cancer—Updated 06/1999. National Cancer Institute. Available at: http://oncolink.upenn.edu/ pdq_html/6/engl/600523.html. Accessed summer 2001.
9. Brosman SA. Prostatic intraepithelial neoplasia (PIN). eMedicine.com, Inc; 2001. Available at: http://www.emedicine.com/ med/topic3056.htm. Accessed summer 2001.
10. The burden of prostate cancer. Centers for Disease Control and Prevention. Available at: http://www.cdc.gov/cancer/prostate/ prostate.htm. Accessed summer 2001.
11. What is prostate cancer? Mayo Foundation for Medical Education and Research; 2001. Available at: http://www.mayohealth. org/home?id=DS00043. Accessed summer 2001.

Menopause

1. About estrogen and estrogen dominance. Progesterone Advocates Network; 1999–2000. Available at: http://www. progestnet.com/documents/estrogen.html. Accessed summer 2001.
2. Basic facts about menopause. The North American Menopause Society; 2001. Available at: http://www.menopause.org/ aboutm/facts. html. Accessed summer 2001.
3. Endocrinology and menopause. The Endocrine Society; 2001. Available at: http://216.205.53.178/endo/pubrelations/ patientinfo/menopause.htm. Accessed summer 2001.
4. Estrogen dominance–Parts 1-6. InSpired Health Solutions; 1999–2001. Available at: http://www.thyrodine.com/estrogen/index. htm. Accessed summer 2001.
5. Kolb L. Estrogen dominance. 2000. Available at: http://altnature.com/library/ estrogen.htm. Accessed summer 2001.
6. Menopause. American Heart Association; 2000. Available at:: http://www.american-heart.org/ Heart_and_Stroke_A_Z_ Guide/menop.html. Accessed summer 2001.
7. NCI fact sheet: Menopausal hormone replacements therapy—Updated 04/2000. National Cancer Institute. Available at: http://oncolink. upenn.edu/pdq_html/ 6/engl/600310.html. Accessed summer 2001.
8. Statistical facts and figures. North American Menopause Society; 2001. Available at: http://www.menopause.org/aboutm/ stats.html. Accessed summer 2001.
9. Luzuy F, Campana A. The menopause. Available at: http://matweb.hcuge.ch/ matweb/endo/Reproductive_health/ Menopause.html. Accessed summer 2001.

Pelvic Inflammatory Disease

1. Abbuhl S. Pelvic inflammatory disease. eMedicine.com, Inc; 2001. Available at: http://www. emedicine.com/emerg/ topic410.htm. Accessed summer 2001.

2. Pelvic inflammatory disease (PID). Authors and The University of Iowa; 1992–2001. Available at: http://www.vh.org/Patients/ IHB/IntMed/ Infectious/STDs/PID.html. Accessed summer 2001.

3. Pelvic inflammatory disease. Board of Trustees of the University of Illinois; 1999. Available at: http://www.mckinley.uiuc. edu/health-info/womenhlt/pid.html. Accessed summer 2001.

4. Pelvic inflammatory disease. National Institute of Allergy and Infectious Diseases, National Institutes of Health. Available at: http://www. niaid.nih.gov/factsheets/ stdpid.htm. Accessed summer 2001.

5. McLaughlin E. Salpingitis. Healthanswers. com. Available at:http://www. healthanswers.com/library/MedEnc/enc/ 2096.asp. Accessed summer 2001.

Pregnancy

1. Diseases that can complicate pregnancy. Merck & Co., Inc; 1995–2001. Available at: http://www.merck.com/pubs/mmanual_ home/sec22/246.htm. Accessed summer 2001.

2. Gestational diabetes: What it means for me and my baby. American Academy of Family Physicians; 2000. Available at: http:// familydoctor.org/handouts/075.html. Accessed summer 2001.

3. Valley VT. Ectopic pregnancy. eMedicine.com, Inc; 2001. Available at: http://www.emedicine. com/emerg/ topic478.htm. Accessed summer 2001.

4. Toth PP, Jothivijayarani A. Obstetrics: Hypertension in pregnancy, preeclampsia, and eclampsia. Author and The University of Iowa; 1992–2001. Available at: http://www.vh.org/Providers/ClinRef/ FPHandbook/Chapter08/10-8.html. Accessed summer 2001.

Premenstrual Syndrome

1. Barnard ND. Nutritional factors in menstrual pain and premenstrual syndrome. Physician's Committee for Responsible Medicine. Available at: http://www.pcrm. org/research/menstrual. html. Accessed summer 2001.

2. Phalen KF. Treatment of choice. *The Washington Post*. August 1. 2000:Z19. Available at: http://www.washingtonpost.com/ wp-dyn/articles/A14785-2000Aug1.html. Accessed summer 2001.

3. Premenstrual syndrome (PMS). MedicineNet, Inc.; 1996–2001. Available at: http://www.medicinenet.com. Accessed summer 2001.

4. Pre-menstrual syndrome (PMS). The Board of Trustees of the University of Illinois; 2001. Available at: http://www.mckinley.uiuc.edu/ health-info/womenhlt/ pms.html. Accessed summer 2001.

5. Dietary suggestions for premenstrual syndrome. Mayo Foundation for Medical Education and Research; 2000. Available at: http://www.mayohealth.org/mayo/pted/ htm/pms_sb.htm. Accessed summer 2001.

6. What is premenstrual syndrome (PMS)? Internet Health Library; 1999–2001. Available at: http://www.internethealthlibrary. com/Health-problems/Premenstrual%20 Syndrome%20(PMS).htm. Accessed summer 2001.

Miscellaneous Conditions

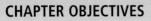

11

CHAPTER OBJECTIVES

After reading this chapter, the reader should be able to . . .

- Name the most common variety of cancer reported.
- Name the leading cause of death among cancers.
- Name three carcinogenic chemicals.
- Name five of the seven leading signs or symptoms of cancer.
- Briefly define Stages 0 through IV in cancer staging.
- Name a caution for massage when a client is receiving radiation treatment.
- Name a caution for massage when a client is receiving chemotherapy treatment.
- Name a caution for massage when a client has had some lymph nodes removed for staging purposes.
- Name three types of cysts.
- Name two cautions for massage and recent open surgery.

INTRODUCTION

Miscellaneous Conditions

Cancer, General

Cysts

Fatigue

Postoperative Situations

Miscellaneous Conditions

Cancer, General

Definition: What Is It?

Cancer is a variety of more than 100 different diseases that have one thing in common: normal body cells mutate slightly and begin to replicate uncontrollably into masses of cells called tumors. At some point in the process, some cells may break off the initial growth and travel elsewhere in the body where they colonize new tissue.

Demographics: Who Gets It?

One-half of all men and one-third of all women in the United States will develop some sort of cancer in their lifetime.[a] Cancer kills more than 550,000 people in the United

---

[a]Cancer: what is it? American Cancer Society; 2000. Available at: http://www3.cancer.org/cancerinfo/load_cont.asp?st=wi&ct=1&language=english. Accessed summer 2001.

States every year. Overall, both the incidence of new cases and the death rate of most cancers have begun to decline. This is probably due to a number of issues including slowing tobacco use, better education about the risks of sunlight exposure, more sensitive screening procedures, and better chances of finding cancers in early stages. Nonetheless, the improvement in cancer statistics also reflects inequities in health care access. The incidence and death rates of cancer are better among White upper-income citizens than they are among non-White citizens who have lower incomes. Currently, the overall survival rate for cancer is 80%. It is estimated that if all persons had appropriate access to early screening processes, that survival rate would be closer to 95%.[b]

Skin cancer is the most common variety of cancer reported (and these statistics do not even reflect the countless moles that are removed as a safeguard against melanoma development), but lung cancer is the leading cause of death by cancer for both men and women. Other leading causes of death include breast and ovarian cancer for women, prostate cancer for men, and cancer of the pancreas, colon, and rectum for both genders.

Etiology: What Happens?

No one is positive about what causes a healthy cell to change into a malignant cell. One thing that all cancers have in common is that the DNA of a cell mutates in a way that the cell acquires certain growth properties. As researchers learn more about the process of metastasis, new ways to interrupt the process and limit the ability of cancer cells to invade and destroy healthy tissue are being discovered.

The following is a simplified version of the process of metastasis, as it is currently understood:

- *Oncogene activation.* An oncogene is a gene that initiates malignant characteristics within a cell. Oncogene activation is the beginning of the changes that cause certain cells to become malignant. The trigger for activation may be toxic environmental exposures, diet, or a genetic predisposition, but it is often not clear.

- *Proliferation.* The mutated cells proliferate without control, often piling up into distinct masses. As they do this they may secrete specific enzymes that allow them to survive a normal immune system attack against perceived invaders.

- *Angiogenesis.* This is the growth of blood vessels to supply the tumor. Any growth of more than 1 or 2 cm³ requires a specific blood supply. Some cancer cells seem well supplied with the chemical messengers that command the body to build new capillaries. The more highly invested a tumor is with blood vessels, the more likely it is to have metastasized.

CANCER IN BRIEF

What is it?
Cancer is the mutation of normal cells into cells with particular characteristics, including the tendency to proliferate into distinguishable growths and to spread through the body to other areas where they may colonize new tissues.

How is it recognized?
In early stages many cancers are difficult to detect. Later signs depend on what part of the body is being affected, but can include things like unusual bleeding, susceptibility to infection, changes in skin lesions, a persistent cough or hoarseness, changes in bladder or bowel habits, painless lumps or swellings, or pain where tumors have grown to the point that they compress or erode into delicate tissue.

Is massage indicated or contraindicated?
The decision about whether to include massage as part of a treatment plan with cancer is a complicated one. Some types of bodywork are said to boost circulatory and lymph flow, which could be interpreted as increasing the risk of metastasis. Research shows, however, that it takes up to 9 years for many tumors to reach a palpable size. In light of this, it seems unlikely that a 60-minute session could have a serious impact on this disease process.

Many cancer patients seek massage as a way to help them cope with the challenges of cancer treatments. Massage and other bodywork modalities offered in this context can be beneficial, as long as the risks of working with clients who are undergoing surgery, chemotherapy, radiation, or other procedures are respected, and the therapist works as part of a well-informed health care team.

METASTASIS
Meta means "beyond" (e.g., the metacarpals are beyond the carpals). *Stasis* means "staying the same." Meta-stasis, then, means "beyond staying the same," or in other words, *changing what should not be changed.*

[b]Cancer: what is it? American Cancer Society; 2000. Available at: http://www3.cancer.org/cancerinfo/load_cont.asp?st=wi&ct=1&language=english. Accessed summer 2001.

- *Invasion.* As a tumor grows, it must convince the local extracellular matrix to make room for it without stimulating an inflammatory response. Again, special enzymes secreted by cancer cells are at the center of this process. These enzymes help to dissolve the connective tissue that provides the support for epithelium, where most cancers grow.

- *Migration.* Some cancer cells break off the primary tumor and travel through the lymphatics or circulatory capillaries to new areas. This is a complicated process involving the penetration of capillary walls to enter them and a second penetration to exit them.

- *Colonization.* When cancer cells land in a new target tissue, they must begin the process over again, starting with proliferation. This requires that the cells be able to adhere to the new tissue and that they can secrete the correct enzymes to suppress an immune system attack, create new blood vessels, and erode the extracellular matrix. The first tumor that grows in the disease process is called the primary tumor; other tumors that grow from metastasis of the primary tumor are called secondary tumors. In other words, a tumor in the bladder that metastasized from the ovary is not bladder cancer—it is secondary ovarian cancer in the bladder.

It is unclear how often cells become malignant in an average human life. It may be a fairly common occurrence, which simply is not successful as long as immune system mechanisms prevent the growth of abnormal new cells. This raises some interesting questions about the connections among cancer, stress, and immune system efficiency.

Causes

Triggers for oncogene activation vary by tissue type and individual. Causes of cancer are slowly being narrowed to some identifiable factors. These are generally discussed as internal or external factors.

Internal Factors Every cell in the body has a built-in capacity for self-destruction. This is a natural and healthy process called *apoptosis* or *programmed cell death*. A specific gene in some cancer cells has been found to inhibit apoptosis. Therefore, some cancers may be as much caused by cells that *refuse to die* as it is by new cells coming to life.

Some cancers are brought about by or connected to inherited characteristics. This means an inherited gene is likely to cause cellular mutations sometime in the future (such genes have been identified for a small percentage of breast and colon cancers). It could also mean that a person may have a genetic susceptibility to factors that would not be a threat to someone else. Some inborn hormonal problems or immune system dysfunctions can also increase the risk for developing cancer.

External Factors Carcinogens are chemical or environmental agents that have been identified as cancer-causers. The hydrocarbons in cigarette smoke are carcinogens, as is ultraviolet radiation from the sun, especially for fair-skinned people. Radiation from excessive x-rays and exposure to certain substances such as asbestos, benzene, nickel, cadmium, uranium, and vinyl chloride have also been found to be carcinogenic.

Some viruses can cause certain types of cancer. Others simply have a strong statistical link with the development of various cancers, but the cause-and-effect relationship has not been defined. Some cancer-related viruses include:

- *Human immunodeficiency virus (HIV).* This virus can cause Kaposi's sarcoma, a type of skin cancer (see *HIV/AIDS*, Chapter 5).

- *HTLV-1.* This is a virus in the same family as HIV, has been linked to *leukemia* and *lymphoma* (Chapter 5).

- *Hepatitis B (HBV).* This has been linked to liver cancer (see *hepatitis,* Chapter 7).

- *Epstein–Barr virus (EBV).* This has been linked to Burkitt's lymphoma and *Hodgkin's disease* (Chapter 5).

- *Human papilloma virus (HPV).* This is implicated in nearly all cases of *cervical cancer* (Chapter 10).

- *Herpes simplex type II (genital herpes).* This has been linked to cervical and uterine cancer.

It is often a combination of external and internal factors that tip the scales in favor of developing cancer. Exposure to carcinogens in certain combinations can also be dangerous. For example, heavy smoking combined with excessive alcohol consumption is an especially potent combination for developing cancers of the mouth or upper gastrointestinal tract. Very often many years, even decades, may pass between the initial exposure to a carcinogen and the development of distinguishable tumors. This makes it difficult to pin down precise causes of cancer that will be consistent from person to person.

Signs and Symptoms

Symptoms of cancer vary widely, depending on the site. One of the most insidious features of this disease is that it is often painless until it is too late to do anything about it. Tumors will begin to cause pain when they place pressure on nerve endings, or when they cause a blockage in a tube or duct that will in turn put pressure on nerve endings. The American Cancer Society has compiled a list of common signs that are red flags for the possibility of cancer.[c] They include:

- A change in bowel or bladder habits.

- A sore that does not heal.

- Unusual bleeding or drainage.

- Thickening or lump in the breast or elsewhere.

- Indigestion or swallowing difficulty.

- A change in a wart or mole.

- Persistent cough or hoarseness.

Diagnosis

Cancers are found by a variety of methods, depending on the affected part of the body. Many cancers are found by either self or clinical examinations; this is true for breast, cervical, rectal, and prostate cancers. Other tumors are found by imaging techniques such as radiographs, computed tomography (CT) scans, magnetic resonance imaging (MRI), endoscopies, and ultrasound. Barium swallows and enemas can reveal tumors in the gastrointestinal tract.

If suspicious changes are noted, tissue samples are taken and analyzed for the presence of malignant cells; this is called a biopsy. If these tests are positive, further examinations of the patient will follow to determine how far the cancer has developed.

[c]UPHS PENNHealth tip: "Cancer warning signs." Trustees of the University of Pennsylvania 1994–2001. Available at: http://cancer.med.upenn.edu/causeprevent/screening/tip1016.html. Accessed summer 2001.

Staging

Most types of cancer develop in predictable enough patterns that they can be staged, or given a label that indicates how far the cancer has advanced. Two widely recognized systems are used for staging cancer. They can be used independently or together to rate the degree of progression and aggressiveness of the disease.

The TNM classification system rates tumors by:

- Tumor size *(T)*.

- Nodal involvement *(N)*.

- Extent of metastasis *(M)*.

The numerical staging system gives a number to indicate the degree of progression:

- *Stage 0* means some abnormal cells are present and they may be malignant. However, they are isolated and show no signs of spreading. Stage 0 cancer is sometimes called cancer *in situ*.

- *Stage I* cancer involves a small tumor.

- *Stage II* means the tumor may be larger, or signs of metastasis to nearby lymph nodes could be present.

- *Stage III* indicates larger tumors and further signs of metastasis.

- *Stage IV* generally means that the cancer has metastasized to distant parts of the body. A general convention states that when a cancer has metastasized to the other side of the diaphragm from where it started, it is in Stage IV.

Staging may be further qualified by the use of "A" and "B" delineations. For instance, breast cancer in Stage II-A means the tumor is small but has spread to the axillary lymph nodes, *or* the tumor may be slightly larger but has *not* spread to the axillary nodes. Stage II-B means the tumor is up to 5 cm and has spread into the axillary nodes, *or* it is larger than 5 cm and has *not* spread to the axillary nodes.

Cancers of the lymph nodes and bone marrow (lymphoma and leukemia) have a different growth pattern than other cancers. Because they do not involve primary tumors, their staging systems refer to blood counts and symptoms.

The purpose of staging is to evaluate the progression of the disease, with the intention of predicting how successful the malignant cells could be when they try to colonize new tissues. This allows the health care team to design a treatment program best suited to the individual patient.

Treatment

Decisions for how to treat cancer depend on the stage it is in, the age and general health of the patient, and what kind of cancer is present. Within each tumor different kinds of cells may require different modes of attack. This makes the successful treatment of cancer a matter of finding the correct combination of surgery, chemotherapy, hypothermia, radiation, hormones, and biological therapies.

- *Surgery.* Cancer surgeries are performed to remove malignant tumors and a margin of healthy tissue around them, when possible. A sample of nearby lymph nodes is often taken as well to examine them for signs of metastasis. If a "sentinel" node can be identified (this is a node through which most or all of the lymph entering an area passes before going on to other nodes), it can be taken alone for examination. This refinement has led to a reduction in some of the side effects of cancer surgery.

- *Chemotherapy.* A variety of cytotoxic drugs have been developed for use in cancer treatment. These drugs specifically target any fast-growing cells in the body, so in addition to killing cancer cells they may also attack the skin (resulting in hair loss), the gastrointestinal tract (leading to chronic nausea and mouth sores), and the blood cells (causing easy bruising and bleeding disorders as well as white blood cell suppression).

- *Autologous bone marrow transplant.* This is a procedure in which some healthy bone marrow is harvested from the patient and stored. Then a very extreme course of cytotoxic drugs is administered. This kills the cancer cells but kills most white blood cells too. After chemotherapy, the stored bone marrow is replanted in the patient, where it replaces the immune system cells killed by chemotherapy. This procedure is for use only in very extreme cases; it has a number of dangerous side affects and serious complications, but it can be a life-saver if nothing else works.

- *Radiation.* With this type of therapy high-energy rays are focused on tumors to kill them or at least slow their growth. The radiation may be applied from an external machine, which requires daily outpatient visits for several weeks, or it may come from small radioactive pellets that are temporarily implanted close to the tumor.

- *Hormones.* Breast and prostate cancer tumors both depend on the presence of certain hormones to grow. Therapies to limit the secretion of these hormones or to change the way they affect the body are used in the treatment of these cancers.

- *Hypothermia.* In some cases, specifically with cervical cancer and actinic keratosis (see *skin cancer*, Chapter 1), potentially malignant cells may be killed by freezing them off the affected structure.

- *Biologic therapy.* Recently found weaknesses in the process of metastasis have led to the development of more refined cancer treatments. Cancer cells are able to limit immune system responses because of their particular enzyme secretions, but that could be overcome with specialized treatments that enhance an immune system response to cancer cell antigens (cellular markers that identify "non-self" cells). Several cancer "vaccines" are currently being explored to sensitize immune system agents to these antigens. An exciting aspect of this research is that it targets *only* cancer cells, which could keep the side effects of treatment to a minimum. These highly specialized treatments may eventually reach the same prevalence as traditional cancer treatments.

- *Stem cell implantation.* The implantation of stem cells specifically for leukemia patients carries promise as an effective cancer treatment. These "cellular blanks" have the potential to grow into whatever kinds of cells the body needs to replace.

Prevention

In looking at who gets cancer and some of the causes involved, the Cancer Research Foundation of America has published a list of suggestions for how to stay cancer-free.[d]

---

[d]Cancer prevention guide. Cancer Research Foundation of America. Available at: http://www.preventcancer.org. Accessed spring 2002.

Not surprisingly, this list could be applied to any number of disorders.

- Eat more fruit, vegetables, and whole grain breads and cereals while controlling dietary fat.
- Exercise regularly.
- Use sunscreen or clothing to protect the skin.
- Stop smoking and other tobacco use.
- Use alcohol moderately.
- Practice safe sex. (Note: this is as a precaution against contracting human papilloma virus, which is associated with cervical cancer. Research shows, however, that barrier methods such as condoms do *not* protect against the spread of this virus.[e] Therefore, "safe sex" in this context means to have relations with an uninfected partner.)
- Use early cancer screening methods.

Massage?

For many years it has been assumed that circulatory types of massage carry the risk of aiding the process of metastasis by boosting blood and lymph flow. Research shows, however, that cancerous growths can take years to become established before they are detectable by palpation. It seems farfetched to suppose that a 60-minute massage could contribute to that process any more significantly than a brisk walk around the block or a long hot shower. Nonetheless, it is obviously inappropriate to rub on a tumor or any undiagnosed swelling or thickening of tissue.

Massage for persons undergoing cancer treatment, however, has a vital and useful role. It can assist in pain control, decrease perceived stress levels, and create a general parasympathetic state through reduced blood pressure and decreased muscle tension. It can improve appetite and the quality of sleep. Perhaps most of all, it provides for a basic human need: nurturing, caring, informed touch at a time when many cancer patients feel isolated and dehumanized.

It is important, however, to bear in mind the complications associated with various cancer treatments, because they can have serious implications for the choices of bodywork modalities, especially when multiple treatments are employed.

- *Surgery.* The most obvious caution for recent cancer surgery to remove tumors and lymph nodes is the open scar and risk of infection that goes along with it. Other complications of surgery can include nerve damage and lymphedema (a situation in which the affected limb cannot drain its accumulations of lymph because nodes have been removed). Lymphedema can occur shortly following a surgery or at any time after if the affected limb is traumatized by an injury or local infection. Lymphedema contraindicates Swedish and circulatory types of massage but can be treated by practitioners trained in lymph movement techniques.
- *Chemotherapy.* Chemotherapy has many serious side effects, including a drastically impaired immune system, nausea, fatigue, and ulcers in the mouth and mucous membranes. Chemotherapy is usually administered in stages, so a patient will undergo a course of treatment, take some time to recover, and then have another

[e]Human papillomavirus (HPV). American Cancer Society; 2000. Available at: http://www3.cancer.org/ cancerinfo/load_cont.asp?ct=8&doc=84&Language=English. Accessed summer 2001.

course. Massage therapists working with clients undergoing chemotherapy must be especially conscious of their own health so as not to expose their clients to dangerous pathogens. Some experts recommend that patients receive massage during breaks between chemotherapy treatments; others suggest that therapists might want to use gloves if they are working with clients who are suffused with cytotoxic drugs. These decisions must be made on a case-by-case basis. It would be wise to share any such concerns with the client's health care team.

Cancer Screening— Who, What, Where, When, Why?

The science of early cancer detection is far from fully developed or universally accepted. A survey of several different medical agencies yields significantly different guidelines for individuals to follow in the attempt to be vigilant against early signs of cancer. Screening recommendations are further complicated by differences for low-risk and high-risk populations.

The following is a brief synopsis of the leading ideas about early cancer detection. Any of these is subject to change as research reveals whether specific testing procedures actually reduce the mortality rate from the types of cancer they target.[f]

TYPE OF CANCER	RECOMMENDATIONS FOR LOW-RISK POPULATIONS	RECOMMENDATIONS FOR HIGH-RISK POPULATIONS
Breast cancer	*Self-exam.* Monthly from age 20 onward *Clinical exam.* Every 3 years from ages 20–39 and annually from 40 onward *Mammogram.* Opinions vary, but most suggest exams every 1–3 years from age 40 or 50 onward	High-risk populations include women with the identified breast cancer genes, women who have first-degree relatives with breast cancer, or women who have had breast cancer or other types of cancer before Screening schedules need to be matched to individual case
Cervical cancer	When a woman becomes sexually active, she should have a yearly pelvic exam and Pap test; when she has had three normal tests in a row, she can cut back on frequency to once every 3 years, or by her doctor's recommendation, for as long as she has a cervix Some studies suggest that testing can be suspended after age 65	High-risk populations for cervical cancer are women who have shown signs of cervical dysplasia in pelvic exams or Pap tests Screening should continue on a yearly basis until patients have three normal tests in a row Screening can be discontinued if a patient has had a hysterectomy, *unless* the surgery was related to cervical cancer
Skin cancer	Several agencies recommend a monthly self-exam for changes in skin, with a clinical visual exam every 3 years from age 20 to 40, and annually from age 40 onward; counseling for avoiding sun exposure and the use of sunblock is also a part of skin cancer prevention and early detection	High-risk populations include persons previously diagnosed with any type of skin cancer or precancerous condition; clinical exams should be scheduled on an as-needed basis
Lung, ovarian, and endometrial cancer	No effective noninvasive screening measures have been developed to detect these cancers in early stages; therefore, it is not practical to make recommendations for low-risk populations	Some screening techniques may find these cancers, but they tend to be invasive procedures that are reserved for patients with a high risk for developing them

[f]Zoorob R. Cancer screening guidelines. American Academy of Family Physicians; 2001. Available at: http://www.aafp.org/afp/20010315/ 1101.html. Accessed fall 2001.

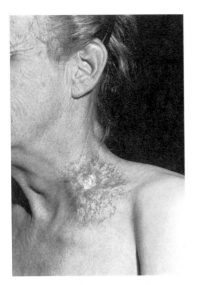

Figure 11-1. Radiation burn

- *Radiation.* Externally applied radiation can result in burns on the skin as well as fatigue, impaired immunity, and lymphedema if lymph nodes are destroyed in the process. Massage therapists must avoid skin lesions and the possibility of sharing pathogens with clients who have very limited capacity to fight back. Radiation can cause significant burns on the skin, which of course must be avoided (Fig. 11-1, Color Plate 40).

- *Other cautions.* The side effects of other cancer treatments are variable. Applications of liquid nitrogen to freeze off actinic keratosis lesions can injure the skin. Tamoxifen, a hormone-like drug for breast cancer, is associated with an increased risk of blood clotting. The potential side effects of biologic cancer treatments and stem cell implants have yet to be discovered.

No matter what kind of cancer or cancer treatments a person is going through, it is vital for his or her massage therapist to keep in communication with the rest of the client's health care team to provide the best benefits that bodywork has to offer with minimum risks.

CYSTS IN BRIEF

What are they?
Cysts are layers of connective tissue that surround and isolate something that should not be in the body (e.g., a piece of shrapnel or a localized infection).

How are they recognized?
Palpable cysts are generally small, painless, distinct masses that move slightly under the skin.

Is massage indicated or contraindicated?
Cysts locally contraindicate massage.

Cysts
Definition: What Are They?

When something that does not really belong gets inside or grows inside the body, a remarkable reaction occurs. Like an oyster covering a grain of sand with layers of pearl, humans cover their "grains of sand" with layers of connective tissue, making an easily discernible and isolated *cyst*. The notable exception to this habit is *cancer* (this chapter).

Etiology: What Happens?

A wide variety of cysts may develop in the body. *Baker's cysts* (Chapter 3) are outpouchings of the synovial joint in the popliteal fossa. *Ganglion cysts* (Chapter 3) are pouches formed by tendinous sheaths. *Ovarian cysts* (Chapter 10) are usually harmless self-limiting growths on the ovaries at the site of egg release. Layers of connective tissue also form around any foreign material that gets into the body. Unremoved shrapnel will be encysted, for example, as will localized infections of *tuberculosis* (Chapter 6).

The most common kinds of cysts that massage therapists encounter are *sebaceous cysts*, which are the focus of the rest of this discussion. Sebaceous cysts are a bit like a pimple gone bad (see *acne*, Chapter 1). A sebaceous gland fills up with sebum and waste, but instead of draining or being consumed by macrophages, the debris from this localized infection is walled off and "removed" from the body by a tough layer of dense connective tissue. There it will generally stay until it is surgically removed or the body eventually (and this can take months or years) gets around to reabsorbing it.

Signs and Symptoms

Sebaceous cysts are small, usually painless bumps under the skin that may move slightly, depending on the mobility of the fascia. They are most common on the scalp, neck, or shoulders (sites of acne infections).

Complications

Staphylococcus bacteria can sometimes attack sebaceous cysts, resulting in an acute infection. Other cysts are generally not vulnerable to infection but may be situated in a place to become snagged or irritated by normal day-to-day activities.

Treatment

Most cysts require no treatment unless they are in a place that causes pain or they are removed for cosmetic reasons. If the connective tissue wrapping has isolated the cyst adequately, it can generally be removed with simple surgery. Infected sebaceous cysts are treated with systemic antibiotics.

Massage?

Cysts locally contraindicate massage. In the extremely unlikely event that a massage therapist could pop one, its contents could cause a dangerous immune reaction. It is more likely, though, that massage would simply irritate the surrounding tissues and cause soreness. If a client has a questionable or new cyst that has not been diagnosed, the therapist should recommend that the client have it diagnosed before the next appointment. Most painless bumps under the skin are not dangerous, but diagnosis is not within the scope of practice of massage therapy.

Fatigue

Definition: What Is It?

Here is a condition with which most people are familiar. Fatigue is a state in which the body does not function at its best levels because of lack of recovery time. For the purposes of simplicity, the world of fatigue will be divided here into two types: *mental/emotional* fatigue and *physical* fatigue brought about by overexertion.

Etiology: What Happens?

The two varieties of fatigue are usually inextricably blended with each other. For example, living in chronic stress (mental/emotional fatigue) can throw the neck muscles into an ongoing contraction (physical fatigue). This person will always feel more tired than if those muscles were able to release their unnecessary tension. The feeling of always being tired is a self-fulfilling prophecy; the perception that a person is tired will cause him or her to move less efficiently, which exacerbates that loss of energy.

> **FATIGUE IN BRIEF**
>
> **What is it?**
> Fatigue is a state of having less than optimal energy as a result of inadequate rest and recovery time. Fatigue can be brought about by mental or physical exertion or by any combination of both.
>
> **How is it recognized?**
> A person living with mental or physical fatigue feels tired, moves inefficiently, and may be more prone to injury.
>
> **Is massage indicated or contraindicated?**
> In the absence of other conditions, fatigue indicates massage.

Complications

Fatigue is often related to *sleep disorders* (Chapter 3), which can create long-lasting problems in the body. Fatigue can cause a person to move inefficiently or clumsily, thus increasing the chance of accident or injury. Fatigue that is not relieved with a reasonable amount of rest and recovery time may be a warning sign of some other conditions. *Chronic fatigue syndrome* (Chapter 5) is a possibility, as are *anemia* (Chapter 4) and *hypothyroidism* (Chapter 8).

Massage?

As long as more serious pathologies are ruled out, physical and emotional fatigue both indicate massage. After a good session a client can get off the table and feel like he or she has just been infused with several hours' worth of sleep. That is the extra measure of energy available when it is not being wasted on counterproductive muscular contractions. Massage can also provide an hour-long vacation from the stress that was stimulating the contractions.

For fatigue brought on by mental or emotional stress, massage can re-establish the lost balance between sympathetic and parasympathetic reactions. Massage sessions provide a rare opportunity for a client to listen and pay attention to what is happening in his or her body, which provides tools for avoiding similar problems in the future.

For physical fatigue from exhaustion or overexertion, massage works on a mechanical level by reducing hypertonicity, flushing out waste products, improving local circulation, and speeding recovery time.

Ultimately, ongoing fatigue is a reflection of the continuous circle between emotions that are expressed in bodies through muscular tension and muscular tension that interferes with rest and recovery and thus causes emotional upset. For massage therapists, it is a chicken-or-the-egg proposition, and frankly, it does not matter which came first. The bodyworker's job is to address whatever symptoms are present and to be sensitive to the more subtle signals about underlying tensions that may exacerbate those symptoms.

POSTOPERATIVE SITUATIONS IN BRIEF

What are they?
Postoperative situations are conditions in which clients are recovering from any kind of surgery.

How is it recognized?
Surgeries may be major and invasive, or they may be conducted through tiny holes in the abdomen or through long tubes inserted into blood vessels to get to a destination far away.

Is massage indicated or contraindicated?
Massage can be appropriate for persons recovering from surgery, depending on the reason for the surgery and the danger of possible complications.

Postoperative Situations
Definition: What Is It?

Not so very long ago most surgeries involved systemic anesthesia, large incisions, and major trauma to the body. These were followed by prolonged hospital stays and a wide variety of possible complications ranging from infection, to blood clots, to the discovery that a sponge or clamp had been left inside the body.

Today the whole world of surgery has changed with lasers, balloons, and procedures that are conducted with microscopic tools through tiny incisions in the skin. Many surgeries that used to involve general anesthesia and hospital stays are now being performed on an outpatient basis.

Massage?

The rapid development of new less invasive surgical techniques is good news for massage therapists, because the risks involved with major surgery are very serious and frequently make doing many kinds of bodywork impractical. Obviously, the appropriateness of massage for someone recovering from any kind of surgery depends on the scope and predisposing cause of the surgery and how much of the body has been affected.

The two major cautions for massage with major surgery are immunosuppressant drugs and blood clots (see *thrombophlebitis/deep vein thrombosis*, Chapter 4). Immunosuppressant drugs are usually used with a client recovering from an organ transplant or cancer surgery. A client taking these medications is at risk for infection from anyone else's pathogens.

Blood clots are a lurking threat for anyone who has just been through major surgery, especially surgery involving the leg, hip, or pelvis. A safe plan is to avoid circulatory types of bodywork until the threat of clotting has passed. The therapist should consult with the client's health care team to identify when that might be (6 weeks is a commonly suggested waiting period). Reflexive and energetic work up until then will not only be safe and appropriate, but very welcomed as well.

In the absence of contraindications, carefully applied frictions around the edges of a new scar can have positive influence on the localized healing process. It is important not to stretch the skin beyond tolerance or to work near an open wound. Therapists can also teach their clients how to mobilize their own scar tissue to minimize hypertrophy and adhesions.

Chapter Review Questions: Miscellaneous Conditions

1. Briefly describe the staging process for cancer. What are the stages, and what do they mean?

2. What are the possible risks of massaging a client who is living with cancer?

3. What are the possible benefits of massaging a client who is living with cancer?

4. Name three external factors that may contribute to the risk of developing cancer.

5. Describe the circular relationship between mental/emotional fatigue and physical fatigue.

6. How have recent innovations in surgical techniques changed the way massage applies to postoperative patients?

7. Name two important risks to bear in mind for patients recovering from open surgery.

8. A client has a small (5 cm) undiagnosed lump on her upper back. It is dense but not painful and moves slightly on palpation. What is it most likely to be, and what should a responsible massage therapist do about it?

Bibliography, Miscellaneous Conditions

General References, Reproductive System

1. de Dominico G, Wood E. *Beard's Massage.* Philadelphia, Pa: WB Saunders; 1997

2. Damjanou I. *Pathology for the Health-Related Professions.* Philadelphia, Pa: WB Saunders; 1996.

3. Travell J, Simons DG. *Myofascial Pain and Dysfunction: The Trigger Point Manual.* Baltimore, Md: Williams & Wilkins; 1983.

4. Clemente CD. *Anatomy: A Regional Atlas of the Human Body.* 3rd ed. Baltimore, Md: Urban & Schwarzenburg; 1987.

5. Tortora GJ, Anagnostakos NP. *Principles of Anatomy and Physiology.* 6th ed. New York, NY: Harper & Row; 1990.

6. *Taber's Cyclopedic Dictionary.* 14th ed. Philadelphia, Pa: FA Davis; 1981.

7. *Stedman's Medical Dictionary.* 26th ed. Baltimore, Md: Williams & Wilkins; 1995.

8. Memmler RL, Wood DL. *The Human Body in Health and Disease.* 5th ed. Philadelphia, Pa: JB Lippincott; 1983.

9. Juhan D. *Job's Body: A Handbook for Bodywork.* Barrytown, NY: Station Hill Press; 1987.

10. Mulvihill ML. *Human Diseases: A Systemic Approach.* 2nd ed. Norwalk, CT: Appleton & Lange; 1987.

11. Kunz JRM, Finkel AJ, eds. *The American Medical Association Family Medical Guide.* New York, NY: Random House; 1987.

12. Marieb EM. *Human Anatomy and Physiology.* Redwood City, CA: Benjamin/Cummings; 1989.

13. Field T. *Touch Therapy.* London: Churchill, Livingstone; 2000.

14. Sapolsky RM. *Why Zebras Don't Get Ulcers: An Updated Guide to Stress, Stress-Related Disease, and Coping.* New York, NY: W.H. Freeman; 1998.

Cancer, General

1. Report to the nation: Cancer incidence and deaths decline overall during past decade. American Cancer Society; 2000. Available at: http://www2.cancer.org/zine/index.cfm?sc=001&fn=001_06062001_0. Accessed summer 2001.

2. King MW. Growth factors and cytokines. Indiana State University of Medicine. Available at: http://web.indstate.edu/thcme/mwking/growth-factors.html. Accessed summer 2001.

3. Cancer facts. Question and answers about complementary and alternative medicine in cancer treatment. National Cancer Institute, Office of Cancer Complementary and Alternative Medicine (OCCAM). Available at: http://cis.nci.nih.gov/fact/9_14.htm. Accessed summer 2001.

4. Cancer invasion and metastasis. State University of New York at Stony Brook. Available at: http://www.path.sunysb.edu/courses/im/. Accessed summer 2001.

5. Cancer prevention guide. Cancer Research Foundation of America. Available at: http://www.preventcancer.org. Accessed spring 2002.

6. Coping with cancer. National Cancer Institute. Available at: http://www.nci.nih.gov/cancer_information/coping/. Accessed spring 2002.

7. History of cancer. American Cancer Society; 2000. Available at: http://www3.cancer.org/cancerinfo/load_cont.asp?ct=1&doc=3&Language=English. Accessed summer 2001.

8. Lymphedema (PDQ) supportive care—Patients. National Cancer Institute. Available at: http://cancernet.nci.nih.gov/cgi-bin/srchcgi.exe?DBID=pdq&TYPE=search&SFMT=pdq_statement/1/0/0&Z208=208_00442P. Accessed spring 2002.

9. Summary of American Cancer Society recommendations for the early detection of cancer in asymptomatic people. American Cancer Society; 2000. Available at: http://www3.cancer.org/cancerinfo/sitecenter.asp?ct=1&ctid=8&scp=8.3.10.40038&scs=4&scss=20&scdoc=41255&pnt=2&language=english. Accessed summer 2001.

10. UPHS PENNHealth tip: "Cancer warning signs." Trustees of the University of Pennsylvania; 1994–2001. Available at: http://cancer.med.upenn.edu/causeprevent/screening/tip1016.html. Accessed summer 2001.

11. Cancer: What is it? American Cancer Society; 2000. Available at: http://www3.cancer.org/cancerinfo/load_cont.asp?st=wi&ct=1&language=english. Accessed summer 2001.

12. Zoorob R. Cancer screening guidelines. American Academy of Family Physicians; 2001. Available at: http://www.aafp.org/afp/20010315/1101.html. Accessed fall 2001.

13. Walton T. Clinical thinking and cancer. *Massage Ther J*. 2000;39(3):66.

14. Curties D. Could massage therapy promote cancer metastasis? *Massage Ther J*. 2000;39(3):83.

15. Malloy J. Do the benefits of massage outweigh the risks? *Massage Ther J*. 2001;39(4):60.

16. MacDonald G. How cancer spreads. *Massage Ther J*. 2001;39(4):74.

17. Curties D. Cancer therapies. *Massage Ther J*. 2001;39(4):80.

18. Chapman C. Lymphedema 101: What every therapist should know. *Massage Ther J*. 2001;39(4):86.

Cysts

1. Cysts. New Zealand Dermatological Society; 1997–1999. Available at: http://www.dermnet.org.nz. Accessed summer 2001.

2. Sebaceous cysts. InteliHealth Inc.; 1996–2001. Available at:: http://www.intelihealth.com/IH/ihtIH/WSIHW000/9339/10649.html. Accessed summer 2001.

COLOR PLATES

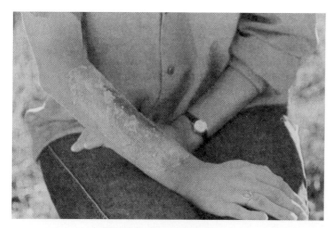

Color Plate 28. 3rd degree burn.

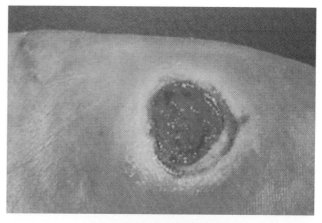

Color Plate 29. Decubitus ulcer

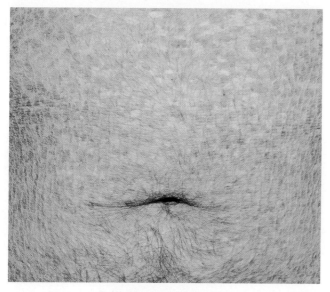

Color Plate 30. Ichthyosis.

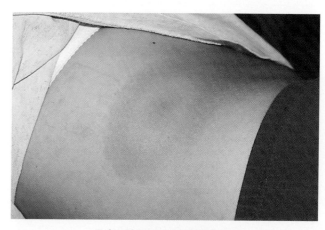

Color Plate 31. Lyme disease.

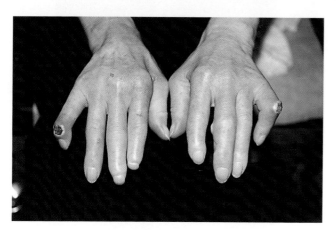

Color Plate 32. Scleroderma.

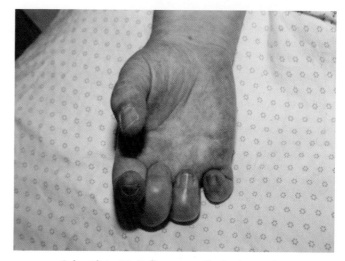

Color Plate 33. Reflex sympathetic dystrophy.

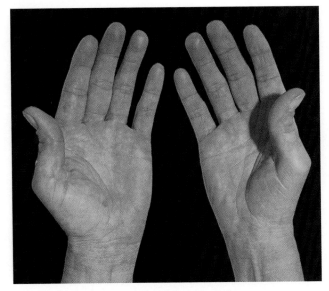

Color Plate 34. Raynaud's syndrome.

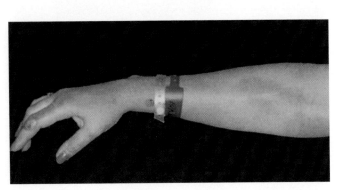

Color Plate 35. Lymphangitis: an infection of lymph capillaries.

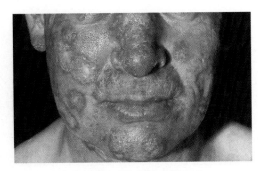

Color Plate 36. Discoid lupus.

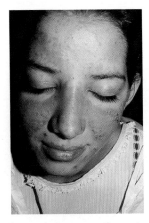

Color Plate 37. Systemic lupus erythematosus: malar rash.

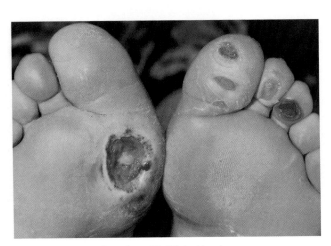

Color Plate 38. Diabetic ulcers.

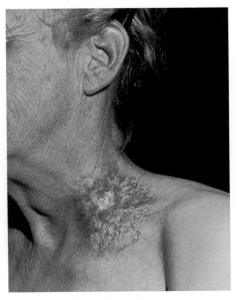

Color Plate 39. Radiation burn.

Taking a Client History

Taking a thorough client health history is a delicate art, especially if it is to be done in less than 1 hour. Many people have uncomplicated backgrounds and simple complaints and disorders, but as massage moves into the medical mainstream, therapists will need to be prepared to deal responsibly and professionally with clients whose lists of diseases, conditions, accidents, surgeries and medications can make a person's head swim.

Massage therapists go to school to learn how to touch people in ways that are beneficial to their health. They also go to massage school to learn whom *not* to touch, or at least not to touch in certain ways. The health history is the first conversation a therapist has with a potential client about his or her body; this is the time to make that all-important judgment about the appropriateness of massage. The time will come for most therapists when they will have to turn someone away, at least temporarily. It is not easy to do, but knowing that it is, above all, for the client's safety and benefit, makes it an easier task.

A successful client-therapist relationship is a partnership in which both parties work together toward specific goals. The most important quality for massage therapists to cultivate as they learn how to establish this relationship is careful, patient listening. This skill is a rare one, but it is critical for a successful practice. Massage therapy clients put themselves in very vulnerable, intimate relationships with virtual strangers. If massage therapists are good listeners and show understanding about clients' experiences, the relationship can be one of warmth, safety, and productivity rather than disconnection or even anxiety.

What follows is a sample client history form that might be used in a massage clinic specializing in circulatory-based bodywork. Relevant questions are discussed to see how some answers might influence the decision-making process. Finally, some ideas for creating possible treatment plans are offered.

This is a longer, more detailed intake form than many therapists use. Nevertheless, it can provide a great deal of valuable information not only about a client's present status, but about his or her past experiences and current attitudes about health. It is often a good idea to schedule an extra-long appointment for a therapist and client to go through this form together.

It is utterly impossible to create a comprehensive guideline for taking client histories; there are simply too many variables. The way some conditions connect to or hint at others; whether a client is taking various kinds of medications; a client's occupation, working conditions, and living conditions; and the way sleep, diet, and exercise habits can influence overall health all influence the decision about whether certain types of massage may be appropriate, or if, perhaps, the client should seek help elsewhere.

Sample Client History Form

Name

Address

Billing Information

General Information:

Age

Occupation

Describe your exercise habits:

Describe your general diet:

Describe how well you sleep:

Describe your general health:

Health History:

Have you ever had any surgery or hospitalization?

    More than 10 years ago:

    5 to 10 years ago:

    Less than 5 years ago:

Have you ever been involved in an injury or an accident?

    More than 10 years ago:

    5 to 10 years ago:

    Less than 5 years ago:

What kind of care did you receive?

Do you consider that you have recovered from these events?

Do you have any chronic, ongoing conditions that you deal with on a regular basis? Explain.

Are you taking any medication? Explain.

Are you currently seeing a doctor for any reason? Explain.

Do you have any skin rashes or other skin problems right now?

Check off any of the following conditions that you have experienced:

Skin
Boils
Fungal infections
Herpes simplex
Warts
Eczema
Psoriasis
Skin cancer

Musculoskeletal
Fibromyalgia
Rheumatoid arthritis
Osteoarthritis
TMJ dysfunction
Strains, sprains or tendinitis
Carpal tunnel syndrome
Thoracic outlet syndrome

Nervous
Depression
Multiple sclerosis
Post polio syndrome
Headaches
Stroke
Seizure disorders
Reduced sensation
Sleep disorders
Chemical dependency

Circulatory
Anemia
Thrombophlebitis
Deep vein thrombosis
High blood pressure
Heart disease
Varicose veins
Clotting disorders

Lymph/Immune
Edema
Leukemia/lymphoma
HIV/AIDS
Chronic fatigue syndrome
Lupus
Other auto-immune disorders

Respiratory
Asthma
Emphysema
Sinusitis
Tuberculosis

Digestive
GERD (reflux)
Ulcers
Crohn's disease
Ulcerative colitis
Irritable bowel syndrome
Gallstones
Cirrhosis
Hepatitis

Endocrine
Diabetes
Hypothyroidism
Hyperthyroidism

Urinary
Kidney stones
Renal failure

Reproductive
Breast cancer
Endometriosis
Ovarian cysts
Prostate cancer
Painful menstruation
Are you pregnant?

Other:
Explanation:

Treatment goals:
Why are you here? What do you hope to accomplish?

Please indicate where you have pain:

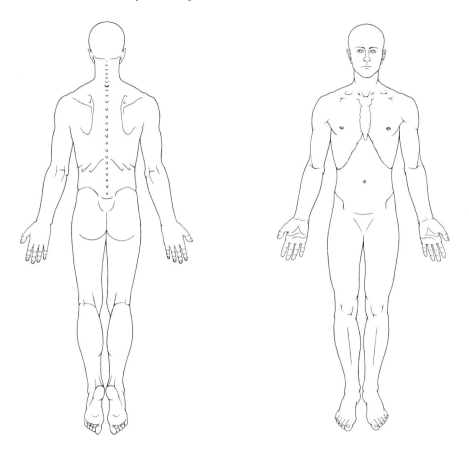

Describe what you do that causes pain, and what activities tend to make it worse:

Do you have any questions about massage?

Disclaimer

General Questions:

Age

Age is a pertinent question because some conditions are particularly prevalent in certain age groups. Of course, it's fairly easy to tell if a client is within a reasonable age expectation for these conditions just by sight, but it's a good idea to get it in writing anyway.

Occupation

This is a key piece of information, particularly for clients who come in with specific pain patterns or injuries that they want to address. This question can lead to a brief discussion of the physical demands that a job may place on a person. The massage therapist should not hesitate to try to "act out" any repetitive or stressful motions a client describes, in an attempt to understand how these activities might contribute to pain and dysfunction.

Exercise, sleeping, eating habits

These descriptions can reveal how a client sees her health efforts. This is not the time to pass judgment or make recommendations; it's just a chance to add information to the whole picture.

General health description

Many people will describe themselves as basically healthy, but some will come seeking massage to help them cope with ongoing difficult physical situations. How a client perceives her own health is a useful piece of information.

Health History

Surgeries and hospitalizations

For convenience, these are broken into three time periods. It's useful to know about long-ago events, because they may influence what's currently happening. However, it's usually much more crucial to know what has been going on in more recent history.

Injuries and accidents

As with surgeries and hospitalizations, recent events are usually more pertinent than ancient history, but the complete picture can reveal important patterns. This question should elicit information about on-the-job injuries, sports injuries, car accidents and any other kinds of trauma that caused significant pain or loss of function.

Care and recovery

The follow-up questions about accidents and injuries give information about the client's perspective of her healing process.

Ongoing, chronic conditions

This question will be asked again in a different way with the check-off list of diseases, but it's always good to give clients an extra chance to reveal important information.

Seeing a doctor

If a client is under a doctor's care, she probably has at least a moderately serious condition that massage may influence for better or worse. It is never a bad idea to inform a primary care physician that a particular patient wishes to include massage as part of her health care.

Taking medication

If the answer to this question is yes, it is vitally important to know *why*. If a client is unsure why, then a consultation with the primary care physician is called for.

Medications for cardiovascular problems, high blood pressure, kidney dysfunction, antibiotics, pain killers, muscle relaxants and anti-depressants all have implications for massage. A discussion of why a client may need them and how to fit massage into the picture will keep both client and therapist on safe ground.

Skin rashes

This is a self-defensive question for massage therapists, as well as an important part of the health picture. If the answer is yes, again it's important to know *why*. A skin rash may be just a local caution, or it may suggest that a client needs to reschedule.

Check-off list

If everything has gone well, nothing will appear on this list that hasn't already been discussed. This is by no means a complete list of every condition a person is likely to encounter, but the conditions included here are either chronic, ongoing or repetitive situations, or they have special significance to massage therapists. This list is simply a suggestion. As therapists develop their own client history forms they may have other conditions they wish to include, and some they prefer to leave out.

Disclaimer

Many people recommend including a disclaimer explaining that a massage therapist does not diagnose conditions or treat them medically, and that it is the client's responsibility to seek medical care appropriately and to keep the therapist updated on her health status.

Treatment Plan

The difference between an outstanding massage therapist and a so-so one is intention. Good massage therapists always know why they're doing what they're doing, and though those goals and methods may change from moment to moment, the consciousness of working with purpose should always be present. Treatment plans are important tools for therapists and clients. They provide a basis for "before and after" comparisons and reminders of intentions for future work. Even clients who are just seeking massage as a once-in-a-while treat can benefit from the clarification of goals that a treatment plan can offer.

Having a human figure that a client can mark with painful spots is a useful visual guide that will accompany a therapist's own sensitivities. Some people recommend that a client mark this figure with numbers from 1 to 10, indicating how painful certain areas might be.

Problems areas can change, move and even disappear. Treatment goals may also change as a person's health status evolves. Having clients redo this portion of the history form every few appointments can provide useful progress reports for the client-therapist team.

Some massage therapists use a standard "SOAP" format to accompany the general health information with a client history. It can be used with each appointment, or updated as needed. This format is as follows:

Subjective findings: That is, what does the client report—what hurts, where, when, and under what circumstances.

Objective findings: That is, what does the therapist find—are there different areas from the client's description that are painful? Does the tissue have varying qualities of elasticity and resilience in different areas? Are there hot spots? Cold areas? Limited range of motion?

Assessment: This is the therapist's interpretation of findings. It is *not* a diagnosis, but rather a pulling together of information to create an understanding of why a client is experiencing her symptoms.

Plan: This is the strategy the client and therapist will use together to achieve their goals. It might be as simple as "Swedish massage for relaxation of muscles, improved circulation and pain relief in upper back" or as complex as "Cross fiber friction to specific tendon insertions with range of motion gymnastics followed by ice and a referral to a physical therapist for strengthening exercises in order to overcome a chronic tendinitis."

An example of a client intake form is included here. This client is a real person, whose long-ago problems have recurring influence on her everyday living.

Sample Client History Form

Name *Janet M.*

General Information

Age *34*

Occupation: *Accounting. I sit at the computer and on the phone for 8 hours a day. I have a cordless headset.*

Describe your exercise habits: *I walk two times a day, for fifteen minutes. Some days are more vigorous than others. From July to October I coach cheerleading, and I never ask the girls to do something I'm not willing to do.*

Describe your general diet: *I have a quick breakfast: a bagel or something like that. Lunch depends on how busy I am. It could be some yogurt, or a microwave meal, Sometimes I have leftovers from last night's supper. Dinner is always a sit-down meal. We eat lots of fruit and veggies.*

Describe how well you sleep: *I usually sleep for six hours, but I never feel rested. I can always remember my dreams. I never seem to get past the dream stage.*

Describe your general health: *It's pretty good. I seldom get sick, although it's happened more this year than ever before. I have to make myself do a lot of things—I have very low energy. And depression is a factor in all of this too.*

Health History

Describe any surgery or hospitalization:

More than 10 years ago:
1988: childbirth, followed by cryosurgery for dysplasia.

5 to 10 years ago:
1990: I had a kidney stone while I was pregnant. I finally passed it, soon before my daughter was born. If I hadn't, they would have taken it out right after labor.

Less than 5 years ago:
Four years ago I had two surgeries for thoracic outlet syndrome. In the first one they went in through the axilla on the left side. They took out the cervical rib and the first rib. A month later they did the same thing on the right side, but they only took the first rib. The cervical rib was too small to worry about.

Describe any injuries or an accidents:

More than 10 years ago:
I was in a VW in the middle of a 5-car pile up. My little car ended up looking like an accordion.

5 to 10 years ago:

Less than 5 years ago:

What kind of care did you receive?

No care for the whiplash following the car wreck. Lots of physical therapy following my surgeries.

Do you consider that you have recovered from these events? Please explain:

Oh, yes. Before I had surgery, I couldn't even hold my hands above my shoulders.

Do you have any chronic, ongoing conditions that you deal with on a regular basis? Explain.

Sure. I have pain, fatigue, stress, depression. Several months ago I was diagnosed with fibromyalgia.

Are you taking any medication? Please explain:

I take Zoloft, an anti-depressant.

Are you currently seeing a doctor for any reason? Please explain:

Yes, I see an MD for fibromyalgia and a chiropractor as needed.

Do you have any skin rashes or other skin problems right now?

No.

Check off any of the following conditions that you have experienced:

Skin	**Musculoskeletal**	**Nervous**
Boils	✔ Fibromyalgia	Depression
Fungal infections	Rheumatoid arthritis	Multiple sclerosis
Herpes simplex	Osteoarthritis	Post polio syndrome
Warts	TMJ dysfunction	✔ Headaches
Eczema	Strains, sprains or tendinitis	Stroke
Psoriasis	Carpal tunnel syndrome	Seizure disorders
Skin cancer	✔ Thoracic outlet syndrome	Reduced sensation
		Sleep disorders
		Chemical dependency
Circulatory	**Lymph/Immune**	**Respiratory**
Anemia	Edema	Asthma
Thrombophlebitis	Leukemia/lymphoma	Emphysema
Deep vein thrombosis	HIV/ AIDS	Sinusitis
High blood pressure	✔ Chronic fatigue syndrome	Tuberculosis
Heart disease	Lupus	
Varicose veins	Other auto-immune disorders	
Clotting disorders		
Digestive	**Endocrine**	**Urinary**
GERD (reflux)	Diabetes	✔ Kidney stones
Ulcers	Hypothyroidism	Renal failure
Crohn disease	Hyperthyroidism	Ulcerative colitis
✔ Irritable bowel syndrome		
Gallstones		
Cirrhosis		
Hepatitis		
Reproductive		
Breast cancer		
Endometriosis		
Ovarian cysts		
Prostate cancer		
Painful menstruation		
Are you pregnant?		

Other: *My hands swell up at night. I had severe dizziness and headaches for several months at the onset of the fibromyalgia.*

Explanation: *The chronic fatigue and irritable bowel syndrome are part of the fibromyalgia.*

Treatment Goals:

Why are you here? What do you hope to accomplish?
I was told this would help with stress and muscle pain.

Please indicate where you have pain:

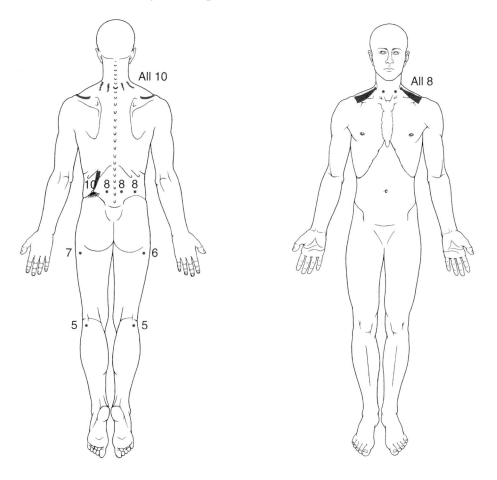

Describe what you do that causes pain, and what activities tend to make it worse:
At the onset of my fibromyalgia I was working full time, I went to school two nights a week, I was on the PTA and helped to run Brownies. I've found that overdoing in general makes everything much worse, but so does doing nothing. I also have to be careful about over-exercising.

What questions do you have about massage or this massage session?
How bad is it going to hurt, and how often should I do it?

Subjective findings

These are recorded on the image of the human body, above.

Objective findings

Janet's tissues are generally mobile and elastic superficially, although there is a sense of brittleness or fragility when the deeper layers are palpated. Circulation is good. The area over and above the scapula on the right side is particularly unyielding; it feels like a piece of cardboard under skin. By the end of our time together it had begun to give, but just a little.

When she lies supine, Janet's shoulders rise up off the table by several inches. The tissue on the anterior aspect of the shoulder girdle is tender and not clearly definable through touch.

Assessment

I suspect that as a result of Janet's thoracic outlet surgery, her pectoralis minor and major are bound up with significant scar tissue. This accounts for the rolling of the shoulders anteriorly, and the chronic pain she feels in her upper back—she marked these areas with "10"s on her chart. I wouldn't be at all surprised if her diagnosis of fibromyalgia related to the muscular imbalances caused by her surgeries, although the headaches and dizziness she experienced may be connected to a different aspect of that disease.

Plan

I recommend regular sessions (every week or every other week, depending on time constraints) of gentle Swedish massage, focussing on the muscular relationships surrounding the shoulder girdle: pec minor and major, the deltoid, trapezius, rhomboids, levator scapulae, etc.

I encourage Janet to do the exercises taught by her physical therapist to stretch the anterior shoulder girdle muscles.

I plan to focus on the paraspinals and quadratus lumborum, perhaps in relationship to the ilio-psoas, in future appointments.

I plan to work slowly and conservatively, and to encourage Janet to drink a lot of water following each appointment so that she can minimize any soreness that may follow.

Hygienic Methods for Massage Therapists

Massage therapists work with a physical intimacy unmatched by practically any other health care profession. How many health professionals, outside of surgeons, spend an hour or more devoting the total of their concentration and focus, as well as their touch, to the well-being of their clients?

Working in physically intimate circumstances carries the risk of spreading infection. Infection can move from the therapist to the client, but also from the client to the therapist (who can transfer it to the next client, and so on). For this reason, massage therapists have to be very familiar with the most common types of infectious agents to recognize them when possible and to guard against them always.

The guidelines provided here are probably more conservative than most practicing therapists observe. Massage is a quickly growing profession, however, and massage therapists will be increasingly at risk for professional liability if stringent standards of cleanliness and professionalism are not followed.

This discussion focuses on three aspects of keeping therapists and clients healthy: the infectious agents to guard against, methods by which to keep free of infection, and practical implications for massage therapists.

Infectious Agents

Millions of pathogens can make people sick. The main groups discussed here are not a comprehensive list, but cover the agents that are most common in industrialized countries. They include bacteria, viruses, fungi, and animal parasites.

Bacteria

These are divided into saprophytes (the "good guys" that live off dead material) and parasites (the "bad guys" that live off living material—like human bodies).

Parasitical bacteria include the following groups:

- Cocci (round-shaped bacteria), which appear in these configurations:

  - *Staphylococcus* bacteria are shaped like bunches of grapes. They are responsible for most local skin infections, boils, and acne.

  - *Streptococcus* bacteria are in chains. They are involved in many systemic infections like strep throat and blood poisoning.

  - *Gonococcus* bacteria cause gonorrhea.

  - *Diplococcus* bacteria cause bacterial pneumonia.

Everybody has colonies of bacteria growing on their skin. Hosts do not usually become sick because their immune system can develop resistance to resident pathogens. However, clients, especially clients who are in any way immune-suppressed, will not be so resistant to a therapist's personal colonies of bacteria. This why it is so important to avoid touching areas where the skin is not intact: these lesions are an infection waiting to happen.

Staphylococcus and streptococcus are the two most important bacteria to know about. These have mutated into thousands of tough varieties that can be difficult to treat.

Other types of bacteria are less common, but it is a good idea to be familiar with them. They include:

- *Bacilli*. These rod-shaped bacteria are the spore-makers. They have a tough outer shell that protects them from the environment and many chemicals that would kill other bacteria. Bacilli bacteria are responsible for anthrax, tuberculosis, typhoid, tetanus, and diphtheria.

- *Spirochetes*. These spiral-shaped bacteria cause syphilis and Lyme disease and contribute to the development of peptic ulcers.

Viruses

Viruses are not, technically speaking, alive. They are tiny (much smaller than bacteria) collections of proteins with genetic coding. Once inside a host cell, the virus changes the function of that cell to be a virus factory. When that factory is full of inventory, it ruptures, releasing the new viruses to search for new host cells.

Viruses outside bodies usually disintegrate fairly quickly. Some of them, however, are tougher to get rid of than others. The two main adversaries of massage therapists are herpes simplex and hepatitis B.

- *Herpes simplex*. This is the virus that causes oral and genital herpes. It is a sturdy virus that can linger on tables, doorknobs, and other surfaces for several hours. It is highly contagious in the acute (blistering) stage. If a client has fever blisters or suspicious sores around their thighs and buttocks, consider them at least locally contraindicated and isolate sheets, face pads, or other equipment in a special laundry container for bleaching.

- *Hepatitis B*. This virus is not easy to catch (it requires some sort of intimate contact or fluid exchange), but it has a serious impact on the body and is strongly associated with liver cancer. Hepatitis B is transmissible through shared fluid, including saliva, lymph, and blood. The virus is extremely sturdy and very virulent. It is the leading killer of nurses in the United States. In some places, it is considered to be an epidemic.

  A vaccine for hepatitis B has been developed. People who are in blood-exposure professions are required to get it, and massage therapists can, too.

Fungi

The chief enemies here are dermatophytes, specifically the fungi that cause tinea corporis (body ringworm), tinea capitis (head ringworm), tinea cruris (jock itch), or tinea pedis (Athlete's foot). Tinea lesions look like red, slightly raised rings on the skin. They are very common and very contagious, especially for people with weak immune systems.

Fungal infections can have a gestation period of 2 to 3 weeks, during which time the infected person can transmit the fungus to others.

Animal Parasites

Three main species comprise the majority of animal parasites that can spread from one person to another.

- *Head lice.* These are arthropods that live on the scalp. They spread from one person to another very easily, either by jumping from one head to the next or by lurking on coat hooks, chair backs, or in shared hats. Lice are often identified by the presence of nits—lice eggs—that are white and cling to hair shafts.

- *Body lice.* These are close relatives of head lice. They usually live in pubic hair but can also be found in body hair, eyebrows, and eyelashes. They drink blood and cause a great amount of itching. Body lice usually spread through intimate contact, as in sharing a bed or massage sheets.

- *Scabies.* These are lesions caused by microscopic mites that burrow under the skin, drinking blood, laying eggs, and leaving irritating wastes. They can be hard to diagnose because actual bugs are not always picked up in skin samples. Scabies lesions are itchy, especially at night, and they often appear in warm, sweaty places like the groin, armpits, crooks of elbows and knees, and between fingers and toes.

Consider the sheets and other linens of any client who shows signs of parasitical infestation as "hot." Separate them from other sheets and wash them in hot water with extra bleach.

Aseptic Methods: Keeping Free from Infection

Asepsis means absence of infection. Aseptic methods are techniques to keep massage therapists and their clients as free as possible from infectious agents.

Antiseptics

Antiseptic substances are the weakest of the aseptic methods. They create a hostile environment for many bacteria, although they may not actually kill them. Antiseptics are ineffective against bacteria that are encased in spores and many viruses. Antiseptics are safe to use on skin. Some antiseptics (rubbing alcohol, iodine, hydrogen peroxide) used to be considered disinfectants (a stronger class of germ-killer) but now, because germs have become so much tougher, they can no longer dependably kill what they used to.

Antiseptics include:

- *Hand soap.* Some hand soaps include special germ-killers in their formulae. These may increase the soap's effectiveness at killing easily accessible pathogens, but this does not mean that hands washed with special antiseptic soap are completely germ-free.

- *Rubbing alcohol.* Rubbing alcohol works best in a 70% solution (as it is packaged) because a 100% solution makes the germs' membranes thicker and less permeable. Rubbing alcohol is effective against bacteria but not viruses or spores.

- *Hydrogen peroxide.* This is a mild antiseptic that is used in 3% solution for skin and mucous membranes.

Disinfectants

These are agents that should be effective against all viruses and bacteria except those with spores. Many disinfectants are marketed with target pathogens. They can also be called *germicides* or *bactericides.*

Disinfectant techniques are too strong to be used on skin, but as a rule, they *do not* kill spores.

Examples include:

- *Bleach.* A 10% solution is used for surfaces, and 1 cup/wash is used for laundry. Bleach is effective against staphylococcus, streptococcus, fungus, hepatitis, HIV, and herpes. It is still the industry standard for disinfecting most surfaces.

- *Phenol.* A 10% solution of phenol can be used for surfaces. It is caustic to skin and lungs. Phenol is effective against bacteria, fungus, herpes, and flu virus.

- *Quaternary ammonium compounds (Quats).* These substances are available through medical or janitorial supply outlets. Although they are useful for killing pathogens, they do not necessarily remove dirt or other debris. Quats are used for "cold sterilization" of items that cannot be subjected to an autoclave.

Sterilization

These methods kill every living thing within a field. Massage therapists cannot sterilize themselves or their clients, but they can sterilize some of their tools and work surfaces, if absolutely necessary.

Some sterilization methods include:

- *Baking.* At 350°F for 1 hour.

- *Boiling.* The item should be completely immersed in water at 212°F for 20 minutes.

- *Autoclave (steam cabinet).* Items should be under 15 psi, at 250°F for 30 minutes.

Microwave ovens do not sterilize items because the heat is unevenly distributed.

Practical Applications for Massage Therapists

Massage therapists should be especially aware of the dangers of pathogens and parasites. They carry the risks of contracting disease themselves and of spreading disease from client to client. It is important for massage therapists to use aseptic methods wisely and regularly.

Personal Cleanliness

- *Washing hands.* It is impossible to say this too often. Hands should be washed between clients and after handling tissues or other bodily fluid-bearing items. Remember that cold and flu viruses are transmitted by hands far more efficiently than by floating randomly in the air. The friction of hands rubbing together is the most important part of handwashing.

- *Keep fingernails short and clean.* Imagine getting a massage from someone with longish or slightly dirty nails. How relaxed could a person be, imagining all those cooties crawling around on the skin?

- *Attend to clothing.* Uniforms, jackets, or aprons should be scrupulously clean. If a style of massage is practiced where the client's skin comes in contact with the therapist's clothing (e.g., when arms are being treated), then that clothing should be treated in the same way as sheets. Care should be taken so that one client does not come in contact with cloth or materials that may have been contaminated by a previous client.

- *Broken skin.* Broken skin is an open invitation to infection. Massage therapists should avoid it on their clients and keep it covered on themselves. Rubber "finger cots" are extremely useful items when a therapist has a scraped knuckle or a hangnail.

Linen

Laws regarding linen storage for health care professionals vary from state to state. Some states require professionals to store their dirty linen in closed containers and clean linen in closed cabinets. It is a good idea to have a second container available for "hot" sheets that need to be treated with special care. In addition to sheets, a massage therapist's laundry may include uniforms or aprons, pillowcases, face hole covers, heating pad covers, towels, bolster covers, and anything else that contacts a client's skin.

Beware of stuffing oily sheets into baskets or boxes and letting them sit. Oil will go rancid and smell, or it has been known to spontaneously combust. The moral: wash sheets promptly!

Some massage therapists or clinics hire a laundry service to take care of their linens. In this case sheets will probably be rented from the service. These sheets are typically washed and rinsed repeatedly at 180°F. They are bleached and then subjected to antibleachers to reduce the chemical aftermath. Even so, some people may have a reaction to the chemicals left in the fabric.

Extra blankets, mattress pads, sheepskins, etc., do not need to be washed unless they come in contact with clients. It is a good idea to wash them once a month or so anyway, just for freshness.

Storage and Dispensation of Oil, Lotion, and Creams

All lubricants need to be kept in clean containers and dispensed in a way that prevents contamination. For instance, if a therapist has a tub of coconut oil, he or she must dip out what is going to be used into a paper cup (using a spatula, not the fingers). Then the therapist must *not* put the leftovers back into the tub—it is contaminated and must be thrown away.

Remember that if a client has a contagious condition—herpes, for example—the therapist may transmit the virus to the outside of the oil bottle. That same oil bottle may be used for the next client, and the virus is lurking on the surface just waiting for a chance to get on another potential host's skin. In other words, it is a good idea to wash oil bottles at the same time as washing hands.

Care of Massage Tables and Other Equipment

If a client who shows signs of a communicable disease has been on a table, it is time to swab. A 70% concentration of rubbing alcohol is the standard, although it is drying to vinyl and of questionable impact against sturdy viruses like herpes and hepatitis B. (It will remove those annoying oily hand prints, though.) Regardless, it is a good habit to swab the table once a week or so, especially the face cradle.

Any other surfaces that clients contact should be cleaned regularly. Most things like heat or cold packs are probably covered by cloth that can be laundered, but therapists must be ever-vigilant against possible contaminated surfaces.

Client Endangerments

Endangerments are sites where massage therapists can cause damage to some of the body's most delicate tissues. Structures particularly at risk are nerves, blood vessels, organs, and lymph nodes. This list covers the most basic endangerments, although if a massage therapist tries hard enough he or she could cause injury to almost any part of the body.

Nerves

Pinning or compressing nerves can bruise, irritate, or otherwise damage them. Clients can experience sharp shooting, tingling, electric, or hot sensations when this happens. It is important to know the pathways of the most vulnerable nerves because, unfortunately, massage therapists cannot always count on clients, some of whom expect massage to hurt, to give accurate feedback about whether the pain they are feeling is "good" pain or bad pain.

Blood Vessels

The general risk of arterial entrapment is the blocking of circulation, causing numbness, discomfort, and even blackouts. Entrapment of veins, since they are weaker, can injure them, creating varicosities, hemorrhages, or clots.

Organs

There are a few organs that can be trapped and impaired by massage therapy. They are generally at risk because they are close to the surface or they are anchored in a way that makes them vulnerable to being pinned or compressed.

Lymph Nodes

Lymph nodes are epithelial cells within a connective tissue framework. They are especially palpable when they are inflamed; being able to feel lymph nodes, especially around the neck or the back of the head, often indicates that they are working overtime and the client may be fighting off an infection.

Head and Face Endangerments

- *Eyes.* Obviously, eyes are a local caution for massage. Special care must also be taken with clients who wear contact lenses. If a client wears hard contacts, the therapist should suggest that they be removed during a treatment (potential problems include drying out and lacerations to the sclera). If a client wears soft or extended wear contacts, removing them probably will not be an issue. Some therapists keep a bottle of distilled water and a lens case in their office, just in case a client decides to remove their contact lenses.

- *Nerve foramina.* Three pairs of foramina allow the mental, the infraorbital, and the supraorbital nerves to exit from the skull. These nerves supply the face with sensation and motor control. Heavy pressure on these spots can be extremely painful and may even damage the nerves as they emerge (Fig. 1).

- *Temporomandibular joint (TMJ).* Branches of both the trigeminal and the facial nerves are accessible near the TMJ. Whether massage therapy could actually cause an attack of Bell's palsy or trigeminal neuralgia is not clear, but it is the responsibility of every therapist to know how to avoid even the possibility of putting a client at risk for these problems.

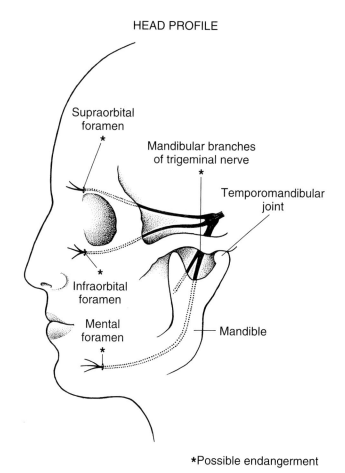

HEAD PROFILE

*Possible endangerment

Figure 1. Head profile

This is not to say that the whole TMJ area and jaw muscles are off-limits to massage. On the contrary, massage can be an important part of reducing habitual muscle tone in persons prone to jaw-clenching. Nevertheless, massage practitioners who work in this area must know where the nerves are vulnerable and how to avoid putting them at risk (Fig. 1).

Anterior Trunk and Neck Endangerments

For all structures in the anterior triangle of the neck and the anterior trunk, see Figure 1.

- *Anterior triangle of the neck.* The anterior triangle of the neck is defined by the sternal fibers of the left and right sternocleidomastoid muscles and the mandible. Many structures contained in this area are vulnerable to damage, and not much musculature that is easily accessible for massage. Some therapists make a specialty of working on the muscles of the anterior neck with good results, but they, along with all other massage practitioners, must be very familiar with the complicated anatomy of this area in order to stay out of harm's way. Structures in the anterior triangle of the neck that must be respected include:

  - *Common carotid artery*
    This huge artery runs deep to the sternocleidomastoid muscles and carries most of the blood supply to the head. About level with the thyroid cartilage, the common carotid artery splits into the internal and external carotid artery. The point of division, the carotid sinus, is equipped with special sensory nerves that measure blood pressure to maintain appropriate blood flow to the head. External pressure applied here can alter that blood flow, leading to dizziness and faintness. Atherosclerotic plaque can also accumulate in the carotid artery, making this area a local contraindication for clients with a high risk of cardiovascular disease.

  - *Jugular vein*
    The jugular vein lies superficial to the common carotid. It is less vulnerable to damage but still does not need to be stretched or compressed in any way.

  - *Trachea*
    This cartilaginous tube is part of the respiratory system and leads to the lungs. It is quite strong and resilient, but pressure directly on the tube will cause a choking feeling for the client.

  - *Thyroid cartilage*
    The thyroid cartilage is a moveable piece of material that bobs up and down with the swallowing reflex. The most prominent part of the thyroid cartilage is the laryngeal prominence, or Adam's apple.

  - *Thyroid gland*
    The thyroid gland is a butterfly-shaped piece of epithelium that wraps around the trachea. It is an endocrine gland, secreting hormones that control metabolism. Embedded within the thyroid gland are much smaller parathyroid

ANTERIOR TRUNK

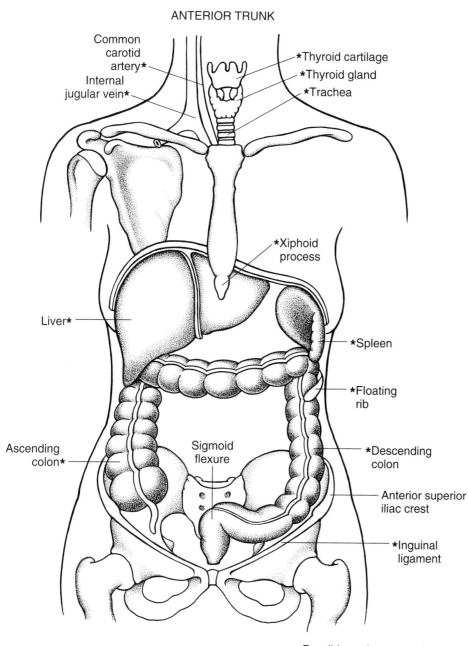

Common
carotid
artery*

Internal
jugular vein*

*Thyroid cartilage
*Thyroid gland
*Trachea

*Xiphoid
process

Liver*

*Spleen

*Floating
rib

Ascending
colon*

Sigmoid
flexure

*Descending
colon

Anterior superior
iliac crest

*Inguinal
ligament

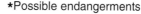

*Possible endangerments

Figure 2. Anterior trunk

glands. This whole structure is primarily epithelial, with little connective tissue protection.

- *Brachial plexus: neck and shoulder.* The brachial plexus is made up of spinal nerves C5 to T1. They criss-cross and interweave with each other before separating into the different nerves that supply the arm. Most of this interweaving happens between the neck and the shoulder. The nerves run between the medial and posterior scalene muscles, under the clavicle and coracoid process, and then wrap around the humerus. They are larger than they seem; coming out of the neck they are actually about the same thickness as shoelaces. They can be pinned against several different bones or other tissues on their way to the arm, so massage therapists should be very familiar with the pathways of the brachial plexus nerves.

- *Xiphoid process.* The inferior edge of the sternum has a small piece of bone that protrudes out over the liver. This prominence, the xiphoid process, can be broken off if sharp, downward pressure is exerted on it.

- *Floating ribs.* Massage is unlikely to actually damage floating ribs. Tracing or outlining the ribcage can cause ticklishness or even pain if a therapist does not know exactly where the floating ribs are and how to avoid pinning soft tissue against them.

- *Liver.* A massage therapist would have to be working much too deep and hard than is usually called far to bruise a healthy liver. However, it is good to know both where it is located and how big it is. Clients with enlarged livers due to hepatitis, jaundice, cirrhosis, or other problems may be particularly sensitive in this area.

- *Spleen.* The spleen is tucked up way under the left ribs. For most people the spleen is not a significant endangerment, but if it is enlarged for any reason the whole area can be uncomfortable.

- *Colon.* The colon is at special risk for entrapment and bruising because it is anchored at the flexures and cannot simply move out of the way like the small intestine can. Care must be taken, when doing deep abdominal work, to respect both that the colon can be pinned, and that material should move through it in a clockwise direction. Pressure should not be exerted contrary to this direction of flow.

- *Ovaries.* The ovaries are normally located so low and central in the pelvis that they are inaccessible to massage therapists. Sometimes, though, endometriosis, an ovarian cyst, or other anomaly can cause the ovaries to move into areas where they may be pinned and bruised.

Posterior Trunk and Neck Endangerments

For all structures in the posterior trunk and neck, see Figure 3.

- *Kidneys.* The kidneys are vulnerable to damage because they are only partially protected by the rib cage. The right kidney sits a bit lower than the left. An easy way to remember this is that it looks like the right kidney is pushed downward by the liver. Both can be bruised if vigorous tapotement is performed over the mid-back area.

- *Spinous processes.* These are listed as endangerments because massage therapists can cause pain by pressing or frictioning paraspinal muscles in toward the spinous processes, rather than out and away from them. Pressure toward the spine can be appropriate, as long as soft tissues are not being impaled or ground into hard ones.

POSTERIOR TRUNK

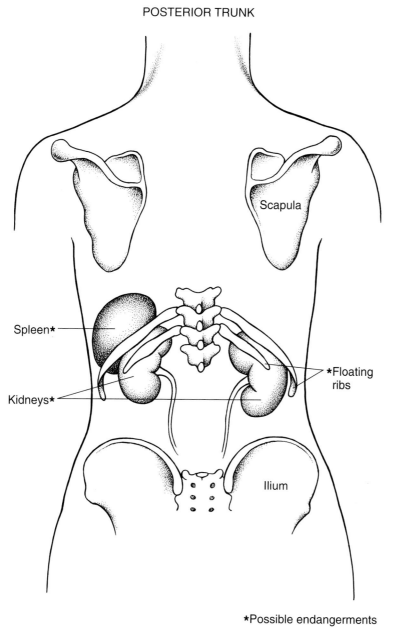

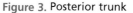

*Possible endangerments

Figure 3. Posterior trunk

Arm Endangerments

For structures in the arms, see Figures 4 and 5.

- *Brachial plexus: arm.* By the time the brachial plexus has reached the arm it has separated into its five different components: the axillary nerve, the musculocutaneous nerve, and the radial, median, and ulnar nerves. It is useful to know the basic pathways of all these structures, although they may vary slightly from one person to another. Specific endangerment spots include the axilla, the medial aspect of the upper arm, and the cubital fossa. The ulnar nerve is vulnerable medial to the olecranon: it causes the "funny bone" sensation when it is knocked or irritated.

- *Axillary lymph nodes.* Lymph nodes should not be specifically isolated or massaged. They have the important job of filtering pathogens from the blood, and should be left alone.

- *Cephalic and basilic veins.* Veins, perhaps more than any other structure discussed here, run in pathways that are unique from one person to the next, so it is impossible to state categorically where they might be vulnerable. One thing that is consistent, however, is that they run at least part way up the medial side of the upper arm.

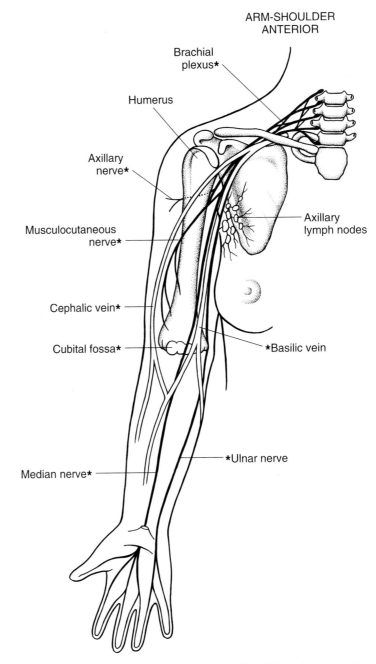

Figure 4. Anterior arm/shoulder

Conveniently, this is already an area to avoid because some of the brachial plexus nerves are also vulnerable here. The cephalic vein can also be trapped where it runs along the edges of the anterior deltoid and pectoralis major.

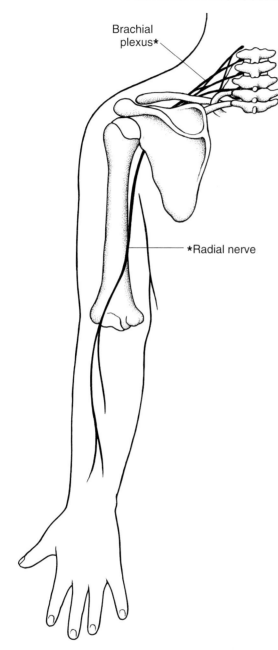

POSTERIOR ARM/SHOULDER

Brachial plexus*

*Radial nerve

Figure 5. Posterior arm/shoulder

Leg Endangerments

For structures of the legs, see Figures 6, 7, 8, and 9.

- *Femoral triangle.* The femoral triangle, defined by the inguinal ligament and the sartorius muscle, is a particularly rich area for vulnerable structures. The femoral artery and vein are both accessible here, as are the inguinal lymph nodes and the femoral nerve. Deep, specific work on the adductors must be conducted with special care to avoid damaging these structures (Fig. 6).

- *Sciatic nerve.* The sciatic nerve, the thickest nerve in the body, runs through the deep lateral rotators and down the back of the leg, where it splits into the common peroneal nerve and the tibial nerve. The sciatic nerve is difficult to pin or damage because the musculature surrounding it is so thick, but if the nerve is irritated for any reason, massage may exacerbate the situation (Fig. 7)

- *Popliteal fossa.* The popliteal fossa is the area on the posterior aspect of the knee that is defined by the heads of the gastrocnemius below, and the edges of the biceps femoris and the semitendinosus above. In this hollow area there are several structures to know about, including the small saphenous vein, the popliteal vein, the popliteal artery, and the lower branches of the sciatic nerve: the tibial and common peroneal nerves (Fig. 7).

- *Great saphenous vein.* The great saphenous vein runs up the medial side of the calf where there is little to protect it from being pinned to the tibia. On the upper leg the vein runs along the edge of the sartorius, but the quadriceps are bulky enough that pinning the great saphenous to the femur is not generally possible (Fig. 8).

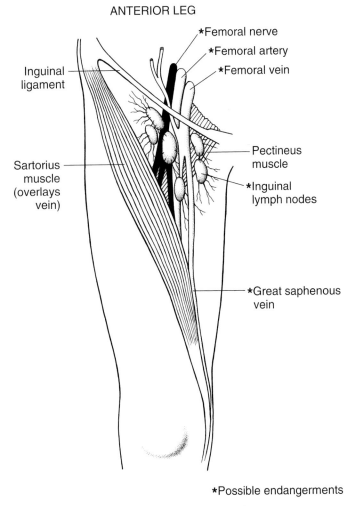

ANTERIOR LEG

*Femoral nerve
*Femoral artery
*Femoral vein

Inguinal ligament

Pectineus muscle

Sartorius muscle (overlays vein)

*Inguinal lymph nodes

*Great saphenous vein

*Possible endangerments

Figure 6. Anterior leg

POSTERIOR LEG

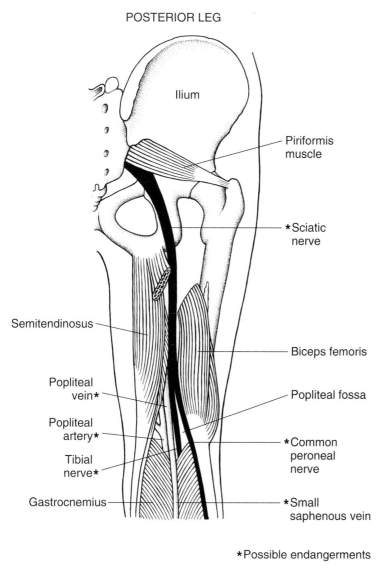

Ilium

Piriformis muscle

*Sciatic nerve

Semitendinosus

Biceps femoris

Popliteal vein*

Popliteal fossa

Popliteal artery*

*Common peroneal nerve

Tibial nerve*

Gastrocnemius

*Small saphenous vein

*Possible endangerments

Figure 7. Posterior leg

- *Common peroneal nerve.* The common peroneal nerve is vulnerable for a short distance just inferior to the head of the fibula. Specific pressure or friction on the peroneus longus can sometimes irritate this nerve, which will send shocky, electrical sensations down into the foot (Fig. 9).

MEDIAL LEG   LATERAL LEG

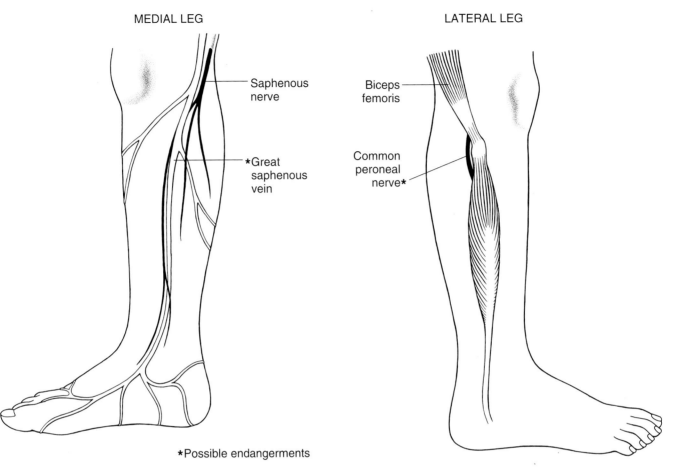

Saphenous
nerve

*Great
saphenous
vein

Biceps
femoris

Common
peroneal
nerve*

*Possible endangerments

Figure 8. Medial leg

Figure 9. Lateral leg

Quick Reference Charts

Read This First!

This appendix provides a reference for massage students and practitioners who need fast answers to simple questions. It is *not* intended as a substitute for reading the complete article for each condition, and will not provide enough information to make a well-informed decision without that background. Some conditions listed here, however, are not detailed in the text. These have been marked with an *.

Several things are important to remember while using these quick reference charts:

- The label "indicated" does *not* mean that a condition will always be improved by massage. It means that massage will not make the situation worse, and the support and comfort massage gives can certainly be beneficial to the client, if not to the particular condition.
- The term "massage" refers to circulatory-based massage that has a direct effect on blood and lymph flow. If a condition is labeled "contraindicated," it's usually because the influence of massage on circulation would have a negative impact on the client. This does not necessarily rule out touch altogether, however, and many conditions that contraindicate vigorous circulatory massage are perfectly appropriate for less mechanically based bodywork modalities.
- When massage is considered appropriate or indicated, it is a systemic recommendation. When massage is contraindicated, guidelines for whether those cautions are local or systemic have been provided.
- The specific kind of impact that massage may have on various conditions is discussed in the complete articles rather than here in the abbreviated version.

The most important thing to remember is that it is impossible to make a foolproof judgement about whether massage is a good choice strictly from a book. Every client is different; every practitioner has a different kind of approach. These recommendations are just that: *recommendations* that may help to shape well-informed decisions about the appropriateness of massage.

CONDITION NAME	WHAT IS IT/ WHAT ARE THEY?	HOW IS IT RECOGNIZED/ HOW ARE THEY RECOGNIZED?	IS MASSAGE INDICATED OR CONTRAINDICATED?
ABORTION, SPONTANEOUS AND ELECTIVE IN BRIEF (page 454)	Spontaneous and elective abortions are pregnancies that are ended, unintentionally or intentionally, before the fetus is born naturally.	Generalized or pelvic pain may be present, along with vaginal bleeding. Often, however, no outward signs may show that a woman is recovering from a spontaneous or elective abortion.	Massage is locally contraindicated (no deep abdominal work) for women recovering from a recent spontaneous or elective abortion until her bleeding has stopped and she is free of any signs of infection. Bodywork elsewhere can be supportive and helpful.
ACNE IN BRIEF (page 18)	Acne is a bacterial infection of sebaceous glands usually found on the face, neck, and upper back. It is closely associated with adolescence or liver dysfunction that results in excess testosterone in the system.	It looks like raised, inflamed pustules on the skin, sometimes with white or black tips.	Acne locally contraindicates massage, because of the risk of spreading infection, causing pain, and exacerbating the symptoms with the application of an oily lubricant.
ACROMEGALY IN BRIEF (page 418)	Acromegaly is a condition involving the excessive secretion of growth hormone, often related to a benign tumor on the pituitary gland.	This disorder usually begins in middle age, when patients find that their hands, feet, and face have gradually grown and become distorted. Joint pain with bony deformation is common. Debilitating headaches, visual problems, or cranial nerve damage may occur if the tumor presses on sensitive tissue in the central nervous system. Ultimately, cardiovascular weakness will develop as the heart tries to pump blood to new tissues.	The primary risk for most acromegaly patients is that their cardiovascular system cannot keep up with the demands of their suddenly growing bodies. High blood pressure, enlargement of the heart, and heart failure are common complications of this disorder. As long as those concerns are respected and the therapist does not challenge the circulatory system of the client too vigorously, massage may be appropriate for acromegaly patients, who also experience joint pain. Massage therapists should work with these clients as part of a well-informed health care team.
ACUTE BRONCHITIS IN BRIEF (page 332)	Acute bronchitis is an infection and inflammation of the bronchiole tree, anywhere between the trachea and the bronchioles. If inflammation extends into the bronchioles and alveoli, it is called bronchopneumonia.	The hallmark of acute bronchitis is a persistent productive cough along with sore throat, nasal congestion, fatigue, and possibly low fever. Whereas other symptoms generally subside within 10 days, the cough may last for several weeks while the bronchi heal.	Acute bronchitis, like all acute infections, contraindicates circulatory massage. If the infection has passed and the cough is the only lingering symptom, massage may be appropriate as long as the client is comfortable on the table.
ALZHEIMER'S DISEASE IN BRIEF (page 160)	Alzheimer's disease is a degenerative disorder of the brain involving shrinkage and death of neural tissue.	Alzheimer's disease is difficult to diagnose definitively in a living person, but signs and symptoms include progressive memory loss, deterioration of language and cognitive skills, disorientation, and lack of ability to care for oneself.	If an Alzheimer's disease patient feels comfortable and nurtured while receiving touch, then massage is very much indicated. If the patient feels disoriented and threatened, the therapist will have to change tactics. Alzheimer's patients may not be able to communicate verbally, so therapists must be sensitive to nonverbal cues.

CONDITION NAME	WHAT IS IT/ WHAT ARE THEY?	HOW IS IT RECOGNIZED/ HOW ARE THEY RECOGNIZED?	IS MASSAGE INDICATED OR CONTRAINDICATED?
AMYOTROPHIC LATERAL SCLEROSIS IN BRIEF (page 163)	Amyotrophic lateral sclerosis (ALS) is a progressive disease that begins in the central nervous system. It involves the degeneration of motor neurons and the subsequent atrophy of voluntary muscles.	Symptoms of ALS include weakness, fatigue, and muscle spasms. It appears most frequently in patients between 40 and 70 years of age.	ALS indicates massage, with caution, when a massage therapist works as part of a health care team.
ANEMIA IN BRIEF (page 249)	Anemia is a symptom rather than a disease itself. It indicates a shortage of red blood cells, or of hemoglobin, or both.	Symptoms of anemia include pallor, shortness of breath, fatigue, and poor resistance to cold. Other symptoms may accompany specific varieties of anemia.	Anemia that is idiopathic or due to nutritional deficiency may indicate massage, as long as no neurologic damage has occurred. Anemia related to bone marrow suppression (i.e., cancer), chronic disease or inlammation, or premature destruction of red blood cells may contraindicate rigorous bodywork, although some types of energy work may be appropriate.
ANEURYSM IN BRIEF (page 267)	An aneurysm is a bulge or out-pouching in a vein, artery, or the heart. They usually occur in the thoracic or abdominal aorta or in the arteries at the base of the brain.	Symptoms of aneurysms are determined by their location. Thoracic aneurysms may cause chronic hoarseness; abdominal aneurysms may cause local discomfort, reduced urine output, or severe backache. Cerebral aneurysms may be silent or may cause extreme headache when they are at very high risk for rupture.	If a client has been diagnosed with an aneurysm, circulatory massage will probably be contraindicated. Massage is also strongly cautioned for clients who fit the profile for aneurysms but have not been diagnosed.
ANKYLOSING SPONDYLITIS IN BRIEF (page 82)	Ankylosing spondylitis (AS) is progressive inflammatory arthritis of the spine.	It generally begins as stiffness and pain around the sacrum, with occasional referred pain down the back of the buttocks and into the legs. It has acute and subacute episodes. In advanced AS the vertebrae fuse together in a flexed position.	Massage is indicated in the subacute stages of AS, when along with exercise and physical therapy it may be useful in maintaining flexibility.
ANXIETY DISORDERS IN BRIEF (page 185)	Anxiety disorders are a group of mental disorders that have to do with exaggerated, irrational fears and the attempts to control those fears. Some anxiety disorders come and go, some are chronic progressive problems, and others reach a peak and then sometimes recede or remain stable. All anxiety disorders begin as emotional responses that create inappropriate sympathetic reactions.	Although triggers for individual cases may vary, many anxiety disorders involve sympathetic reactions in the body, including fast heart rate, sweating, dizziness, faintness, nausea, and other symptoms. In addition, some disorders bring about feelings of impending death, a sense of physical detachment, unwelcome or frightening thoughts, and other reactions.	If the stimulus of bodywork is perceived as something safe and welcome, then massage can have a useful place in dealing with a variety of anxiety disorders.
APPENDICITIS IN BRIEF (page 381)	Appendicitis is inflammation of the vermiform appendix. It is usually a result of infection following a blockage at the opening of the appendix. The blockage may be caused by a hardened piece of fecal matter or by lymphatic inflammation.	The symptoms of appendicitis are widely variable but include general abdominal pain that gradually settles in the lower right quadrant. Rebound pain is usually severe. Fever, nausea, vomiting, food aversion, constipation, and diarrhea may be present.	Acute appendicitis contraindicates massage. This condition may complicate into peritonitis if it is neglected.

CONDITION NAME	WHAT IS IT/ WHAT ARE THEY?	HOW IS IT RECOGNIZED/ HOW ARE THEY RECOGNIZED?	IS MASSAGE INDICATED OR CONTRAINDICATED?
ASTHMA IN BRIEF (page 348)	Asthma is the result of spasmodic constriction of bronchial smooth muscle tubes in combination with chronic local inflammation and excess production of mucus.	Asthma attacks are sporadic episodes involving coughing, wheezing, and difficulty with breathing, especially exhaling.	Massage is a good idea for anyone with asthma, as long as he or she is not in the throes of an attack. Between episodes massage can be useful to reduce stress and deal with some of the muscular problems that accompany difficulty with breathing.
ATHEROSCLEROSIS IN BRIEF (page 270)	Atherosclerosis is a condition in which the arteries become inelastic and brittle due to atherosclerotic plaques.	Atherosclerosis has no symptoms until it is very advanced. However, it is connected to several other types of circulatory problems, including hypertension, arrhythmia, coronary artery disease, cerebrovascular disease, and peripheral vascular disease.	Advanced atherosclerosis systemically contraindicates rigorous circulatory massage, but other modalities may offer many benefits with a minimum of risks.
BAKER CYSTS IN BRIEF (page 111)	Baker cysts are fluid-filled extensions of the synovial membrane at the knee. They protrude into the popliteal fossa, usually on the medial side.	Baker cysts are usually painless sacs that are palpable deep to the superficial fascia in the popliteal fossa. They may cause pain or a feeling of tightness in the knee in flexion.	Massage is locally contraindicated in the popliteal fossa anyway, especially if a Baker cyst is present. In addition, if any signs of circulatory disruption (coldness, clamminess, edema) are visible distal to the cyst, that whole area is a contraindication, and the client needs to be cleared of the possibility of thrombosis.
BELL'S PALSY IN BRIEF (page 205)	Bell's palsy is a flaccid paralysis of one side of the face caused by inflammation or damage to cranial nerve VII, the facial nerve.	Symptoms of Bell's palsy include drooping of the muscles on the affected side, difficulty with drinking and eating, and difficulty in closing the eye on one side. Pain, headaches, hypersensitivity to sound, and drooling may also occur.	Bell's palsy indicates massage to maintain flexibility and good circulation in the affected muscles. It is important, however, to rule out causes for the nerve damage that may contraindicate massage.
BENIGN PROSTATIC HYPERPLASIA IN BRIEF (page 478)	Benign prostatic hyperplasia (BPH) is a condition in which the prostate gland of a mature man begins to grow for the first time since the end of puberty. It is not related to cancer, which is why this condition is called "benign."	The primary symptoms of BPH have to do with mechanical obstruction of the urethra. This leads to problems with urination, including an increased need to urinate, difficulties with initiating flow, leaking, and the sensation that the bladder is never emptied. Many men with BPH never develop these symptoms, however. For them, BPH is a silent condition.	BPH is a common condition among mature men, and it does not usually involve cancer or infection. Massage is perfectly appropriate for these clients, as long as no signs of urinary tract infection or kidney disorders are present.

CONDITION NAME	WHAT IS IT/ WHAT ARE THEY?	HOW IS IT RECOGNIZED/ HOW ARE THEY RECOGNIZED?	IS MASSAGE INDICATED OR CONTRAINDICATED?
BOILS IN BRIEF (page 4)	Boils are localized bacterial infections of the skin. The causative agent is usually *Staphylococcus aureus*.	Boils involve painful, red, hot pustules on the skin. They may occur singly or in interconnected clusters called carbuncles.	Boils contraindicate massage at least locally, and care should be taken to make sure the infection is not systemic (the client should be screened for other symptoms such as swelling, fever, or discomfort other than at the site of the lesion). The bacteria that cause boils are extremely virulent and communicable. The sheets of a client with boils should be isolated and treated with bleach.
BLADDER CANCER IN BRIEF (page 442)	Bladder cancer is the growth of malignant cells in the urinary bladder. Most bladder cancer starts in the superficial layer of transitional epithelium.	The earliest sign of bladder cancer is the appearance of blood in the urine, which may be red or rust colored. Bladder cancer is painless at this point. In later stages the bladder may become irritable. Painful urination, reduced urination, or decreased urinary frequency may all occur.	As with most varieties of cancer, massage with its parasympathetic effects and immune system support has a place in the recovery process. Bladder cancer has a high recurrence rate and most patients undergo surgery at some point. As long as these issues are respected and the massage therapist works as part of a well-informed health care team, bodywork may be appropriate for these patients.
BREAST CANCER IN BRIEF (page 465)	Breast cancer is the growth of malignant tumor cells in breast tissue; these cells can invade skin and nearby muscles and bones. If they invade lymph nodes, they can metastasize to the rest of the body.	The first sign of breast cancer is a small painless lump or thickening in the breast tissue or near the axilla. The lump may be too small to palpate, but may show on a mammogram. Later the skin may change texture, the nipple may change shape, and discharge from the nipple may be present.	Many breast cancer patients undergo treatment options that are extremely taxing on general health and physical and emotional well-being. As long as bodywork choices are made that respect these challenges, massage can be a wonderful, supportive, important coping mechanism for many breast cancer patients.
BUNIONS IN BRIEF (page 113)	A bunion is a protrusion at the metatarsal-phalangeal joint of the great toe that occurs when the toe is laterally deviated.	Bunions are recognizable by the large bump on the medial aspect of the foot. When they are inflamed they are red, hot, and possibly edematous.	The point of a bunion locally contraindicates massage, especially when or if it is inflamed. Massage elsewhere on the foot or body is very much appropriate within pain tolerance to help with compensation patterns that occur when it is difficult to walk.
BURNS IN BRIEF (page 37)	Burns are caused by damage to the skin that causes the cells to die. They can be caused by fire, overexposure to the sun, dry heat, wet heat, electricity, radiation, extreme cold, and toxic chemicals.	First-degree burns involve mild inflammation. Second-degree burns also involve blistering and damage at the deeper levels of the epidermis. Third-degree burns go down into the dermis itself and often show white or black charred edges. In the post-acute stage, serious burns often involve shrunken, contracted scar tissue over the area of skin that has been affected.	Burns contraindicate massage (except, perhaps, mild sunburns) in the acute stage. In the subacute and post-acute stages, massage may be performed around the damaged area within pain tolerance of the client.

CONDITION NAME	WHAT IS IT/ WHAT ARE THEY?	HOW IS IT RECOGNIZED/ HOW ARE THEY RECOGNIZED?	IS MASSAGE INDICATED OR CONTRAINDICATED?
BURSITIS IN BRIEF (page 115)	A bursa is a fluid filled-sack that acts as a protective cushion at points of recurring pressure, eases the movement of tendons and ligaments moving over bones, and cushions points of contact between bones. Bursitis is the inflammation of a bursa.	Acute bursitis is painful and is aggravated by both passive and active motion. Muscles that tighten around the affected joint may severely limit range of motion. It may be hot or edematous if the bursa is superficial enough to be palpated.	Acute noninfectious bursitis locally contraindicates massage. Massage elsewhere on the body during an acute phase, and directly on the muscles of the affected joint (within pain limits) in a subacute phase, is perfectly appropriate.
CANCER IN BRIEF (page 497)	Cancer is the mutation of normal cells into cells with particular characteristics, including the tendency to proliferate into distinguishable growths and to spread through the body to other areas where they may colonize new tissues.	In early stages many cancers are difficult to detect. Later signs depend on what part of the body is being affected, but can include things like unusual bleeding, susceptibility to infection, changes in skin lesions, a persistent cough or hoarseness, changes in bladder or bowel habits, painless lumps or swellings, or pain where tumors have grown to the point that they compress or erode into delicate tissue.	The decision about whether to include massage as part of a treatment plan with cancer is a complicated one. Some types of bodywork are said to boost circulatory and lymph flow, which could be interpreted as increasing the risk of metastasis. Research shows, however, that it takes up to 9 years for many tumors to reach a palpable size. In light of this, it seems unlikely that a 60-minute session could have a serious impact on this disease process. Many cancer patients seek massage as a way to help them cope with the challenges of cancer treatments. Massage and other bodywork modalities offered in this context can be beneficial, as long as the risks of working with clients who are undergoing surgery, chemotherapy, radiation, or other procedures are respected, and the therapist works as part of a well-informed health care team.
CANDIDIASIS IN BRIEF (page 406)	Candidiasis is a condition in which the normally occurring *Candida albicans* fungi that colonize the gastrointestinal tract become invasive and disrupt normal function of the digestive system and other systems in the body.	Signs and symptoms of candidiasis can be severe and acute, involving mouth and skin lesions as well as systemic blood infections, or subtle and chronic, involving fatigue, impaired mental ability, food and chemical sensitivities, and several other symptoms in varying degrees of severity.	Chronic candidiasis indicates massage, but therapists should understand that many acute candidiasis patients experience compromised immune system function and so should take care to protect clients from the threat of infection.
CARPAL TUNNEL SYNDROME IN BRIEF (page 136)	Carpal tunnel syndrome (CTS) is irritation of the median nerve as it passes under the transverse carpal ligament into the wrist. It can have several different causes.	CTS can cause pain, tingling, numbness, and weakness in the part of the hand supplied by the median nerve. Pain may also radiate proximally up the forearm.	Depending on the underlying factors, some CTS cases may respond well to massage. Work on or around the wrist must stop immediately if any symptoms are elicited. It is necessary to get a medical diagnosis to know which type of CTS is present.

CONDITION NAME	WHAT IS IT/ WHAT ARE THEY?	HOW IS IT RECOGNIZED/ HOW ARE THEY RECOGNIZED?	IS MASSAGE INDICATED OR CONTRAINDICATED?
CEREBRAL PALSY IN BRIEF (page 207)	Cerebral palsy (CP) is an umbrella term used to refer to a variety of central nervous system injuries that may occur prenatally, at birth, or in early infancy. These injuries usually result in motor impairment but may also lead to sensory and cognitive problems as well.	CP is usually diagnosed early in infancy when voluntary motor skills are expected to begin to develop. CP patients may have hyper- or hypotonic muscles, suppressed or extreme reflexes, poor coordination, and they may show random, involuntary movement.	As long as sensation is intact and the patient is able to communicate with the therapist in some way, massage is appropriate and potentially very useful for persons with CP, as they work to maintain muscular elasticity and improve motor skills.
CERVICAL CANCER IN BRIEF (page 455)	Cervical cancer is the development of cancerous cells in the lining of the cervix. These may spread to affect the whole cervix, the rest of the uterus, and other pelvic organs.	Early stages of cervical cancer are virtually silent; this disease is detected by Pap tests before symptoms develop. Later signs and symptoms include bleeding or spotting outside a normal menstrual period, vaginal discharge, and pelvic pain.	Most cases of cervical cancer are caught and eradicated before the woman is in serious danger of metastasis. These patients are good candidates for any kind of bodywork. For a woman dealing with advanced stages of cervical cancer, the massage therapist must make adjustments for the radiation, chemotherapy, or surgical procedures that may be part of her experience.
CHEMICAL DEPENDENCY IN BRIEF (page 189)	Chemical dependency is the use of material in methods or dosages that result in damage to the user and people whom the user contacts. The issue of chemical dependency covers the use of both legal and illegal substances.	Specific symptoms of chemical dependency are determined by what substances are being consumed. Generally speaking, the symptoms of dependence include a craving for the substance in question, an inability to voluntarily limit use, unpleasant or dangerous withdrawal symptoms, and increasing tolerance of the substance's effects.	People who are recovering from chemical dependency can benefit from massage, as long as no contraindicating conditions have developed as part of the abuse. Massage is contraindicated for people who are intoxicated at the time of their appointment.
CHRONIC BRONCHITIS IN BRIEF (page 351)	Chronic bronchitis is one of the lung disorders classified as chronic obstructive pulmonary disease. It involves long-term inflammation of the bronchi with or without infection, leading to permanent changes in the bronchial lining. Chronic bronchitis frequently occurs as a prelude to or simultaneously with emphysema.	Chronic bronchitis is diagnosed when a person experiences a productive cough that occurs most days for 3 months or more for at least 2 consecutive years. Other common signs are a susceptibility to respiratory tract infections, cyanosis, and pulmonary edema.	Massage can be appropriate for chronic bronchitis patients, as long as they are not fighting acute respiratory infection at the time, and as long as heart function is not compromised.
CHRONIC FATIGUE SYNDROME IN BRIEF (page 309)	Chronic fatigue syndrome (CFS) is a collection of signs and symptoms that affect many systems in the body and result in debilitating fatigue.	The central symptom of CFS is fatigue that is not restored by rest. It may be accompanied by swollen nodes, slight fever, muscular and joint aches, headaches, excessive pain after mild exercise, and non-restorative sleep.	CFS indicates massage; it can be a very helpful part of a treatment plan.

CONDITION NAME	WHAT IS IT/ WHAT ARE THEY?	HOW IS IT RECOGNIZED/ HOW ARE THEY RECOGNIZED?	IS MASSAGE INDICATED OR CONTRAINDICATED?
CIRRHOSIS IN BRIEF (page 394)	Cirrhosis is a condition in which normal liver cells become disorganized and dysfunctional; many of them are replaced or crowded out by scar tissue. Cirrhosis is often the final stage of chronic or acute liver diseases.	Early symptoms of cirrhosis include loss of appetite, nausea, vomiting, and weight loss. Later complications may include muscle wasting, jaundice, ascites, vomiting blood, and mental and personality changes.	Advanced cirrhosis involves difficulties with fluid flow in the body. Bodywork that challenges this ability may not be appropriate. Some cirrhosis patients experience muscle wasting as their ability to metabolize proteins diminishes. Exercise and physical therapy are recommended for these patients for maintenance of strength and function, and massage as part of a health care team may have a role in this process as well.
COLORECTAL CANCER IN BRIEF (page 383)	Colorectal cancer is the development of malignant tumors in the colon or rectum. Growths can block the bowel and/or metastasize to other organs, particularly the liver.	Colorectal cancer creates different symptoms depending on what part of the bowel is affected. The most dangerous symptoms are extreme changes in bowel habits, including diarrhea or constipation lasting more than 10 days. Other symptoms include blood in the stool, iron-deficiency anemia, and unintentional weight loss.	If a client is diagnosed with colon or rectal cancer in the early stages, some types of massage may be a useful supportive therapy to help deal with the side effects of cancer treatment. Colorectal cancer survivors are good candidates for massage, although the presence of a colostomy bag may require some specialized adjustments.
COMMON COLD IN BRIEF (page 333)	The common cold (or upper respiratory tract infection) is a viral infection from any of about 200 different types of viruses.	The symptoms of colds are nasal discharge, sore throat, mild fever, dry coughing, and headache. Symptoms last anywhere from 2 days to 2 weeks.	Colds indicate circulatory massage only when the acute stage has passed, and even then massage may exacerbate symptoms as the healing process may be accelerated.
CROHN'S DISEASE IN BRIEF (page 370)	Crohn's disease is a progressive inflammatory condition that may affect any part of the gastrointestinal tract. It involves the development of deep ulcers, blockages, and the formation of abnormal passageways (fistulas) in the small and large intestine.	The primary symptom of Crohn's disease is abdominal pain, especially in the lower right quadrant (the distal end of the ileum). Cramping, diarrhea, and pain at the anus may also accompany active flares of this disease.	Massage is appropriate for Crohn's disease patients when their condition is in remission. During flares they may also benefit from noncirculatory work, but abdominal work will be uncomfortable.
CYSTS IN BRIEF (page 504)	Cysts are layers of connective tissue that surround and isolate something that should not be in the body (e.g., a piece of shrapnel or a localized infection).	Palpable cysts are generally small, painless, distinct masses that move slightly under the skin.	Cysts locally contraindicate massage.
DECUBITUS ULCERS IN BRIEF (page 39)	Bedsores, also called decubitus ulcers, are caused by impaired circulation to the skin. Lack of blood supply leads to irreversible tissue death.	Unlike other sores, ulcers do not crust over; they remain open wounds that are highly vulnerable to infection.	Bedsores indicate massage only *before* they develop. Once the tissue has been damaged it is too late, and they locally contraindicate massage until they have completely healed over.

CONDITION NAME	WHAT IS IT/ WHAT ARE THEY?	HOW IS IT RECOGNIZED/ HOW ARE THEY RECOGNIZED?	IS MASSAGE INDICATED OR CONTRAINDICATED?
DEPRESSION IN BRIEF (page 193)	Depression is an umbrella term covering a number of mood disorders that can result in persistent feelings of sadness, guilt, and/or hopelessness.	Symptoms vary according to the type of depression and the individual, but they usually include a loss of enjoyment derived from usual hobbies and activities, disappointment with oneself, hopelessness, irritability, and a change in sleeping habits.	Most types of depression indicate massage, which can work in several ways to alleviate symptoms both temporarily and in the long run.
DERMATITIS/ECZEMA IN BRIEF (page 21)	Dermatitis is an umbrella term for inflammation of the skin. Eczema is a type of *atopic* dermatitis: a noncontagious skin rash usually brought about by an allergic reaction. Contact dermatitis is an inflammation brought about by irritation or allergic responses in the skin.	Dermatitis presents itself in various ways, depending on what type of skin reactions are elicited. Exposure to poison oak or poison ivy results in large inflamed wheals; metal allergies tend to be less inflamed and more isolated in area. Eczema usually appears as very dry and flaky skin (seborrheic eczema) or blistered, weepy skin (dyshidrotic eczema).	The appropriateness of massage depends completely on the source of the problem and the condition of the skin. If the skin is very inflamed or has blisters or other lesions, it contraindicates massage at least locally until the acute stage has passed. If the skin is not itchy and the affected area is highly isolated, as with a metal allergy to a watchband or earrings, massage is only a local caution.
DIABETES MELLITUS IN BRIEF (page 419)	Diabetes is a group of metabolic disorders characterized by glucose intolerance and disturbances in carbohydrate, fat, and protein metabolism.	Early symptoms of diabetes include frequent urination, chronic thirst, and increased appetite, along with weight loss, nausea, and vomiting. These symptoms are often so subtle that the first signs of disease are the complications it can cause: peripheral neuropathy, impaired vision, kidney dysfunction, or other problems.	Diabetes indicates massage as long as tissues are healthy and circulation is unimpaired. Many people with advanced or poorly treated diabetes experience numbness, cardiovascular problems, and/or kidney failure. Circulatory massage in these situations is not appropriate.
DISLOCATIONS IN BRIEF (page 83)	Dislocations are traumatic injuries to joints where the articulating bones are forcefully separated.	Acute (new) dislocations are extremely painful. The bones may be visibly separated and the joint may lose all function.	Dislocations indicate massage in the subacute stage, as long as work is conducted within pain tolerance. As the area heals, massage may be useful for managing scar tissue accumulation and muscle spasm around the affected joint.
DIVERTICULAR DISEASE IN BRIEF (page 387)	Diverticulosis is the development of small pouches that protrude from the colon. Diverticulitis is the inflammation that happens when these pouches become infected. Collectively these disorders are known as diverticular disease.	Diverticulosis is generally silent, or symptomless. When inflammation (diverticulitis) is present, lower left side abdominal pain, cramping, bloating, constipation, or diarrhea may occur.	Deep abdominal massage is locally contraindicated if the client knows diverticula have developed. Acute infection of diverticula systemically contraindicates circulatory massage.
DUPUYTREN'S CONTRACTURE IN BRIEF (page 117)	Dupuytren's contracture is an idiopathic shrinking and thickening of the fascia on the palm of the hand.	This is a painless condition that usually affects the ring and little fingers, pulling them into permanent flexion.	Dupuytren's contracture indicates massage as long as sensation is present, although massage may do little to reverse the process if it has gone too far.

CONDITION NAME	WHAT IS IT/ WHAT ARE THEY?	HOW IS IT RECOGNIZED/ HOW ARE THEY RECOGNIZED?	IS MASSAGE INDICATED OR CONTRAINDICATED?
DYSMENORRHEA IN BRIEF (page 458)	Dysmenorrhea is the technical term for menstrual pain that is severe enough to interfere with and limit the activities of women of childbearing age. It may be a primary problem or secondary to some other pelvic pathology.	The symptoms of dysmenorrhea are dull aching or sharp severe lower abdominal pain preceding and/or during menstruation. Nausea and vomiting may accompany very severe symptoms. Secondary dysmenorrhea may create pelvic pain outside normal periods as well.	Massage is appropriate for primary dysmenorrhea, although the abdomen locally contraindicates deep work during days of heavy menstrual flow. The appropriateness of bodywork for secondary dysmenorrhea depends of the type of pathology involved, along with stage, severity, and other variables.
EATING DISORDERS IN BRIEF (page 201)	Eating disorders are a group of psychological problems involving compulsions around food and weight gain or loss. Anorexia, bulimia, and compulsive overeating are each distinct problems, although overlap between them frequently occurs.	Signs and symptoms of anorexia and bulimia may be hard to recognize in early stages, since these behaviors are usually done in private. Long-term consequences include esophageal and colon damage, tooth damage, arrhythmia and low cardiac stroke volume, electrolyte imbalance, hormonal disturbance, osteoporosis, and many other problems. Compulsive overeating is recognizable by eating habits in combination with significant weight gain, often in a short period.	Massage may be very supportive and appropriate for all types of eating disorders, as long as the body's chemistry can keep up with the changes bodywork brings about. If a client is in an advanced stage of anorexia or bulimia, bodywork choices may need to change in order to respect the delicacy of the body's system.
EDEMA IN BRIEF (page 300)	Edema is the retention of interstitial fluid because of electrolyte or protein imbalances, or because of mechanical obstruction in the circulatory or lymphatic systems.	Edematous tissue is puffy or boggy. It may be hot, if associated with local infection, or quite cool, if it is cut off from local circulation.	Most edemas contraindicate circulatory massage. This is especially true of pitting edema, in which the tissue does not immediately spring back from a touch. Edemas that indicate massage include those due to subacute soft tissue injury or temporary immobilization caused by some factor that does *not* contraindicate massage.
EMBOLISM, THROMBUS IN BRIEF (page 253)	Thrombi are stationary clots; emboli are clots that travel through the circulatory system. Emboli are usually composed of blood, but may also be fragments of plaque, fat globules, air bubbles, tumors, or bone chips.	If venous thrombi break loose or *embolize,* they can only land in the lungs, causing pulmonary embolism (PE). Symptoms of PE include shortness of breath, chest pain, and coughing up sputum that is streaked with blood. Many venous thrombi and pulmonary emboli are silent, that is, they cause no symptoms until the damage has been done. Clots that form on the arterial side of the system can lodge anywhere their artery carries them. Some of the most common (and dangerous) locations for arterial clots to land are in the coronary arteries (heart attack), the brain (transient ischemic attack or stroke), and the kidneys (renal infarction).	Any disorder than involves the potential for lodged or traveling clots contraindicates circulatory massage.

CONDITION NAME	WHAT IS IT/ WHAT ARE THEY?	HOW IS IT RECOGNIZED/ HOW ARE THEY RECOGNIZED?	IS MASSAGE INDICATED OR CONTRAINDICATED?
EMPHYSEMA IN BRIEF (page 354)	Emphysema is a condition in which the alveoli of the lungs become stretched and inelastic. They merge with each other, decreasing surface area, destroying surrounding capillaries, and limiting oxygen-carbon dioxide exchange.	Symptoms of emphysema include shortness of breath with mild or no exertion, a chronic dry cough, rales, cyanosis, and susceptibility to secondary respiratory infection.	Emphysema indicates massage with caution for circulatory complications, secondary infection, and positioning the client for maximum comfort.
ENCEPHALITIS IN BRIEF (page 176)	Encephalitis is inflammation of the brain usually brought about by a viral infection.	Signs and symptoms of encephalitis include fever, headache, confusion, and personality and memory changes. In rare cases, encephalitis may cause permanent neurologic damage or even death.	Acute encephalitis contraindicates massage. If encephalitis is part of a client's history but there are no signs of present infection or neurologic damage, massage is acceptable.
ENDOMETRIOSIS IN BRIEF (page 460)	Endometriosis is the implantation and growth of endometrial cells in the peritoneal cavity (and possibly elsewhere) that swell and decay with the menstrual cycle.	Endometriosis may have no symptoms. When it does, they generally include pelvic and abdominal pain, difficulties with urination or defecation, painful intercourse, and other problems, depending on which tissues have been affected. Symptoms worsen during menstruation. Infertility is a frequent complication of endometriosis.	If a client knows she has endometriosis, deep abdominal or pelvic work may be painful, especially when it is close to her menstrual cycle. The supportive effects of massage, however, can be an important part of the coping mechanisms women with this disorder must develop.
ERYSIPELAS IN BRIEF (page 6)	Erysipelas is a streptococcus infection that kills skin cells, leading to painful inflammation of the skin. It usually occurs on the face or lower leg.	This condition is marked by a distinct margin between the reddened, affected area and the surrounding unaffected areas. When it occurs on the face it often creates a red "butterfly" shape over the cheeks and bridge of the nose. It can be accompanied by fever and signs of systemic infection.	This is a bacterial infection that can invade both the lymph and circulatory systems. It systemically contraindicates massage until the infection has completely passed.
FATIGUE IN BRIEF (page 505)	Fatigue is a state of having less than optimal energy as a result of inadequate rest and recovery time. Fatigue can be brought about by mental or physical exertion or by any combination of both.	A person living with mental or physical fatigue feels tired, moves inefficiently, and may be more prone to injury.	In the absence of other conditions, fatigue indicates massage.
FEVER IN BRIEF (page 312)	Fever is a controlled increase in core temperature, usually brought about by immune system reactions, often in response to pathogenic invasion.	Fever is identifiable by readings on a thermometer.	Most fever contraindicates massage, as it is an indication that the body is fighting an infection, and should be allowed to do its work undisturbed.
FIBROID TUMORS IN BRIEF (page 463)	Fibroid tumors are benign growths in the muscle or connective tissue of the uterus.	Fibroid tumors are often asymptomatic. Some, however, cause heavy menstrual bleeding or may put mechanical pressure on other structures in the pelvis.	Large, diagnosed fibroid tumors contraindicate deep abdominal massage. However, most fibroids are quite small and virtually symptomless, and massage will not affect them. In these cases massage can benefit the client, although it will not change the state of her fibroid tumors.

CONDITION NAME	WHAT IS IT/ WHAT ARE THEY?	HOW IS IT RECOGNIZED/ HOW ARE THEY RECOGNIZED?	IS MASSAGE INDICATED OR CONTRAINDICATED?
FIBROMYALGIA IN BRIEF (page 53)	Fibromyalgia syndrome (FMS) is a chronic pain syndrome involving the development of a predictable pattern of tender points.	FMS is diagnosed when other diseases have been ruled out, and when 11 active tender points are found distributed among all quadrants of the body.	FMS indicates massage. Care must be taken not to overtreat, however, because clients are extremely sensitive to pain and may have accumulations of waste products in the tissues that are difficult to flush out adequately.
FRACTURES IN BRIEF (page 73)	A fracture is any kind of broken or cracked bone.	Most fractures are painful and involve loss of function at the nearest joints, but some may be difficult to diagnose without an x-ray or other imaging techniques.	Acute fractures locally contraindicate massage, but work done on the rest of the body can yield reflexive benefits. Later stages of fracture recovery indicate massage.
FUNGAL INFECTIONS IN BRIEF (page 7)	Fungal infections of human skin, also called mycoses, are caused by fungi called dermatophytes. When dermatophytes colonize the skin, the characteristic lesions are called tinea. Thus, within this heading several different types of tinea are listed.	Most tinea lesions begin as one reddened, circular, itchy patch. Scratching the lesions may help to spread them to other parts of the body. As they get larger, they tend to clear in the middle and keep a red ring around the edges. Athlete's foot, another type of mycosis, usually involves moist blisters and cracking between the toes. If it affects the nails they will become yellow, thickened, and pitted.	Fungal infections contraindicate massage at least locally in all phases. If the affected areas are very limited (e.g., only the feet are involved or only one or two small, covered lesions are present), massage may be administered to the rest of the body. If a large area is involved, and especially if the infection is acute (i.e., not yet responding to treatment), then massage is a systemic contraindication.
GALLSTONES IN BRIEF (page 397)	Gallstones are crystallized formations of cholesterol or bile pigments in the gallbladder. They can be as small as grains of sand or as large as a golf ball.	Most gallstones do not cause symptoms. When they do, pain that may last several hours develops in the upper right side of the abdomen. Pain may refer to the back between scapula and the right shoulder. Gallstones stuck in the ducts of the biliary system may cause jaundice or pancreatitis.	Silent (symptomless) gallstones have little impact on overall health and function, so massage for these clients is certainly appropriate, although draining strokes over the liver and costal angle are not a good idea. Clients recovering from gallbladder surgery may need some special considerations. A client with a history of gallstones but no present symptoms is a fine candidate for massage.
GANGLION CYSTS IN BRIEF (page 118)	Ganglion cysts are small fluid-filled synovial sacks that are attached to tendinous sheaths, or joint capsules.	Ganglion cysts form small bumps that usually appear on the hand, wrist, or ankle. They are not usually painful unless they are in a place to be injured by normal wear and tear.	Ganglion cysts locally contraindicate massage. Friction or direct pressure do not make them go away and may irritate them by stimulating excessive fluid flow.
GASTROENTERITIS IN BRIEF (page 368)	Gastroenteritis is any form of gastrointestinal inflammation. This may be due to a viral or bacterial infection, a parasite, fungus, food intolerance, or other cause.	The symptoms of gastroenteritis are nausea, vomiting, and diarrhea. Fever, blood in the stools, and other signs may be present, depending on the cause.	Acute gastroenteritis contraindicates massage, especially when it is caused by an infectious agent. Chronic situations may be appropriate for bodywork, as long as the etiology of the problem is clearly understood.

CONDITION NAME	WHAT IS IT/ WHAT ARE THEY?	HOW IS IT RECOGNIZED/ HOW ARE THEY RECOGNIZED?	IS MASSAGE INDICATED OR CONTRAINDICATED?
GASTROESOPHAGEAL REFLUX DISEASE IN BRIEF (page 373)	Gastroesophageal reflux disease (GERD) is a condition involving a weak or impaired esophageal sphincter and the chronic splashing of acidic stomach secretions into the unprotected esophagus.	Most people experience occasional "heartburn": the sensation of having corrosive gastric juices enter the esophagus. GERD is diagnosed when heartburn symptoms have been present long enough to cause structural changes to the esophageal lining, which could lead to serious complications.	People with GERD often find that lying down exacerbates their symptoms, especially if it is within a couple of hours of eating. Clients may therefore wish to use bolsters that allow them to be in a reclining position, to have the head-end of the table elevated by several inches, or to sit in a massage chair.
GLOMERULONEPHRITIS IN BRIEF (page 434)	Glomerulonephritis is a condition in which the glomeruli (small structures that are part of the nephron-capillary unit) become inflamed and cease to function efficiently.	Early symptoms of glomerulonephritis include dark or rust-colored urine, foamy urine, or blood in the urine. Later symptoms indicate chronic renal failure: systemic edema, fatigue, headaches, decreased urine output, rashes and discoloration of the skin, and general malaise.	Symptomatic glomerulonephritis systemically contraindicates circulatory massage. This is an inflammatory condition that impairs the body's ability to manage fluid exchanges. Bodywork that does not significantly impact circulation may be appropriate.
GOUT IN BRIEF (page 85)	Gout is an inflammatory arthritis caused by deposits of sodium urate (uric acid) in and around joints, especially in the feet.	Acute gout causes joints to become red, hot, swollen, shiny, and extremely painful. It usually has a sudden onset.	Gout systemically contraindicates massage when it is acute. Gouty joints locally contraindicate massage at all times.
GUILLAIN-BARRÉ SYNDROME IN BRIEF (page 222)	Guillain-Barré syndrome (GBS) is a demyelinating disorder of peripheral nerves. It usually begins in the feet and moves proximally. It is probably autoimmune in nature, but the specific triggers have not been identified.	GBS is marked by sudden onset (symptoms usually begin quickly and peak within 2 weeks) followed by gradual remission (most patients have full or nearly full recovery within 18 months). Furthermore, GBS affects limbs symmetrically and moves proximally toward the trunk, which distinguishes it from other peripheral nerve problems.	When a person has reached the peak of his or her GBS attack, physical and occupational therapy are often used to speed recovery and prevent muscle atrophy. Massage may be useful at this stage to improve circulation and to reduce fatigue and anxiety.
HEADACHES IN BRIEF (page 224)	Headaches are pain caused by any number of sources. Muscular tension, vascular spasm and dilation, and chemical imbalances can all contribute to headache. Headaches only rarely indicate a serious underlying disorder.	Tension-type headaches are usually bilateral and steadily painful. Vascular headaches are often unilateral and have a distinctive "throbbing" pain from blood flow into the head. Headaches brought about by central nervous system injury or disease are extreme, severe, and prolonged. They can have a sudden or gradual onset	Headaches due to infection or central nervous system injury contraindicate massage. Persons experiencing vascular headaches generally avoid stimuli like massage, but tension-type headaches definitely indicate massage.
HEART ATTACK IN BRIEF (page 284)	A heart attack, or myocardial infarction, is damage to the myocardium caused by a sudden obstruction in blood flow through the coronary arteries, which results in permanent myocardial damage.	Symptoms of most heart attacks include a sensation of great pressure on the chest, spreading pain, and lightheadedness, dizziness, and nausea. Sometimes symptoms vary, and occasionally a minor heart attack may occur with no symptoms at all.	Patients recovering from recent heart attacks are not candidates for circulatory massage. After they have completely recovered they *may* be able to receive massage, depending on the rest of their cardiovascular health.

CONDITION NAME	WHAT IS IT/ WHAT ARE THEY?	HOW IS IT RECOGNIZED/ HOW ARE THEY RECOGNIZED?	IS MASSAGE INDICATED OR CONTRAINDICATED?
HEART FAILURE IN BRIEF (page 287)	Heart failure is a condition in which the heart no longer can function well enough to keep up with the needs of the body. It is usually slowly progressive, developing over a number of years before any changes in function may be noticeable.	Different symptoms will be present depending on which side of the heart is working inefficiently. Left-sided heart failure results in fluid congestion in the lungs with general weakness and shortness of breath. Right-sided heart failure results in fluid back-ups throughout the system, which show as edema especially in the ankles and legs. Both varieties of heart failure will lead to chest pain; cold, sweaty skin; a fast, irregular pulse; coughing, especially when the person is lying down; and very low stamina.	Circulatory massage in inappropriate for clients with heart failure, as it has the goal of pushing fluid through a system that is incapable of adjusting to those changes. Energy or noncirculatory modalities are more appropriate to help clients lower stress and cope with the challenges of severely restricted circulation.
HEMATOMA IN BRIEF (page 255)	A hematoma is a deep bruise (leakage of blood) between muscle sheaths.	Superficial hematomas are simple bruises. Deep bleeds may not be visible but will be painful. If extensive bleeding has occurred, a characteristic "gel-like" feel will develop in the affected tissue.	Massage is at least locally contraindicated for acute hematomas because of the possibility of blood clots and pain. In the subacute stage (at least 2 days after the injury has occurred) when the surrounding blood vessels have been sealed shut and the body is in the process of breaking down and reabsorbing the debris, gentle massage around the perimeter of the area and hydrotherapy can be helpful.
HEMOPHILIA IN BRIEF (page 256)	Hemophilia is a genetic disorder in which certain clotting factors in the blood are either inactive or missing.	Hemophilia can cause superficial bleeding that persists for longer than normal, or internal bleeding into joint cavities or between muscle sheaths with little or no provocation.	Severe cases of hemophilia contraindicate bodywork that can mechanically stretch, manipulate, or accidentally injure delicate tissues. Milder cases of hemophilia may be safer for circulatory massage.
HEPATITIS IN BRIEF (page 400)	Hepatitis is inflammation of the liver, usually due to viral infection.	All types of hepatitis produce the same symptoms, with variable severity. Symptoms, when any occur at all, include fatigue, abdominal pain, nausea, diarrhea, and jaundice.	Acute hepatitis contraindicates circulatory massage. For clients with chronic hepatitis, the appropriateness of massage depends on their general health.
HERNIA IN BRIEF (page 119)	A hernia is a hole or rip in the abdominal wall or the inguinal ring through which the small intestines may protrude.	Abdominal hernias usually show some bulging and mild to severe pain, depending on whether a portion of the small intestine is trapped.	Untreated hernias locally contraindicate massage. If the hernia is accompanied by fever or other signs of infection, it systemically contraindicates massage. Recent hernia surgeries fall under the category of postsurgical situations. Massage is acceptable for sites of old hernia surgeries with no complications.
HERNIATED DISC IN BRIEF (page 140)	A herniated disc is a situation in which the nucleus pulposus or the surrounding annulus fibrosis of an intervertebral disc protrudes in such a way that it puts pressure on nerve roots, the cauda equina, or the spinal cord itself.	The symptoms of nerve pressure include radiculopathy (shooting, electrical pain along the dermatome), specific muscle weakness, paresthesia (tingling, "pins and needles"), reduced sensation, and numbness.	Herniated discs that are not acutely painful indicate massage.

CONDITION NAME	WHAT IS IT/ WHAT ARE THEY?	HOW IS IT RECOGNIZED/ HOW ARE THEY RECOGNIZED?	IS MASSAGE INDICATED OR CONTRAINDICATED?
HERPES SIMPLEX IN BRIEF (page 9)	Herpes simplex is a viral infection resulting in cold sores or fever blisters on the face or around the mouth, or blisters around the genitals, thighs, or buttocks.	Herpes simplex outbreaks are often preceded by 2 to 3 days of tingling, itching, or pain. Then blisters appear gathered around a red base. The blisters gradually crust and disappear, usually within 2 weeks.	Any kind of herpes simplex in the acute stage locally contraindicates massage. Massage is also inappropriate if the client is showing any signs of systemic infection. The sheets of clients with active herpes simplex must be isolated and bleached. Massage for clients with a history of herpes but no active or prodromic symptoms may be appropriate, but therapists should be aware that no visible lesions need to be present for the virus to be present on the skin.
HERPES ZOSTER IN BRIEF (page 179)	Herpes zoster, or shingles, is a viral infection of sensory neurons from the same virus that causes chickenpox.	Shingles creates rashes and extremely painful blisters unilaterally along the affected dermatomes. The trunk or buttocks are the most common areas, but it occasionally affects the trigeminal nerve.	This is an extraordinarily painful condition and contraindicates massage in the acute stage. After the blisters have healed and the pain has subsided, massage is appropriate.
HIV/AIDS IN BRIEF (page 314)	Acquired immune deficiency syndrome (AIDS) is a disease caused by the human immunodeficiency virus (HIV), which attacks and disables the immune system. This leaves a person vulnerable to a host of diseases that are usually not a threat to uninfected people.	Most people with HIV experience a week or two of flu-like symptoms within a few weeks of being infected, followed by an interval with no symptoms. When the virus has successfully inactivated the immune system, infection by opportunistic pathogens like cytomegalovirus or *Pneumocystis carinii* will occur.	All stages of HIV infection indicate massage as long as the practitioner is healthy and does not pose any risk to the client, and the client is able to keep up with the changes that massage brings about in the body.
HIVES IN BRIEF (page 25)	Hives are an inflammatory skin reaction to an allergen or emotional stressor.	Hives range from small red spots to large wheals, which are warm to the touch and itchy. Individual lesions generally subside within a few hours, but successive hives may appear; the cycle can continue for several weeks at a time.	Hives contraindicates massage at least locally. If the lesions cover a large portion of the body, this may be a systemic contraindication. Bringing even more circulation to the skin only makes a bad situation worse.
HYPERTHYROIDISM IN BRIEF (page 424)	Hyperthyroidism is a condition in which the thyroid gland produces too much of its hormones that stimulate metabolism of fuel into energy. It is usually related to an autoimmune attack against the whole thyroid gland, but it can be caused by small, localized hyperactive nodules or infection.	Signs and symptoms of hyperthyroidism involve too much production of energy from available fuel and include restlessness, sleeplessness, irritability, dry skin and hair, rapid heartbeat, tremor, unintended weight loss, and for women, irregularity of menstrual periods. Some hyperthyroid patients experience complications involving eye problems or skin rashes. A severe and acute episode of hyperthyroidism is called a thyroid storm.	Most people with hyperactive thyroid glands respond well to massage, which may help, at least temporarily, to ameliorate some of the stress-related symptoms that they experience. Massage on or around the thyroid gland itself, however, may trigger a thyroid storm, so the anterior neck is a local contraindication.

CONDITION NAME	WHAT IS IT/ WHAT ARE THEY?	HOW IS IT RECOGNIZED/ HOW ARE THEY RECOGNIZED?	IS MASSAGE INDICATED OR CONTRAINDICATED?
HYPERTENSION IN BRIEF (page 276)	Hypertension is the technical term for high blood pressure.	High blood pressure has no dependable symptoms. The only way to identify it is by taking several blood pressure measurements over time.	For borderline or mild high blood pressure massage may be useful as a tool to control stress and increase general health, but other pathologies having to do with kidney or cardiovascular disease must be ruled out. High blood pressure that requires medication may be inappropriate for circulatory massage, but may respond well to other modalities.
HYPOGLYCEMIA IN BRIEF (page 426)	Hypoglycemia is the condition of having abnormally low levels of blood glucose, so cells have no access to important fuel.	Signs and symptoms of a hypoglycemic episode include dizziness, confusion, chills and sweating, hunger, headache, and pallor. Symptoms pass when a person eats or drinks something with quickly available glucose.	A person in a hypoglycemic episode needs to replace glucose first, get a massage second. Once the symptoms have passed, bodywork is a fine choice. If a person experiences ongoing hypoglycemic symptoms or frequent acute episodes, he or she should find out why.
HYPOTHYROIDISM IN BRIEF (page 427)	Hypothyroidism is a condition in which the thyroid gland produces an inadequate supply of the hormones that regulate metabolism of fuel into energy. Some cases of hypothyroidism are the result of an autoimmune attack on the thyroid gland, but others are related to the long-term complications of treatment for hyperthyroidism or other factors.	Symptoms of hypothyroidism are subtle and often missed. They include fatigue, weight gain, depression, intolerance of cold, and for women, heavy menstrual periods.	One of the complications of hypothyroidism, especially in elderly patients, is the accelerated development of atherosclerosis. As long as this condition is recognized and respected, massage can be a supportive and positive experience for hypothyroidism patients.
ICHTHYOSIS IN BRIEF (page 43)	Ichthyosis is pathologically dry skin that is much more severe than average dry skin.	Ichthyosis creates distinctive diamond-shaped "scales" on the skin, usually on the lower legs.	When ichthyosis appears independently of other conditions, it certainly indicates massage. Massage probably will not provide a permanent solution to this problem, but massage can make it better in the short run. Areas where deep cracking may expose the blood supply should be avoided.
IMPETIGO IN BRIEF (page 12)	Impetigo is a bacterial (staphylococcus or streptococcus) infection of the skin.	Impetigo is marked by a rash with fluid-filled blisters and honey-colored crusts. It usually begins somewhere on the face but can appear anywhere on the body.	Until the lesions have completely healed, this highly contagious condition strictly contraindicates massage.
INFLAMMATION IN BRIEF (page 319)	Inflammation is a protective device in response to injury or infection. It involves localized vascular, cellular, and chemical reactions to isolate the area and to resolve the damage through immune system response.	The signs of inflammation are redness, pain, swelling, heat, and loss of function. These can be localized or systemic.	Acute inflammation contraindicates circulatory massage, but bodywork may be appropriate for subacute situations, depending on the causative factors. Inflammation due to infection obviously carries a higher risk to the client and the practitioner than inflammation in response to musculoskeletal injury.

CONDITION NAME	WHAT IS IT/ WHAT ARE THEY?	HOW IS IT RECOGNIZED/ HOW ARE THEY RECOGNIZED?	IS MASSAGE INDICATED OR CONTRAINDICATED?
INFLUENZA IN BRIEF (page 335)	Influenza ("flu") is a viral infection of the respiratory tract.	The symptoms of flu include high fever and muscle and joint achiness that may last for up to 3 days, followed by a runny nose, coughing, sneezing, and general malaise.	Flu indicates circulatory massage during the subacute stage only.
INTERSTITIAL CYSTITIS IN BRIEF (page 445)	Interstitial cystitis (IC) is a chronic inflammation of the bladder involving scar tissue, stiffening, decreased capacity, pinpoint hemorrhages, and sometimes ulcers in the bladder walls.	Symptoms of IC are very much like those of urinary tract infections: burning, increased frequency, and urgency of urination; decreased capacity of the bladder; and pain, pressure, and tenderness.	IC is a poorly understood condition that seems to be exacerbated by stress. Bodywork may be a helpful and supportive choice for IC patients, although it probably will not do anything to reverse the situation.
IRRITABLE BOWEL SYNDROME IN BRIEF (page 390)	Irritable bowel syndrome (IBS) is a collection of signs and symptoms that indicate a functional problem with the digestive system, specifically with the colon. It is aggravated by stress and diet.	The symptoms of IBS include alternating bouts of constipation and diarrhea, bloating or abdominal distension, and moderate to severe crampy abdominal pain that is relieved with defecation.	IBS indicates massage as long as bodywork does not exacerbate symptoms.
JAUNDICE IN BRIEF (page 404)	Jaundice is a symptom of liver dysfunction, involving the presence of excess bilirubin in the blood. The bilirubin is then distributed and dissolved in subcutaneous fat, mucous membranes, and the sclera of the eyes.	Jaundice gives the skin, eyes, and mucous membranes a yellowish cast.	The presence of jaundice is not enough information on which to base a decision about bodywork. The underlying cause for the jaundice must be understood before a decision can be made, based on the comparative risks and benefits of bodywork in the context of that condition.
KIDNEY STONES IN BRIEF (page 436)	A kidney stone is a solid deposit of crystalline substances inside the kidney.	Small stones may create no symptoms at all, but when larger stones enter the ureters, they can cause extreme pain called renal colic. Renal colic may be accompanied by nausea and vomiting. Fever and chills indicate that infection is part of the problem. Pain may refer from the back into the groin.	Acute renal colic contraindicates massage, although any kind of bodywork is appropriate for people with a history of stones but no current symptoms.
LEUKEMIA IN BRIEF (page 258)	Leukemia is a collection of blood disorders involving the production of non-functioning white blood cells in bone marrow.	Different types of leukemia have slightly different profiles, but all varieties include signs brought about by interference with the production of normal blood cells: anemia, easy bruising from lack of platelets, and low resistance to infection.	Leukemia is usually treated with chemotherapy. Both the disease and the treatment wreak havoc with the immune system. While some types of bodywork may be supportive during this time, care must be taken to protect the client from any threat of infection. People who have survived leukemia for 5 years without any signs of remission are considered "cured" and are perfectly fine candidates for massage.

CONDITION NAME	WHAT IS IT/ WHAT ARE THEY?	HOW IS IT RECOGNIZED/ HOW ARE THEY RECOGNIZED?	IS MASSAGE INDICATED OR CONTRAINDICATED?
LICE AND MITES IN BRIEF (page 13)	Lice and mites are tiny animals that drink blood. They are highly contagious and spread through close contact with skin or infested sheets or clothing.	• The mites that cause scabies are too small to see, but they leave itchy trails where they burrow under the skin. They prefer warm, moist places such as the axillae or between fingers. • Head lice are easy to see, but they can hide. A more dependable sign is their eggs: nits are small white rice-shaped flecks that cling strongly to hair shafts. • Pubic lice look like tiny white crabs. All three of these parasites create a lot of itching.	All three infestations contraindicate massage, until the parasites have been completely eradicated. If a massage therapist is exposed to any of these animals, every client he or she works on subsequently is also exposed, even before the therapist shows any symptoms. Parasitic infestations are something every massage therapist fears. Bodyworkers are so very vulnerable to whatever is crawling around on clients' skins. Here, as in all things fearful, the best defense is information.
LUPUS IN BRIEF (page 323)	Lupus is an autoimmune disease in which antibodies attack various types of tissue throughout the body. Three distinct types of lupus exist, but systemic lupus erythematosus (SLE) is both the most common and the most serious.	Eleven specific criteria have been determined for a diagnosis of lupus. They include, among other things, arthritis in two or more joints, pleurisy, pericarditis, kidney, and nervous system dysfunction.	When lupus is in a state of acute flare, circulatory massage could exacerbate symptoms. When the condition is in remission, bodywork of any kind could be very helpful to reduce pain and anxiety and to help maintain flexibility.
LUNG CANCER IN BRIEF (page 358)	Lung cancer is the development of malignant cells in the lungs. These cells have easy access to blood and lymph vessels, and quickly spread to other organs in the body.	The early symptoms of lung cancer are virtually indistinguishable from normal irritation from cigarette smoke: a chronic cough, blood-stained sputum, and recurrent bronchitis or pneumonia.	Sadly, most people diagnosed with lung cancer do not survive. Massage has a place in cancer recovery care and in terminal care, but these situations call for specific precautions to achieve maximum benefit with minimal risk.
LYME DISEASE IN BRIEF (page 89)	Lyme disease is a bacterial infection spread by the bites of specific species of ticks. The immune response to the bacteria causes inflammation of large joints, along with neurologic and cardiovascular symptoms.	The hallmark early symptom of Lyme disease is a circular "bull's eye" rash at the site of the tick bite. The skin may be red, itchy, and hot, but it is not usually raised or scaly. The rash may be accompanied by fever, fatigue, and joint pain. Later symptoms may include acute intermittent inflammation of one or more large joints, numbness, poor coordination, Bell's palsy, and irregular heart beat.	The inflammation associated with Lyme disease runs in acute and subacute phases. During subacute phases massage may be appropriate to maintain joint function and relieve pain. In this situation it is important to be working as part of a health care team for the maximum benefit and minimum risk to the infected person.
LYMPHANGITIS IN BRIEF (page 301)	Lymphangitis is an infection of lymph capillaries. If it gets into the nodes, it is called lymphadenitis. If it gets past the lymphatic system, it is called blood poisoning (septicemia) and it can be life threatening.	Lymphangitis has all the signs of local infection: pain, heat, redness, and swelling. It may also show red streaks from the site of infection running toward the nearest lymph nodes.	Lymphangitis contraindicates circulatory massage until the infection has been completely eradicated.

CONDITION NAME	WHAT IS IT/ WHAT ARE THEY?	HOW IS IT RECOGNIZED/ HOW ARE THEY RECOGNIZED?	IS MASSAGE INDICATED OR CONTRAINDICATED?
LYMPHOMA IN BRIEF (page 303)	Lymphoma is any variety of cancer that grows in lymph nodes. Several types have been identified, some of which are aggressive and very threatening, others of which may progress more slowly.	Painless swelling of lymph nodes is the cardinal sign of lymphoma, along with the possibility of anemia, fatigue, low-grade fever, night sweats, itchiness, abdominal pain, and loss of appetite, all of which last for 2 weeks or more.	Rigorous circulatory massage is generally not recommended for a person who is fighting lymphoma, although this may be a case-by-case decision. Persons who have been free from lymphoma for 5 years or more are considered "cured." Noncirculatory types of massage may be appropriate for lymphoma patients, although it is recommended that the therapist participate as part of an integrated health care team.
MARFAN'S SYNDROME IN BRIEF*	Marfan's syndrome is a genetic disorder that can affect the musculoskeletal system, the circulatory system, and the eye.	Symptoms of Marfan's syndrome include abnormally long, thin fingers; systemic ligament laxity; and tall stature. Cardiovascular symptoms include mitral valve prolapse and the regurgitation of blood through the mitral valve. Symptoms in the eye include subluxation of the lens and myopia.	If cardiovascular problems are addressed, a patient with Marfan's syndrome has a virtually normal life expectancy. Therefore, with medical clearance, massage is appropriate for most Marfan's syndrome patients who have normal heart function.
MENINGITIS IN BRIEF (page 180)	Meningitis is an infection of the meninges, specifically the pia mater and the arachnoid layers.	Symptoms of acute meningitis include very high fever, rash, photophobia, headache, and stiff neck. Symptoms are not always consistent, however; they may appear in different combinations for different people.	Meningitis, a contagious and inflammatory disease, strictly contraindicates massage in the acute phase. People who have recovered from meningitis with no lasting damage are perfectly fine to receive massage.
MENOPAUSE IN BRIEF (page 483)	Menopause refers to the moment when functioning ovaries become nonfunctioning ovaries. Although this usually happens as a normal part of aging, menopause can be induced through surgery, radiation, or medication.	The symptoms associated with a decline in ovarian function ("perimenopause") include night sweats, hot flashes, insomnia, mood swings, decreased sex drive, vaginal itchiness or dryness, and poor concentration and memory. Longer-term symptoms include an increased risk for osteoporosis and cardiovascular disease.	Bodywork is highly appropriate for a woman who is going through the transition of losing ovarian function. While for some women this is a liberating, exciting time, for others it involves radical and not always welcome changes in self-definition and self-perception. Massage gives powerful positive feedback about physical experience and can help to ameliorate some of the psychological and physical disruptions that menopause can trigger.
MOLES IN BRIEF (page 26)	Moles are isolated areas where the pigment cells in the epidermis have produced excess melanin.	Moles can range in color from light tan to blackish-blue. Their color is usually uniform throughout. Moles are usually circular or oval.	Massage does not help or hurt moles, but massage therapists may be able to see changes in a mole that a client cannot see.

CONDITION NAME	WHAT IS IT/ WHAT ARE THEY?	HOW IS IT RECOGNIZED/ HOW ARE THEY RECOGNIZED?	IS MASSAGE INDICATED OR CONTRAINDICATED?
MONONUCLEOSIS IN BRIEF (page 306)	Mononucleosis is an infection, usually with the Epstein–Barr virus but occasionally with cytomegalovirus or other agents. The virus attacks epithelial tissue in the salivary glands and throat first and then invades B-cells and lymph nodes.	The three leading symptoms for mononucleosis are fever, swollen lymph nodes, and sore throat. Other symptoms may include fatigue, low stamina, enlarged spleen, and enlarged liver.	Mononucleosis contraindicates circulatory massage in the acute stage when the body is fighting hard to beat back this viral attack. In later stages, as long as circulation is healthy and the spleen and liver are not congested, circulatory massage may improve recovery time, although abdominal work should be avoided. Non-circulatory types of bodywork may be appropriate, as long as the possibility of lymphatic congestion is considered.
MULTIPLE SCLEROSIS IN BRIEF (page 165)	Multiple sclerosis (MS) is an idiopathic disease that involves the destruction of myelin sheaths around both motor and sensory neurons in the central nervous system.	MS has many symptoms, depending on the nature of the damage. These can include fatigue, eye pain, spasticity, tremors, and a progressive loss of vision, sensation, and motor control.	Subacute stages of MS, when the client is in remission, indicate massage. Circulatory or other vigorous types of bodywork should be avoided during periods of flare.
MUSCULAR DYSTROPHY IN BRIEF (page 61)	Muscular dystrophy is a group of related inherited disorders all of which involve the degeneration and wasting of muscle tissue.	Different varieties of muscular dystrophy destroy different areas of skeletal muscles. The age of onset, initial symptoms, and long-term prognosis depend on what kind of genetic problem is present.	The early signs of muscular dystrophy often involve muscles that become tight and constrictive. Physical therapy is often used to prevent or minimize contractures as long as possible; massage can fit in this context as well, as long as the massage therapist is working as part of a health care team.
MYASTHENIA GRAVIS IN BRIEF (page 145)	Myasthenia gravis (MG) is a neuromuscular disorder in which an autoimmune attack is launched against acetylcholine receptors at the neuromuscular junction. This makes it difficult to stimulate a muscle to contract, leading to fatigue and weakness.	MG can develop at any age, but is most common in women in their 20s and in men in their 50s. It often begins with weakness in facial muscles and in the muscles used in speaking, eating, and swallowing. MG is a progressive disease, but it is usually treatable with medical intervention.	Massage can be appropriate for persons with MG, because this disease does not affect sensation. Massage may not affect acetylcholine uptake in any positive way but it will not make it worse. Care must be taken to respect the side effects that accompany medications used to treat MG.
MYOFASCIAL PAIN SYNDROME IN BRIEF (page 58)	Myofascial pain syndrome (MPS) is a collection of signs and symptoms that indicate trauma to muscles that leads to a cycle of chronic spasm, ischemia, and pain.	MPS is recognized mainly through the development of trigger points in predictable locations in affected muscles. Trigger points are highly painful both locally and in specific patterns of referred pain.	MPS indicates massage, which can "break through" the pain-spasm cycle and help to eradicate the irritating metabolic wastes that accumulate around trigger points.
MYOSITIS OSSIFICANS IN BRIEF (page 63)	This is the growth of a calcium deposit in soft tissues. It usually follows trauma that involves significant leakage of blood between fascial sheaths.	A radiograph is the best way to see this problem, but it is palpable as a dense mass where, anatomically, no such thing should be.	Massage is always a local contraindication for myositis ossificans, but work around the edges of the area may stimulate the reabsorption of the bone tissue without doing further damage.

CONDITION NAME	WHAT IS IT/ WHAT ARE THEY?	HOW IS IT RECOGNIZED/ HOW ARE THEY RECOGNIZED?	IS MASSAGE INDICATED OR CONTRAINDICATED?
OPEN WOUNDS AND SORES IN BRIEF (page 41)	Open wounds and sores are skin injuries that have not completely healed.	Unhealed lesions may be marked by bleeding, crusts, exuding pus, or other signs of regenerative activity.	Any opening in the skin is an open invitation for infection. At the very least, open wounds and sores locally contraindicate massage. They may systemically contraindicate massage if they appear as a sign of serious systemic disease.
OSGOOD-SCHLATTER DISEASE IN BRIEF (page 121)	Osgood-Schlatter disease is the result of chronic or traumatic irritation at the insertion of the quadriceps tendon, in combination with adolescent growth spurts.	When Osgood-Schlatter disease is acute, the tibial tuberosity is hot, swollen, and painful. The bone may grow a large protuberance at the site of the tendinous insertion.	An acute flare of Osgood-Schlatter disease locally contraindicates circulatory massage, which could exacerbate inflammation. Techniques for reducing lymphatic retention and work elsewhere on the body are certainly appropriate. A client with a history of Osgood-Schlatter disease but no current inflammation at the knee may benefit from the pain relief and reduction in quadriceps muscle tone that massage can supply.
OSTEOARTHRITIS IN BRIEF (page 92)	This is joint inflammation brought about by wear and tear causing cumulative damage to articular cartilage.	Affected joints are stiff, painful, and occasionally palpably inflamed. Osteoarthritis most often affects knees, hips, and distal joints of the fingers.	Arthritis contraindicates massage if it is acutely inflamed. It indicates massage in the subacute stage when bodywork can contribute to muscular relaxation and mobility of the affected joint.
OSTEOGENESIS IMPERFECTI IN BRIEF*	This is a large group of inherited conditions that involve abnormally fragile bones. These bones can break with very minimal trauma.	Signs and symptoms of osteogenesis imperfecti include deformity of long bones, unusually lax ligaments, and a bluish tint to the sclerae of the eye.	Depending on the severity of the condition, vigorous massage may be contraindicated for osteogenesis imperfecti. Therapists will need to work with primary care physicians to make case-by-case decisions for clients who have this condition.
OSTEOPOROSIS IN BRIEF (page 74)	This is loss of bone mass and density brought about by endocrine imbalances and poor metabolism of calcium.	Osteoporosis in the early stages is identifiable only by radiographic and bone density tests. In later stages compression or spontaneous fractures of the vertebrae, wrists, or hips may be present. Kyphosis brought about by compression fractures of the vertebrae is a frequent indicator of osteoporosis.	Gentle massage is indicated for persons with osteoporosis, with extra caution for the comfort and safety of the client. Massage does not affect the progression of the disease once it is present, but may significantly reduce associated pain. Acute fractures, however, contraindicate massage.
OVARIAN CANCER IN BRIEF (page 472)	Ovarian cancer is the development of malignant tumors on the ovaries that may metastasize to other structures in the pelvic or abdominal cavity.	Symptoms of ovarian cancer are generally extremely subtle until the disease has progressed to life-threatening levels. Early symptoms include a feeling of heaviness in the pelvis, vague abdominal discomfort, occasional vaginal bleeding, and weight gain or loss.	As with all cancers, the appropriateness of massage depends on what treatment measures the client is going through. Massage therapists working with clients who have ovarian cancer should be part of a fully informed health care team.

CONDITION NAME	WHAT IS IT/ WHAT ARE THEY?	HOW IS IT RECOGNIZED/ HOW ARE THEY RECOGNIZED?	IS MASSAGE INDICATED OR CONTRAINDICATED?
OVARIAN CYSTS IN BRIEF (page 475)	Most ovarian cysts are fluid-filled growths on the ovaries. Some types of cysts are associated with ovarian cancer or other reproductive disorders, but the cysts discussed here are benign.	The symptoms of ovarian cysts may be nonexistent or may cause a disruption in the menstrual cycle. Constant or intermittent pain in the pelvis, pain with intercourse, or symptoms similar to early pregnancy may arise from different types of ovarian cysts.	Ovarian cysts that have been diagnosed locally contraindicate massage.
PAGET'S DISEASE IN BRIEF (page 78)	This is a chronic bone disorder in which healthy bone is rapidly reabsorbed and replaced with fibrous connective tissue that never fully calcifies.	Paget's disease is often silent. When it does cause symptoms they usually include deep bone pain, local heat, and sometimes visible deformation of the affected bones. The risk of fractures is also high.	Paget's disease is often treated with exercise and physical therapy to maintain flexibility. Massage may fit into this context as well, with caution for the extreme fragility of the affected bones.
PARKINSON'S DISEASE IN BRIEF (page 170)	Parkinson's disease is a degenerative disease of the substantia nigra cells in the brain. These cells produce the neurotransmitter dopamine, which helps the basal ganglia to maintain balance, posture, and coordination.	Early symptoms of Parkinson's include general stiffness and fatigue; resting tremor of the hand, foot or head; stiffness; and poor balance. Later symptoms include a shuffling gait, a "mask-like" appearance to the face, and a monotone voice.	Parkinson's disease indicates massage, with caution. Care must be taken for the physical safety of these clients who cannot move freely or smoothly.
PATELLOFEMORAL SYNDROME IN BRIEF (page 95)	Patellofemoral syndrome (PFS) is an overuse disorder that can lead to damage of the patellar cartilage.	PFS causes pain at the knee, stiffness after immobility, and discomfort in walking down stairs.	PFS indicates massage, as long as the knee is not acutely inflamed. Massage may not be useful to correct this problem, but it will certainly do no harm and can address issues of muscle tightness and imbalance.
PELVIC INFLAMMATORY DISEASE IN BRIEF (page 486)	Pelvic inflammatory disease (PID) is an infection of female reproductive organs. It starts at the cervix and can move up to infect the uterus, fallopian (uterine) tubes, ovaries, and entire pelvic cavity.	The symptoms of acute PID include abdominal pain, fever, chills, headache, nausea, and vomiting. Chronic PID may produce no symptoms or may involve chronic pain, lassitude, and pain during urination and intercourse.	Acute PID systemically contraindicates massage until all signs of infection have subsided. Chronic PID may be appropriate for massage if the woman is aware of her condition and is treating it appropriately. Deep work in the lower abdomen and/or pelvis is not appropriate for women with PID.
PERIPHERAL NEUROPATHY IN BRIEF (page 174)	Peripheral neuropathy is damage to peripheral nerves, usually of the hands and feet, often as a result of some other underlying condition such as alcoholism, diabetes, or lupus.	Sensory damage, motor damage, or both may be present. Symptoms include burning or tingling pain beginning distally and slowly moving proximally, loss of movement or control of movement, hyperesthesia, and eventual numbness.	Peripheral neuropathy contraindicates massage when numbness interferes with the client's ability to give accurate feedback. In other cases, therapists will need to make case-by-case judgments about whether massage fits in the context of the underlying factors.
PERITONITIS IN BRIEF (page 408)	Peritonitis is inflammation, usually due to bacterial infection, of the peritoneal lining of the abdomen.	Acute peritonitis shows the signs of systemic infection: fever and chills, along with abdominal pain, distension, nausea, and vomiting.	Acute peritonitis is a medical emergency and contraindicates massage.

CONDITION NAME	WHAT IS IT/ WHAT ARE THEY?	HOW IS IT RECOGNIZED/ HOW ARE THEY RECOGNIZED?	IS MASSAGE INDICATED OR CONTRAINDICATED?
PES PLANUS IN BRIEF (page 122)	This is the medical term for flat feet.	Flat feet lack well-defined arches. Pronation of the ankle may also be present.	Pes planus indicates massage. In some cases the health of intrinsic foot muscles and ligaments can be improved to the point where alignment in the foot is also improved. In cases where the ligaments are lax through genetic or other problems, massage may not correct the situation but it will not make it worse.
PLANTAR FASCIITIS IN BRIEF (page 123)	Plantar fasciitis is the pain and inflammation caused by injury to the plantar fascia of the foot.	Plantar fasciitis is acutely painful after prolonged immobility. Then the pain recedes but comes back with extended use. It feels sharp and bruise-like, usually at the anterior calcaneus or deep in the arch, but the pain can appear almost anywhere the plantar fascia goes.	Plantar fasciitis indicates massage. It can help release tension in deep calf muscles that put strain on the plantar fascia; it can also help to affect the development of scar tissue at the site of the tear.
POLIO IN BRIEF (page 182)	Polio is a viral infection, first of the intestines and then (for about 1% of exposed people) the anterior horn cells of the spinal cord.	The destruction of motor neurons leads to degeneration, atrophy, and finally paralysis of skeletal muscles.	The polio virus does not affect sensation or cognition. Therefore, massage is very appropriate for polio survivors, as long as acute phase of the infection has passed.
POSTOPERATIVE SITUATIONS IN BRIEF (page 506)	Postoperative situations are conditions in which clients are recovering from any kind of surgery.	Surgeries may be major and invasive, or they may be conducted through tiny holes in the abdomen or through long tubes inserted into blood vessels to get to a destination far away.	Massage can be appropriate for persons recovering from surgery, depending on the reason for the surgery and the danger of possible complications.
POST POLIO SYNDROME IN BRIEF (page 184)	Post polio syndrome (PPS) is a group of signs and symptoms common to polio survivors, particularly those who experienced significant loss of function in the acute stage of the disease.	Symptoms of PPS include a sudden onset of fatigue, achiness, and weakness. Breathing and sleeping difficulties may also occur.	PPS indicates massage.
POSTURAL DEVIATIONS IN BRIEF (page 80)	Postural deviations are overdeveloped thoracic or lumbar curves (kyphosis and lordosis) or an S-curve in the spine (scoliosis).	Extreme curvatures are easily visible, although radiographs are used to pinpoint exactly where the problems begin and end.	All postural deviations indicate massage as long as other underlying pathologies have been eliminated. Bodywork may not be able to reverse any damage, but it can certainly provide relief for the muscular stress that accompanies spinal changes.
PNEUMONIA IN BRIEF (page 339)	Pneumonia is an infection in the lungs brought about by bacteria, viruses, or other pathogens.	The symptoms of pneumonia include coughing that may be dry or productive, high fever, pain on breathing, and shortness of breath. Extreme cases may show cyanosis, or a bluish caste to the skin and nails.	Depending on the causative factor and the general resiliency of the person, pneumonia may indicate massage in the subacute stage.

CONDITION NAME	WHAT IS IT/ WHAT ARE THEY?	HOW IS IT RECOGNIZED/ HOW ARE THEY RECOGNIZED?	IS MASSAGE INDICATED OR CONTRAINDICATED?
PREGNANCY IN BRIEF (page 487)	Pregnancy is the state of carrying a fetus.	The symptoms of advanced pregnancy are obvious, but symptoms that specifically pertain to massage include loose ligaments, muscle spasms, clumsiness, and fatigue.	All stages of uncomplicated pregnancy indicate massage, with specific cautions relating to each trimester.
PREMENSTRUAL SYNDROME IN BRIEF (page 490)	Premenstrual syndrome (PMS) is a collection of many signs and symptoms that occur in the time between ovulation and menstruation and then subside after menstruation begins. It may have several different causes and triggers.	Signs and symptoms of PMS are often divided into physical and emotional features. Physical symptoms include breast tenderness, bloating, digestive upset, fatigue, changes in appetite, backache, and many others. Emotional signs include irritability, anxiety, depression, mood swings, and other possible problems.	Although the specific causes of PMS are not clearly understood, it is clear that this condition is not related to infection, structural problems, or neoplasm. Therefore, PMS indicates bodywork, which may help to reestablish balance in the endocrine and nervous systems.
PROSTATE CANCER IN BRIEF (page 480)	Prostate cancer is the growth of malignant cells in the prostate gland, which may then metastasize, usually to nearby bones or into inguinal lymph nodes.	The symptoms of prostate cancer include problems with urination: weak stream, increased frequency, urgency, nocturia, and other problems arising from constriction of the urethra.	Prostate cancer patients may face any combination of surgery, radiation, chemotherapy, and hormonal therapy to deal with their disease. Bodywork that accommodates for these challenges while minimizing risks can be helpful and supportive, as long as the massage therapist is working as part of a fully informed health care team.
PSORIASIS IN BRIEF (page 28)	Psoriasis is a non-contagious chronic skin disease involving the excessive production of new skin cells that pile up into isolated lesions.	The most common variety of psoriasis looks like pink or reddish patches, sometimes with a silvery scale on top. It occurs most frequently on elbows and knees, but it can develop anywhere.	The acute stage of psoriasis locally contraindicates massage, because the extra stimulation and circulation massage provides can make a bad situation worse. In subacute stages, massage is appropriate as long as the skin is intact.
PYELONEPHRITIS IN BRIEF (page 438)	Pyelonephritis is an infection of the kidney and/or renal pelvis.	Symptoms of acute pyelonephritis include burning pain with urination, back pain, fever, chills, nausea, and vomiting. Chronic infections may show no symptoms.	Kidney infections systemically contraindicate circulatory massage until the infection has been completely eradicated.
RAYNAUD'S SYNDROME IN BRIEF (page 280)	Raynaud's syndrome is defined by episodes of vasospasm of the arterioles, usually in fingers and toes, and occasionally in the nose, ears, and lips.	Affected areas will often go through marked color changes of white or ashy gray for dark-skinned people, to blue to red. Attacks can last for less than 1 minute or several hours. Numbness and/or tingling may follow during recovery.	Massage is indicated for Raynaud's syndrome that is *not* associated with underlying pathology. Otherwise, guidelines for the precipitating condition should be followed.

CONDITION NAME	WHAT IS IT/ WHAT ARE THEY?	HOW IS IT RECOGNIZED/ HOW ARE THEY RECOGNIZED?	IS MASSAGE INDICATED OR CONTRAINDICATED?
REFLEX SYMPATHETIC DYSTROPHY SYNDROME IN BRIEF (page 210)	Reflex sympathetic dystrophy syndrome (RSDS) is a chronic pain condition in which an initial trauma causes pain that is more severe and longer lasting than is reasonable to expect. The pain can become a self-sustaining phenomenon that becomes a lifelong affliction.	RSDS moves in stages, although symptoms may overlap. In early stages it involves redness, heat, sweating, and severe burning pain. In later stages the skin may turn bluish, and the nearby joints and muscles may atrophy. Bones in the area thin and become vulnerable to breakage. Late stage RSDS can involve irreversible changes to the affected area and symptoms that spread to other parts of the body.	Most RSDS patients have little or no tolerance for touch of any kind, at least in the area where the pain syndrome began. Physical therapy is often recommended to keep the affected joints moveable and functioning; massage may help to relieve some of the pain associated with this therapy. Massage within tolerance in other parts of the body may be welcome and supportive.
RENAL FAILURE IN BRIEF (page 440)	Renal failure is a situation in which the kidneys are incapable of functioning at normal levels. It may be an acute or a chronic problem, but it is often life-threatening.	Symptoms of acute and chronic renal failure differ in severity and type of onset, but some things they have in common are reduced urine output, systemic edema, and changes in mental state brought about by the accumulation of toxins in the blood.	Acute and chronic renal failure systemically contraindicate circulatory massage.
RHEUMATOID ARTHRITIS IN BRIEF (page 96)	Rheumatoid arthritis (RA) is an autoimmune disease in which immune system agents attack synovial membranes, particularly of the joints in the hands and feet. Other structures, such as muscles, tendons, and blood vessels, may also be affected.	In the acute phase affected joints are red, swollen, hot, and painful. They often become gnarled and distorted. It tends to affect the body symmetrically and is not determined by age.	Only the subacute stage of RA indicates massage. At that point bodywork may be used to re-establish mobility and to reduce the stresses that can trigger another flare.
SCAR TISSUE IN BRIEF (page 41)	Scar tissue refers to the new tissue that is created to replace damaged and dead cells at the site of an injury. Scar tissue on the skin has some different characteristics than scar tissue that develops in deeper layers of fascia and muscle.	Scar tissue on the skin often lacks pigmentation and hair follicles.	The acute stage of any injury in which the skin has been damaged contraindicates massage. In the subacute stage massage may improve the quality of the healing process.
SCLERODERMA IN BRIEF (page 125)	Scleroderma is a chronic autoimmune disorder involving damage to small blood vessels that leads to abnormal accumulations of scar tissue in the skin. Internal organs may also be affected.	Scleroderma can have many varied symptoms, depending on which tissues are involved. The most common outward signs are edema followed by hardening and thickening of the skin, usually of the hands and face.	Scleroderma may indicate massage if circulatory and kidney damage is not advanced. Clients whose systems are not capable of keeping up with the changes circulatory massage brings about may benefit from bodywork with less mechanical impact.
SEIZURE DISORDERS IN BRIEF (page 229)	Seizure disorders are any condition that causes seizures. They are often related to some kind of neurologic damage (tumors, head injuries, or infection), although it may be impossible to delineate exactly what that damage is. Epilepsy is a subtype of seizure disorder.	Seizures may take very different forms for different people; they range from barely noticeable to life-threatening. Seizure disorders are diagnosed through physical examination, a description of symptoms, computed tomography scans, magnetic resonance imaging scans, and electroencephalograms.	Seizure activity itself contraindicates massage, but bodywork is certainly appropriate for patients with most kinds of seizure disorders at any other time.

CONDITION NAME	WHAT IS IT/ WHAT ARE THEY?	HOW IS IT RECOGNIZED/ HOW ARE THEY RECOGNIZED?	IS MASSAGE INDICATED OR CONTRAINDICATED?
SEPTIC ARTHRITIS IN BRIEF (page 100)	Septic arthritis is joint inflammation caused by infection inside the joint capsule.	This conditions shows the cardinal signs of inflammation: pain, heat, redness, and swelling, although these symptoms may be mild. It is often accompanied by fever.	Massage is contraindicated for septic arthritis until the infection is completely gone from the joint. At that time massage may be useful to help restore function.
SHIN SPLINTS IN BRIEF (page 65)	"Shin splints" refers to a collection of lower leg injuries including muscle tears, periostitis, hairline fractures, and other problems. They are usually brought about by overuse and/or misalignment at the ankle.	Pain along the tibia may be superficial or deep, mild or severe. The pattern of pain differs with the specific structures that are injured.	Muscle injuries indicate massage, but it is advised with caution for periostitis or stress fractures, and is contraindicated entirely for acute exertional compartment syndrome.
SINUSITIS IN BRIEF (page 342)	Sinusitis is inflammation of the paranasal sinuses from allergies, infection, or physical obstruction.	Symptoms include headaches, localized tenderness over the affected area, runny or congested nose, facial or tooth pain, fatigue, and, if it is related to an infection, thick opaque mucus, fever, and chills.	Acute infections contraindicate massage, but chronic or noninfectious situations can be appropriate for bodywork as long as the client is comfortable on the table.
SKIN CANCER IN BRIEF (page 30)	Skin cancer is cancer in the stratum basale of the epidermis (basal cell carcinoma [BCC]), cancer of the keratinocytes in the epidermis (squamous cell carcinoma [SCC]), or cancer of the melanocytes (pigment cells) of the epidermis (malignant melanoma).	For BCC and SCC, one should look for the cardinal sign: sores that never heal. These are the clearest indication of BCC or SCC. These sores can resemble blisters, warts, pimples, or simple unexplained bumps and abrasions. They are usually painless but may bleed or become slightly itchy as the cells become active. For malignant melanoma, one should look for a mole that exhibits the ABCDE's of melanoma.	For BCC, which does not tend to metastasize, massage is a local contraindication, as long as the lesion has been diagnosed by a dermatologist. SCC and malignant melanoma carry the risk of metastasis. Therefore, any decisions about massage must be made according to the treatments the client is having, weighing possible benefits with possible risks.
SLEEP DISORDERS IN BRIEF (page 232)	Sleep disorders are a collection of problems including insomnia, sleep apnea, restless leg syndrome, narcolepsy, and circadian rhythm disruption that make it difficult to get enough sleep or to wake up feeling rested and refreshed.	The primary symptom of sleep disorders is excessive daytime sleepiness. If this continues for a prolonged period, a weakened immune system, memory and concentration loss, and an increased risk of automotive or on-the-job accidents may be the result.	Sleep disorders indicate massage. Bodywork may not correct a mechanical or psychological dysfunction that leads to sleep deprivation, but it can improve the quality of sleep and can reduce the mental and physical stresses that may interfere with sleep.
SPASMS, CRAMPS IN BRIEF (page 68)	Spasms and cramps are involuntary contractions of skeletal muscle. Spasms are considered to be low-grade, long-lasting contractions, whereas cramps are short-lived, very acute contractions.	Cramps are extremely painful with visible shortening of muscle fibers. Long-term spasms are painful and may cause inefficient movement, but may not have acute symptoms.	Acutely cramping muscle bellies do not invite massage, although stretching and origin/insertion work can trick the proprioceptors into letting go. Muscles that have been cramping respond well to massage, which can reduce residual pain and clean up chemical wastes. Underlying cramp-causing pathologies must be ruled out before massage is applied. Long-term spasm indicates massage because it can break through the ischemia-spasm-pain cycle to reintroduce circulation to the area as well as reduce muscle tone and flush out toxins.

CONDITION NAME	WHAT IS IT/ WHAT ARE THEY?	HOW IS IT RECOGNIZED/ HOW ARE THEY RECOGNIZED?	IS MASSAGE INDICATED OR CONTRAINDICATED?
SPINAL CORD INJURY IN BRIEF (page 212)	Spinal cord injury is a situation in which some or all of the fibers in the spinal cord have been damaged, usually by trauma but occasionally from other problems such as tumors or bony growths in the spinal canal.	The signs and symptoms of spinal cord injury vary with the nature of the injury. Loss of motor function follows destruction of motor neurons, but that paralysis may be flaccid or spastic depending on the injured area. Loss of sensation follows the destruction of sensory pathways. If the injury is not complete, some motor or sensory function may remain in the affected tissues.	Mechanical types of massage are appropriate only where sensation is present and no underlying pathologies may be exacerbated by the work. Areas without sensation contraindicate massage that intends to manipulate and influence the elasticity of tissue.
SPONDYLOSIS IN BRIEF (page 102)	Spondylosis is osteoarthritis of the spine.	It is identifiable on a radiograph, which shows a characteristic thickening of the affected vertebral bodies, facets, and ligamentum flava. Pain is present only if pressure is exerted on nerve roots, which also causes numbness, paresthesia, and specific muscle weakness. Otherwise, the only sign of spondylosis may be slow, progressive loss of range of motion in the spine.	Spondylosis indicates massage with caution. Muscle splinting to protect against movement that may be dangerous is often a feature of this condition; massage therapists should not interfere with this mechanism.
STOMACH CANCER IN BRIEF (page 376)	Stomach cancer is the development of malignant tumors in the stomach, which may then metastasize directly to other abdominal organs or through blood and lymph flow to distant places in the body.	Symptoms of stomach cancer include a feeling of fullness after only a little food, heartburn, unintentional weight loss, vague abdominal pain above the navel, and occasionally vomiting, constipation, or diarrhea.	The prognosis for stomach cancer, which is rarely found before metastasis, is generally not promising. Most clients who know that they have stomach cancer will probably be undergoing a series of treatments including surgeries, chemotherapy, and radiation. Bodywork to alleviate the discomforts of cancer treatment may be appropriate, as long as the risks involved with each type of intervention are respected.
SPONDYLOLISTHESIS IN BRIEF* (page 104)	Spondylolisthesis is a condition in which the vertebral body of one of the lumbar vertebrae is anterior of the rest of the lumbar vertebrae.	Spondylolisthesis causes irritation at the joints between the affected vertebrae, resulting in symptoms of spondylosis, or arthritis of the spine.	Massage can be indicated for spondylolisthesis; the same guidelines as those for spondylosis must be followed.
SPRAINS IN BRIEF (page 105)	Sprains are injured ligaments. Injuries can range from a few traumatized fibers to a complete rupture.	In the acute stage pain, redness, heat, swelling, and loss of joint function will be evident. In the subacute stage these symptoms will be abated, although perhaps not entirely absent. Passive stretching of the affected ligament will be painful until all inflammation has subsided.	Subacute sprains indicate massage. Bodywork can influence the healthy development of scar tissue and reduce swelling and damage due to edematous ischemia. Therapists must take care to rule out bone fractures or other injuries that sprains may temporarily mask.
STRAINS IN BRIEF (page 69)	Strains are injuries to muscles.	Pain, stiffness, and occasionally palpable heat and swelling are all signs of muscle strain. Pain may be exacerbated by passive stretching or resisted contraction of the affected muscle.	Muscle strains indicate massage, which can powerfully influence the production of useful scar tissue, reduce adhesions and edema, and reestablish range of motion.

CONDITION NAME	WHAT IS IT/ WHAT ARE THEY?	HOW IS IT RECOGNIZED/ HOW ARE THEY RECOGNIZED?	IS MASSAGE INDICATED OR CONTRAINDICATED?
STROKE IN BRIEF (page 216)	A stroke is damage to brain tissue caused either by a blockage in blood flow or by an internal hemorrhage.	The symptoms of stroke include paralysis, weakness, and/or numbness on one side; blurry or diminished vision on one side with asymmetrically dilated pupils; dizziness and confusion; difficulty in speaking or understanding simple sentences; sudden extreme headache; and possibly loss of consciousness.	Most people who survive strokes are at high risk for other cardiovascular problems. Rigorous circulatory massage should probably be avoided with this group, although they may certainly benefit from other types of bodywork to augment their rehabilitative physical therapy.
TEMPOROMANDIBULAR JOINT DISORDERS IN BRIEF (page 107)	Temporomandibular joint (TMJ) disorders arise when constant strain, stress, and malocclusion of the jaw lead to pain and loss of function of the TMJ.	Symptoms of TMJ disorder include head, neck, and shoulder pain; ear pain; mouth pain; clicking or locking in the jaw; and loss of range of motion in the jaw.	Massage can be useful for TMJ problems, if intervention is begun before bony deformation begins. However, this condition can be difficult to diagnose, so it is important to be working with other medical professionals in these situations.
TENDINITIS IN BRIEF (page 127)	Tendinitis is inflammation of a tendon, usually due to injury at the tenoperiosteal or musculotendinous junction.	Pain and stiffness are usually present, and in acute stages palpable heat and swelling will occur. Pain is exacerbated by resisted exercise of the injured muscle-tendon unit.	Tendinitis indicates massage. In the acute stage, lymph drainage techniques may help to limit and resolve inflammation. In the subacute stage, massage may influence the production of useful scar tissue, reduce adhesions and edema, and re-establish range of motion.
TENOSYNOVITIS IN BRIEF (page 128)	Tenosynovitis is the inflammation of a tendon and/or its surrounding tenosynovial sheath. It can happen wherever a tendon passes through a sheath, but is especially common in the wrist and hand.	Pain, heat, and stiffness mark the acute stage of tenosynovitis. In the subacute stage only stiffness and pain may be present. The tendon may feel or sound gritty as it moves through the sheath. It is difficult to bend fingers with tenosynovitis, but even harder to straighten them.	Tenosynovitis contraindicates massage in the acute stage of inflammation and indicates massage when the swelling has subsided.
THORACIC OUTLET SYNDROME IN BRIEF (page 147)	Thoracic outlet syndrome (TOS) is a collection of signs and symptoms brought about by occlusion of nerve and blood supply to the arm.	Depending on what structures are compressed, TOS shows shooting pains, weakness, numbness, and paresthesia ("pins and needles") along with a feeling of fullness and possible discoloration of the affected arm from impaired circulation.	This depends on the source of the problem. TOS from muscle tightness indicates massage. TOS symptoms due to muscle degeneration or some other disorder such as spondylosis or herniated disc will not respond well to massage.
THROMBOPHLEBITIS, DEEP VEIN THROMBOSIS IN BRIEF (page 263)	Thrombophlebitis and deep vein thrombosis (DVT) are inflammations of veins due to blood clots.	Symptoms of thrombophlebitis may include pain, heat, redness, swelling, and local itchiness as well as a hard cord-like feeling at the affected vein. Symptoms for DVT may be nonexistent or can be more extreme: possibly pitting edema distal to the site, often with discoloration, and intermittent or continuous pain that is exacerbated by activity or standing still for a long period.	Thrombophlebitis and DVT contraindicate any kind of bodywork that may disrupt clots, which could lead to pulmonary embolism.

CONDITION NAME	WHAT IS IT/ WHAT ARE THEY?	HOW IS IT RECOGNIZED/ HOW ARE THEY RECOGNIZED?	IS MASSAGE INDICATED OR CONTRAINDICATED?
TORTICOLLIS IN BRIEF (page 130)	Torticollis is a unilateral spasm of neck muscles. It can be caused by a variety of factors, including mild musculoskeletal injury, congenital abnormalities, or central nervous system problems.	Flexion and rotation of the head are the main symptoms. The spasm may be constant or intermittent. Torticollis may also cause pain in the neck, shoulders, and back.	This depends on the cause of the problem. Simple wryneck from trigger points, cervical misalignment, ligament sprain, or trauma may be appropriate for massage if no acute inflammation is present. Spasmodic torticollis patients may benefit from pain relief offered by massage, but work should be done in cooperation with the patient's health care team. If symptoms do not improve or if signs of systemic infection are present, a more thorough diagnosis should be sought.
TREMOR IN BRIEF (page 175)	Tremor is rhythmic, involuntary muscle movement. It can be a primary disorder (unrelated to other problems) or it can be a symptom of other neurologic diseases.	Tremor is identified through uncontrolled fine or gross motor movements.	Tremor may indicate massage as long as no contraindicating conditions are contributing factors.
TRIGEMINAL NEURALGIA IN BRIEF (page 220)	Trigeminal neuralgia (TN) is a condition involving sharp electrical or stabbing pain along one or more branches of the trigeminal nerve (cranial nerve V), usually in the lower face and jaw.	TN pain is very sharp and severe. Patients report stabbing, electrical, or burning sensations that occur in brief episodes but repeat with or without identifiable triggers. A muscular tic is often present as well.	TN is intensely painful, and even very light touch may trigger an attack. It therefore contraindicates massage on the face, unless the client specifically guides the therapist into what feels safe and comfortable. Massage elsewhere on the body is appropriate, although TN clients may prefer not to be face down.
TUBERCULOSIS IN BRIEF (page 345)	Tuberculosis is a bacterial infection that usually begins in the lungs but may spread to bones, kidney, lymph nodes, or elsewhere in the body. It is a highly contagious airborne disease.	Infection with the tuberculosis bacterium may produce no initial symptoms. If the infection turns into the active disease, symptoms may include coughing, bloody sputum, fatigue, weight loss, and night sweats.	Active tuberculosis disease systemically contraindicates massage, unless the client has been consistently taking medication for several weeks and has medical clearance. Massage for clients with tuberculosis infection but no disease is fine, but these people should be under medical supervision as well.
ULCERATIVE COLITIS IN BRIEF (page 392)	Ulcerative colitis is a condition in which the mucosal layer of the colon becomes inflamed and develops shallow ulcers.	Symptoms of acute ulcerative colitis include abdominal cramping pain, chronic diarrhea, blood and pus in stools, weight loss, and mild fever.	Acute ulcerative colitis contraindicates circulatory massage at least locally; the presence of fever systemically contraindicates massage. In subacute situations gentle abdominal massage may be helpful, but only within the tolerance of the client.
ULCERS IN BRIEF (page 378)	Ulcers are sores that for various reasons do not go through a normal healing process; they remain open and vulnerable to infection. Peptic ulcers occur in the stomach or duodenum (the proximal portion of the small intestine).	The symptoms of peptic ulcers include general burning or gnawing abdominal pain between meals that is relieved by taking antacids or eating. Other symptoms can include bloating, burping, gas, and consistent vomiting after meals.	Specific work on the abdomen may exacerbate symptoms of peptic ulcers, so they are at least a local contraindication for mechanical types of bodywork. Other modalities and massage away from the upper abdomen are certainly appropriate for ulcer patients.

CONDITION NAME	WHAT IS IT/ WHAT ARE THEY?	HOW IS IT RECOGNIZED/ HOW ARE THEY RECOGNIZED?	IS MASSAGE INDICATED OR CONTRAINDICATED?
URINARY TRACT INFECTION IN BRIEF (page 447)	A urinary tract infection (UTI) is an infection of the urinary tract, usually from bacteria that live in the digestive tract.	Symptoms of UTIs include pain and burning sensations during urination, increased urinary frequency, urgency, and cloudy or blood-tinged urine. In the acute stage, fever and general malaise may be present.	Acute UTIs contraindicate circulatory massage, as do all acute infections. Massage may be appropriate in the subacute stage, although deep work on the abdomen is still locally cautioned until all signs of infection are gone.
VARICOSE VEINS IN BRIEF (page 281)	Varicose veins are distended veins, usually in the legs, caused by vascular incompetence and a reflux of blood returning to the heart.	Varicose veins are ropey, slightly bluish, elevated veins that twist and turn out of their usual course. They happen most frequently in branches of the saphenous veins on the medial side of the calf, although they are also found on the posterior aspects of the calf and thigh.	Massage is locally contraindicated for extreme varicose veins and anywhere distal to them. Mild varicose veins contraindicate deep, specific work, but are otherwise safe for massage.
WARTS IN BRIEF (page 16)	Warts are neoplasms that arise from the keratinocytes in the epidermis; they are caused by extremely slow-acting viruses.	Typical warts (verruca vulgaris) look like hard, cauliflower-shaped growths. They usually occur on the hands. They can affect anyone, but teenagers are especially prone to them.	Massage is a local contraindication for warts. The virus is contained in the blood and shedding skin cells, and it is possible to get warts from another person.
WHIPLASH IN BRIEF (page 133)	Whiplash is an umbrella term referring to a collection of soft tissue injuries that may occur with cervical acceleration/deceleration. These injuries include sprained ligaments, strained muscles, damaged cartilage and joint capsules, and temporomandibular joint problems. Although whiplash technically refers to soft-tissue injury, damage to other structures including vertebrae, discs, and the central nervous system frequently occurs at the same time.	Symptoms of whiplash vary according to the nature of the injuries. Pain at the neck and referring into the shoulders and arms along with chronic headaches are the primary indicators.	An acute whiplash injury contraindicates circulatory or mechanically based massage. In the subacute and mature phases of scar tissue formation, however, massage along with chiropractic or manipulation can contribute greatly to a positive resolution of the problem.

Glossary of Terms

Ablate: To remove or destroy function.

Abrasion: A scrape involving injury to the epithelial layer of the skin or mucous membranes.

Absence seizure: A type of seizure characterized by lack of activity with occasional clonic movements.

Acute: A stage of injury or infection: short term, severe.

Acyclovir: An antiviral agent often used in the treatment of herpes simplex.

Adenoma: A benign neoplasm, usually occurring in epithelial tissue.

Adhesion: The adhering or uniting of two surfaces. Layers of connective tissue may adhere, which limits movement and increases the risk of injury.

Adhesive capsulitis: A condition involving inflammatory thickening of a joint capsule, usually at the shoulder, leading to loss of range of motion. Also known as "frozen shoulder."

Adson's test: A test for thoracic outlet syndrome. The patient is seated with his or her head extended and rotated toward the affected side. With deep inspiration there is a diminution or total loss of radial pulse on that side.

Adventitia: The outermost connective tissue layer that covers organs and vessels.

Aerobic metabolism: Metabolism that occurs in the presence of adequate oxygen, which reduces the overall production of toxic waste products.

Albumin: Any of several naturally occurring blood proteins, some of which contribute to blood clotting capacity.

Aldosterone: A hormone manufactured in the adrenal cortex. It helps to maintain appropriate fluid balance by influencing sodium reabsorption in the kidneys. The principal mineralocorticoid.

Allergen: A substance that produces an allergic reaction.

Alpha-1 antitrypsin: A protein that protects the inner lining of alveoli.

Alveolus, alveoli: A small cavity or socket. Specifically, the terminal epithelial structures in the lungs where gaseous exchange takes place.

Amantadine: An antiviral agent sometimes used to treat influenza.

Ambulatory: Able to walk about; not confined to bed or a wheelchair.

Amenorrhea: Absence or abnormal cessation of menses.

Amine: A positively charged ion found only in association with negatively charged ions; amines combine with acids to form salts.

Amino acid: An organic acid in which one of the hydrogen atoms on a carbon atom has been replaced by NH_2. A building block of proteins.

Amphiarthrosis: A form of joint in which the two bones are joined by fibrocartilage.

Anaerobic metabolism: Metabolism that takes place without adequate supplies of oxygen, which may result in the excessive build up of toxic waste products.

Anaphylactic shock: Am immediate, transient allergic reaction characterized by contraction of smooth muscle and dilation of capillaries.

Androgen: A hormone that stimulates activity of sex organs.

Angina: A severe, often constricting pain. Usually refers to *angina pectoris.*

Angiogenesis: Development of new blood vessels.

Angiogram: Radiograph of blood vessels after the injection of contrast material.

Angioneurotic edema: A situation in which hives appear on the face and neck and swelling occurs to the point that breathing becomes difficult.

Angioplasty: Recanalization of a blood vessel, usually by means of balloon dilation and/or the placement of a stent.

Annulus fibrosis: Fibrous ring of tissue in an intervertebral disc.

Anoxia: Absence of oxygen.

Antibody: A immunoglobulin molecule produced by B-cells and designed to react with specific antigens.

Anticoagulant: An agent that prevents or inhibits coagulation of the blood.

Antigen: Any substance that, as a result of coming into contact with appropriate cells, elicits a state of immune response.

Antrectomy: Removal of the antrum (distal half) of the stomach in treatment of peptic ulcer.

Aphtha, aphthae: Small ulcer on a mucous membrane, usually in the mouth.

Aplastic: Referring to conditions characterized by defective regeneration (i.e., varieties of cancer).

Apnea: Absence of breathing.

Apoptosis: Programmed cell death.

Arachnoid: A delicate membrane of spider-web–like filaments that lies between the dura mater and the pia mater.

Arrhythmia: Irregularity of the heartbeat.

Arteriogram: Radiographic demonstration of an artery after the injection of a contrast medium.

Arteriole: A minute artery continuous with a capillary network.

Ascites: The accumulation of serous fluid in the peritoneal cavity.

Asphyxia: Impaired or absent exchange of carbon dioxide and oxygen in the respiratory system.

Ataxia: Inability to coordinate muscle activity for smooth movement.

Atelectasis: Absence of gas from a part or whole of the lung; pulmonary collapse.

Athetoid: Referring to slow, writhing, involuntary movement of fingers and hands, sometimes of toes and feet.

Atopic: Relating to an allergic reaction.

Atrium, atria: A chamber or cavity connected to other cavities. Specifically, the superior chambers of the heart.

Atrophy: A wasting of tissues from a number of causes, including diminished cellular proliferation, ischemia, malnutrition, and death.

Auscultation: Listening to sounds made by various body parts as a diagnostic tool.

Autogenic transplant: The transplant of a substance that originated within the patient's body, as in bone marrow cells. Also called autologous transplant.

Autoimmune: Arising from and directed against the individual's tissues.

Avascular: Without blood or lymphatic vessels.

Avulsion: A tearing away or forcible separation.

Axon: The process of a nerve cell that conducts impulses away from the cell body.

Babesiosis: An infection with a species of protozoan parasites, transferred to humans by tick bites.

Barrel chest: An occasional symptom of emphysema, in which the intercostal muscles hold the rib cage out as wide as possible.

Barrett esophagus: Chronic ulceration of the lower esophagus, often associated with gastroesophageal reflux disorder (GERD); sometimes a precursor to adenocarcinoma of the esophagus.

Basal ganglia: Large masses of gray matter at the base of the cerebral hemispheres.

Basal layer: Also called the *stratum basale:* the deepest layer of the epidermis.

Basophil: A phagocytic leukocyte.

Bell's law: The ventral spinal roots are motor, while the dorsal spinal roots are sensory.

Benign: Denoting the mild character of an illness or nonmalignant character of a neoplasm.

Benign prostate hypertrophy (BPH): A nodular hyperplasia of the prostate; the gland thickens in a way that may obstruct the urethra.

Benzene: A highly toxic hydrocarbon from light coal tar oil, used as a solvent.

Beta blocker: A type of drug that limits sympathetic reactions, specifically as they relate to the cardiovascular system.

Beta cell: Cell in the pancreas that secretes insulin.

Bile: Yellowish-brown or green fluid produced in the liver, stored in the gallbladder, and released into the duodenum to aid in the digestion of fats.

Biliary colic: Intense spasmodic pain felt in the right upper quadrant of the abdomen from impaction of a gallstone in the cystic duct.

Bilirubin: A dark bile pigment formed from the hemoglobin of dead erythrocytes.

Bipolar disease: Synonym for manic depression.

Bismuth: A metallic element used in several medicines, specifically in those designed to affect stomach acidity.

Blood–brain barrier: A selective filter that prevents or inhibits the passage of ions or large compounds from the blood to the brain tissue; located in a continuous layer of endothelial cells connected by tight junctions.

Bone scan: A diagnostic test to look for bone cancer or infections, to evaluate unexplained pain, or to diagnose fractures

Borrelia burgdorferi: A species of bacteria that causes Lyme disease; transferred to humans through tick bites.

Bowman's capsule: The beginning of a nephron that surrounds the glomerulus.

Bradykinesia: A decrease in the spontaneity of movement.

Bronchiectasis: Chronic dilation of the bronchi or bronchioles, often as a consequence of inflammatory disease or obstruction.

Bruxism: Jaw clenching that results in rubbing and grinding of teeth, especially during sleep.

Bulla, bullae: A bubble-like structure, specifically the air-filled blisters on the lung formed by fused alveoli in emphysema.

Calcitonin: A hormone that increases the deposition of calcium and phosphate in bone.

Calcium channel blockers: A class of medications that prevents the passage of calcium through membranes; used to treat hypertension, angina pectoris, and arrhythmia.

Callus: A thickening of the keratin layer of the epidermis as a result of repeated friction or intermittent pressure.

Candida: A genus of yeast-like fungi.

Carbuncle: A group of localized infections of hair follicles, with the formation of connecting sinuses. A group of boils.

Catheter atherectomy: Removal of atherosclerotic plaque through a catheter; usually applied to carotid arteries.

Cauda equina: Bundle of spinal nerve roots that runs through the lumbar cistern; it comprises the roots of all the spinal nerves below L_1. From Latin, "horse tail."

Celiac sprue: Chronic inflammation and atrophy of the mucosa of the small intestine, related to an allergy to gluten.

Cellular immunity: Also called *cell-mediated immunity*. Immune responses that are initiated by T-cells and mediated by T-cells, macrophages, or both.

Cervical rib: An abnormally wide transverse process of a cervical vertebra, or a supernumerary rib that articulates with a cervical vertebra, but does not articulate with the sternum. C_7 is the vertebra most often affected.

Chemonucleolysis: Injection of chymopapain into the nucleus pulposus of a herniated disc.

Chemotherapy: The treatment of disease by chemical means (i.e., drugs).

Chlamydia: A genus of bacteria that is a causative factor for pelvic inflammatory disease and other infections; the chief agent of bacterial sexually transmitted diseases in the United States.

Cholangitis: Inflammation of the bile duct or biliary tree.

Cholecyst: Synonym for gallbladder.

Choledocholithiasis: Presence of a gallstone in the common bile duct.

Cholelithiasis: Presence of stones in the gallbladder or bile ducts.

Cholinesterase inhibitors: Class of drugs that improves myoneural function; used for myasthenia gravis.

Chondroitin sulfate: One of the substances present in the extracellular matrix of connective tissue.

Christmas disease: Synonym for hemophilia B, involving a deficiency in clotting factor IX.

Chronic: Referring to a health-related state: low intensity, lasting a long time.

Chyme: Semifluid mass of partly digested food in the stomach or small intestine.

Cilium, cilia: Hair-like extension of the surface of certain epithelial cells.

Circadian rhythm: Relating to biological variations or rhythms that last approximately 24 hours. From Latin *circa* (about) and *dies* (day).

Clonic spasm: Alternating involuntary contraction and relaxation of a muscle.

Cognitive-behavioral therapy: A technique in psychotherapy that uses guided self-discovery, imaging, self-instruction, and other elicited cognitions as the principal mode of treatment.

Colic: An abnormal contraction of smooth muscle, particularly in the digestive tract.

Collagen: A major protein forming the white fibers of connective tissue.

Colonoscopy: A visual examination of the internal surface of the colon by means of a colonoscope.

Colostomy: The establishment of an artificial opening from the skin to the colon.

Colposcopy: Examination of the vagina and cervix by means of an endoscope.

Comedo: A dilated hair follicle filled with bacteria; the principal lesion of acne vulgaris.

Complement: A combination of many serum proteins that react with each other in various ways to disable antigens and assist immune system response.

Complex regional pain syndrome: A term used to describe a chronic pain syndrome; sometimes called reflex sympathetic dystrophy syndrome.

Condyle: A rounded articular surface at the extremity of a bone.

Congenital: Referring to mental or physical traits that exist at birth.

Consolidation: Solidification into a firm, dense mass, specifically with cellular exudate in the lungs during pneumonia.

Constriction: A narrowed portion of a luminal structure.

Contact inhibition: The tendency of basal cells involved in healing to stop reproducing when they encounter cells from the other side of the wound.

Cor pulmonale: Right-sided ventricular hypertrophy, often arising from diseases of the lungs.

Corticosteroid injection: An injection of a specific steroid into an injured area for its anti-inflammatory and/or connective tissue dissolving properties.

Cortisol: A glucocorticoid secreted by the adrenal cortex. It acts on carbohydrate metabolism and influences the growth and nutrition of connective tissue.

Cortisone: A form of cortisol that may be injected into specific areas to act as an anti-inflammatory or to help dissolve connective tissue.

Coxsackie virus: A group of viruses first isolated in Coxsackie, New York. They may be responsible for several human diseases, including meningitis and juvenile diabetes.

Creatine kinase: An enzyme used in muscle contraction that allows the transformation of adenosine diphosphate (ADP) into adenosine triphosphate (ATP) and creatine; levels of creatine kinase are sometimes elevated following a heart attack.

Crepitus: A crackling sound resembling the noise heard on rubbing hair between the fingers.

Crisis: A sudden change, usually for the better, in the course of an acute disease.

Crust: A hard outer covering; a scab.

Cyanosis: A bluish or purplish coloration of the skin and mucous membranes due to deficient oxygenation of the blood.

Cystadenoma: A benign neoplasm from glandular epithelium.

Cystine: A type of acid that can create deposits of crystals in the urine or in the kidneys.

Cystoscope: A lighted tubular endoscope for examining the interior of the bladder.

Cytokine: Hormone-like proteins secreted by many different cells, involved in cell-to-cell communication.

Cytomegalovirus: A group of viruses in the Herpesviridae family infecting humans and animals.

Cytotoxic drug: A drug that is detrimental or destructive to certain cells.

Debridement: Excision of dead tissue and foreign matter from a wound.

Degeneration: A retrogressive pathologic change in tissues, in consequence of which their functions may be impaired or destroyed.

Dementia: The loss, usually progressive, of cognitive and intellectual functions, without impairment of perception or consciousness.

Dendrite: The process of a nerve cell that carries impulses toward the cell body.

De Quervain tenosynovitis: Inflammation of the tendons of the first dorsal compartment of the wrist, which includes the extensor pollicis brevis and the abductor pollicis longus.

Dermabrasion: Procedure to remove acne scars or pits from the skin using sandpaper, rotating wire brushes, or other abrasive materials.

Dermatome: The area of skin supplied by cutaneous branches from a single spinal nerve.

Dermatophyte: A fungus that causes superficial infections of the skin, hair, and nails.

Diaphoresis: Perspiration.

Diaphysis: The shaft of a long bone.

Diarthrosis: Also called *synovial joint*. A joint in which articulating surfaces are covered by articular cartilage and held together by a capsular ligament which is lined with a synovial membrane. Some degree of freedom of movement is possible with diarthrotic joints.

Diastole: Normal post-systolic dilation of the heart cavities, during which they fill with blood.

Diffusion: Random movement of small particles in solution to a uniform distribution within a closed space.

Dihydrotestosterone (DHT): An androgenic hormone with the same uses and actions as testosterone. Elevated levels are associated with an increased risk of benign prostatic hyperplasia.

Dilation: The enlargement of a hollow structure or opening.

Dimethyl sulfoxide (DMSO): A penetrating solvent enhancing absorption of therapeutic agents through the skin.

Dioxin: A contaminate in some herbicides, associated with toxicity, some forms of cancer, and birth defects.

Diplegia: Paralysis of corresponding parts on both sides of the body.

Diuretic: A chemical agent that increases urine output.

Diverticulum/diverticula: A pouch or sac opening from a tubular or saccular organ (e.g., the colon or urinary bladder).

Dopamine: A neurotransmitter present in the basal ganglia.

Dura mater: A tough, fibrous membrane forming the outer covering of the central nervous system.

Dyshidrosis: A skin eruption involving blisters and itching that usually appears on the volar surface of the hands or feet.

Dyspepsia: "Upset stomach," resulting in pain, burning, nausea, and gas.

Dysphagia: Difficulty in swallowing.

Dysplasia, dysplastic: Abnormal tissue development.

Dyspnea: Shortness of breath.

Dysthymia: Chronic mood disorder involving long-term, low-grade depression.

Dystonia: A state of abnormal (too much or too little) muscle tone.

Dystrophin: A protein found in the sarcolemma of normal muscle tissue; it is missing in individuals with some forms of muscular dystrophy.

Ecchymosis: A purplish patch caused by blood leaking into the skin; a bruise.

Eclampsia: The occurrence of one or more convulsions not attributable to other cerebral conditions. In this case, related to pregnancy-induced hypertension.

Edema: An accumulation of an excessive amount of watery fluid in cells, tissues, or serous membranes.

Ehrlichiosis: A tick-borne bacterial infection of humans and dogs.

Elastin: A yellow, elastic fibrous protein that contributes to the connective tissue of elastic structures.

Electroencephalogram (EEG): A recording of electrical potentials of the brain, derived from electrodes attached to the scalp.

Electrolyte: Any compound that, in solution, conducts electricity and is decomposed by it.

Electromyography (EMG): A recording of electrical activity in muscle tissue.

Emollient: An agent that softens the skin or soothes irritation of the skin.

Endarterectomy: Excision of the diseased layers of an artery along with atherosclerotic plaques.

Endo-: A prefix indicating *within, inner, absorbing,* or *containing.*

Endogenous: Originating or produced within the organism or one of its parts.

Endometritis: Inflammation of the endometrium.

Endometrium: The inner layers of the uterine wall.

Endomysium: The connective tissue sheath surrounding muscle fibers.

Endosteum: A layer of cells lining the inner surface of bone in the central medullary cavity of long bones.

Enterovirus: Any of a diverse group of viruses that attack the intestines.

Enzyme: A protein that acts as a catalyst to induce chemical changes in other substances while remaining unchanged itself.

Eosinophil: A class of phagocytic white blood cells with anti-parasitic functions.

Ephelis, ephelides: Freckles.

Epi-: Prefix indicating *upon, following,* or *subsequent to.*

Epicondylitis: Infection or inflammation of an epicondyle.

Epidermis: The superficial epithelial portion of the skin.

Epimysium: The connective tissue membrane surrounding a skeletal muscle.

Epinephrine: The chief hormone of the adrenal medulla; a potent stimulant of the sympathetic response.

Epithelium: A purely cellular avascular layer covering all free surfaces including skin, mucous, and serous glands.

Epstein–Barr virus: A herpesvirus that causes infectious mononucleosis and is implicated in Burkitt's lymphoma.

Erythema: Redness of the skin due to capillary dilation.

Erythema migrans: A type of rash, usually seen as an early symptom of Lyme disease.

Erythrocyte: A mature red blood cell.

Erythropoietin (EPO): A hormone secreted by the kidneys and possibly other tissues that stimulates the formation of red blood cells.

Essential: Of unknown etiology, specifically in reference to hypertension.

Estradiol: The most potent naturally occurring estrogen in mammals.

Estriol: Estrogenic metabolite of estradiol; usually the predominant estrogenic metabolite found in urine, especially during pregnancy.

Estrogen: A group of hormones secreted by the ovaries, placenta, testes, and possibly other tissues. Estrogens influence secondary sexual characteristics and the menstrual cycle.

Estrogen replacement therapy (ERT): A treatment for the prevention or slowing of osteoporosis by replacing some of the hormones that are lost or diminished with the onset of menopause.

Estrone: A metabolite of estradiol.

Exenteration: Removal of internal organs and tissues, usually performed to ablate cancer.

Exogenous: Originating or produced outside the organism.

Exophthalmus: Protrusion of one or both eyeballs.

External scar tissue: Scar tissue that develops outside of the injured structure, often binding that structure to other nearby structures in adhesions.

Extracorporeal shockwave lithotripsy: Breaking up of renal or ureteral calculi by focused ultrasound energy.

Exudate: Any fluid that has seeped out of a tissue or its capillaries because of inflammation or injury.

Fascicle, fasciculi: A band or bundle of fibers, specifically muscle fibers.

Fasciculation: Involuntary contractions or twitchings of fasciculi.

Fecalith: A hard mass composed of solidified or petrified feces.

Festinating gait: Gait in which the trunk is flexed, legs are stiff but flexed at the knees and hips, and the steps are short and progressively more rapid.

Fetal alcohol syndrome: A specific pattern of fetal malformation and health problems among offspring of mothers who are chronic alcoholics.

Fibrillation: Exceedingly rapid contractions or twitching of muscular fibrils.

Fibrin: An elastic filamentous protein that aids in coagulation of the blood.

Fibroblast: A cell capable of forming collagen fibers.

Filtration: The process of passing a liquid or gas through a filter.

Fimbria, fimbriae: Any fringe-like structure. Ovarian fimbriae extend over the ovaries.

Fistula: An abnormal passage from one epithelial surface to another.

Fixation: The condition of being firmly attached or set. In regard to the spine, being excessively limited in movement between individual vertebrae.

Flaccid paralysis: Paralysis with a loss of muscle tone, although sensation is present.

Folate: A form of folic acid.

Folic acid: Member of the vitamin B complex necessary for the normal formation of red blood cells.

Frozen shoulder: See *adhesive capsulitis*.

Fundoplication: Suture of the fundus of the stomach around the esophagus to prevent reflux with hiatal hernia.

Furuncle: A localized bacterial infection in a hair shaft. A boil.

Gamma-aminobutyric acid (GABA): A principal inhibitory neurotransmitter.

Gamma globulin: A preparation of proteins of human plasma, containing the antibodies of normal adults.

Gastrostomy: Establishment of a new opening into the stomach.

Glomerulus: A tuft of capillary loops surrounded by the Bowman's capsule at the beginning of each nephric tubule in the kidney.

Glucagon: A hormone secreted by the liver, which elevates blood sugar concentration.

Glucocorticoid: Any steroid-like compound capable of influencing metabolism; also exerts an anti-inflammatory effect. Cortisol is the most potent of the naturally occurring glucocorticoids.

Glycogen: A substance found primarily in the liver and muscles that is easily converted into glucose.

Goiter: Chronic enlargement of the thyroid gland not due to a neoplasm. May be related to both hyperthyroidism and hypothyroidism.

Golgi tendon organ: A proprioceptive sensory nerve ending embedded in tendon fibers. It is activated by changes in tendon tension.

Grand mal: Also called *generalized tonic clonic seizure*. Characterized by a sudden onset of tonic contraction of the muscles, giving way to clonic convulsive movements.

Granulocyte: A mature granular leukocyte.

Greater omentum: A fold of peritoneum holding fat cells that hangs like an apron in front of the intestines.

Growth hormone (GH): See *somatotrophin.*

Hallux valgus: A deviation of the great toe toward the lateral side of the foot.

Haustrum, haustra: One of a series of sacs or pouches, as seen in the colon.

Helicobacter pylori: Species of bacteria associated with peptic ulcers.

Hematuria: Any condition in which the urine contains blood or red blood cells.

Heme: The oxygen-carrying, color-bearing group of hemoglobin.

Hemiplegia: Paralysis of one side of the body.

Hemo-: A prefix denoting anything to do with blood.

Hemodialysis: Dialysis of soluble substances and water from the blood by diffusion through a semipermeable membrane.

Hemoglobin: Red protein of erythrocytes which binds to oxygen.

Hemolytic: Destructive to blood cells.

Hemoptysis: Expectoration of blood derived from the lungs or bronchi as a result of pulmonary or bronchial hemorrhage.

Hemorrhage: An escape of blood through ruptured vessels.

Hepatorenal syndrome: Occurrence of acute renal failure in patients with disease of the liver or biliary tract, apparently due to decreased renal blood flow.

Heterotopic ossification: The formation of calcium deposits in soft tissues, particularly seen with spinal cord injury patients.

High-density lipoprotein (HDL): A compound in plasma containing both lipids and proteins; HDLs are associated with a reduced risk of cardiovascular disease.

Histamine: A secretion of some cells that is a powerful stimulant of gastric secretion, a constrictor of bronchial smooth muscle, and a vasodilator.

Hobnailed liver: Characteristically knobby, bumpy appearance of a liver with advanced cirrhosis.

Homans' sign: A pain at the back of the knee or calf when the ankle is slowly dorsiflexed with the knee bent. This test indicates incipient or established thrombosis in the veins of the leg.

Homeostasis: A state of equilibrium in the body with respect to various functions and the chemical compositions of fluids and tissues.

Human papilloma virus (HPV): Class of DNA viruses that cause genital and cutaneous warts.

Humoral immunity: Immunity associated with circulating antibodies, as opposed to cellular immunity.

Hunner ulcer: A focal and often multiple star-shaped lesion involving all layers of the bladder wall; a sign of interstitial cystitis.

Hyaluronic acid: A gelatinous material in tissue spaces that acts as a lubricant and shock absorbant.

Hyper-: A prefix denoting *excessive, above normal.*

Hyperacusis: Abnormal acuteness of hearing due to irritability of sensory nerves.

Hyperglycemia: An abnormally high concentration of glucose in the circulating blood.

Hyperkinesia: Excessive muscular activity.

Hyperplasia: An increase in the number of cells in a tissue or organ, outside of tumor formation.

Hyperreflexia: A condition in which the deep tendon reflexes are exaggerated.

Hypersensitivity: An exaggerated response to the stimulus of a foreign agent.

Hyperthermia: High body temperature; fever.

Hypertonic: Having a greater degree of tension.

Hypertrophic scar: An elevated scar resembling a keloid but which does not spread into surrounding tissues.

Hyperuricemia: Enhanced blood concentrations of uric acid.

Hypnic myoclonia: The startling sensation that a person is about to fall; it often occurs while nearly asleep.

Hypo-: A prefix denoting *deficient, below normal.*

Hypoglycemia: An abnormally low concentration of glucose in circulating blood.

Hypokinesia: Diminished or slowed movement.

Hypotonic: Having a lesser degree of tension.

Hypoxia: Below normal levels of oxygen.

Idiopathic: Denoting a disease of unknown cause.

In situ: At the site only; refers to early stages of cancer development.

Incision: A cut or surgical wound.

Infarction: Sudden insufficiency of arterial or venous blood supply due to emboli, thrombi, vascular torsion, or necrosis.

Inflammatory bowel disease: Umbrella term for Crohn's disease and ulcerative colitis.

Infundibulum: Funnel-shaped structure or passage; the link between the pituitary gland and the hypothalamus.

Insulin: A hormone secreted by beta cells in the pancreas that promotes the utilization of glucose in tissue cells.

Integumentary: Relating to the skin.

Interferon: A class of proteins with anti-viral properties.

Interleukin-1: A cytokine that enhances the proliferation of T-helper cells and the growth and differentiation of B-cells.

Internal scar tissue: Scar tissue that accumulates within the injured structure (e.g., tendon, muscle, or ligament).

Interstitial: Relating to spaces within a tissue or organ but excluding such spaces as body cavities or potential space.

Intrinsic factor: A mucoprotein in the stomach necessary for the absorption of vitamin B_{12}.

Iritis: Inflammation of the iris of the eye.

Ischemia: Local anemia due to a mechanical obstruction of the blood supply.

Ixodes: A genus of hard ticks, many of which are parasitic to humans and which may be the vector for the spread of some diseases.

Keloid scar: A nodular mass of scar tissue that may occur after surgery, a burn, or cutaneous diseases.

Keratin: A substance present in cuticular structures (e.g., hair, nails, and horns).

Keratinocyte: A cell of the epidermis that produces keratin.

Ketoacidosis: Acidosis caused by the enhanced production of ketonic acids.

Ketogenic: Giving rise to ketones in metabolism.

Ketone: A potentially toxic product of metabolism; the most recognized ketone is acetone.

Klebsiella: A genus of bacteria that may or may not be pathogenic, depending on the individual type.

Kupffer cells: Specialized phagocytes found in the liver.

Kyphosis: A deformity of the spine, characterized by extensive flexion.

Laceration: A torn or jagged wound.

Lactobacilli: A genus of bacteria that are part of the normal flora of the mouth, intestinal tract, and vagina.

Laparoscopy: Examination of the abdominal contents with a scope passed through the abdominal wall.

Laparotomy: Incision into the abdominal wall.

Leiomyoma: A benign neoplasm derived from smooth muscle tissue.

Lentigo: A brown macule or spot, resembling a freckle.

Lesion: A wound or injury; a pathogenic change in tissues.

Leukocyte: A type of blood cell formed in several different types of tissues, involved in immune reactions. A white blood cell.

Levodopa: The biologically active form of dopa; a precursor of dopamine.

Levulose: Fructose: fruit sugar.

Lhermitte's sign: Sudden electric-like shocks extending down the spine on flexion of the head.

Ligamentum flava: A pair of yellow elastic fibrous structures that bind the laminae of adjoining vertebrae.

Limbic system: A group of brain structures and their connections that exert important influence on the endocrine and autonomic nervous systems. The limbic system is association with motivational and mood states.

Linea alba: Fibrous band that runs vertically from the xiphoid process to the pubis; site of attachment for abdominal muscles.

Lithium: An element of the alkali metal group, used to treat depression and other mood disorders.

Lordosis: A deformity of the spine, characterized by excessive extension.

Low-density lipoprotein (LDL): A compound in plasma containing both lipids and proteins; LDLs are associated with an increased risk of cardiovascular disease.

Lumen: The space in the interior of a tubular structure.

Lymphadenitis: Inflammation of a lymph node or nodes.

Lymphangion: A lymphatic vessel.

Lymphocyte: A white blood cell formed in lymphatic tissues.

Lymphokines: A group of hormone-like substances, released by lymphocytes, that mediate immune responses.

Macrophage: A type of phagocytic white blood cell.

Magnetic resonance imaging (MRI): A diagnostic modality in which the magnetic nuclei of a patient are aligned in a strong, uniform magnetic field. The signals they emit are converted into images that permit three-dimensional reference to soft tissues.

Malaise: A feeling of general discomfort or uneasiness.

Malar rash: A rash of the cheeks or cheekbones, often associated with lupus or erysipelas.

Malignant: Having the property of locally invasive and destructive growth and metastasis.

Malocclusion: Any deviation from a physiologically acceptable contact of opposing dentitions.

Marfan syndrome: A connective tissue disorder characterized by long fingers and limbs and cardiovascular weakness.

Mast cell: A white blood cell found in connective tissue that contains heparin and histamine.

Matrix: The intercellular substance of a tissue.

Melanin: Dark brown to black pigment formed in the skin and some other tissues.

Melanocyte: A pigment-producing cell located in the basal layer of the epidermis.

Melatonin: A substance secreted by the pineal gland that suppresses some glandular function; associated with circadian rhythm.

Menarche: A woman's first menstrual period.

Menses: Periodic hemorrhage from the uterine mucosa; usually preceded by ovulation but not by fertilization.

Mesentery: A double layer of peritoneum attached to the abdominal wall and enclosing a portion of the abdominal viscera.

Metabolite: Any product of metabolism, especially catabolism.

Metastasis: The spread of a disease process from one part of the body to another, as with the spread of cancer.

Microaerophilic: Referring to a type of bacteria that requires oxygen, although less than is available in the air.

Microbe: Any very minute organism.

Micrographia: Handwriting that grows progressively smaller and more cramped.

Mineralocorticoid: One of the steroids from the adrenal cortex that influence salt metabolism.

Mittelschmerz: Abdominal pain occurring at the time of ovulation.

Monoamine oxidase inhibitor (MAOI): A class of antidepressants that inhibit the breakdown of certain neurotransmitters.

Monocyte: A relatively large leukocyte; normally comprises 3 to 7% of the leukocytes in circulating blood.

Mononeuropathy: Disorder involving a single nerve.

Muscle spindle: Proprioceptor that wraps around specialized muscle fibers to relay information about the relative length of the muscle fibers.

Myalgic encephalomyelitis: Inflammation of the brain and spinal cord characterized by muscle pain.

Mycoplasma: A specialized type of bacteria that do not possess a true cell wall but are bound by a three-layered membrane.

Mycosis: Any disease caused by a fungus.

Myelin: A membrane composed of fat and protein molecules that surrounds nerve fibers.

Myeloid cell: Any cell that develops into a granulocyte of blood; also refers to any bone marrow cell.

Myofibril: One of the fine longitudinal fibers occurring in skeletal or cardiac muscle fiber.

Myotonia: Delayed relaxation of a muscle after a strong contraction.

Myxedema coma: A state of profound unconsciousness related to extreme hypothyroidism.

Narcolepsy: A sleep disorder involving recurring episodes of sleep during the day and interrupted sleep at night.

Necrosis: Pathologic death of one or more cells or of a portion of tissue or organ.

Neuralgia inducing cavitational osteonecrosis (NICO): A recently recognized problem in which there is tissue death at the site of extracted teeth, which causes pain in the face. Also called *osteomyelitis*.

Neoplasm: An abnormal tissue that grows by cellular proliferation, more rapidly than normal, and continues to grow after the stimuli that initiated the new growth cease.

Nephrolithiasis: Presence of renal calculi.

Nephron: A long convoluted tubular structure; the functional unit of the kidney.

Nerve growth factor: A protein that helps to control the development of sympathetic neurons and other nerve tissue; associated with heightened pain sensitivity.

Neurilemma: A cell that enfolds one or more axons of the peripheral nervous system.

Neurofibrillary tangle: Intraneural accumulations of filaments with twisted, contorted patterns; associated with Alzheimer's disease.

Neuron: The functional unit of the nervous system consisting of the nerve cell body, the dendrites, and the axon.

Neutrophil: A type of mature white blood cell formed in the bone marrow.

Nevus, nevi: A malformation of the skin, colored by hyperpigmentation or increased vascularity.

Nit: The ovum of a head or body louse.

Nociceptor: A peripheral nerve organ or mechanism for the reception and transmission of painful or injurious stimuli.

Nocturia: Urinating at night.

Nonsteroidal anti-inflammatory drug (NSAID): Aspirin, ibuprofen. Any collection of anti-inflammatory drugs that do not include steroidal compounds. Examples include aspirin, acetaminophen, ibuprofen, and naproxen.

Norepinephrine: A hormone produced in the adrenal medulla, secreted in response to hypotension and physical stress.

Nosocomial: Denoting a new disorder that develops while being treated in a hospital; specifically applied to some varieties of pneumonia.

Noxious: Injurious, harmful.

Nucleus pulposus: The soft fibrocartilage central portion of an intervertebral disk.

Numb-likeness: A condition characterized by reduced sensation but not total numbness.

Oncogene: Any of a family of genes that may foster malignant processes if mutated or activated by certain viruses.

Onychomycosis: Fungal infection of the nails.

Oocyte: The female sex cell.

Oophorectomy: Surgical removal of the ovaries.

Organic brain syndrome: A group of behavioral and/or psychological signs and symptoms caused by transient or permanent dysfunction of the brain; associated with chronic alcoholism.

Orthotics: The science concerned with the making and fitting of orthopedic appliances. Also used to refer to orthopedic appliances that are made to adjust the alignment and weight-bearing stress in the feet.

Osteoblast: A bone-forming cell.

Osteoclast: A cell functioning in the absorption and removal of osseus tissue.

Osteomalacia: A disease characterized by progressive softening and bending of the bones.

Osteomyelitis: Inflammation of the bone marrow and adjacent bone tissue.

Osteophyte: A bony outgrowth or protuberance.

Osteotomy: Cutting bone, usually using a saw or chisel.

Oxygen free radical: An atom or atom group carrying an unpaired electron and no charge. They may promote heart disease, cancer, Alzheimer's disease, and other progressive disorders.

Pain-spasm cycle: Self-perpetuating cycle of pain, which causes spasm, which increases pain, ad infinitum.

Palliative: Denoting the alleviation of symptoms without curing the underlying disease.

Palpable: Perceptible to touch.

Palpitation: Forcible or irregular pulsation of the heart perceptible to the patient, usually with an increase in frequency or force, with or without an irregularity in rhythm.

Pap test: Microscopic examination of cells scraped (usually from the uterine cervix) and stained with Papanicolaou stain to look for signs of cancer.

Paraplegia: Paralysis of both lower extremities and generally the lower trunk.

Parathyroid hormone (PTH): A hormone secreted by the parathyroid glands that raises serum calcium levels by causing bone resorption.

Paresis: Partial or incomplete paralysis.

Paresthesia: An abnormal sensation, such as burning, prickling, tickling, or tingling.

Pathogen: Any virus, microorganism, or substance causing disease.

Pediculosis: The state of being infested with lice.

Peptide: A compound of two or more amino acids.

Percutaneous nephrolithotomy: Incision through the skin directly to the kidney for the removal of a renal calculus.

Percutaneous transluminal coronary angioplasty (PCTA): A surgical procedure for enlarging a narrowed coronary vessel by inflating and withdrawing through the narrowed region a balloon on the tip of a catheter.

Perforation: Abnormal opening in a hollow organ.

Perfusion: The forcing of fluid to flow through the vascular bed of a tissue or through the lumen of a hollow structure.

Peri-: Prefix denoting *around*, *about*, or *near*.

Pericarditis: Inflammation of the pericardium.

Perimenopause: The 3- to 5-year period before the final cessation of the menstrual cycle, during which estrogen levels begin to drop.

Perimysium: The fibrous sheath enveloping each of the primary bundles of skeletal muscle fibers.

Periosteum: The thick fibrous membrane covering every surface of a bone except the articular cartilage.

Petit mal: A brief seizure characterized by arrest of activity and occasional clonic movements.

Phalen maneuver: Maneuver in which the wrist is maintained in flexion for 60 seconds or more; the sensation of paresthesia or other symptoms may indicate carpal tunnel syndrome.

Phlebectomy: Excision of a segment of a vein, especially to treat varicose veins.

Phlegm: Abnormal amounts of mucus, especially as expectorated from the mouth.

Photosensitivity: Abnormal sensitivity to light, especially of the eyes.

Phyto-: Having to do with plants.

Pia mater: A delicate fibrous membrane firmly adherent to the brain and spinal cord.

Pitting edema: Edema that retains for a time the indentation produced by pressure.

Plasmapheresis: Removal of whole blood from the body, separation of its cellular elements, and reinfusion of them suspended in saline or another plasma substitute.

Plaque: A small differentiated area on a surface; atheromatous plaques form well-defined yellow areas or swellings on the intimal surface of an artery.

Platelet: An irregularly shaped fragment of a megakaryocyte that aids in blood clotting.

Pleurisy: Inflammation of the pleurae.

Plexus: A network or interjoining of nerves, blood vessels, or lymphatic vessels.

Polyarteritis nodosa: A disease involving segmental inflammation and necrosis of medium- and small-sized arteries.

Polycythemia: An increase above normal in the number of red cells in the blood.

Polydipsia: Excessive thirst that is relatively prolonged.

Polyneuropathy: A disease process involving a number of peripheral nerves.

Polyphagia: Excessive eating.

Polysomnography: Continuous monitoring of normal and abnormal physiologic functioning during sleep.

Polyuria: Excessive excretion of urine.

Prednisone: An analogue of cortisol; used as a steroidal anti-inflammatory.

Preeclampsia: Development of hypertension with proteinuria or edema, or both, due to pregnancy.

Pretibial myxedema: A rash that occurs in the tibial region, specifically associated with hyperthyroidism.

Prodromic: Relating to the early or premonitory symptom of a disease, especially herpes simplex.

Proliferants: Injected substances that are designed to stimulate the growth of new collagen fibers which, with appropriate stretching and exercise, will lay down in alignment with the original fibers.

Prophylaxis: Prevention of a disease or of a process that can lead to a disease.

Proprioceptor: Sensory end organs that relay information about position and muscle tension.

Proptosis: Protruding eyes; see *exophthalmus*.

Prostaglandin: Several substances present in many tissues with effects such as vasodilation, vasoconstriction, and stimulation of smooth muscle tissue.

Prostate-specific antigen (PSA): A glycoprotein found in normal seminal fluid and produced in prostate epithelial cells. Elevated levels of PSA are associated with prostatic enlargement and an increased risk of prostate cancer.

Prostatitis: Inflammation of the prostate.

Protease inhibitor: A group of acquired immune deficiency syndrome (AIDS) drugs that work to interrupt the maturing phase of the virus.

Pseudogout: Acute episodes of synovitis caused by calcium pyrophosphate crystals as opposed to urate crystals, as in true gout.

Psychodynamic therapy: Therapy based on the psychological forces that underlie human behavior.

Pustule: A small, circumscribed elevation of the skin containing purulent material.

Pyelogram: A radiograph of the kidneys and ureters following the injection of a contrast medium.

Pyrogen: A fever-inducing agent that causes a rise in temperature.

Quadriplegia: Paralysis of all four limbs.

Radiation: The sending forth of light, short radio waves, ultraviolet or x-rays, or any other waves for treatment, diagnosis, or other purpose.

Radicular pain: Pain felt along the pathway of a spinal nerve.

Radiculopathy: Any disorder of the spinal nerve roots.

Rales: Term for an extra sound heard on auscultation of breath sounds.

Reduction: The restoration, by surgical or manipulative procedures, of a part to its normal anatomic relation.

Reed–Sternberg cells: Large transformed lymphocytes, indicative of Hodgkin's disease.

Reiter's syndrome: A combination of symptoms, including urethritis, cutaneous lesions, arthritis, and diarrhea. One or more of these symptoms may recur at intervals, but the arthritis may be persistent.

Relaxin: A hormone secreted during pregnancy that allows the softening and lengthening of the pubis symphysis, along with other connective tissues.

Repetitive stress injury: Any injury related to wear-and-tear brought about by repeated, especially percussive, movements.

Renal calculus: A stone or pebble formed in the kidney collection system.

Renal colic: Severe pain caused by the impaction or passage of a calculus in the ureter or renal pelvis.

Renin: An enzyme produced by the kidneys that is involved in vasoconstriction and hypertension.

Restless leg syndrome: A sense of uneasiness, twitching, or restlessness that occurs in the legs after going to bed; associated with sleep disorders.

Reticulocyte: An immature red blood cell.

Retinoid: A class of keratolytic drugs derived from retinoic acid and used for treatment of severe acne and psoriasis.

Retinopathy: Non-inflammatory degenerative disease of the retina.

Retrovirus: A virus in the family of Retroviridae. They possess RNA, which serves as a template for the synthesis of DNA in the host cell.

Rimantadine: An antiviral agent that closely resembles amantadine but is often better tolerated.

Ringworm: A fungal infection of the keratin component of hair, skin, or nails. Tinea.

Rodent ulcer: A slowly enlarging ulcerated basal cell carcinoma, usually on the face.

Salpingitis: Inflammation of the fallopian (uterine) tube.

Sarcomere: The segment of a myofibril between Z lines; the functioning contractile unit of striated muscle.

Schwann cells: Cells forming a continuous envelope around each fiber of peripheral nerves.

Scoliosis: Abnormal lateral curve of the vertebral column.

Seasonal affective disorder (SAD): A depressive disorder that is exacerbated by reduced daylight hours and subsides in spring and summer.

Sebaceous gland: Gland in the dermis that usually opens into hair follicles and secretes an oily semi-fluid: sebum.

Seborrhea: Overactivity of the sebaceous glands resulting in an excessive amount of sebum.

Seborrheic keratosis: Superficial benign skin lesions of proliferating epithelial cells.

Sebum: The secretion produced by sebaceous glands.

Selective serotonin reuptake inhibitor (SSRI): A class of drugs used in the treatment of depression that selectively prevent the reuptake of serotonin in the brain.

Self-limiting: Denoting a disease that tends to cease after a period of time.

Sentinel lymph node: The first lymph node to receive lymph drainage from a malignant tumor; if it is found clear of metastasis, all the other nearby nodes are clear also.

Septicemia: Systemic disease caused by the spread of microorganisms and their toxins in the circulating blood.

Serotonin: A chemical found in many different tissues. In the brain it is a neurotransmitter associated with mood disorders; in the body it can be a vasoconstrictor, it can stimulate smooth muscle contraction, and it can inhibit gastric secretion.

Sigmoidoscopy: An inspection, through an endoscope, of the sigmoid flexure of the colon.

Sinoatrial node: The mass of specialized cardiac fibers that act as the "pacemaker" for the heart.

Sjögren's syndrome: An autoimmune disorder with a collection of signs and symptoms, including conjunctivitis, dryness of mucous membranes, and bilateral enlargement of the parotid glands.

Sodium urate: Uric acid.

Somatotrophin: A hormone produced in the anterior pituitary that promotes body growth, fat mobilization, and the inhibition of glucose utilization.

Sonogram: A diagnostic technique that uses ultrasound waves to create a computerized image.

Spastic paralysis: Central nervous system damage resulting in permanent muscle contraction; combines aspects of hypertonia, hypokinesia, and hyperreflexia.

Spasticity: A state of increased muscle tone with exaggerated muscle tendon reflexes.

Specific immunity: The immune state in which there is an altered reactivity directed solely against the antigens that stimulated it.

Specific muscle weakness: Degeneration and weakening of muscles supplied by specifically damaged motor neurons; as opposed to *general muscle weakness*, which may not be drelated to nerve damage.

Sphincter: A muscle that encircles a duct, tube, or orifice.

Sphygmomanometer: Blood pressure cuff.

Spina bifida: A birth defect in which one or more vertebral arches do not completely fuse.

Spirochete: A type of bacteria shaped like undulating spiral-shaped rods.

Spirometry: A test to measure respiratory gases using a spirometer.

Splenomegaly: Enlargement of the spleen.

Spondylolisthesis: Forward movement of the body of one of the lumbar vertebrae on the vertebra below it, or on the sacrum.

Spondylolysis: Degeneration of the articulating part of the vertebra.

Sporadic: Occurring irregularly, haphazardly.

Sputum: Expectorated matter, especially mucus or mucopurulent matter expectorated in diseases of the air passages.

Squamous: Relating to or covered with scales.

Staging: The classification of distinct phases or periods in the course of a disease.

Staphylococcus: A type of bacteria formed of spherical cells that divide to make irregular clusters.

Starling's equilibrium: Also called Starling's hypothesis: the principle that the amount of fluid squeezed out of circulatory capillaries should be almost equal to the amount being drawn into lymphatic capillaries.

Stenosis: A stricture of any canal.

Stent: A device to hold tissue in place or provide support.

Steroids: A large group of chemical compounds including some hormones and drugs of a particular molecular composition. Some steroids include gonadal and adrenal hormones.

Strabismus: A lack of parallelism in the visual axes of the eyes.

Streptococcus: A type of bacteria formed of spherical cells that occur in pairs or in long or short chains.

Stroma: The framework, usually made of connective tissue, of an organ, gland, or other tissue.

Struvite: A compound of magnesium ammonium phosphate, found in some renal calculi.

Subacute: Between acute and chronic, denoting a mild duration or severity.

Subcutaneous: Beneath the skin.

Subluxation: An incomplete dislocation; although a relationship is altered, contact between joint surfaces remains.

Substance P: A neurotransmitter that is primarily involved in pain transmission and is one of the most potent compounds affecting smooth muscle tissue.

Substantia nigra: A large mass composed of pigmented cells located in the brainstem. The site of dopamine synthesis.

Superficial fascia: A loose fibrous envelope of connective tissue under the skin containing fat, blood vessels, and nerves.

Superior vena cava syndrome: Obstruction of the superior vena cava by benign or malignant lesions that cause the engorgement of the blood vessels of the face, neck, and arms; sometimes seen with lung cancer.

Sympathectomy: Excision of a section of a sympathetic nerve or one or more of the sympathetic ganglia.

Synarthrosis: A fibrous joint, sometimes said to be immovable.

Synovectomy: The excision of part or all of the synovial membrane of a joint.

Synovial joint: A diarthrosis or freely moveable joint.

Systole: The contraction of the heart, specifically of the ventricles.

Tachycardia: Rapid heart beat, usually applied to rates greater than 100 beats per minute.

Tamoxifen: An anti-estrogen agent used in the treatment of breast cancer.

Tau: A protein that helps to maintain the structure of the cytoskeleton; found in the plaques of persons with Alzheimer's disease.

Telangiectasia: Dilation of previously existing small vessels, most commonly in the skin.

Tender point: One of many predictable bilateral pairs of points that produce a painful response with a minimum of pressure (4 kg); used to help diagnose fibromyalgia.

Teratoma: A neoplasm that contains tissues not normally found in the tissue in which it arises; usually found as benign ovarian cysts in women and malignant testicular growths in men.

Testosterone: A naturally occurring androgen found in testes and other tissues.

Tetraplegia: Quadriplegia.

Thenar: Referring to the fleshy mass on the lateral side of the palm; the ball of the thumb.

Thermal capsulorraphy: The use of heat to shrink and repair a joint capsule, specifically at the shoulder, to prevent future dislocations.

Thermography: The making of a regional temperature map of the body, obtained by using an infrared sensing device.

Thrombocyte: Platelet.

Thrombosis: Formation or presence of a clot.

Thymoma: A neoplasm originating in the thymus; usually benign.

Thymosin: A hormone that restores thymus function.

Tic douloureux: A synonym for trigeminal neuralgia.

Tinea: A fungal infection of the keratin component of hairs, skin, or nails.

Tinel's sign: Distally radiating pain or tingling caused by tapping over the site of a superficial nerve, indicating inflammation or entrapment of that nerve; a test used to help identify carpal tunnel syndrome.

Tinnitus: A sensation of noises (ringing, whistling, booming) in the ears.

Tissue plasminogen activator (tPA): A genetically engineered protein that acts as a powerful thrombolytic ("clot-busting") agent.

Tonic/clonic seizure: The sudden onset of tonic contraction of muscles, giving way to clonic convulsive movements. Grand mal seizure.

Tonic spasm: Continuous involuntary spasm of skeletal muscle.

Tophus, tophi: Deposits of uric acid and urates in tissue around joints and other areas, seen with gout.

Toxic megacolon: Acute nonobstructive dilation of the colon.

Transcriptase: An enzyme that converts RNA to DNA in the acquired immune deficiency syndrome (AIDS) virus.

Transcutaneous: Denoting the passage of substances through unbroken skin.

Tricyclic antidepressants: A chemical group of drugs that share a three-ringed nucleus (e.g., amitriptyline, imipramine).

Trigger point: A small area in which muscle fibers have suffered injury and not gone through a normal healing process. Pressure on a trigger point elicits moderate to severe pain in specific referring patterns.

Trophic: Relating to or dependent on nutrition.

Trophic ulcer: Ulcer resulting from cutaneous sensory denervation.

Tubercle: A nodule or bump; may refer to bony prominences, elevations on the skin or other tissues, or to the lesions caused by infection with *Mycobacterium tuberculosis*.

Tumor: Any swelling, usually denoting a neoplasm.

Tunica intima: The innermost coat of a blood or lymphatic vessel.

Tunica media: The middle, usually muscular coat of a blood vessel or lymphatic vessel.

Tyrosine: An amino acid present in most proteins.

Unilateral: Confined to one side only.

Uremia: An excess of urea and other nitrogenous waste in the blood.

Ureterolithiasis: A kidney stone lodged in the ureter.

Urticaria: An eruption of itching wheals; synonym for hives.

Vagotomy: Division of the vagus nerve.

Varix, varices: A dilated vein.

Vasculitis: Inflammation of a blood or lymphatic vessel.

Venography: A radiographic demonstration of a vein after the injection of a contrast medium.

Ventricle: A normal cavity, specifically in the brain or heart.

Venule: A venous branch continuous with a capillary.

Verruca: A wart composed of a thickened keratinic layer of the epidermis.

Vesicle: A small, circumscribed fluid-filled elevation of the skin, a blister.

Villus, villi: A projection from the surface, especially of a mucous membrane.

Virulent: Extremely toxic, denoting a markedly pathogenic microorganism.

von Willebrand disease: A disease characterized by the tendency to bleed primarily from the mucous membranes and prolonged bleeding time.

Wheal: A reddened, itchy, changeable edematous area of the skin that is caused by exposure to an allergenic substance in a susceptible individual.

Wolff's law: A law stating that every change in the form and/or function of a bone is followed by changes in internal and external architecture of the bone.

Wright's test: A thoracic outlet syndrome test in which the hand is placed over the head, and the head is turned toward the affected side. If this exacerbates symptoms or reduces the strength of the pulse of the affected side, impingement to the axillary artery and lower brachial plexus nerves is suspected.

Xeroderma: Excessively dry skin; a mild form of ichthyosis.

Yuppie flu: Vernacular for a set of signs and symptoms that may be diagnosed as chronic fatigue syndrome.

Zygapophyseal joint: Relating to a zygapophysis or articular process of a vertebra.

Illustration Credits

Illustration Credits
Color Plates

Color Plate 1. Reprinted with permission from Rassner G. *Atlas of Dermatology.* 3rd ed. Philadelphia, PA: Lea & Febiger; 1994:228.

Color Plate 2. Reprinted with permission from Rassner G. *Atlas of Dermatology.* 3rd ed. Philadelphia, PA: Lea & Febiger; 1994:228.

Color Plate 3. Reprinted with permission from Rassner G. *Atlas of Dermatology.* 3rd ed. Philadelphia, PA: Lea & Febiger; 1994:51.

Color Plate 4. Reprinted with permission from Willis MC. *Medical Terminology: The Language of Health Care.* 1st ed. Baltimore: Williams & Wilkins, 1996:100. Courtesy of Laurence J, and Richard D. Underwood, Mission Viejo, CA.

Color Plate 5. Reprinted with permission from Goodheart HP. *A Photoguide of Common Skin Disorders: Diagnosis and Management.* Baltimore, MD: Williams & Wilkins; 1999:132.

Color Plate 6. Reprinted with permission from Rassner G. *Atlas of Dermatology.* 3rd ed. Philadelphia, PA: Lea & Febiger; 1994:65.

Color Plate 7. Reprinted with permission from Rassner G. *Atlas of Dermatology.* 3rd ed. Philadelphia, PA: Lea & Febiger; 1994:42.

Color Plate 8. Reprinted with permission from Goodheart HP. *A Photoguide of Common Skin Disorders: Diagnosis and Management.* Baltimore, MD: Williams & Wilkins; 1999:90.

Color Plate 9. Reprinted with permission from Rassner G. *Atlas of Dermatology.* 3rd ed. Philadelphia, PA: Lea & Febiger; 1994:49.

Color Plate 10. Reprinted with permission from Goodheart HP. *A Photoguide of Common Skin Disorders: Diagnosis and Management.* Baltimore, MD: Williams & Wilkins; 1999:246.

Color Plate 11. Reprinted with permission from Rassner G. *Atlas of Dermatology.* 3rd ed. Philadelphia, PA: Lea & Febiger; 1994:46.

Color Plate 12. Reprinted with permission from Rassner G. *Atlas of Dermatology.* 3rd ed. Philadelphia, PA: Lea & Febiger; 1994:47.

Color Plate 13. Reprinted with permission from Rassner G. *Atlas of Dermatology.* 3rd ed. Philadelphia, PA: Lea & Febiger; 1994:241.

Color Plate 14. Reprinted with permission from Goodheart HP. *A Photoguide of Common Skin Disorders: Diagnosis and Management.* Baltimore, MD: Williams & Wilkins; 1999:44.

Color Plate 15. Reprinted with permission from Rassner G. *Atlas of Dermatology.* 3rd ed. Philadelphia, PA: Lea & Febiger; 1994:101.

Color Plate 16. Reprinted with permission from Willis MC. *Medical Terminology: The Language of Health Care.* 1st ed. Baltimore, MD: Williams & Wilkins; 1996:A5. Courtesy of American Academy of Dermatology, Schamburg, Ill.

Color Plate 17. Reprinted with permission from Rassner G. *Atlas of Dermatology.* 3rd ed. Philadelphia, PA: Lea & Febiger, 1994:196.

Color Plate 18. Reprinted with permission from Goodheart HP. *A Photoguide of Common Skin Disorders: Diagnosis and Management.* Baltimore, MD: Williams & Wilkins; 1999:49.

Color Plate 19. Reprinted with permission from Rassner G. *Atlas of Dermatology.* 3rd ed. Philadelphia, PA: Lea & Febiger; 1994:173.

Color Plate 20. Reprinted with permission from Rassner G. *Atlas of Dermatology.* 3rd ed. Philadelphia, PA: Lea & Febiger; 1994:169.

Color Plate 21. Reprinted with permission from Rassner G. *Atlas of Dermatology.* 3rd ed. Philadelphia, PA: Lea & Febiger; 1994:170.

Color Plate 22. Reprinted with permission from Rassner G. *Atlas of Dermatology.* 3rd ed. Philadelphia, PA: Lea & Febiger; 1994:171.

Color Plate 23. Reprinted with permission from Rassner G. *Atlas of Dermatology.* 3rd ed. Philadelphia, PA: Lea & Febiger; 1994:176.

Color Plate 24. Reprinted with permission from Rassner G. *Atlas of Dermatology.* 3rd ed. Philadelphia, PA: Lea & Febiger; 1994:319.

Color Plate 25. Reprinted with permission from Rassner G. *Atlas of Dermatology.* 3rd ed. Philadelphia, PA: Lea & Febiger; 1994:207.

Color Plate 26. Reprinted with permission from Judd RL, Ponsell PP. *Mosby's First Responder.* 2nd ed. St. Louis, MO: Mosby-Year Book; 1988.

Color Plate 27. Reprinted with permission from Rassner G. *Atlas of Dermatology.* 3rd ed. Philadelphia, PA: Lea & Febiger; 1994:82.

Color Plate 28. Reprinted with permission from Judd RL, Ponsell PP. *Mosby's First Responder.* 2nd ed. St. Louis, MO: Mosby-Year Book; 1988.

Color Plate 29. Reprinted with permission from Willis MC. *Medical Terminology: The Language of Health Care.* 1st ed. Baltimore, MD: Williams & Wilkins; 1996:A5.

Color Plate 30. Reprinted with permission from Rassner G. *Atlas of Dermatology.* 3rd ed. Philadelphia, PA: Lea & Febiger; 1994:25.

Color Plate 31. Reprinted with permission from Goodheart HP. *A Photoguide of Common Skin Disorders: Diagnosis and Management.* Baltimore, MD: Williams & Wilkins; 1999:145.

Color Plate 32. Reprinted with permission from Goodheart HP. *A Photoguide of Common Skin Disorders: Diagnosis and Management.* Baltimore, MD: Williams & Wilkins; 1999:366.

Color Plate 33. Photo courtesy of Robert Schwartzmann, MD, Philadelphia, PA.

Color Plate 34. Reprinted with permission from Rassner G. *Atlas of Dermatology.* 3rd ed. Philadelphia, PA: Lea & Febiger; 1994:271.

Color Plate 35. Reprinted with permission from Fitzpatrick J, Aeling J. *Dermatology Secrets in Color.* 2nd ed. Philadelphia, PA: Hanley & Belfus; 2000; 191, Figure 8.

Color Plate 36. Reprinted with permission from *Stedman's Medical Dictionary.* 27th ed. Baltimore, MD: Lippincott Williams & Wilkins; 2000:1036.

Color Plate 37. Reprinted with permission from Goodheart HP. *A Photoguide of Common Skin Disorders: Diagnosis and Management.* Baltimore, MD: Williams & Wilkins; 1999:356, Figure 25-20.

Color Plate 38. Reprinted with permission from Rassner G. *Atlas of Dermatology.* 3rd ed. Philadelphia, PA: Lea & Febiger; 1994:302.

Color Plate 39. Reprinted with permission from Rassner G. *Atlas of Dermatology.* 3rd ed. Philadelphia, PA: Lea & Febiger; 1994:84.

Chapter 1

Figure 1-1. Reprinted with permission from Willis MC. *Medical Terminology: The Language of Health Care.* 1st ed. Baltimore, MD: Williams & Wilkins, 1996:90.

Figure 1-2. Reprinted with permission from Rassner G. *Atlas of Dermatology.* 3rd ed. Philadelphia, PA: Lea & Febiger; 1994:228.

Figure 1-3. Reprinted with permission from Rassner G. *Atlas of Dermatology.* 3rd ed. Philadelphia, PA: Lea & Febiger; 1994:228.

Figure 1-4. Reprinted with permission from Rassner G. *Atlas of Dermatology.* 3rd ed. Philadelphia, PA: Lea & Febiger; 1994:51.

Figure 1-5. Reprinted with permission from Willis MC. *Medical Terminology: The Language of Health Care.* 1st ed. Baltimore: Williams & Wilkins, 1996:100. Courtesy of Laurence J, and Richard D. Underwood, Mission Viejo, CA.

Figure 1-6. Reprinted with permission from Goodheart HP. *A Photoguide of Common Skin Disorders: Diagnosis and Management.* Baltimore, MD: Williams & Wilkins; 1999:132.

Figure 1-7. Reprinted with permission from Rassner G. *Atlas of Dermatology.* 3rd ed. Philadelphia, PA: Lea & Febiger; 1994:65.

Figure 1-8. Reprinted with permission from Rassner G. *Atlas of Dermatology.* 3rd ed. Philadelphia, PA: Lea & Febiger; 1994:42.

Figure 1-9. Reprinted with permission from Goodheart HP. *A Photoguide of Common Skin Disorders: Diagnosis and Management.* Baltimore, MD: Williams & Wilkins; 1999:90.

Figure 1-10. Reprinted with permission from Rassner G. *Atlas of Dermatology.* 3rd ed. Philadelphia, PA: Lea & Febiger; 1994:49.

Figure 1-11. Reprinted with permission from Goodheart HP. *A Photoguide of Common Skin Disorders: Diagnosis and Management.* Baltimore, MD: Williams & Wilkins; 1999:246.

Figure 1-12. Reprinted with permission from Goodheart HP. *A Photoguide of Common Skin Disorders: Diagnosis and Management.* Baltimore, MD: Williams & Wilkins; 1999:246.

Figure 1-13. Reprinted with permission from Willis MC. *Medical Terminology: The Language of Health Care.* 1st ed. Baltimore, MD: Williams & Wilkins; 1996:100.

Figure 1-14. Reprinted with permission from Willis MC. *Medical Terminology: The Language of Health Care.* 1st ed. Baltimore, MD: Williams & Wilkins; 1996:100.

Figure 1-15. Reprinted with permission from Rassner G. *Atlas of Dermatology.* 3rd ed. Philadelphia, PA: Lea & Febiger; 1994:46.

Figure 1-16. Reprinted with permission from Rassner G. *Atlas of Dermatology.* 3rd ed. Philadelphia, PA: Lea & Febiger; 1994:47.

Figure 1-17. Reprinted with permission from Rassner G. *Atlas of Dermatology.* 3rd ed. Philadelphia, PA: Lea & Febiger; 1994:241.

Figure 1-18. Reprinted with permission from Goodheart HP. *A Photoguide of Common Skin Disorders: Diagnosis and Management.* Baltimore, MD: Williams & Wilkins; 1999:44.

Figure 1-19. Reprinted with permission from Rassner G. *Atlas of Dermatology.* 3rd ed. Philadelphia, PA: Lea & Febiger; 1994:101.

Figure 1-20. Reprinted with permission from Willis MC. *Medical Terminology: The Language of Health Care.* 1st ed. Baltimore, MD: Williams & Wilkins; 1996: A5. Courtesy of American Academy of Dermatology, Schamburg, IL.

Figure 1-21. Reprinted with permission from Rassner G. *Atlas of Dermatology.* 3rd ed. Philadelphia, PA: Lea & Febiger; 1994:196.

Figure 1-22. Reprinted with permission from Goodheart HP. *A Photoguide of Common Skin Disorders: Diagnosis and Management.* Baltimore, MD: Williams & Wilkins; 1999:49.

Figure 1-23. Reprinted with permission from Rassner G. *Atlas of Dermatology.* 3rd ed. Philadelphia, PA: Lea & Febiger; 1994:173.

Figure 1-24. Reprinted with permission from Rassner G. *Atlas of Dermatology.* 3rd ed. Philadelphia, PA: Lea & Febiger; 1994:169.

Figure 1-25. Reprinted with permission from Rassner G. *Atlas of Dermatology.* 3rd ed. Philadelphia, PA: Lea & Febiger; 1994:170.

Figure 1-26. Reprinted with permission from Rassner G. *Atlas of Dermatology.* 3rd ed. Philadelphia, PA: Lea & Febiger; 1994:171.

Figure 1-27. Reprinted with permission from Rassner G. *Atlas of Dermatology.* 3rd ed. Philadelphia, PA: Lea & Febiger; 1994:176.

Figure 1-28. Reprinted with permission from Rassner G. *Atlas of Dermatology.* 3rd ed. Philadelphia, PA: Lea & Febiger; 1994:319.

Figure 1-29. Reprinted with permission from Rassner G. *Atlas of Dermatology.* 3rd ed. Philadelphia, PA: Lea & Febiger; 1994:207.

Figure 1-30. Reprinted with permission from Judd RL, Ponsell PP. *Mosby's First Responder.* 2nd ed. St. Louis, MO: Mosby-Year Book; 1988.

Figure 1-31. Reprinted with permission from Rassner G. *Atlas of Dermatology.* 3rd ed. Philadelphia, PA: Lea & Febiger; 1994:82.

Figure 1-32. Reprinted with permission from Judd RL, Ponsell PP. *Mosby's First Responder.* 2nd ed. St. Louis, MO: Mosby-Year Book; 1988.

Figure 1-33. Reprinted with permission from Willis MC. *Medical Terminology: The Language of Health Care.* 1st ed. Baltimore, MD: Williams & Wilkins; 1996:A5.

Figure 1-34. Reprinted with permission from Rassner G. *Atlas of Dermatology.* 3rd ed. Philadelphia, PA: Lea & Febiger; 1994:25.

Chapter 2

Figure 2-1. Reprinted with permission from Travell JG, Simons DG. *Myofascial Pain and Dysfunction: The Trigger Point Manual. Volume 1: The Upper Extremities.* 1st ed. Baltimore, MD: Williams & Wilkins; 1983:33.

Figure 2-2. Commissioned from Sandra Dean.

Figure 2-3. Commissioned from Kimberly Battista.

Figure 2-4. Reprinted with permission from Travell JG, Simons DG. *Trigger Point Pain Patterns: Wall Charts.* 1st ed. Baltimore, MD: Williams & Wilkins; 1996.

Figure 2-5. Reprinted with permission from Travell JG, Simons DG. *Myofascial Pain and Dysfunction: The Trigger Point Manual. Volume 1: The Upper Extremities.* 1st ed. Baltimore, MD: Williams & Wilkins; 1983:60.

Figure 2-6. Reprinted with permission from *Stedman's Concise Illustrated.* 4th ed. p.653.

Figure 2-7. Reprinted with permission from Clemente CD. *Anatomy: A Regional Atlas of the Human Body.* 4th ed. Baltimore, MD: Williams & Wilkins; 1997:Plate 349.

Figure 2-8. Commissioned from Sandra Dean.

Figure 2-9. Commissioned from Sandra Dean.

Figure 2-10. Reprinted with permission from Willis MC. *Medical Terminology: The Language of Health Care.* 1st ed. Baltimore, MD: Williams & Wilkins; 1996:132.

Figure 2-11. Reprinted with permission from Roentgen EJ. *Diagnosis of Diseases of Bone.* 3rd ed. Baltimore, MD: Williams & Wilkins; 1981;2:841. Courtesy of Herbert M. Stauffer, Temple University Hospital, Philadelphia, PA.

Figure 2-12. Reprinted with permission from Agur, Lee. *Grant's Atlas of Anatomy.* 10 ed. 1999:251.

Figure 2-13. Reprinted with permission from Brant WE, Helms CA. *Fundamentals of Diagnostic Radiology*. 2nd ed. Baltimore, MD: Williams &Wilkins; 1999:1058.

Figure 2-14. Reprinted with permission from Willis MC. *Medical Terminology: The Language of Health Care*. 1st ed. Baltimore, MD: Williams & Wilkins; 1996:135.

Figure 2-15. Reprinted with permission from Macnab I, McCulloch J. *Neck Ache and Shoulder Pain*. 1st ed. Baltimore, MD: Williams & Wilkins; 1994:201.

Figure 2-16. Reprinted with permission from Baker CL. *The Hughston Clinic Sports Medicine Book*. 1st ed. Baltimore, MD: Williams & Wilkins; 1995:534.

Figure 2-17. Reprinted with permission from Baker CL. *The Hughston Clinic Sports Medicine Book*. 1st ed. Baltimore, MD: Williams & Wilkins; 1995:365.

Figure 2-18. Reprinted with permission from Barker LR, Burton JR, Zieve, PD. *Principles of Ambulatory Medicine*. 4th ed. Baltimore, MD: Williams & Wilkins; 1995:935.

Figure 2-19. Reprinted with permission from Koneman EW. *Color Atlas and Textbook of Diagnostic Microbiology*. 5th ed. Philadelphia, PA: Lippincot-Raven; 1997:Figure E.

Figure 2-20. Reprinted with permission from Goodheart HP. *A Photoguide of Common Skin Disorders: Diagnosis and Management*. Baltimore, MD: Williams & Wilkins; 1999:145.

Figure 2-21. Commissioned from Sandra Dean.

Figure 2-22. Reprinted with permission from Harris JH Jr, Harris, WH, Novelline RA. *The Radiology of Emergency Medicine*. 3rd ed. Baltimore, MD: Williams & Wilkins; 1993:440.

Figure 2-23. Reprinted with permission from Macnab I, McCulloch J. *Neck Ache and Shoulder Pain*. 1st ed. Baltimore, MD: Williams & Wilkins; 1994:45.

Figure 2-24. Reprinted with permission from Macnab I, McCulloch J. *Neck Ache and Shoulder Pain*. 1st ed. Baltimore, MD: Williams & Wilkins; 1994:45.

Figure 2-25. Reprinted with permission from Travell JG, Simons DG. *Myofascial Pain and Dysfunction: The Trigger Point Manual. Volume 1: The Upper Extremities*. 1st ed. Baltimore, MD: Williams & Wilkins; 1983:175.

Figure 2-26. Reprinted with permission from Barker LR, Burton JR, Zieve, PD. *Principles of Ambulatory Medicine*. 4th ed. Baltimore, MD: Williams & Wilkins; 1995:946.

Figure 2-27. Reprinted with permission from Barker LR, Burton JR, Zieve, PD. *Principles of Ambulatory Medicine*. 4th ed. Baltimore, MD: Williams & Wilkins; 1995:946.

Figure 2-28. Commissioned from Sandra Dean.

Figure 2-29. Reprinted with permission from Salter RD. *Textbook of Disorders and Injuries of the Musculoskeletal System*. 2nd ed. Baltimore, MD: Williams & Wilkins; 1983:Figure 6-125.

Figure 2-30. Reprinted with permission from Basmajian JV. *Primary Anatomy*. 8th ed. Baltimore, MD: Williams & Wilkins; 1982:Figure 6-46.

Figure 2-31. Reprinted with permission from Moore KL, Agur AMR. *Essential Clinical Anatomy*. 1st ed. Baltimore, MD: Williams & Wilkins; 1995:326.

Figure 2-32. Reprinted with permission from Bickley LS. *Bates' Guide to Physical Examination and History Taking*. 7th ed. Baltimore, MD: Lippincott Williams & Wilkins; 1999:548.

Figure 2-33. Reprinted with permission from *Stedman's Medical Dictionary*. 27th ed. Baltimore, MD: Lippincott Williams & Wilkins; 2000:813.

Figure 2-34. Reprinted with permission from Yochum TR, Rowe LJ. *Essentials of Skeletal Radiology*. 2nd ed. Baltimore, MD: Lippincott Williams & Wilkins; 1996;2:1291, Figure 13-59B.

Figure 2-35. Reprinted with permission from Benninghoff, Goerttler. *Lehrbuch der Anatomie des Menschen*. Ferer H, Staubesand J, eds. Munich: Urban & Schwarzenberg. As seen in Clemente CD. *Anatomy: A Regional Atlas of the Human Body*, 3rd ed. Munich: Urban & Schwarzenberg; 1987:Figure 506.

Figure 2-36. Reprinted with permission from Baker CL. *The Hughston Clinic Sports Medicine Book*. 1st ed. Baltimore, MD: Williams & Wilkins; 1995:604.

Figure 2-37. Reprinted with permission from Goodheart HP. *A Photoguide of Common Skin Disorders: Diagnosis and Management*. Baltimore, MD: Williams & Wilkins; 1999:366.

Figure 2-38. Reprinted with permission from Clemente CD. *Anatomy: A Regional Atlas of the Human Body*. 4th ed. Baltimore, MD: Williams & Wilkins; 1997:Plate 63.

Figure 2-39. Reprinted with permission from Moore KL. *Clinically Oriented Anatomy*. 3rd ed. Baltimore, MD: Williams & Wilkins; 1992:791.

Figure 2-40. Reprinted with permission from Foreman SM, Croft, AC. *Whiplash Injuries: The Cervical Acceleration/ Deceleration Syndrome*. 2nd ed. Baltimore, MD: Williams & Wilkins; 1995:295.

Figure 2-41. Reprinted with permission from Clemente CD. *Anatomy: A Regional Atlas of the Human Body*. 4th ed. Baltimore, MD: Williams & Wilkins; 1997:Plate 68.

Figure 2-42. Reprinted with permission from Macnab I, McCulloch J. *Neck Ache and Shoulder Pain*. 1st ed. Baltimore, MD: Williams & Wilkins; 1994:459.

Figure 2-43. Reprinted with permission from Moore KL. *Clinically Oriented Anatomy*. 3rd ed. Baltimore, MD: Williams & Wilkins; 1992:327.

Figure 2-44. Reprinted with permission from Willis MC. *Medical Terminology: The Language of Health Care*. 1st ed. Baltimore, MD: Williams & Wilkins; 1996:133.

Figure 2-45. Reprinted with permission from Travell JG, Simons DG. *Myofascial Pain and Dysfunction: The Trigger Point Manual. Volume 1: The Upper Extremities*. 1st ed. Baltimore, MD: Williams & Wilkins; 1983: 604.

Chapter 3

Figure 3-1. Commissioned from Sandra Dean.

Figure 3-2. Commissioned from Sandra Dean.

Figure 3-3. Reprinted with permission from Rosdahl CB. *Book of Basic Nursing*. 7th ed. Philadelphia, PA: Lippincott-Raven; 1999:1063, Figure 77-3.

Figure 3-4. Reprinted with permission from Rassner G. *Atlas of Dermatology*. 3rd ed. Philadelphia, PA: Lea & Febiger; 1994:44.

Figure 3-5. Reprinted with permission from Sobotta. *Atlas der Anatomie des Meschen*. Ferner H, Staubesand J, eds. Munich: Urban & Schwarzenberg. As seen in Clemente CD. *Anatomy: A Regional Atlas of the Human Body*. 3rd ed. Munich: Urban & Schwarzenberg; 1987:Figures 404, 406.

Figure 3-6. Reprinted with permission from Clemente CD. *Anatomy: A Regional Atlas of the Human Body*. 4th ed. Baltimore, MD: Williams & Wilkins; 1997:Plate 463.

Figure 3-7. Reprinted with permission from Moore KL, Agur AMR. *Essential Clinical Anatomy*. 1st ed. Baltimore, MD: Williams & Wilkins; 1995:353.

Figure 3-8. Photo courtesy of Robert Schwartzmann, MD, Philadelphia, PA.

Figure 3-9. Reprinted with permission from Yochum TR, Rowe LJ. *Essentials of Skeletal Radiology*. 2nd ed. Baltimore, MD: Lippincott Williams & Wilkins; 1996; 1:398, Figure 6-38.

Figure 3-10. Reprinted with permission from Davis RL, Robertson, DM. *Textbook of Neuropathology*. 3rd ed. Baltimore, MD: Williams & Wilkins; 1997:758.

Figure 3-11. Reprinted with permission from Benninghoff, Goerttler. *Lehrbuch der Anatomie des Menschen*. Ferer H, Staubesand J, eds. Munich: Urban & Schwarzenberg. As seen in Clemente CD. Anatomy: *A Regional Atlas of the Human Body*. 3rd ed. Munich: Urban & Schwarzenberg; 1987:Figure 611.

Figure 3-12. Reprinted with permission from Travell, JG, Simons, DG. *Myofascial Pain and Dysfunction: The Trigger Point Manual*. Baltimore, MD: Williams & Wilkins; 1983:323, Figure 17.2.

Chapter 4

Figure 4-1. Reprinted with permission from Willis MC. *Medical Terminology: The Language of Health Care.* 1st ed. Baltimore, MD: Williams & Wilkins; 1996:A16. White blood cells. *Wintrobe's Clinical Hematology.* 9th ed. Philadelphia, PA: Lea & Febiger; 1993.

Figure 4-2. Reprinted with permission from Willis MC. *Medical Terminology: The Language of Health Care.* 1st ed. Baltimore, MD: Williams & Wilkins; 1996:162.

Figure 4-3. Reprinted with permission from McKenzie SB. *Textbook of Hematology.* 2nd ed. Baltimore, MD: Williams & Wilkins; 1996:155, Figure D.

Figure 4-4. Reprinted with permission from Willis MC. *Medical Terminology: The Language of Health Care.* 1st ed. Baltimore, MD: Williams & Wilkins; 1996:164.

Figure 4-5. Commissioned from Sandra Dean.

Figure 4-6. Reprinted with permission from Willis MC. *Medical Terminology: The Language of Health Care.* 1st ed. Baltimore, MD: Williams & Wilkins; 1996:165.

Figure 4-7. Reprinted with permission from Willis MC. *Medical Terminology: The Language of Health Care.* 1st ed. Baltimore, MD: Williams & Wilkins; 1996:171.

Figure 4-8. Reprinted with permission from Rassner G. *Atlas of Dermatology.* 3rd ed. Philadelphia, PA: Lea & Febiger; 1994:271.

Figure 4-9. Reprinted with permission from Sheldon H. *Boyd's Introduction to the Study of Disease.* 11th ed. Philadelphia, PA: Lea & Febiger; 1992:90.

Figure 4-10. Reprinted with permission from Willis MC. *Medical Terminology: The Language of Health Care.* 1st ed. Baltimore, MD: Williams & Wilkins; 1996:172.

Chapter 5

Figure 5-1. Commissioned from Sandra Dean.

Figure 5-2. Reprinted with permission from Fitzpatrick J, Aeling J. *Dermatology Secrets in Color.* 2nd ed. Philadelphia, PA: Hanley & Belfus; 2000; 191, Figure 8.

Figure 5-3. Reprinted with permission from Bickley LS. *Bates' Guide to Physical Examination and History Taking.* 7th ed. Baltimore, MD: Lippincott Williams & Wilkins, 1999:660.

Figure 5-4. Reprinted with permission from Mindel A. *AIDS: A Pocket Book of Diagnosis and Management.* 1st ed. Baltimore, MD: Urban & Schwarzenberg; 1990:116.

Figure 5-5. Commissioned from Sandra Dean.

Figure 5-6. Reprinted with permission from *Stedman's Medical Dictionary.* Baltimore, MD: Lippincott Williams & Wilkins; 27th ed. 2000:1036.

Figure 5-7. Reprinted with permission from Goodheart HP. *A Photoguide of Common Skin Disorders: Diagnosis and Management.* Baltimore, MD: Williams & Wilkins; 1999:356, Figure 25.20.

Chapter 6

Figure 6-1. Reprinted with permission from Willis MC. *Medical Terminology: The Language of Health Care.* 1st ed. Baltimore, MD: Williams & Wilkins; 1996:A18.

Figure 6-2. Reprinted with permission from Willis MC. *Medical Terminology: The Language of Health Care.* 1st ed. Baltimore, MD: Williams & Wilkins; 1996:A18.

Figure 6-3. Reprinted with permission from Fletcher CDM, McKee PH. *An Atlas of Gross Pathology.* 1st ed. London: Gower Medical Publishing; 1987.

Figure 6-4. Reprinted with permission from Willis MC. *Medical Terminology: The Language of Health Care.* 1st ed. Baltimore, MD: Williams & Wilkins; 1996:233.

Figure 6-5. Commissioned from Sandra Dean.

Figure 6-6. Reprinted with permission from Roche Lexikon Medizin, 3.Auflage, Urban & Schwarzenberg. Munich, Germany.

Chapter 7

Figure 7-1. Commissioned from Sandra Dean.

Figure 7-2. Reprinted with permission from Rosdahl CB. *Textbook of Basic Nursing.* 7th ed. Philadelphia, PA: Lippincott-Raven; 1999:1265, Figure 87-7.

Figure 7-3. Commissioned from Sandra Dean.

Figure 7-4. Reprinted with permission from Willis, MC. *Medical Terminology: The Language of Health Care.* 1st ed. Baltimore, MD: Williams & Wilkins; 1996:374.

Figure 7-5. Reprinted with permission from Willis, MC. *Medical Terminology: The Language of Health Care.* 1st ed. Baltimore, MD: Williams & Wilkins;1996:371. From *West J Med.* 1981;134:415.

Figure 7-6. Reprinted with permission from Willis MC. *Medical Terminology: The Language of Health Care.* 1st ed. Baltimore, MD: Williams & Wilkins; 1996:377.

Figure 7-7. Reprinted with permission from *Stedman's Medical Dictionary.* Baltimore, MD: Lippincott Williams & Wilkins; 27th ed. 2000:277.

Figure 7-8. Reprinted with permission from Moore KL, Agur AMR. *Essential Clinical Anatomy.* 1st ed. Baltimore, MD: Williams & Wilkins; 1995:97.

Chapter 8

Figure 8-1. Reprinted with permission from Rassner G. *Atlas of Dermatology.* 3rd ed. Philadelphia, PA: Lea & Febiger; 1994:302.

Figure 8-2. Reprinted with permission from *Stedman's Medical Dictionary.* Baltimore, MD: Lippincott Williams & Wilkins; 27th ed. 2000:C15.

Chapter 9

Figure 9-1. Reprinted with permission from Willis MC. *Medical Terminology: The Language of Health Care.* Baltimore, MD: Williams & Wilkins; 1996:407.

Figure 9-2 Reprinted with permission from Massry SG, Glassock T. *Textbook of Nephrology.*1st ed. Baltimore, MD: Williams & Wilkins; 1983;2:6.281.

Chapter 10

Figure 10-1 Commissioned from Sandra Dean.

Figure 10-2 Reprinted with permission from Beckmann CRB. *Obstetrics and Gynecology for Medical Students.* 1st ed. Baltimore, MD: Williams & Wilkins; 1992:306.

Figure 10-3. Reprinted with permission from Beckmann CRB. *Obstetrics and Gynecology for Medical Students.* 1st ed. Baltimore, MD: Williams & Wilkins; 1992:398.

Figure 10-4. Reprinted with permission from Mitchell GW. *The Female Breast and Its Disorders.* 1st ed. Baltimore, MD: Williams & Wilkins; 1990:140.

Figure 10-5. Commissioned from Sandra Dean.

Figure 10-6. Reprinted with permission from Moore KL, Agur AMR. *Essential Clinical Anatomy.* 1st ed. Baltimore, MD: Williams & Wilkins; 1995:163.

Figure 10-7. Commissioned from Sandra Dean.

Chapter 11

Figure 11-1. Reprinted with permission from Rassner G. *Atlas of Dermatology.* 3rd ed. Philadelphia, PA: Lea & Febiger; 1994:84, Figure 3.6.

Appendix 1

Figure 1. Reprinted with permission from Travell JG, Simons DG. *Myofascial Pain and Dysfunction: The Trigger Point Manual. Volume 1: The Upper Extremities.* 1st ed. Baltimore, MD: Williams & Wilkins; 1983:48.

Figure 2. Reprinted with permission from Travell JG, Simons DG. *Myofascial Pain and Dysfunction: The Trigger Point Manual. Volume 1: The Upper Extremities.* 1st ed. Baltimore, MD: Williams & Wilkins; 1983:47.

Index

Page numbers in *italics* denote figures;
Those followed by a "t" denote tables.